The HEALING POWER of
Rainforest
HERBS

A Guide to Understanding and Using Herbal Medicinals

LESLIE TAYLOR, ND

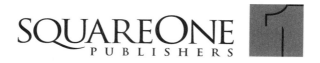

SQUAREONE
PUBLISHERS

This book is not intended to provide medical advice and is sold with the under-standing that the publisher and the author are not liable for the misconception or misuse of information provided. The author and Square One Publishers shall have neither liability nor responsibility to any person or entity with respect to any loss, damage, or injury caused or alleged to be caused directly or indirectly by the information contained in this book, or the use of any substances mentioned. Readers should always check with a qualified health practitioner before begin-ning any herbal medicine treatment.

Cover Designers: Phaedra Mastrocola and Jacqueline Michelus
In-House Editor: Elaine Weiser
Typesetter: Gary A. Rosenberg

Square One Publishers
115 Herricks Road
Garden City Park, NY 11040
(877) 900-BOOK • (516) 535-2010
www.squareonepublishers.com

Library of Congress Cataloging-in-Publication Data

Taylor, Leslie.
    The healing power of rainforest herbs : a guide to understanding and using herbal medicinals / Leslie Taylor.
        p. cm.
    Includes bibliographical references and index.
    ISBN 0-7570-0144-0
1. Rain forest plants—Therapeutic use. 2. Herbs—Therapeutic use. I. Title.

RM666.H33T388 2005
615'.321—dc22
           2004022843

CONTENTS

PART THREE

Medicinal Plants of the Amazon

To the Indigenous Peoples of the Amazon Rainforest.

WE, THE INDIGENOUS PEOPLES, *have been an integral part of the Amazon Biosphere for millennia. We used and cared for the resources of that biosphere with respect, because it is our home, and because we know that our survival and that of our future generations depend on it. Our accumulated knowledge about the ecology of our home, our models for living within the Amazonian Biosphere, our reverence and respect for the tropical forest and its other inhabitants, both plant and animal, are the keys to guaranteeing the future of the Amazon Basin, not only for our peoples, but also for all humanity.*

Our experience, especially during the past 100 years, has taught us that when politicians and developers take charge of our home, they are capable of destroying it because of their short-sightedness, their ignorance, and their greed.

We are concerned that the Amazon peoples, and in particular the Indigenous Peoples, have been left out of the environmentalists' vision of the Amazonian Biosphere. The focus of concern of the environmental community has typically been the preservation of the tropical forests and its plant and animal inhabitants. Little concern has been shown for its human inhabitants who are also part of that biosphere.

We are concerned that the Indigenous Peoples and their representative organizations have been left out of the political process, which is determining the future of our homeland. The environmentalist community has at times lobbied on our behalf; it has spoken out and written in the name of the Amazonian Indians. While we appreciate these efforts, it should be made clear that we never delegated this power to the environmentalist community nor to any individual or organization within that community.

The most effective defense of the Amazonian Biosphere is the recognition and defense of the territories of the region's Indigenous Peoples and the promotion of their models for living within that biosphere and for managing its resources in a sustainable way.

Coordinating Body for the Indigenous Organizations of the Amazon Basin (COICA), adapted from COICA's "To the Community of Concerned Environmentalists" (1989)

"To the center of the world you have taken me
Great Spirit and showed me the goodness and the beauty
and the strangeness of the greening earth,
the only mother—and there the spirit shapes of things,
as they should be, you have shown me
and I have seen."

—Susan Seddon Boulet
From her book, *Shaman*

INTRODUCTION

A tall, fair-skinned blonde woman traveling down the Amazon River and into the remote areas of the Amazon rainforest is an oddity of sorts. However, for most of my life I've been told that I'm odd. Admittedly, trekking through jungles, studying the plant knowledge of indigenous Indian shamans and South American herbal healers, getting harassed in airport customs with a suitcase full of strange-looking murky liquids, bark, leaves, and roots, and running a large corporation in the process, is pretty unusual. However, it never really was a goal of mine to just be "usual."

Most people who first meet me often ask: "How did you ever get into a profession like this?" Looking back, a series of journeys seems to have redirected the course of my life and shaped it into what it is today. I have to go back about twenty years to my most memorable journey, which started me onto this odd path where I find myself today.

I first became interested in herbal medicine and alternative health when, in my mid-twenties, I was diagnosed with acute myeloblastic leukemia (AML). Conventional medicine gave up on me after two years of traditional chemotherapy and cancer treatments and sent me home to die. I was twenty-four years old and was told I wouldn't see my twenty-fifth birthday. But being the odd, determined, stubborn, rebellious individual that most people described me as even back then, I didn't give up.

Twenty years ago it was even harder than it is now to access accurate information on herbs and alternative therapies. But you might say that I had a "dying need to know," and I began studying alternative health with a vengeance. With a combination of herbal medicine, diet, nutrition, and other natural healing modalities, I was diagnosed as cancer-free eighteen months later. Not only was my cancer gone, but the extensive damage that was done to my body and internal organs from the conventional cancer treatments was healed or on the mend. Another real oddity, I was told. My oncologist, who scoffed at anything herbal or unconventional, believes that I was simply too stubborn to die. I know there is some truth in that statement, but I also believe that herbal medicine went a long way in curing my cancer and healing my body.

What I didn't understand then (or now, really) is why they call chemotherapy and today's modern medicine "conventional medicine" and refer to herbal medicine as "alternative." My personal journey showed me that herbal medicine was much more conventional. It dates back literally centuries in time, with the less-than-100-year-old pharmaceutical industry offering the "alternatives" to the plant medicines we've used since before human beings even learned how to chronicle their uses. At least for me, herbal medicine was much more effective than the "alternatives" conventional medicine offered me in my personal battle with cancer.

After winning this battle, I continued on in my business career in Texas, starting companies in several different industries and selling them when I became bored with their day-to-day management. In business I was considered "successful," and that success resulted in a ballistic, workaholic lifestyle. I continued studying herbal medicine and alternative health as a hobby, choosing to use herbs and natural health rather than drugs for my and my family's health. They thought I was pretty odd too, but they accepted the strange herbal potions and nutritional remedies I gave them when they were sick.

Then, in 1989, I took a much-needed vacation that changed the course of my life yet again. Maybe it was just the first time I had taken a breath or a break in many years, but a journey to the wilds of Africa somehow reconnected me to the land, nature, and wildlife. It showed me that I needed to make a change in the hectic, harried life I had created, which was involved in the ego of success and the power of money and which wasn't really personally fulfilling. So, when I returned from Africa, I sold my companies, bought a ranch in the hill country of Texas, and "retired."

There—in a conventional, sort of backwards, rural Texas community north of Austin—I quickly became "the odd woman at Clear Creek Ranch" to the local farmers and ranchers. I grew weird plants, herbs, and vegetables, raised a motley menagerie of teenage boys and exotic animals (which hardly ever acted like they were supposed to), had too much land that was "unproductive," and was obviously in dire need of a husband to make her do things right. Leastwise, that's what the local farmers and ranchers would tell you. That didn't keep them from dropping by to tell me about their aches and pains to see what kind of odd concoction of plants I might pick out of the gardens and give them, and which somehow mysteriously worked. Often, they'd just drop by to see what odd thing I was up to that day.

Wanting to give something back (and a bit bored with farm life), I started a small consulting company there on the ranch. The company (me) researched and collected information on cancer and AIDS therapies that were being used in other places in the world and taught cancer patients how they could access them. My personal mission was to compile all the research on alternative therapies and to make the information available to those faced with the same struggle that I had once confronted. It had been a great source of frustration and a committed struggle for me to try to access this type of information when I had cancer, especially at a time when I had little enough energy to just get through a day.

It was during this research that I came across an herbal extract that was sold as an herbal drug in Europe for cancer and AIDS patients, with some interesting results. When I determined that it was a simple extract of a natural plant that could be sold here as an herbal supplement (for a lot less money than the European company was charging), I decided to go to the source where the plant grew. My mission then was to try to import the plant into the United States. The plant was called cat's claw (*Uncaria tomentosa*), and the source was the Amazon rainforest in Peru. This new journey into the Amazon rainforest changed the course of my life yet again.

On that first journey into the rainforest, I fell in love. I fell in love with the jungle, the people, the culture, the lifestyle and attitude, the plants and trees, the incredible rivers . . . all of which make up the Amazon rainforest. I also saw, on that first trip, the incredible amount of destruction that was happening in the Amazon. I saw that it was possible that the whole thing could go up in smoke and be wiped off the face of the Earth, conceivably in my lifetime. Waiting for my flight home in the Lima airport in Peru, I sat there sunburned, bug-bit, tired, and excited and decided that not only did I want to start a new company in the States to begin importing this wonderful plant called cat's claw but that I also had to try to make a difference to help stop the destruction of the Amazon rainforest. I didn't quite know how then, but I knew that an odd, determined, stubborn, rebellious sort of person such as myself had as good a chance as anyone else did.

That was the beginning of a group of companies that I founded in my thoughts sitting in the Lima airport, and officially two days later in Austin, Texas. I came out of "retirement" and began importing cat's claw into the United States shortly thereafter. Through my ongoing work with the company and the many subsequent trips to the Amazon, I learned more and more about the other medicinal plants that were used as natural medicines by the indigenous peoples in the rainforest and began importing those as well. My company quickly outgrew Clear Creek Ranch and it was time to sell it and move back into the city as the journey, which now seemed to have a life of its own, continued forward.

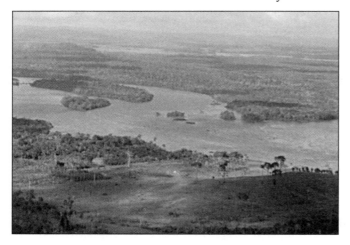

Xingu River in the Amazon rainforest outside of Altamira, Brazil.

In my work with the Raintree group of companies which I founded in 1995, I have been setting up plant harvesting programs with Indian tribes and rural Amazon communities, that are today, sustainably harvesting more than sixty medicinal plants from Peru, Brazil, Ecuador, and Colombia. My ongoing research on medicinal plants continues to take me into the heart of the rainforest, where I work side by side with indigenous tribal shamans and medicine men, rural village herbalists and local "doctors" called curanderos, as well as North and South American herbalists, plant chemists, and universities.

Traveling through the remote areas of the Amazon where medicines, hospitals, and doctors are virtually non-existent has brought an opportunity to learn as a practitioner how to treat illnesses and diseases that I would never encounter in the United States . . . malaria, diphtheria, yellow fever, typhoid, and leprosy, just to name a few (not to mention the incredible bacterial, parasitic and fungal infections I've seen!). As a practitioner or healer in the jungle, I am called "jaguar-woman," white witch, shaman, an Indian phrase that translates to "big mother in charge," or curandera (healer) by the remote villages and Indians I visit and work with. I use their ancient knowledge of their plants and combine it with western research and science, so my "potions" are different, yet familiar, to their shamans and healers. Again, they think I'm pretty odd too, but many have never seen a very tall blonde woman with blue eyes and freckles (which many shamans have tried to cure me of!). As a board certified naturopath here in the States, I enjoy working on the many hard cases that get referred to me—people who have exhausted all other therapies and are willing to try some unusual jungle remedy for their cure. It seems my life has come full circle in the last twenty years, and I now find myself helping many cancer patients in my practice, when it was once me that was faced with this deadly disease so many years ago.

Oddly enough, of all the businesses I have founded and managed in my career, this is the only one that I've never had to determinedly push, market, make work, or direct. Since they were created, I have literally been running behind them trying to keep up. They seem to have a life, path, and purpose of their own; and I have never worked so hard, had so much fun and adventure, and been as personally fulfilled as I am today. It has certainly been a grand adventure. However odd it is, I feel I am truly blessed to be on the path I find myself on today.

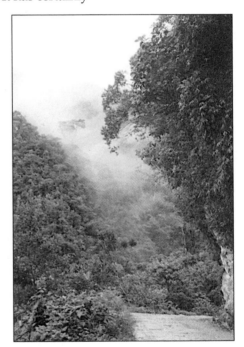

My journey has just recently been redirected yet again: this year, I've moved myself and company—lock, stock, and barrel—to Carson City, Nevada. It seems that it was time for me to focus on helping some North American Indian tribes, much in the same manner that I've been assisting the South American Indians over the years. If this new venture/adventure is successful, my next book may well be on North American Indian medicinal plants and the need to put our own Native Americans back onto their ancestral lands (now owned and controlled by our government's forestry agencies) as caretakers of the land in sustainable plant harvesting programs. What an adventurous journey that will be! Believe it or not, I haven't been bored—not once—in the last nine years; that doesn't look like it will be changing any time soon, either!

Before I became known as "the white witch of the Amazon," I was (and am) a businesswoman first and foremost. When I first arrived in the Amazon, I approached the rainforest and rainforest conservation in a business-like manner and began to look for business solutions to rainforest destruction. This was odd to the activists and conservationists I came across, but again, I was used to being called odd. I believed then and now that, wherever you are in the world, basic business strategies still apply. Greed is greed and profits are profits, even in the remote jungles. If you want someone to do something, make it profitable for them to do and it's not so hard to convince them. So I set

A cloud forest in the high elevations of the Peruvian jungle.

about showing people in the rainforest how they could make more money sustainably harvesting medicinal plants like cat's claw than they could make at timber harvesting, grazing livestock, agriculture, or subsistence cropping—practices that destroy the forest. It sounds almost too simple, but it's effective and it works.

The only component left to make this business strategy work is to create the market demand for these sustainable forest resources so that it can result in profits for those participating. That's not as hard as it sounds either. The alternative health and natural/herbal products industry in the United States is growing at an unprecedented rate. Recent statistics show that consumers have spent more out-of-pocket funds on alternative health and alternative

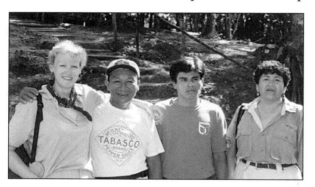

The author with shaman Don Antonio Monteviero, his assistant, and Yvone Meija, director of ACEER research center.

health products and supplements than they have for conventional medicine over the past few years. And the rainforest does provide a wealth of beneficial natural products and highly effective medicinal plants for that industry.

This book represents almost ten years of my personal research and documentation on these important medicinal plants in the Amazon rainforest during my journeys into the South American jungles and in my journey with Raintree. I firmly believe that medicinal plants, such as those discussed in this book, are the true wealth of the rainforest and the means by which it can be saved from destruction. They have for centuries positively affected the health and well-being of the inhabitants of the forest. Through their sustainable harvesting, they can and will positively affect the health, well-being, and continuance of the rainforest itself.

It is my sincere hope that you, the reader of this book, will learn an appreciation of the rainforest and why it is so important to be saved; learn more about the wealth of beneficial medicinal plants it provides us; and learn how you can take part in positively affecting your health and the health of the rainforest with these wonderful plants.

May your own journeys and adventures be prosperous!

Yours in health,
Leslie Taylor, ND

HOW TO USE
THIS BOOK

his book is divided into three main sections. The first chapter provides an introductory discussion on the rainforest, the Amazon rainforest in particular, and the issues involved in its destruction and preservation. Part One: Rainforest Herbal Primer provides information on herbal medicine principles in general, the similarities and differences between using herbs and drugs, methods of preparing herbal remedies, and some recipes for rainforest remedies. Part Two: Quick Guides to Medicinal Plants of the Amazon includes helpful at-a-glance references to essential information on rainforest herbs. If you are interested in finding the best herbs to take for producing a desired effect—for example, stimulating the immune system or producing a laxative effect—turn to Properties and Actions of Rainforest Plants. This table includes the technical terms and definitions of the functions and actions that are attributed to various herbs; the plants most widely used by herbalists for achieving such results; a list of those plants that have been researched and scientifically validated; and those that have been traditionally used by indigenous peoples. If you are searching for the plants to use for the treatment of a specific disorder, go to Herbal Treatment of Specific Diseases and Disorders, which matches an extensive list of various diseases with the rainforest plants used as treatment. The Plant Data Summary is a section that offers a quick look at each of the rainforest herbs discussed in this book. Essential information is listed, such as the main actions of the herb; its primary preparation method; its main uses; which actions have been documented by scientific research or traditionally used; and any cautions to using the herb. This summary, which has been conveniently condensed, guides the reader as to which plants to read about in greater detail in Part Three: Medicinal Plants of the Amazon.

Part Three provides extensive information on seventy-four medicinal plants, trees, vines, and herbs of the rainforest. You will find the following information on each plant: family, genus, and species; common names; parts used; properties and actions; main text on the plant; worldwide uses of the herb; and plant chemical information. The main text provides well-referenced information about each plant. This information includes:

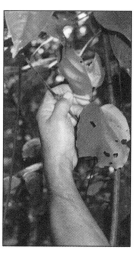

Rainforest plant clavo huasca.

- what the plant looks like

- where and how it grows

- the history of its uses by rainforest inhabitants and in herbal medicine

- its chemicals and their properties

- its biological activities and clinical research

- its current practical uses

- the traditional preparation methods for remedies and dosages

- its contraindications and possible drug interactions

PLANT CHEMICAL INFORMATION

Often, the plant's effective uses or actions are closely tied to specific chemicals found in the plant, chemicals that have been tested and documented to have specific biological activities. In other words, knowledge of the chemicals in the plants can help explain why the plant works for certain disorders. It can also help determine if a plant may have any contraindications, drug interactions, or other cautions. Many readers will just skim over this sort of information, especially the list of chemicals. However, it is very difficult to access this information, and many medical professionals, pharmacists, botanists, researchers, scientists, and alternative health professionals will value this information.

The plant chemical data provided is a summary of chemicals that have been documented to exist in the plant. It does not include every known chemical in the plant, and no distinction has been made as to which chemicals are found in the different parts of the plant (leaves, fruit, bark, and so on). Therefore, the chemical data may or may not be all-inclusive or complete. It is provided as a general reference for the more experienced reader.

BIOLOGICAL ACTIVITIES AND CLINICAL RESEARCH

An overview of scientific laboratory research and clinical data or research about each plant is provided. Complete citations of the studies that are referenced in the text are found in the References section in the back of the book. You also will see the distinction as to whether the research was performed *in vivo* or *in vitro*. *In vivo* studies refer to research that has been performed in animals or humans to determine the effects of a particular chemical/herb/drug. *In vitro* studies refer to research conducted "in the test tube."

Studies performed to determine antibacterial activity provide good examples of the differences between the two terms. In an *in vitro* study, bacteria would be placed in a test tube or a petri dish, along with a plant (or some form of extract of the plant) to determine if the plant and/or extract kills the bacteria or stops its growth. In an *in vivo* study, an animal would be inoculated with bacteria and then administered the plant or extract to determine if the plant is effective in treating the bacterial infection, and at what dosage. Clearly, *in vivo* studies are much more effective in verifying a plant's uses and how they might affect a specific disease or you.

Yet, this is just a point of reference as well: how a plant might affect a rat or mouse does not always relate to how it will affect humans. Readers should also understand that scientific research is in no manner standardized, and different results will be demonstrated based on the methods employed by the researcher. As stated earlier, wherever possible, the summary of research provided will differentiate whether the study was performed *in vitro* or *in vivo* and will give information on the types of methods or extracts that were used.

TRADITIONAL PREPARATIONS

Traditional dosage amounts for plants have been included in the plant information, provided in Part Three, for a reason. These dosage amounts are based on the long history of the plant's use and should be followed within reason. They've been calculated for an average-weight adult person of 120 to 150 pounds and should be generally adjusted up or down based on body weight. Take less if you weigh under 120 pounds and more if you weigh more than 150 pounds (up to double the recommended dosage if you weigh 300 pounds or more). If you plan on taking more than one and one-half times the dosages indicated for your weight, it is best to check with a qualified herbalist, naturopath, or physician who has experience with the particular plant you are choosing to take.

CONTRAINDICATIONS AND DRUG INTERACTIONS

Some of the plants featured in this book are not without side effects, and for most, there is little data about their suitability and contraindications in combination with the many pharmaceutical drugs that are prescribed in the United States. The history of the medicinal uses of these plants mostly comes from South America and Third World countries that typically do not have access to the types of prescription drugs commonly used in the United States. For this reason, the information that is provided for contraindications and drug interactions is not all-inclusive or complete.

Also, as discussed in Chapter 2, much of the data provided in this book on contraindications and drug interactions is based on the plants' chemistry (and documented effects of those chemicals), rather than on funded human clinical studies proving a drug interaction or a medical contraindication. Drug interaction studies just aren't performed on most medicinal plants anywhere. If you are taking any prescription drug, always check with your doctor first before taking herbal supplements or using any of the plants featured in this book.

WORLDWIDE ETHNOMEDICAL USES TABLE

Ethnic uses of medicinal plants can be very important. If a plant has been used in a specific way for a specific purpose for many years and in many different geographical areas, there certainly is a reason for it: it is probably effective. It is this information that helps scientists target which plants to research first and what to study them for. In fact, the majority of our plant-based drugs or pharmaceuticals were discovered through this documentation process. The Worldwide Ethnomedical Uses table summarizes all the documented ethnic uses of the plant. This information includes specific conditions and illnesses for which the plant has been used by people around the world. It includes tribal or indigenous uses, as well as current uses in herbal medicine. This information summarizes how all parts of the plants are employed, without distinction. The information shown in the table should only be used as a reference, and the main body of the text should be reviewed for more detail.

You must be observant when reviewing the documentation provided in this table. Although a plant may be documented to be anti-inflammatory, the ethnic use may be as a topical inflammatory aid for something such as skin rashes, rather than as an anti-inflammatory taken internally for arthritis or stomach inflammation. Or, many tribal remedies documented and employed by indigenous people call for a specific plant to be placed in bath water for a "bathing remedy," rather than taken internally. Other times, a disease or condition like herpes or malaria may be documented and listed in the Worldwide Ethnomedical Uses table; the text, however, may reveal that the specific plant has been employed as an aid to treat symptoms such as fever or lesions rather than as an antiviral or antimalar-ial aid to directly affect the illness. For these reasons, it is important to read the main text on the plant and use the table only as a general reference.

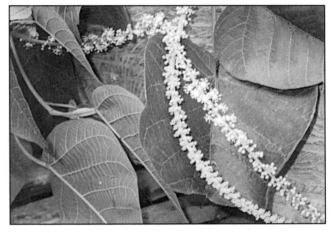

Leaves and flowers of rainforest plant sangre de grado.

Please remember this information is an historical account about how these tropical rainforest plants are employed as natural remedies in South American and Third World countries. This—as well as all of the information found in this book—is not a medical claim or recommendation to use herbs in place of proper medical care. Please always check with a qualified health practitioner before beginning any herbal medicine program on your own—especially if you are taking prescription drugs or have (or think you may have) a serious medical disorder or disease.

At the end of this book, you will find the Rainforest Resources section. Here, you will find valuable information, including: sources for obtaining sustainable rainforest products, nonprofit rainforest organizations, suggested reading on sustainability and rainforest conservation issues, and online resources about rainforest plants and rainforest conservation.

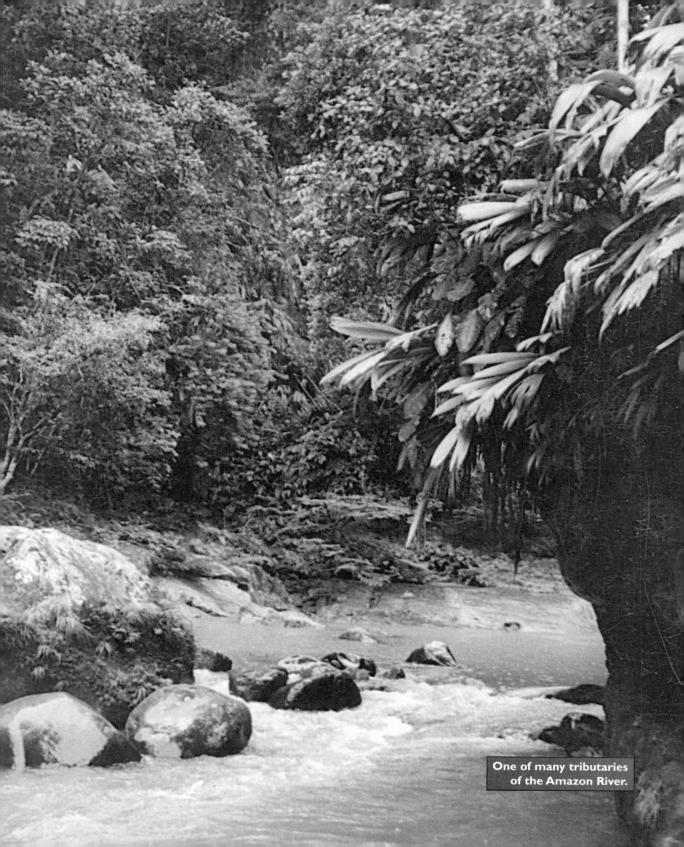

One of many tributaries of the Amazon River.

CHAPTER 1

RAINFOREST DESTRUCTION AND SURVIVAL

The beauty, majesty, and timelessness of a primary rainforest are indescribable. It is impossible to capture on film, to describe in words, or to explain to those who have never had the awe-inspiring experience of standing in the heart of a primary rainforest.

Rainforests have evolved over millions of years to turn into the incredibly complex environments they are today. Rainforests represent a store of living and breathing renewable natural resources that for eons, by virtue of their richness in both animal and plant species, have contributed a wealth of resources for the survival and well-being of humankind. These resources have included basic food supplies, clothing, shelter, fuel, spices, industrial raw materials, and medicine for all those who have lived in the majesty of the forest. However, the inner dynamics of a tropical rainforest is an intricate and fragile system. Everything is so interdependent that upsetting one part can lead to unknown damage or even destruction of the whole. Sadly, it has taken only a century of human intervention to destroy what nature designed to last forever.

THE PROBLEM

The scale of human pressures on ecosystems everywhere has increased enormously in the last few decades. Since 1980 the global economy has tripled in size and the world population has increased by 30 percent. Consumption of everything on the planet has risen—at a cost to our ecosystems. In 2001, The World Resources Institute estimated that the demand for rice, wheat, and corn is expected to grow by 40 percent by 2020, increasing irrigation water demands by 50 percent or more. The Institute further reported that the demand for wood could double by the year 2050; unfortunately, it is still the tropical forests of the world that supply the bulk of the world's demand for wood.

In 1950, about 15 percent of the Earth's land surface was covered by rainforest. Today, more than half has already gone up in smoke. In fewer than fifty years, more than half of the world's tropical rainforests have fallen victim to fire and the chain saw, and the rate of destruction is still accelerating. Unbelievably, more than 200,000 acres of rainforest are burned every day. That is more than 150 acres lost every minute of every day, and 78 million acres lost every year! More than 20 percent of the Amazon rainforest is already gone, and much more is severely threatened as the destruction continues. It is estimated that the Amazon alone is vanishing at a rate of 20,000 square miles a year. If nothing is done to curb this trend, the entire Amazon could well be gone within fifty years.

> The Amazon is being destroyed at an estimated rate of 20,000 square miles a year. If nothing is done to curb this trend, the entire Amazon could be gone within fifty years.

Massive deforestation brings with it many ugly consequences—air and water pollution, soil erosion, malaria epidemics, the release of carbon dioxide into the atmosphere, the eviction and decimation of indigenous Indian tribes, and the loss of biodiversity through extinction of plants and animals. Fewer rainforests mean less rain, less oxygen for us to breathe, and an increased threat from global warming.

But who is really to blame? Consider what we industrialized Americans have done to our own homeland. We converted 90 percent of North America's virgin forests into firewood, shingles, furniture, railroad ties, and paper. Other industrialized countries have done no better. Malaysia, Indonesia, Brazil,

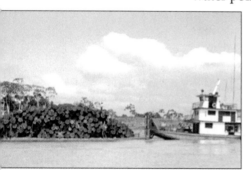

Loggers transporting Amazon timber down the river.

and other tropical countries with rainforests are often branded as "environmental villains" of the world, mainly because of their reported levels of destruction of their rainforests. But despite the levels of deforestation, up to 60 percent of their territory is still covered by natural tropical forests. In fact, today, much of the pressures on their remaining rainforests come from servicing the needs and markets for wood products in industrialized countries that have already depleted their own natural resources. Industrial countries would not be buying rainforest hardwoods and timber had we not cut down our own trees long ago, nor would poachers in the Amazon jungle be slaughtering jaguar, ocelot, caiman, and otter if we did not provide lucrative markets for their skins in Berlin, Paris, and Tokyo.

THE BIODIVERSITY OF THE RAINFOREST

Why should the loss of tropical forests be of any concern to us in light of our own poor management of natural resources? The loss of tropical rainforests has a profound and devastating impact on the world because rainforests are so biologically diverse, more so than other ecosystems (e.g., temperate forests) on Earth.

Consider these facts:

- A single pond in Brazil can sustain a greater variety of fish than is found in all of Europe's rivers.

- A 25-acre plot of rainforest in Borneo may contain more than 700 species of trees—a number equal to the total tree diversity of North America.

- A single rainforest reserve in Peru is home to more species of birds than are found in the entire United States.

- One single tree in Peru was found to harbor forty-three different species of ants—a total that approximates the entire number of ant species in the British Isles.

- The number of species of fish in the Amazon exceeds the number found in the entire Atlantic Ocean.

The biodiversity of the tropical rainforest is so immense that less than 1 percent of its millions of species have been studied by scientists for their active constituents and their possible uses. When an acre of tropical rainforest is lost, the impact on the number of plant and animal species lost and their possible uses is staggering. Scientists estimate that we are losing more than 137 species of plants and animals every single day because of rainforest deforestation.

Surprisingly, scientists have a better understanding of how many stars there are in the galaxy than they have of how many species there are on Earth. Estimates vary from 2 million to 100 million species, with a best estimate of somewhere near 10 million; only 1.4 million of these species have actually been named. Today, rainforests occupy only 2 percent of the entire Earth's surface and 6 percent of the world's land surface, yet these remaining lush rainforests support over half of our planet's wild plants and trees and one-half of the world's wildlife. Hundreds of thousands of these rainforest species are being extinguished before they have even been identified, much less catalogued and studied. The magnitude of this loss to the world

Some scientists believe that there are between 10 million and 30 million yet-to-be-discovered insect species living in rainforest canopy trees.

was most poignantly described by Harvard's Pulitzer Prize-winning biologist Edward O. Wilson over a decade ago:

> The worst thing that can happen during the 1980s is not energy depletion, economic collapses, limited nuclear war, or conquest by a totalitarian government. As terrible as these catastrophes would be for us, they can be repaired within a few generations. The one process ongoing in the 1980s that will take millions of years to correct is the loss of genetic and species diversity by the destruction of natural habitats. This is the folly that our descendants are least likely to forgive us for.

Yet still the destruction continues. If deforestation continues at current rates, scientists estimate nearly 80 to 90 percent of tropical rainforest ecosystems will be destroyed by the year 2020. This destruction is the main force driving a species extinction rate unmatched in 65 million years.

THE AMAZON RAINFOREST . . . THE LAST FRONTIER ON EARTH

The Amazon Rainforest has been described as the "lungs of our planet" because it provides the essential service of continuously recycling carbon dioxide into oxygen.

If Amazonia were a country, it would be the ninth largest in the world. The Amazon rainforest, the world's greatest remaining natural resource, is the most powerful and bioactively diverse natural phenomenon on the planet. It has been described as the "lungs of our planet" because it provides the essential service of continuously recycling carbon dioxide into oxygen. It is estimated that more than 20 percent of Earth's oxygen is produced in this area.

The Amazon covers more than 1.2 billion acres, representing two-fifths of the enormous South American continent, and is found in nine South American countries: Brazil, Colombia, Peru, Venezuela, Ecuador, Bolivia, Guyana, French Guiana, and Suriname. With 2.5 million square miles of rainforest, the Amazon rainforest represents 54 percent of the total rainforests left on Earth.

The Amazon River

The life force of the Amazon rainforest is the mighty Amazon River. It starts as a trickle high in the snow-capped Andes Mountains and flows more than 4,000 miles across the South American continent until it enters the Atlantic Ocean at Belem, Brazil, where it is 200 to 300 miles across, depending on the season. Even 1,000 miles inland it is still 7 miles wide. The river is so deep that ocean liners can travel up its length to 2,300 miles inland.

The Amazon River flows through the center of the rainforest and is fed by 1,100 tributaries, seventeen of which are more than 1,000 miles long. The Amazon is by far the largest watershed and largest river system in the world, occupying over 6 million square kilometers. Over two-thirds of all the fresh water found on Earth is in the Amazon Basin's rivers, streams, and tributaries.

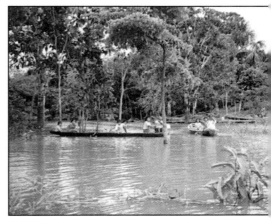

Children of the Peruvian Amazon paddling to school.

With so much water it is not unusual that the main mode of transportation throughout the area is by boat. The smallest and most common boats used today are still made out of hollowed tree trunks, whether they are powered by outboard motors or more often by human-powered paddles. Almost 14,000 miles of Amazon waterway are navigable, and several million miles through swamps and forests are penetrable by canoe. The enormous Amazon River carries massive amounts of silt from runoff from the rainforest floor. Massive amounts of silt deposited at the mouth of the Amazon River has created the largest river island in the world—Marajó Island, which is roughly the size of Switzerland. With this massive freshwater system, it is not unusual that life beneath the water is as abundant and diverse as the surrounding rainforest's plant and animal species. More than 2,000 species of fish have been identified in the Amazon Basin—more species than in the entire Atlantic Ocean.

Over two-thirds of all the fresh water found on Earth is in the Amazon Basin's rivers, streams, and tributaries.

Largest Collection of Plant and Animal Species

The Amazon Basin was formed in the Paleozoic period, somewhere between 500 million and 200 million years ago. The extreme age of the region in geologic terms has much to do with the relative infertility of the rainforest soil and the richness and unique diversity of the plant and animal life. There are more fertile areas in the Amazon River's flood plain, where the river deposits richer soil brought from the Andes, which only formed 20 million years ago.

The Amazon rainforest contains the largest collection of living plant and animal species in the world. The diversity of plant species in the Amazon rainforest is the highest on Earth. It is estimated that a single hectare (2.47 acres) of Amazon rainforest contains about 900 tons of living plants, including more than 750 types of trees and 1,500 other plants. The Andean mountain range and the Amazon jungle are home to more than half of the world's species of flora and fauna; in fact, one in five of all the birds in the world live in the rainforests of the Amazon. To date, some 438,000 species of plants of economic and social interest have been registered in the region, and many more have yet to be catalogued or even discovered.

Scarring and Loss of Diversity

Once a vast sea of tropical forest, the Amazon rainforest today is scarred by roads, farms, ranches, and dams. Brazil is gifted with a full third of the world's remaining rainforests; unfortunately, it is also one of the world's great rainforest destroyers, burning or felling more than 2.7 million acres each year. More than 20 percent of rainforest in the Amazon has been razed and is gone forever. This ocean of green, nearly as large as Australia, is the last great rainforest in the known universe and it is being decimated like the others before it. Why? Like other rainforests already lost forever, the land is being cleared for logging timber, large-scale cattle ranching, mining operations, government road building and hydroelectric schemes, military operations, and the subsistence agriculture of peasants and land-less settlers. Sadder still, in many places the rainforests are burnt simply to provide charcoal to power industrial plants in the area.

THE DRIVING FORCES OF DESTRUCTION

Commercial logging is the single largest cause of rainforest destruction, both directly and indirectly. Other activities also destroy the rainforest, including clearing land for grazing animals and subsistence farming. The simple fact is that people are destroying the Amazon rainforest and the rest of the rainforests of the world because "they can't see the forest for the trees."

Logging for Tropical Hardwoods

Logging tropical hardwoods like teak, mahogany, rosewood, and other timber for furniture, building materials, charcoal, and other wood products is big business and big profits. Several species of tropical hardwoods are imported by developed counties, including the United States, just to build coffins that are then buried or burned. The demand, extraction, and consumption of tropical hardwoods has been so massive that some countries that have been traditional exporters of tropical hardwoods are now importing them because they have already exhausted their supply by destroying native rainforests in slash-and-burn operations. It is anticipated that the Philippines, Malaysia, the Ivory Coast, Nigeria, and Thailand will soon follow, as all these countries will run out of rainforest hardwood timber for export within five years. Japan is the largest importer of tropical woods.

Despite recent reductions, Japan's average tropical timber import of 11 million cubic meters annually is still gluttonous. The demand for tropical hardwood timber is damaging to the ecological, biological, and social fabric of tropical lands and is clearly unsustainable for any length of time.

Behind the hardwood logger come others down the same roads—which were built to transport the timber. The cardboard packing and the wood chipboard industries use 15-ton machines that gobble up the rainforest with 8-foot cutting discs that have eight blades revolving 320 times a minute. These machines that cut entire trees into chips half the size of a matchbox can consume more than 200 species of trees in mere minutes.

Logging rainforest timber is a large economic source, and in many cases, the main source of revenue for servicing the national debt of these developing countries. Logging profits are real to those countries that must attend to their debts, but they are fleeting. Governments are selling their assets too cheaply, and once the rainforest is gone, their source of income will also be gone. Sadly, most of the real profits of the timber trade are made not by the developing countries, but by multinational companies and industrialists of the Northern Hemisphere. These huge, profit-driven companies pay governments a fraction of the timber's worth for large logging concessions on immense tracts of rainforest land—and reap huge profits by harvesting the timber in the most economical manner feasible with little regard to the destruction left in their wake.

Logging concessions in the Amazon are sold for as little as $2 per acre, with logging companies felling timber worth thousands of dollars per acre. Governments are selling their natural resources, hawking for pennies resources that soon will be worth billions of dollars. Some of these government concessions and land deals made with industrialists make the sale of Manhattan for $24 worth of trinkets look shrewd. In 1986, a huge industrial timber corporation bought thousands of acres in the Borneo rainforest by giving 2,000 Malaysian dollars to twelve longhouses of local tribes. This sum amounted to the price of two bottles of beer for each member of the community. Since then, this company and others have managed to extract and destroy about a third of the Borneo rainforest—about 6.9 million acres—and the local tribes have been evicted from the area or forced to work for the logging companies at slave wages.

Fuel Wood and the Paper Industry

In addition to being logged for exportation, rainforest wood stays in developing countries for fuel wood and charcoal. One single steel plant in Brazil making steel for Japanese cars needs millions of tons of wood each year to produce charcoal that can be used in the manufacture of steel. Then, there is the paper industry.

One pulpwood project in the Brazilian Amazon consists of a Japanese power plant and pulp mill. To set up this single plant operation, 5,600 square miles of Amazon rainforest were burned to the ground and replanted with pulpwood trees. This single manufacturing plant consumes 2,000 tons of surrounding rainforest wood every day to produce 55 megawatts of electricity to run the plant. The plant, which has been in operation since 1978, produces more than 750 tons of pulp for paper every twenty-four hours, worth approximately $500,000, and has built 2,800 miles of roads through the Amazon rainforest to be used by its 700 vehicles. In addition, the world's biggest pulp mill is the Aracruz mill in Brazil. Its two units produce 1 million tons of pulp a year, harvesting the rainforest to keep the plant in business and displacing thousands of indigenous tribes. Where does all this pulp go? Aracruz's biggest customers are the United States, Belgium, Great Britain, and Japan. More and more rainforest is destroyed to meet the demands of the developed world's paper industry, which requires a staggering 200 million tons of wood each year simply to make paper. If the present rate continues, it is estimated that the paper industry alone will consume 4 billion tons of wood annually by the year 2020.

> It is estimated that the paper industry alone will consume 4 billion tons of rainforest wood annually by the year 2020.

Once an area of rainforest has been logged, even if it is given the rare chance to regrow, it can never become what it once was. The intricate ecosystem nature devised is lost forever. Only 1 to 2 percent of light at the top of a rainforest canopy manages to reach the forest floor below. Most times when timber is harvested, trees and other plants that have evolved over centuries to grow in the dark, humid environment below the canopy simply cannot live out in the open, and as a result, the plants and animals (that depend on the plants) of the original forest become extinct. Even if only sections of land throughout an area are destroyed, these remnants change drastically. Birds and other animals cannot cross from one remnant of land to another in the canopy, so plants are not pollinated, seeds are not dispersed by the animals, and the plants around the edges are not surrounded by the high jungle humidity they need to grow properly. As a result, the remnants slowly become degraded and die. Rains come and wash away the thin topsoil that was previously protected by the canopy, and this barren, infertile land is vulnerable to erosion. Sometimes the land is replanted in African grasses for cattle operations; other times more virgin rainforest is destroyed for cattle operations because grass planted on recently burned land has a better chance to grow.

Grazing Land

As the demand in the Western world for cheap meat increases, more and more rainforests are destroyed to provide grazing land for animals. In Brazil alone, there are an estimated 220 million head of cattle, 20 million goats, 60 million pigs, and 700 million chickens. Most of Central and Latin America's tropical and temperate rainforests have been lost to cattle operations to meet the world's demand, and still they continue to move southward into the heart of the South American rainforests. To graze one steer in Amazonia takes two full acres. Most of the ranchers in the Amazon operate at a loss, yielding only paper profits purely as tax shelters. Ranchers' fortunes are made only when ranching is supported by government giveaways. A banker or rich landowner in Brazil can slash and burn a huge tract of land in the Amazon rainforest, seed it with grass for cattle, and realize millions of dollars worth of government-subsidized loans, tax credits, and write-offs in return for developing the land. These government development schemes rarely make a profit, as they are actually selling cheap beef to industrialized nations. One single cattle ranch in Brazil that was co-owned by British Barclays Bank and one of Brazil's wealthiest families was responsible for the destruction of almost 500,000 acres of virgin rainforest. The cattle operation never made a profit, but government write-offs sheltered huge profits earned off of logging other land in the Brazilian rainforest owned by the same investors.

> Millions of acres of rainforests have been lost to cattle operations to meet the world's demand for cheap meat.

These generous tax and credit incentives have created more than 29 million acres of large cattle ranches in the Brazilian Amazon, even though the typical ranch could cover less than half its costs without these subsidies. Even these grazing lands do not last forever. Soon the lack of nutrients in the soil and overgrazing degrade them, and they are abandoned for newly cleared land. In Brazil alone, more than 63,000 square miles of land has reportedly been abandoned in this way.

Subsistence Farming

This type of government-driven destruction of rainforest land is promoted by a common attitude among governments in rainforest regions, an attitude that the forest is an economic resource to be harnessed to aid in the development of their countries. The same attitudes that accompanied the colonization of our own frontier are found today in Brazil and other countries with wild and unharnessed rainforest wilderness. These beliefs are exemplified by one Brazilian official's public statement that "not until all

Amazonas is colonized by real Brazilians, not Indians, can we truly say we own it." Were we Americans any different with our own colonization, decimating the North American Indian tribes? Like Brazil, we sent out a call to all the world that America had land for the landless in an effort to increase colonization of our country at the expense of our indigenous Indian tribes. And like the first American colonists, colonization in the rainforest really means subsistence farming.

Subsistence farming has for centuries been a driving force in the loss of rainforest land. And as populations explode in Third World countries in South America and the Far East, the impact has been profound. By tradition, wildlands and unsettled lands in the rainforest are free to those who clear the forest and till the soil. "Squatter's rights" still prevail, and poor, hungry people show little enthusiasm for arguments about the value of biodiversity or the plight of endangered species when they struggle daily to feed their families. These landless peasants and settlers follow the logging companies down the roads they have built to extract timber into untouched rainforest lands, burning off whatever the logging companies leave behind.

The present approach to rainforest cultivation produces wealth for a few, but only for a short time, because farming burned-off tracts of Amazon rainforest seldom works for long. Less than 10 percent of Amazonian soils are suitable for sustained conventional agriculture. However lush they look, rainforests often flourish on such nutrient-poor soils that they are essentially "wet deserts," easier to damage and harder to cultivate than any other soil. Most are exhausted by the time they have produced three or four crops. Many of the thousands of homesteaders who migrated from Brazil's cities to the wilds of the rainforest, responding to the government's call of "land without men for men without land," have already had to abandon their depleted farms and move on, leaving behind fields of baked clay dotted with stagnant pools of polluted water.

However lush they look, rainforests often flourish on such nutrient-poor soils that they are essentially "wet deserts," easier to damage and harder to cultivate than any other soil.

Experts agree that the path to conservation begins with helping these local residents meet their own daily needs. Because of the infertility of the soil, and the lack of knowledge of sustainable cultivation practices, this type of agriculture strips the soil of nutrients within a few harvests, and the farmers continue to move farther into the rainforest in search of new land. They must be helped and educated to break free of the need to continually clear rainforest in search of fresh, fertile land if the rainforest is to be saved.

Leading the Threat: Governments

Directly and indirectly, the leading threats to rainforest ecosystems are governments and their unbridled, unplanned, and uncoordinated development of natural resources. The 2000–2001 World Resources Report put out by the United Nations reported that governments worldwide spend $700 billion dollars a year supporting and subsidizing environmentally unsound practices in the use of water, agriculture, energy, and transportation. In the Amazon, rainforest timber exports and large-scale development projects go a long way in servicing national debt in many developing countries, which is why governments and international aid-lending institutions like the World Bank subsidize them. In the tropics, governments own or control nearly 80 percent of tropical forests, so these forests stand or fall according to government policy; and in many countries, government policies lie behind the wastage of forest resources. Besides the tax incentives and credit subsidies that guarantee large profits to private investors who convert forests to pastures and farms, governments allow private concessionaires to log the national forests on terms that induce uneconomic or wasteful uses of the public domain. Massive public expenditures on highways, dams, plantations, and agricultural settlements, too often supported by multilateral development lending, convert or destroy large areas of forest for projects of questionable economic worth.

Tropical countries are among the poorest countries on Earth. Brazil alone spends 40 percent of its annual income simply servicing its loans, and the per capita income of Brazil's people is less than $2,000 annually. Sadly, these numbers do not even represent an accurate picture in the Amazon because Brazil is one of the richer countries in South America. These struggling Amazonian countries must also manage the most complex, delicate, and valuable forests remaining on the planet, and the economic and technological resources available to them are limited. They must also endure a dramatic social and economic situation, as well as deeply adverse terms of trade and financial relationships with industrial countries. Under such conditions, the possibility of their reaching sustainable models of development alone is virtually nil.

There is a clear need for industrial countries to sincerely and effectively assist the tropics in a quest for sustainable forest management and development if the remaining rainforests are to be saved. The governments of these developing countries need help in learning how to manage and protect their natural resources for long-term profits, while still managing to reduce their debts, and they must be given the incentives and tools to do so. Programs to redefine the timber concessions so there are greater incentives to guard the long-term health of the forest and programs to revive and expand community-based forestry schemes, which ensure more rational use of forests and a better life for the people who live near them, must be developed.

First-World capital must seek out opportunities to partner with organizations that have the technical expertise to guide these programs of sustainable economic development. In addition, programs teaching techniques for sustainable harvesting practices and identifying profitable, yet sustainable, forest products can enable developing countries to improve the standard of living for their people, reduce national debt, and contribute meaningfully to land-use planning and conservation of natural resources.

RAINFORESTS, PHARMACY TO THE WORLD

> Rainforest plants are complex chemical storehouses that contain many undiscovered compounds with unrealized potential for use in modern medicine.

It is estimated that nearly half of the world's approximate 10 million species of plants, animals, and microorganisms will be destroyed or severely threatened over the next quarter-century due to rainforest deforestation. Edward O. Wilson estimates that we are losing 137 plant and animal species every single day. That's 50,000 species a year! Again, why should we in the United States be concerned about the destruction of distant tropical rainforests? Because rainforest plants are complex chemical storehouses that contain many undiscovered biodynamic compounds with unrealized potential for use in modern medicine. We can gain access to these materials only if we study and conserve the species that contain them.

Key to Tomorrow's Cures?

Rainforests currently provide sources for one-fourth of today's medicines, and 70 percent of the plants found to have anti-cancer properties are found only in the rainforest. The rainforest and its immense undiscovered biodiversity hold the key to unlocking tomorrow's cures for devastating diseases. How many cures for devastating disease have we already lost?

Two drugs obtained from a rainforest plant known as the Madagascar periwinkle, now extinct in the wild due to deforestation of the Madagascar rainforest, have increased the chances of survival for children with leukemia from 20 percent to 80 percent. Think about it: eight out of ten children are now saved, rather than eight of ten children dying from leukemia. How many children have been spared and how many more will continue to be spared because of this single rainforest plant? What if we had failed to discover this one important plant among millions before human activities had led to its extinction? When our remaining rainforests are gone, the rare plants and animals will be lost forever—and so will the possible cures for diseases like cancer they can provide.

No one can challenge the fact that we are still largely dependent on plants for treating our ailments. Almost 90 percent of people in developing countries still rely on traditional medicine, based largely on different species of plants and animals, for their primary health care. In the United States, some 25 percent of prescriptions are filled with drugs whose active ingredients are extracted or derived from plants. By 1980 sales of these plant-based drugs in the United States amounted to some $4.5 billion annually. Worldwide sales of these plant-based drugs were estimated at $40 billion in 1990. Currently, 121 prescription drugs sold worldwide come from plant-derived sources from only ninety species of plants. Still more drugs are derived from animals and microorganisms.

More than 25 percent of the active ingredients in today's cancer-fighting drugs come from organisms found only in the rainforest. The U.S. National Cancer Institute has identified more than 3,000 plants that are active against cancer cells, and 70 percent of these plants are found only in the rainforest. In the thousands of species of rainforest plants that have not been analyzed are many more thousands of unknown plant chemicals, many of which have evolved to protect the plants from diseases. These plant chemicals may well help us in our own ongoing struggle with constantly evolving pathogens, including bacteria, viruses, and fungi that are mutating against our mainstream drugs and becoming resistant to them. These pathogens cause serious diseases, including hepatitis, pneumonia, tuberculosis, and HIV, all of which are becoming more difficult to treat. Experts now believe that if there is a cure for cancer and even AIDS, it will probably be found in the rainforest.

> The U.S. National Cancer Institute has identified more than 3,000 plants that are active against cancer cells, and 70 percent of these plants are found only in the rainforest.

Bioprospecting

In 1983, there were no U.S. pharmaceutical manufacturers involved in research programs to discover new drugs or cures from plants. Today, more than 100 pharmaceutical companies, including giants like Merck, Abbott, Bristol-Myers Squibb, Eli Lilly, Monsanto, Smith-Kline Beecham, as well as several branches of the U.S. government, including the National Cancer

Institute, are engaged in plant-based research projects trying to find possible drugs to treat infections, cancer, and AIDS. Most of this research is currently taking place in the rainforest in an industry that is now called "bioprospecting." This new pharmacological industry draws together an unlikely confederacy: plant collectors and anthropologists; ecologists and conservationists; natural product companies and nutritional supplement manufacturers; AIDS and cancer researchers; executives in the world's largest drug companies; and native indigenous shamans. They are part of a radical experiment: to preserve the world's rainforests by showing how much more valuable they are standing than cut down. And it is a race against a clock whose every tick means another acre of charred forest. Yet, it is also a race that pits one explorer against another, for those who score the first big hit in chemical bioprospecting will secure wealth and a piece of scientific immortality.

In November 1991, Merck Pharmaceutical Company announced a landmark agreement to obtain samples of wild plants and animals for drug-screening purposes from Costa Rica's National Biodiversity Institute (INBio); the program is still ongoing today. Spurred by this and other biodiversity prospecting ventures, interest in the commercial value of plant genetic and biochemical resources is burgeoning today. While the Merck-INBio agreement provides a fascinating example of a private partnership that contributes to rural economic development, rainforest conservation, and technology transfer, virtually no precedent exists for national policies and legislation to govern and regulate what amounts to a brand new industry.

Since wealth and technology are as concentrated in most of the North as biodiversity and poverty are in much of the South, the question of equity is particularly hard to answer in ways that satisfy everyone with a stake in the outcome. The interests of bioprospecting corporations are not the same as those of people who live in a biodiversity "hot spot," many of whom are barely eking out a living. As the search for wild species whose genes can yield new medicines and better crops gathers momentum, these rich habitats also sport more and more bioprospectors. Like the nineteenth-century California gold rush or its present-day counterpart in Brazil, this "gene rush" could wreak havoc on ecosystems and the people living in or near them. If it is done properly, however, bioprospecting can bolster both economic and conservation goals while underpinning the medical and agricultural advances needed to combat disease and sustain growing populations.

· The majority of our current plant-derived drugs were discovered by examining the traditional use of plants by the indigenous people who lived where the plants grew and flourished. History has shown that the situation with the rainforest is no different, and bioprospectors now are working side by side with rainforest tribal shamans and herbal healers to learn the wealth of their plant knowledge, and about the many uses of indigenous plants.

UNLOCKING THE SECRETS OF THE RAINFOREST

After the Amerindians discovered America, about twenty millennia before Columbus, all their clothing, food, medicine, and shelter were derived from the forests. Those millennia gave the Indians time to discover and learn empirically the virtues and vices of the thousands of edible and medicinal species in the rainforest. More than 80 percent of the developed world's diet originated in the rainforest and from this indigenous knowledge of the wealth of edible fruits, vegetables, and nuts. Of the estimated 3,000 edible fruits found in the rainforest, only 200 are cultivated for use today, despite the fact that the Indians have used more than 1,500. Many secrets and untold treasures about the medicinal plants used by shamans, healers, and the indigenous people of the rainforest tribes await discovery. Long regarded as hocus-pocus by science, the empirical plant knowledge of the indigenous peoples is now thought by many to be the Amazon's new gold. Their use of the plants provides the bioprospector with the clues necessary to target specific species to research in the race for time before the species are lost to deforestation. More often, the race is defined as being the first pharmaceutical company to patent a new drug utilizing a newly discovered rainforest phytochemical—and, of course, to garner the profits.

Long regarded as hocus-pocus by science, the empirical plant knowledge of the indigenous peoples is now thought by many to be the Amazon's new gold.

Indigenous People, A Valuable Resource

Laboratory synthesis of new medicines is increasingly costly and not as fruitful as companies would like. In the words of one major drug company executive, "Scientists may be able to make any molecule they can imagine on a computer, but Mother Nature . . . is an infinitely more ingenious and exciting chemist." Scientists have developed new technologies to assess the chemical makeup of plants, and they realize that using medicinal plants identified by Indians makes research more efficient and less expensive. With these new trends, drug development has actually returned to its roots: traditional medicine. It is now understood by bioprospectors

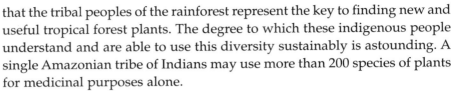

that the tribal peoples of the rainforest represent the key to finding new and useful tropical forest plants. The degree to which these indigenous people understand and are able to use this diversity sustainably is astounding. A single Amazonian tribe of Indians may use more than 200 species of plants for medicinal purposes alone.

A single Amazonian tribe may use more than 200 species of plants for medicinal purposes alone.

Of the 121 pharmaceutical drugs that are plant-derived today, 74 percent were discovered through follow-up research to verify the authenticity of information concerning the medical uses of the plant by indigenous peoples. Nevertheless, to this day, very few rainforest tribes have been subjected to a complete ethnobotanical analysis. Robert Goodland of the World Bank wrote, "Indigenous knowledge is essential for the use, identification and cataloguing of the [tropical] biota. As tribal groups disappear, their knowledge vanishes with them. The preservation of these groups is a significant economic opportunity for the [developing] nation, not a luxury."

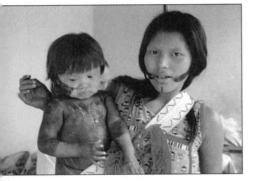

Kayapó tribal woman and child.

Since Amazonian Indians are often the only ones who know both the properties of these plants and how they can best be used, their knowledge is now considered an essential component of all efforts to conserve and develop the rainforest. Since failure to document this lore would represent a tremendous economic and scientific loss to the industrialized world, the bioprospectors are now working side by side with the rainforest tribal shamans and herbal healers to learn the wealth of their plant knowledge. But bioprospecting has a dark side. Indian knowledge that has resisted the pressure of "modernization" is being used by bioprospectors who, like oil companies and loggers destroying the forests, threaten to leave no benefits behind them.

Few Benefits for the Indigenous People

It is a noble idea—the ethnobotanist working with the Indians seeking a cure for cancer or even AIDS, like Sean Connery in the movie *Medicine Man*. Yet behind this lurks a system that, at its worst, steals the Indian knowledge to benefit CEOs, stockholders, and academic careers and reputations. The real goal of these powerful bioprospectors is to target novel and active phytochemicals for medical applications, synthesize them in a laboratory, and have them patented for subsequent drug manufacture and resulting profits. In this process, many active and beneficial plants have been found in the shaman's medicine chest, only to be discarded when it was found

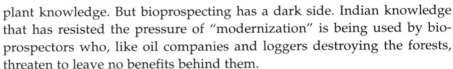

that the active ingredients of the plant numbered too many to be cost effectively synthesized into a patentable drug. It does not matter how active or beneficial the plant is or how long the U.S. Food and Drug Administration (FDA) process might take to approve the new drug; if the bioprospector can not capitalize on it, the public will rarely hear about a plant's newly discovered benefits. The fact is there is a lot of money at stake. In an article published in *Economic Botany*, Dr. Robert Mendelsohn, an economist at Yale University, and Dr. Michael J. Balick, director of the Institute of Economic Botany at the New York Botanical Gardens, estimate the minimum number of pharmaceutical drugs potentially remaining to be extracted from the rainforests. It is staggering! They estimate that there are at least 328 new drugs that still await discovery in the rainforest, with a potential value of $3 billion to $4 billion to a private pharmaceutical company and as much as $147 billion to society as a whole.

> As corporations rush to patent indigenous medicinal knowledge, the originating indigenous communities receive few, if any, benefits.

While the indigenous Indian shamans go about their daily lives caring for the well-being of their tribe, the shaman's rainforest medicines are being tested, synthesized, patented, and submitted for FDA approval in U.S. laboratories thousands of miles away. Soon, children with viral infections, adults with herpes, cancer patients, and many others throughout the world may benefit from new medicines from the Amazon rainforest. But what will the indigenous tribes see of these wonderful new medicines? As corporations rush to patent indigenous medicinal knowledge, the originating indigenous communities receive few, if any, benefits.

LOSING THE KNOWLEDGE

The destruction of the rainforest has followed the pattern of approaching natural land and natural world peoples as resources to be used, and seeing wilderness as idle, empty, and unproductive. Destruction of our rainforests is not only causing the extinction of plant and animal species, it is also wiping out indigenous peoples who live in the rainforest. Obviously, rainforests are not idle land, nor are they uninhabited. Indigenous peoples have developed technologies and resource systems that have allowed them to live on the land, farming, hunting, and gathering in a complex sustainable relationship with the forest. But when rainforests die, so do the indigenous peoples.

In 1500, there were an estimated 6 million to 9 million indigenous people inhabiting the rainforests in Brazil. When Western and European cultures were drawn to Brazil's Amazon in the hopes of finding riches beyond comprehension and artifacts from civilizations that have expired with the

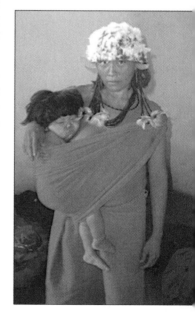

Arawete woman and child—their tribe uses annatto to paint their bodies and color clothing.

passage of time, they left behind decimated cultures in their ravenous wake. By 1900, there were only 1 million indigenous people left in Brazil's Amazon. Although the fabled Fountain of Youth was never discovered, many treasures in gold and gems were spirited away by the more successful invaders of the day, and the indigenous inhabitants of the rainforest bore the brunt of these marauding explorers and conquistadors.

Today there are fewer than 250,000 indigenous people of Brazil surviving this catastrophe, and still the destruction continues. These surviving indigenous people demonstrate the remarkable diversity of the rainforest because they comprise 215 ethnic groups with 170 different languages. Nationwide, they live in 526 territories, which together compose an area of 190 million acres . . . twice the size of California. About 188 million acres of this land is inside the Brazilian Amazon, in the states of Acre, Amapa, Amazonas, Maranhao, Mato Grosso, Para, Rondonia, Roraima, and Tocantins. There may also be fifty or more indigenous groups still living in the depths of the rainforest that have never had contact with the outside world.

Throughout the rainforest, people whose age-old traditions allow them to live in and off the forest without destroying it are losing out to cattle ranching, logging, hydroelectric projects, large-scale farms, mining, and colonization schemes. About half of the original Amazonian tribes have already been completely destroyed. The greatest threat to Brazil's remaining tribal people, most of whom live in the Amazon rainforest, is the invasion of their territory by ranchers, miners, and land speculators and the conflicts that follow. Thousands of peasants, rubber tappers, and indigenous tribes have been killed in Amazonia in the past decade in violent conflicts over forest resources and land.

> The greatest threat to Brazil's remaining tribal people, most of whom live in the Amazon rainforest, is the invasion of their territory by ranchers, miners, and land speculators.

As their homelands continue to be invaded and destroyed, rainforest people and their cultures are disappearing. When these indigenous peoples are lost forever, gone too will be their practical knowledge representing centuries of accumulated knowledge of the medicinal value of plant and animal species in the rainforest. Very few tribes have been subjected to a complete ethnobotanical analysis of their plant knowledge, and most medicine men and shamans remaining in the rainforests today are seventy years old or more. When a medicine man dies without passing his arts on to the next generation, the tribe and the world lose thousands of years of irreplaceable knowledge about medicinal plants. Each time a rainforest medicine man dies, it is as if a library has burned down.

THE SOLUTION: PROFITS WITHOUT PLUNDER

The problem and the solution of the destruction of the rainforest are both economic. Governments need money to service their debts, squatters and settlers need money to feed their families, and companies need to make profits. The simple fact is that the rainforest is being destroyed for the income and profits it yields, however fleeting. Money still makes the world go round—even in South America and even in the rainforest. But this also means that if landowners, governments, and those living in the rainforest today were given a viable economic reason not to destroy the rainforest, it could and would be saved. And this viable economic alternative does exist, and it is working today. Many organizations have demonstrated that if the medicinal plants, fruits, nuts, oils, and other resources like rubber, chocolate, and chicle (used to make chewing gums) are harvested sustainably, rainforest land has much more economic value today and more long-term income and profits for the future than if just timber is harvested or burned down for cattle or farming operations.

In fact, the latest statistics prove that rainforest land converted to cattle operations yields the landowner $60 per acre; if timber is harvested, the land is worth $400 per acre. However, if medicinal plants, fruits, nuts, rubber, chocolate, and other renewable and sustainable resources are harvested, the land will yield the landowner $2,400 per acre. This value provides an income not only today, but year after year, for generations. These sustainable resources—not the trees—are the true wealth of the rainforest.

This is no longer a theory. It is a fact, and it is being implemented today. Just as important, to wild-harvest the wealth of sustainable rainforest resources effectively, local people and indigenous tribes must be employed. Today, entire communities and tribes earn five to ten times more money in wild-harvesting medicinal plants, fruits, nuts, and oils than they can earn by chopping down the forest for subsistence crops. This much-needed income source creates the awareness and economic incentive for this population in the rainforest to protect and preserve the forests for long-term profits for themselves and their children, and is an important solution in saving the rainforest from destruction.

When the timber is harvested for short-term gain and profits, the medicinal plants, nuts, oils, and other important sustainable resources that thrive in this delicate ecosystem are destroyed. The real solution to saving the rainforest is to make its inhabitants see the forest and the trees by creating a consumer demand and consumer markets for these sustainable rainforest products—markets that are larger and louder than today's tropical timber market, markets that will put as much money in their pockets and government coffers as the timber companies do, markets that will give them the economic incentive to protect their sustainable resources for long-term profits, rather than short-term gain.

This is the only solution that makes a real impact, and it can make a real difference. Each and every person in the United States can take part in this solution by helping to create this consumer market and demand for sustainable rainforest products. By purchasing renewable and sustainable rainforest products and resources and demanding sustainable harvesting of these resources using local communities and indigenous tribes of the rainforests, we all can be part of the solution, and the rainforests of the world and their people can be saved.

Tribal Indian elders gathering roots and plants.

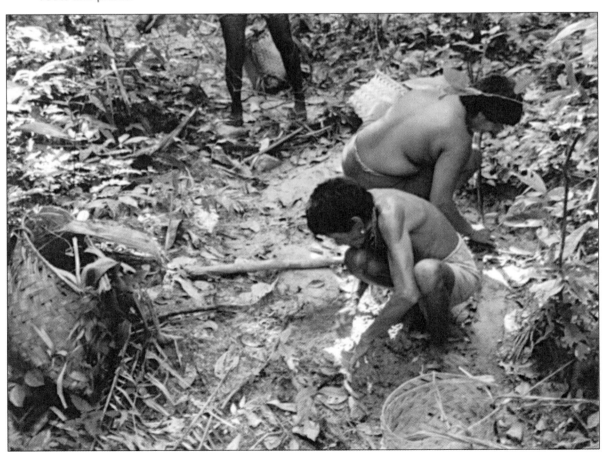

PART ONE

RAINFOREST HERBAL PRIMER

There are currently more than one hundred substances derived from plants in use as drugs throughout the world. Since drugs and active chemicals in plants can have widespread effects when consumed, it is important that people understand the differences and similarities between drugs and medicinal plants. Part One: Rainforest Herbal Primer discusses the use of herbs in health care, pointing out the differences and similarities between drugs and medicinal plants and the need for users to be well informed about the herbs they use (Chapter 2). Basic information about methods for preparing herbal remedies (Chapter 3) and details about rainforest remedies and recipes (Chapter 4) are also discussed.

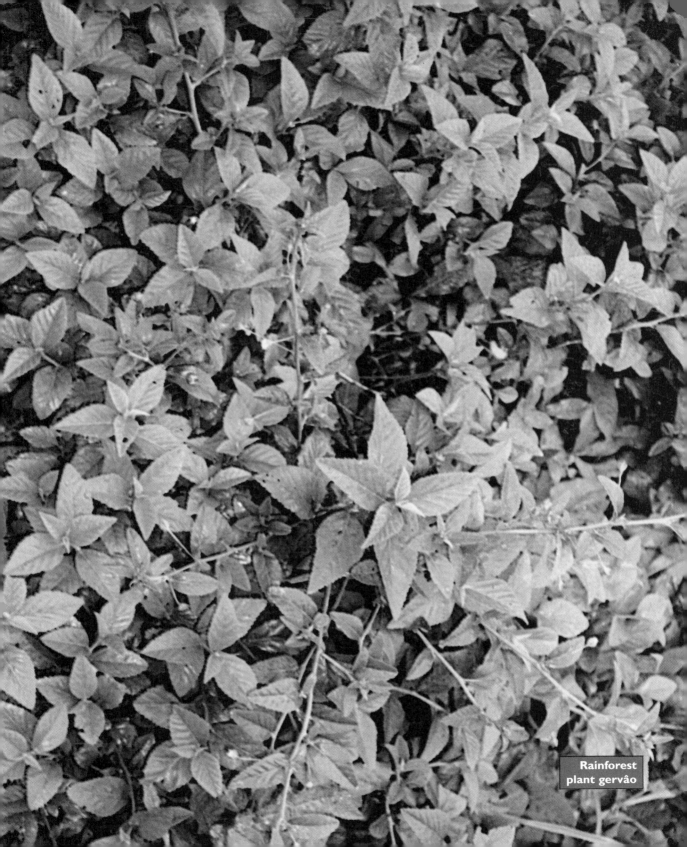

Rainforest
plant gervâo

CHAPTER 2

DIFFERENCES AND SIMILARITIES OF DRUGS AND MEDICINAL PLANTS

Today, there are at least 120 distinct chemical substances derived from plants that are considered important drugs and are currently in use in one or more countries in the world. Some of these drugs are simply a chemical or chemicals extracted from plant materials and put into a capsule, tablet, or liquid. One such example is the plant chemical called *cynarin*, which occurs naturally in the common artichoke plant. In Germany, a cynarin drug is manufactured and sold to treat hypertension, liver disorders, and high cholesterol levels. The drug is simply this single chemical, or an artichoke liquid extract, that has been concentrated and chemically manipulated to contain a specific amount of this one chemical; such a preparation is called a standardized extract. This drug is manufactured by pharmaceutical companies and sold in pharmacies in Germany with a doctor's prescription.

However, in the United States, artichoke extracts are available as natural products and sold in health food stores as "dietary supplements." Some U.S. artichoke products are even standardized to contain a specific amount of cynarin, yet they can still be purchased here as a natural product without a prescription (and for a lot less money than in Germany). There may be little to no difference between the cynarin drug produced in Germany and the artichoke standardized herbal supplement made in the United States considering that the same amount of cynarin is being delivered, dose for dose.

NEED FOR CONSUMER EDUCATION ABOUT HERBAL SUPPLEMENTS AND DRUGS

While American consumers do have more access to less-expensive natural products, such as cynarin-standardized artichoke products, regulations here prohibit the manufacturers to make any claims as to what the products might treat or even be good for, since they must be sold as "foods," not "medicines." Unfortunately, someone looking through the shelves in a health food store for something to help them manage their high blood pressure or high cholesterol might pass by an artichoke extract totally unaware of its status, the research about it, and its uses in Germany and other European countries. Therefore, even though American consumers may have freer access to these less-expensive natural products, they must make an effort to educate themselves about the properties and uses of these herbal substances in order to find the most appropriate natural remedy to meet their needs.

Many American consumers find it very frustrating to sort through a lot of ambiguous information put out by natural product manufacturers who cannot legally label their goods with condition-specific information (and stop them in their tracks in the aisles at the health food store saying, 'Hey, look at me, if you have high cholesterol!'). But, there is another way to look at it. Would you rather pay the much higher price to go to the doctor for the convenience of being told what to take and then spend more money on a prescription, as in Germany? Or would you rather do a little research yourself, skip the doctor's visit (and cost), and purchase a less-expensive natural product at the health food store that the German physician writes a prescription for anyway? Unfortunately, you can not have it both ways—not unless you find a highly knowledgeable naturopath, herbalist, or natural health practitioner who will just tell you (for free) what to buy at the health food store (and finding such a practitioner might take some research effort too!). So get prepared to do some research, take responsibility for your own health and wellness, and educate yourself about which natural remedies and products might be helpful for you.

Get prepared to do some research, take responsibility for your own health and wellness, and educate yourself about which natural remedies and products might be helpful for you.

Another well-known example of how similar a plant and drug can be (but a bit different) is quinine. For well over 100 years, the quinine chemical (an alkaloid) was extracted from the natural bark of Cinchona trees and sold as a prescription drug to treat malaria. American scientists were motivated to try to copy this chemical in the laboratory during World War II when the world's main tropical tree farms fell into the hands of the Japanese and the natural bark was in short supply—during which time American troops in the tropics were dropping like flies to malaria. Scientists were able to make an exact copy of the chemical in the laboratory without using any natural bark to start with, and a synthesized drug was created. Because it was a chemical occurring in nature and not a new one, it could not be patented by any one drug company. Several pharmaceutical companies worldwide began producing and selling synthesized quinine drugs, as they still do today.

While natural quinine-containing bark can be sold in the United States as a natural product, quinine drugs still require a prescription here. In many European countries, even the natural bark is regulated as a drug since it contains naturally occurring and very active quinine alkaloids that are regulated as drugs. This also means that Americans using the bark as a natural remedy should treat it with knowledge and respect due to its very powerful and active ingredient—quinine, which is not without well-documented acute toxicity and side effects. This is yet another reason American consumers need to educate themselves on the properties and actions of plants and their naturally occurring chemicals prior to using them. (Or find a qualified professional to guide them.)

Consumers need to understand that medicinal plants have active plant chemicals which may have therapeutic actions but also have side effects and toxicity at high dosages.

More is Not Always Better: Be Careful About Dosage Amounts

Too many Americans today buy into the idea that herbal products and medicinal plants are like food and are more or less benign and/or safe at any dosage. This is partly a result of legal restrictions stating that these products must be sold as "food supplements" in the United States. Also at play is that old American philosophy of excess: "if some is good, more is better." This idea is also somewhat prevalent in the food and dietary supplements market. While this may be true for some foods and dietary supplements, it is certainly not true for many of the biologically active medicinal plants that are sold here as herbal supplements. It is also not true for many of the rainforest plants discussed in this book.

Traditional dosage amounts for herbal remedies have been included in the plant information provided in Part Three of this book for a reason. These dosage amounts are based on the long history of the plant's use and should be followed within reason. They have been calculated for an average-weight adult person of 120 to 150 pounds and should be generally adjusted up or down based on body weight. Take less if you weigh under

120 pounds, and more if you weigh more than 150 pounds (up to double the recommended dosage if you weigh 300 pounds or more). If you plan on taking more than one and one-half times the dosage that is indicated for your weight, it is best to check with a qualified herbalist, naturopath, or physician who has experience with the particular plant you are choosing to take at higher dosages.

Possible Contraindications and Interactions

Another good reason to learn more about an herbal product or medicinal plant before taking it is possible contraindications and drug interactions. An excellent example of this possible problem is a very active chemical—coumarin—found in many plants and herbal supplements. Unfortunately, there is not enough consumer awareness of this potential interaction yet. Coumarin is a natural plant chemical found in many species of plants in varying amounts—from trace amounts to highly significant amounts. One coumarin-containing plant is the rainforest plant called guaco. It can contain up to 10 percent coumarin.

Coumarin is a very active plant chemical found in many plants that is almost identical to a widely sold prescription blood thinning drug.

In the 1940s, scientists discovered that coumarin was a highly effective blood thinner and went into the laboratory to synthesize or copy the plant chemical and turn it into a prescription drug. They changed the chemical just enough to patent it (basically by adding a type of salt molecule to the natural plant chemical) and renamed it coumadin. Today, coumadin is the eleventh most-prescribed medication in the United States, with annual sales of approximately $500 million in the United States alone. Even though the patent on this blood-thinning drug ran out years ago, it is still produced by just one company (a bit of a controversy) and sold in the United States under the brand name, Warfarin®. (It is manufactured by other companies in other countries and sold at a much cheaper price as coumadin or "generic warfarin.")

The coumadin and coumarin chemicals are very similar in structure, so much so that they are often tested in the laboratory as being the same chemical. When Americans began taking many types of herbal supplements over the last decade, conventional practitioners and surgeons began telling their patients to discontinue any and all herbal supplements prior to and following surgical procedures because of the prevalence of natural coumarin in plants. Since so many plants contained natural coumarin (and it was such an effective blood thinner), the solution was to just tell patients to discontinue everything. No one was really sure which plants contained enough coumarin to increase the risk of bleeding problems during or after a surgical procedure.

This example illustrates yet another reason consumers should be knowledgeable about what type of medicinal plants and herbal products they choose to take and should obtain information and facts from practitioners before launching any self-treatment program with medicinal plants, especially if they routinely take prescription drugs. Someone already taking the prescription drug Warfarin® should be informed that the blood-thinning effects of the drug must be carefully monitored (using blood tests), as excessive thinning of the blood is sometimes associated with fatal bleeding complications, including strokes and hemorrhages in the gastrointestinal tract. More importantly, they should be informed that taking plants high in natural coumarin may increase the blood-thinning effects of the drug and complications could be much more likely. As there are not enough research dollars available to document herb and drug interactions, many common plants that contain natural coumarin have never been officially studied as "blood thinners" in human studies or documented "to potentiate Warfarin® drugs." No warnings are officially published for many of these plants.

So when an interaction between Warfarin® and some herbal product happens, who's at fault? Is it the herbal supplement manufacturer who can not legally make a statement on the label of guaco (or other coumarin-containing plants) that the plant can thin the blood or label the product that it is contraindicated in someone taking Warfarin® in the absence of proven clinical research for that particular plant? Or is it the fault of the drug company that produces Warfarin® since it didn't do research on all the possible interactions between the drug and natural plants (not a legal requirement today)? The doctor who prescribed the Warfarin® drug and didn't ask the patient what herbal supplements he or she was taking or tell the patient which ones to avoid (because the doctor didn't know either)? Or, does the fault lie with the consumer who begins taking herbal supplements without knowing what natural chemicals the supplement contains and fails to check with his or her doctor first? This will probably be a question fought over by trial lawyers for years to come, but it will ultimately be the consumer who always pays the price.

Consumers are the ones experiencing the side effects and health problems, and they ultimately pay the price for litigation through higher insurance and product liability rates. This is also the reason why so many conventional doctors refuse to advise their patients about herbal supple-

Consumers need to take extra care when supplementing with medicinal plants if they routinely take prescription drugs.

ments and many just discourage their use altogether. They simply don't know enough about them, don't have the time to educate themselves properly, and don't want to be in the legal-liability loop for any negative side effect or drug interaction with the drugs they do prescribe and the many herbal supplements available to patients today.

For these reasons, in Part Three, information about contraindications and drug interaction is provided for each plant; this information may, or may not, be officially substantiated by human clinical research. The guaco plant is still a great example. No one has funded any human clinical research to prove that the plant can thin the blood, or that it will potentiate Warfarin® or coumadin drugs, but it has regularly been tested and found to contain highly significant amounts of coumarin. Programs in Brazil are even underway to extract the natural coumarin from this particular plant for the manufacture of Brazilian-made coumadin drugs. Therefore, warnings about contraindications and possible drug interactions with Warfarin® and other coumadin drugs have been provided in the guaco plant data (and for other rainforest plants that contain natural coumarin) in Part Three, based solely on the chemical contents of the plant. While many nonprofessionals may just skim over the chemical information that has been provided for each plant, the information has been recorded and provided to help explain not only why a plant might have a specific biological activity, but also to help you—and your healthcare provider—determine if there may be possible contraindications or drug interactions.

In fact, much of the data provided in this book on contraindications and drug interactions are based on the plants' chemistry or traditional uses in herbal medicine, rather than on funded human clinical studies proving a drug interaction or a medical contraindication. Human studies of this nature are very expensive and just aren't performed on most medicinal plants anywhere. There are too many plants, too many drugs, and not enough money to study all the possible interactions. This also means that the data that is provided in this book should not be considered all-inclusive or complete. It's important to note that much of the history of the medicinal uses of the plants discussed in this book is mainly recorded in tropical Third World countries where the plants grow. The populations of people using plant-based herbal remedies don't regularly take the amount or types of prescription drugs Americans do, and the history of side effects or contraindications when combining the plants with the drugs we use is virtually nonexistent. If you are taking prescription drugs, please always check with your doctor before taking any herbal supplements or medicinal plants, including those you learn about in this book.

NEED FOR CARE IN SELF-MEDICATING WITH HERBAL PRODUCTS

This brings us to yet another common and growing problem in what has been termed the "self-medicating herbal product industry" in the United States. What about the person who is tired of paying the high price for Warfarin® at the pharmacy and wants to try a plant like guaco to replace it? The majority of patients making up the $500 million-a-year market for this particular drug is over 60 years old and lives on a fixed income, so ideas such as this are not so uncommon. Unfortunately, this practice is also fraught with problems, especially in this particular instance. Warfarin® should be taken in very specific dosages, which have been tested to be effective and safe for each patient (dosages can vary from patient to patient) and an individual patient's needs can change over time as his or her medical condition improves or deteriorates. Taking too much or too little can have drastic results. Regular blood tests are administered to ensure the dosage is correct and continues to be correct for each patient.

Since chemical contents in plants can vary, it is difficult to determine the potency of an herbal supplement.

The coumarin content in guaco (and any plant) can change and fluctuate due to where it was grown, how and when it was harvested, climate changes in the growing environment/season, and other natural phenomena. The coumarin content can be 10 percent in one harvest of guaco plants, and as low as 5 percent the following year, even when the same plants are harvested again only a year later. So, in this case, it just would not be a good idea to try to replace the drug with an herbal supplement. Even if one found a "standardized" herbal guaco supplement with a guaranteed potency or content of coumarin, it should only be used under a doctor's supervision, in order to establish the correct dosage for the particular patient (with an obvious medical need) and would require the doctor's ongoing supervision and periodic testing. In most instances, ideally, conventional medicine and traditional medicine should play complementary roles in health care, and one should not replace the other.

PROBLEM OF ONE VS SEVERAL CHEMICALS

While many drugs have originated from biologically active plant chemicals, and many plants' medicinal uses can be attributed to various active chemicals found in them, there is a distinct difference between using a

Ideally, conventional medicine and traditional medicine should play complementary roles in health care, and one should not replace the other.

medicinal plant and a chemical drug. The difference is one that scares most conventionally trained doctors with no training in plants. Drugs usually consist of a single chemical, whereas medicinal plants can contain 400 or more chemicals. It's relatively easy to figure out the activity and side effects of a single chemical, but there is just no way scientists can map all the complex interactions and synergies that might be taking place between all the various chemicals found in a plant, or a traditionally prepared crude plant extract, containing all these chemicals. It is not unusual for a plant to contain a single documented cancer-causing chemical and also maybe five other chemicals that are anticancerous and which may counteract the one "bad" chemical. Overall, the plant extract may even provide some type of anticancerous effect.

In some instances, a particular plant chemical's activity is enhanced or increased when it is combined with another chemical or chemicals that occur naturally in the plant. An example of this is the rainforest plant cat's claw. First, the crude extract of cat's claw was shown to boost immune function. Then, specific alkaloid chemicals in the plant were scientifically documented (and patented) to be the "active constituents" that provided this effect. However, scientists discovered much later that if they extracted just the alkaloids, these alkaloids were less potent at stimulating immune cells than they were when combined with other chemicals (called catechin tannins) that the plant contains. Adding the tannin chemicals to the alkaloids increased the immune-stimulating effect of the alkaloids by almost 40 percent. In this instance, a drug made using only the alkaloids would probably be less effective than a crude extract of the plant that contained both alkaloids and tannins.

The drug industry often misses the boat in this regard. However, their motivations are different. Crude plant extracts cannot be patented or approved as drugs. The drug researcher's goal is to come up with a single chemical with good biological activity—one that can be changed in some way (without losing activity) so that it can be patented as a novel chemical and then be synthetically manufactured into a new patented drug. Sometimes the isolated chemical might not be quite as effective as the crude extract in which it was found, but the researchers have the ability to deliver more of the chemical therapeutically by increasing the dosage of the single chemical. Sometimes, they can even improve on the activity of the plant chemical by modifying it in some way, which also makes it patentable. Even if patents were not an issue, the drug company still would not be able to provide enough scientific data on how so many naturally occurring plant chemicals work individually, much less in combination with one another, to get a crude plant extract approved as a drug under our current drug regulations.

The quinine tree and its quinine alkaloid are again a wonderful example of some of the limitations in this regard. Scientists selected just one single alkaloid from the crude bark extract, the chemical that evidenced the highest antimalarial effect, to turn into a drug. But the crude extract actually had at least fifteen unique chemicals which were individually found to be antimalarial. The crude extract also contained other chemicals that had a different activity: they reduced fever (one of the main symptoms of malaria). Yet even other chemicals were found to be effective regulators of the heart and could be used to treat arrhythmia. (Sometimes very high fevers cause irregular heartbeat or increase the heart rate.) No wonder the crude bark extract was used for hundreds, if not thousands, of years by the indigenous people to treat malaria. It killed the bug that caused the disease, and in the meantime, it treated the symptoms the disease was causing! But similar to the guaco vine, the content of the active chemicals in the quinine tree can fluctuate. Some species of quinine trees can have 1 percent of the main antimalarial alkaloids, while others have up to 7 percent. How would a doctor know if a crude extract contained enough of these main chemicals to be therapeutic or how to prescribe proper dosages if these chemicals varied from extract to extract? For years, this alone has justified the use of the synthesized drug over the natural crude bark extract.

> Crude plant extracts and medicinal plants cannot be patented or approved as drugs. Under U.S. laws these natural plants cannot be marketed as a treatment or remedy for any disease or condition either.

POSSIBLE ANSWER TO DRUG RESISTANCE

Something really interesting has happened with the quinine tree, the quinine drug, and malaria, however. Since we've used this single synthesized drug against malaria for so many years, the malaria-causing organism (a *Plasmodium* protozoa) has mutated to create a defense mechanism against it. Today, we have several different strains of malaria that are completely resistant to our time-honored synthetic quinine drug. Back to the drawing board? Nope. . . back to the crude extract! Even the World Health Organization (WHO) is now revisiting the idea of going back to treating malaria in Third World countries with quinine bark extracts. Preliminary test-tube and animal studies indicate that natural bark extracts can effectively treat the new drug-resistant strains of malaria. Remember those other fourteen antimalarial chemicals in the crude bark extract? Do we know which one is doing the trick—or does it matter?

Many disease-causing organisms have developed resistance to our mainstream single chemical drugs and scientists are now looking at the value of multi-chemical natural plant extracts.

Another very interesting concept is that many disease-causing organisms can easily adapt and mutate to become resistant to a single chemical, but it would be much harder and take much more time for the organisms to create a defense mechanism against fifteen different chemicals simultaneously. Even more interesting: will throwing fifteen different active chemicals against the disease simultaneously speed up the treatment process? Only time will tell, and only if we somehow come up with the money to fund expensive large-scale human studies on unpatentable crude extracts. The pharmaceutical companies can't justify spending these research dollars on a crude plant-based medicine they cannot patent or sell. In this particular case, the WHO and/or large government public health agencies are more likely candidates to come up with the needed research dollars. Worldwide, more than one million people still die every year from malaria, and, unfortunately, this trend is likely to increase as more resistance to our main synthetic quinine drug develops.

The organism causing malaria is not the only evolving disease-causing bug we need to worry about. Bacteria can readily develop defense mechanisms against antibacterial drugs and become drug resistant. Many already have. The common staph bacteria (*Staphylococcus*) has gone through so many mutations over the last thirty years that many different strains have evolved that are now completely resistant to the eight major antibiotic drugs that were once effective against it. Could plants again hold the answer? Very possibly!

SHOTGUN APPROACH, NOT SINGLE BULLET?

An indigenous healer usually selects four to seven plants to combine into a remedy instead of just one. This usually means hundreds, if not thousands of different chemicals are contained in his crude plant extract.

A few years back, scientists evaluated a jungle shaman's "dysentery remedy." It was a crude plant extract that contained seven plants. Now, one must remember, dysentery in the Amazon can be attributed to any number of different bacteria, amebas, and parasites common in the area (and commonly shared in the close communal living environments of indigenous groups). The Indian shaman doesn't have the ability to send blood or stool samples to a laboratory to find out which specific organism is causing the dysentery in his village, but he must still select the appropriate plants to treat his patients. Maybe this is why a shaman usually selects a handful of plants (about four to seven) to brew into a remedy, instead of just one.

When the seven different plants in the dysentery remedy were analyzed, at least twelve different known antibiotic chemicals, five anti-amebic chemicals, and seven antiparasitic chemicals were found between all the plants in the shaman's formula. The twelve different antibiotic chemicals in the extract were found to kill bacteria in at least five different ways; these ways are called biological pathways of action. The shaman didn't really need to know which "bad bug" was the culprit, in what mainstream medicine would call his "shotgun" approach. But does this really matter either? This particular remedy, containing a total of several thousand individual plant chemicals, had at least thirty-one active chemicals that hit the top ten or so main bugs that might cause dysentery. (And, yes, you'd think your doctor was completely nuts if he sent you home with thirty-one prescriptions, so maybe "shotgun" is an appropriate analogy within your doctor's limitations.)

But let's go back to the interesting concept mentioned earlier. If the dysentery bug was an easily-mutating bacteria like staph, how likely would it be that this one organism could survive long enough to create a defense against twelve different antibacterial chemicals coming at it in at least five different ways simultaneously? These drug-resistant strains of bacteria are certainly more prevalent in First World nations in which single-chemical antibiotics are regularly employed than in poor tropical countries in which mainly plant-based remedies are used. Maybe it will take a broadly scattering shotgun to fight these tricky and quickly mutating organisms, instead of a single chemical bullet. Food for thought, for sure!

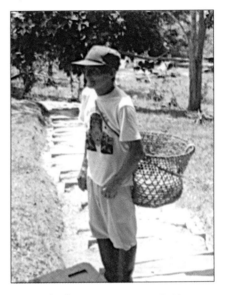

Shaman José Cabberrea, age 87, on his way out to gather medicinal plants.

As more of our gold-standard single-bullet drugs become less effective against newly developing strains of drug-resistant bacteria, viruses, fungi, and parasites, we will probably see more interest and research on medicinal plants, herb-based drugs, and traditional remedies. The rainforests of the world are, and will continue to be, of great importance and one of the main areas where this research will likely take place. Rainforests hold the highest biodiversity and sheer number of novel chemicals on the planet. Acre for acre, they contain more species of plants and animals, and yes, even bacteria, mold, fungi, and virus species than anywhere else on earth.

PLANT'S SURVIVAL INSTINCTS HELPING HUMANKIND

It's also very important to note that all living things have inbred survival instincts. It is literally part of the cellular makeup of all species on earth. In highly mobile species like humans and other animals, the main survival

Rainforest plants contain so many potent and active chemicals since the plants are in a constant battle for survival in an environment literally teeming with life that is constantly evolving.

instinct and mechanism is "flee, fight, or hide." Even bacteria and virus species have learned to flee or hide from immune cells and chemical agents attacking them, as well as to fight them by mutating or changing their own physical structure to defend against them. With stationary plants rooted to the ground and incapable of physically fleeing from danger, their survival instinct is controlled by wonderfully complex and rich chemical defense mechanisms that have evolved over eons. Plants have either created a defense mechanism against what might harm them, or they have succumbed and become extinct.

In the species-rich rainforest, there are many species of fungi, mold, bacteria, viruses, parasites, and insects that attack and kill plants. It is of little wonder that rainforest plants contain so many potent and active chemicals: the plants are in a constant battle for survival in an environment literally teeming with life that is constantly evolving. From soil-borne root rot (a virus) that attacks tender herbaceous plants, to the fungi and mold smothering the life out of huge canopy trees, or to the incredible number of insects devouring any defenseless leaf in the forest, rainforest plants have learned to adapt, create chemical defenses against attack, and survive. Within this rich arsenal of defensive chemicals are antibacterial, antiviral, antifungal, antiparasitic, anti-mold, and insecticidal chemicals with tested potent actions. This is the mechanism the plants use to survive, grow, and flourish as well as to fight the many disease-causing organisms that attack them. It is likely that within these diverse chemicals created to protect the plants from disease, at least a handful or more will be harvested and put to use protecting humans and animals from the same types of disease-causing organisms.

This is yet another reason to respect and value rainforest plants as very active potent herbal remedies and to protect them against humankind's destruction (against which the plants have no defense mechanism). Please respect them—and please help to protect them.

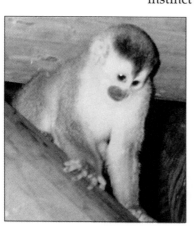

Capuchin monkey— just one example of the Amazon's diversity.

CHAPTER 3

METHODS OF PREPARING HERBAL REMEDIES

In traditional herbal medicine systems, herbal remedies are prepared in several rather standardized ways, which vary based on the plant used and, sometimes, on what condition is being treated. These methods include infusions (hot teas), decoctions (boiled teas), tinctures (alcohol and water extracts), and macerations (cold-soaking), each of which is described in more detail later in this chapter. In indigenous tribal medicine systems in the Amazon, medicine men, or shamans, generally use these same methods in addition to a few others. Other methods include preparing plants in hot baths (in which the patient is soaked or bathed), inhalation of powdered plants (like snuff), steam inhalation of various aromatic plants boiled in hot water, and even aromatherapy (inhaling fragrant essential oils of plants). A well-trained herbalist will always thoroughly review the time-honored method in which a plant has been traditionally prepared, since it holds important information about preparing an effective herbal remedy.

VARIOUS METHODS FOR DIFFERENT PLANTS AND CONDITIONS

The biological or therapeutic activity of a medicinal plant is closely related to the chemicals in the plant. These chemicals can be classified into major groups such as essential oils, alkaloids, acids, steroids, tannins, saponins, and so forth. For each of these classes of chemicals, there may be a preferred method of extraction that facilitates getting the chemicals out of the plant and into the herbal remedy being prepared. For example, some active chemicals found in plants are not soluble in water; therefore preparing a hot tea with the plant or boiling the plant in hot water won't extract these chemicals into the resulting water extract/tea remedy. Generally, if the chemicals aren't soluble in water, they won't be broken down in the digestive process either, so taking the plant in capsule or tablet form won't be much help either. If the active chemicals aren't in the prepared remedy, they probably won't provide any of the benefits attributed to them. However, these same chemicals may be soluble in alcohol, and for this reason, the time-honored way of preparing them as a remedy has been a tincture, or alcohol extract.

The manner in which a plant has been traditionally prepared holds important information about preparing an effective remedy.

Interestingly, this is also the reason why some plants are prepared in one manner to treat one specific condition and in a different way to treat a completely different condition. For example, preparing an infusion/tea of a plant might extract a delicate group of water-soluble anti-inflammatory plant steroids to treat arthritis (and leave behind other non-water soluble chemicals). Yet when the same plant is prepared in alcohol as a tincture, the delicate steroids are degraded or burned up, and antibacterial alkaloids that are only soluble in alcohol are extracted instead. This may explain why a specific plant may be used as a tea to treat arthritis and inflammation but as a tincture to treat various bacterial infections.

The rainforest shamans or rural herbal healers are not trained chemists with high-tech machines and scientific instruments at their disposal to isolate and study plant chemicals. Their knowledge about the best way to prepare medicinal plants into effective herbal remedies has been built over decades of empirical knowledge from trial and error, human experimentation, and even serendipity passed down from generation to generation. Yet, more often than not, plant chemists and scientists generally get around to verifying that these so-called "uneducated" herbal healers have maneuvered through complex chemical differences, reactions, and interactions, and different types of chemicals "unwittingly" developing the most efficient manner to extract and utilize the biological activity of the chemicals. It is usually the shaman's knowledge that the really smart scientists start with; this gives them specific clues as to which types of chemicals might be present.

Rather than enrolling in some organic chemistry class to understand the complex chemical makeup of the plants discussed in this book and how to prepare or use them, simply pay attention to the traditional manner in which they have been prepared. Information about how each plant is concocted when it is used for various conditions and remedies is provided in

Part Three of this book. If the information states that a plant is prepared as a tea to treat one condition but as a tincture to treat something different, there is probably a reason for it.

CHOOSING PRODUCTS

Many of the plants discussed in this book are available in the retail market in dried raw form and/or in manufactured products as capsules, tinctures, extracts, etc. The smart consumer should be prepared to notice whether product manufacturers have followed the traditional preparation methods because the method of preparation makes a difference in the quality of the product and in the results one can expect from use. A good example is the rainforest plant muira puama. Over the last five years, this plant has become popular in the retail market as a male aphrodisiac and libido stimulant, following its long history of use in the Amazon for male sexual dysfunction and as a natural remedy for impotency. As such, it is showing up as an ingredient in many libido- and male sexual health-formulas sold in health food stores. The well-informed consumer would know that most of the chemicals that provide this benefit are soluble only in alcohol, and would pass by the products on the shelf that just put muira puama in a capsule or tablet (and there are quite a few out there!), and choose a prepared alcohol tincture instead.

The smart consumer should be prepared to notice whether product manufacturers have followed the traditional preparation methods because the method of preparation makes a difference in quality and in the results one can expect from use.

It is hard to say if herbal manufacturers are uninformed or just capitalizing on the market created for a popular herb when they ignore traditional preparation methods. Many herbal companies use only one extraction method for every product in their line, regardless of the many medicinal plants they work with and their unique chemical contents. This usually results in some products being effective, while others are not, depending on which active chemicals actually got extracted by the company's one standardized manufacturing method. Unfortunately, it is usually consumers' dollars that determine which are effective. Sadder still, the value and efficacy of the medicinal plants themselves are often judged by these poorly manufactured products. There are many men out there today who claim muira puama just didn't deliver the results (or the value for their money) because they chose some bark capsule product, when, in fact, the plant properly prepared as an alcohol tincture is one of the best natural products available today for male sexual function.

So, as with most industries, the old saying of "let the buyer beware" certainly has a place in the herbal products industry. Before purchasing manufactured herbal products, do some research and pay close attention to traditional methods. Capsules and tablets are certainly more convenient and easier to take, and they don't taste bad, but sometimes they just won't be as effective as a foul-tasting herbal decoction or tincture. There can be some adaptations, however. As a general rule of thumb, many plants that are traditionally prepared as infusions and cold macerations have active chemicals that are soluble in water. This means that the plant can probably be taken in a tablet or capsule form since the chemicals will be broken down and dissolved in the digestive tract.

However, that preparation method will not be recorded as a "traditional" method since herbal healers in the Amazon don't have ready access to tablets and capsules, or the equipment needed to make them. There are a few exceptions, however. Generally, aromatic plants that need heat to release the aromatic essential oils are inhaled when the tea remedy is sipped and better absorbed in the mouth and throat. These adaptations are noted in Chapter 7, the plant summary reference guide. But before buying or preparing a remedy, it is still always best to refer to the complete information in Part Three about the plant, since there may be some differences in methods based on the type of remedy wanted for a specific condition.

PREPARING YOUR OWN REMEDIES

While a bit more trouble and time consuming, making your own natural remedies is usually much more economical than purchasing manufactured products. The remedies can also be much more effective when prepared properly by following time-honored traditional preparation methods.

The first step is finding a good source for the raw plant materials. Most plant materials coming from the Amazon region and other parts of South America will only be available in a dried state in either a cut herb or ground powder form. Find a reputable supplier who exports regularly from the region and please ask questions about their harvesting practices. Many South American plants are harvested unsustainably, causing more rainforest destruction, rather than helping to preserve it. Again, do the research required to find a good supplier, ask questions, and make sure you are obtaining the correct species of plant, and one that has been sustainably harvested.

If you don't plan on using the plant immediately, it is best to keep it unopened, in its original packaging, and away from direct sunlight (just put it in a closed cupboard/cabinet). Many plants will absorb moisture and humidity from the air, so if they are opened, reseal them tightly, or put them into a glass jar with a tight-fitting lid (avoid metal containers). Most plant materials do not require refrigeration or freezing; just keep them at average room temperature (70° to 80° F). Generally, if the plant material is stored properly, the shelf life for optimum freshness will be about a year for dried leaves, or two years for dried barks and roots. If you live in a warm, high-humidity area, it may be impossible to keep moisture out of regularly opened and closed glass containers, and the plants may become moldy. If this happens, discard them and purchase fresh ones. Next time, store them in paper lunch bags so they can "breathe" (although this will reduce the shelf life significantly).

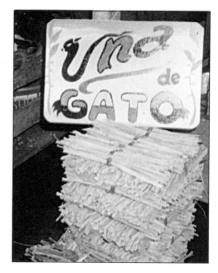

It is not always necessary to find a tea-cut plant to prepare a tea; ground powders can be used to make teas, tinctures, and decoctions just as well. A finely ground plant usually makes a stronger remedy, as more surface area of the plant is available to extract in the liquid. Extra time filtering is normally required when working with plant powders, but many herbalists prefer working with powders instead of bulky cut herbs, since they make stronger extracts. It is also recommended that you use distilled or purified water when extracting medicinal plants. Regular tap water can contain chlorine and other chemicals that might have an interaction or chain reaction with one or more of the many chemicals found in plants.

Local market in Iquitos, Peru selling cat's claw.

Instructions for the main preparation methods used throughout this book in the reference guides and in the main plant section are detailed below.

Infusions

Infusions are typically used for delicate herbs, leaves, and fresh tender plants. Preparing an infusion is much like making a cup of tea. Water is brought just to a boil and then poured over an herb (or combination of herbs), covered, and allowed to sit/steep for ten to fifteen minutes or so. An infusion can be prepared in a drinking cup (by just pouring the heated water over the herb in the cup) or by dropping the herb into the pot in which the water was heated. Empty gauze tea bags are even available at some herb stores; these bags can be filled with herbs and then sealed with an iron. If an infusion is prepared in the heating pan or pot, it is best to use a ceramic pot with a lid (avoid metal pots). Stir the preparation a few times while steeping, especially if you are using cut herbs, and keep the infusion covered.

Do the research required to find a good herbal supplier. Ask questions and make sure you are obtaining the correct species of plant, and one that has been sustainably harvested.

The ratio of herb to water varies depending on the remedy, the plant, and whether cut herb or powdered herb is used. Generally using 1 teaspoon of powdered herb or 2 teaspoons of more bulky cut herb in a 6-to-8-ounce cup of water is sufficient. If you are using a powdered herb, stir once halfway through the steeping time and let the powder settle to the bottom of the cup. Then, drink the infusion off the top (leaving the sediment in the bottom of the cup). If you are using a cut herb, strain the infusion with a tea strainer after steeping.

An herbal infusion is much like preparing a cup of tea.

An infusion is best prepared as needed and taken the same day it is prepared. It can be taken hot, warm, or cold. Standard dosages of infusions are generally 1 teacup (6–8 ounces), two or three times daily. The entire day's dosage can be prepared in the morning (2–3 cups at one time), and the remainder refrigerated until ready to use. The exceptions are the more aromatic plants with active essential oils; these are best prepared in single dosages (by the cupful) as needed and taken immediately while still hot/warm.

Decoctions

Decoctions are usually the method of choice when working with tougher and more fibrous plants, barks, and roots that have water-soluble chemicals. Instead of just steeping the plant part in hot water, the plant material is boiled for a longer period of time to soften the harder woody material and allow it to release its active constituents.

To prepare a decoction, select a ceramic pot with a snug-fitting lid. Measure the amount of herb needed—usually the same ratio of 1 teaspoon powdered herb or 2 teaspoons of cut herb per 8 ounces of water—into the pot and add the proper amount of cold water, depending on how many cups of the decoction you wish to prepare. Turn the heat to medium high and bring to a rolling boil. Place the lid on the pot and reduce the heat to medium or medium-low so that the mixture stays at a good simmer. Simmer it and keep covered for twenty minutes. If you can see steam escaping or smell the aroma of the herb, your lid is not tight enough and valuable essential oils are escaping.

After twenty minutes, remove the pot from the heat and cool slightly. If you are using cut herbs, strain the mixture through a tea strainer into a teacup. When straining, make sure to press on the cut herb pieces in the strainer to get as much liquid/decoction out of the herb as possible. If you are using powdered herb, allow the powder to settle to the bottom of the pot and then pour off the decoction from the top into a teacup (any sediment missed will settle to the bottom of the teacup).

Standard dosages for decoction are generally $\frac{1}{2}$ to 1 cup, two or three times daily. Again, the entire day's dosage can be prepared in the morning (2–3 cups at one time), and the remainder refrigerated until ready to use later in the day.

Strong Decoctions

Depending on the type of plant material used, strong decoctions are prepared in two general ways. The first involves boiling the mixture longer. This is usually indicated when working with larger woody pieces of bark. Longer boiling time, up to two hours or more, is sometimes necessary to break down, soften, and extract the chemicals from the larger pieces. When smaller woody pieces are used but yet a stronger remedy is wanted, the decoction is prepared as above (boiling twenty minutes) and then allowed to sit/soak overnight before the herb is strained out. When straining, again make sure to press on the cut herb pieces in the strainer to get as much moisture/decoction out of the herb pieces as possible.

Tinctures

A tincture is an alcohol and water extract that is used when plants have active chemicals that are not very soluble in water and/or when a larger quantity of the remedy is prepared for convenience and wanted for longer-term storage. Many properly prepared plant tinctures can last several years or more without losing potency. The percentage of alcohol usually helps determine the tincture's shelf life: the more alcohol used, the longer the shelf life. Sometimes the percentage of alcohol and water is unique to the herbs that are used, as some active ingredients are more soluble in alcohol and others more soluble in water. The type of alcohol can vary—vodka, rum, or 90- to 180-proof grain alcohol that is sold as "everclear" in liquor stores and is sometimes cheaper than vodka. Vodka is fine, but remember if it says 40 proof, it is 20 percent alcohol and the rest is water. In the Amazon, a sugar-cane alcohol resembling rum and called *aguardiente* is often used to prepare plant tinctures; it is 40 percent to 50 percent alcohol.

To prepare a tincture with a shelf life of at least one year, plan on using a minimum of 40 percent alcohol and the balance distilled water, unless otherwise noted in the plant information in Part Three. Use a clean glass bottle or jar with a tight-fitting lid or cork. Use a dark-colored bottle (like

> When a plant is prepared in alcohol, it is called a tincture.

Virtually any type of
alcohol can be used to
prepare a tincture.

a recycled green/amber wine bottle) or plan on storing the bottle out of the sunlight. When working with dried plants, use 2 ounces of plant material (cut or powder) for every 8 ounces (1 cup) of liquid. Since many cut herbs can be bulky, measure the amount of cut herb by weight and not volume (most cooks would tell you 2 tablespoons of butter is 1 ounce; however, a lightweight bulky leaf is not as heavy as butter in the same volume or by the tablespoon). A "standard 4:1 tincture" usually means 1 part herb to 4 parts liquid (or as above, 1 ounce herb to 4 ounces of liquid).

To prepare approximately 1 cup of tincture (some of the liquid will be absorbed by the dry plant material), place 2 ounces of the herb (cut up or powdered) into your clean glass container. Pour $\frac{1}{2}$ cup (4 ounces) of distilled water and $\frac{1}{2}$ cup (4 ounces) of 90-proof alcohol into the container (or just use 1 cup of straight 40-proof vodka and no water). Seal the container and store at room temperature away from direct sunlight. Shake the bottle/jar at least once daily. Allow the tincture to soak/extract for at least two weeks (larger woody cut herb pieces may need to soak for four weeks). At the end of two weeks, filter the tincture through a strainer to remove the plant parts (pressing hard on the plant material to get as much liquid out as possible) and pour into a fresh clean glass container and seal. Some people like to pour it through cheesecloth and then use the cheesecloth to more easily wring out the liquid from the plant material. If using a powdered plant for the tincture, stop shaking for three days and the powder will settle to the bottom. Pour the tincture off the top through a piece of cheesecloth to filter it.

Since this method uses a higher ratio of plant to liquid and helps concentrate the chemicals through the use of alcohol, dosages needed for tinctures are usually much less than those for infusions and decoctions. Average dosages for tinctures are about 1–2 milliliters (about 30 to 60 drops) two to three times daily. The tincture can be placed directly in the mouth for immediate absorption, or it can be placed in a small amount of water or juice. If you dislike the alcohol content (or want to give the remedy to a child), place the dosage in about 1–2 ounces of very hot water and most of the alcohol will evaporate in the hot water in a minute or two. (Let cool before taking.) Store the tincture at room temperature and away from direct sunlight.

Macerations

This method of preparation is certainly the easiest. The fresh or dried plant material is simply covered in cool water and soaked overnight. The herb is strained out and the liquid is taken. Normally this is used for very tender plants and/or fresh plants or those with delicate chemicals that might be harmed by heating, or which might be degraded in strong alcohol. This is also the easiest method to adapt to Western methods, since tablets or capsules can be used instead. Alternatively, just stir the ground plant powder into juice, water, or smoothies and drink.

Macerations are prepared when the plant chemicals are sensitive to heat or easily extracted in water.

Poultices and Compresses

Many herbal remedies are applied directly to the skin as poultices, usually on rashes and wounds and as topical pain-relieving remedies. Poultices are prepared in various ways—from the jungle shaman chewing up fresh leaves or roots and spitting them out onto the skin, to mashing up fresh leaves or roots by hand or with a mortar and pestle. Sometimes just enough hot water is poured over dried or fresh plant material to soften them. Then, the wet herbs are placed directly on the skin or between two pieces of cloth and laid on the skin. A light cotton bandage to bind the poultice to the area is generally used. (Or in the jungle, a nice large flexible leaf is commonly employed and tied with a bit of twine.)

To make a compress, simply soak a cloth in a prepared infusion, tincture, or decoction and place the cloth onto the affected part of the body/skin. Since most American readers of this book will only have access to dried plant materials to work with, using compresses instead of poultices will suffice for many of the described indigenous poultice remedies. More specific adaptations and directions are found in Part Three under "Traditional Preparation" where it might say to apply an infusion or decoction topically.

Baths and Bathing Remedies

Quite a few popular jungle remedies that have been used for thousands of years in the Amazon are prepared as vapor baths in which medicinal plants are added to bath water and the patient is soaked in it. This method is not unlike some of the currently evolving dermal delivery systems being employed in conventional medicine for drug absorption. The skin is a wonderful organ capable of absorbing chemicals directly and into the underlying fat tissue, and then into the bloodstream. Since fresh plants are generally used for bathing remedies (chopped or crushed first before adding to the bath water), modifications are not always possible when only dried plant materials are available, as in most of the Western world.

The Indian's bathing remedies are not unlike more complex skin-delivery systems employed with some dermal patch drugs.

An alternative approach is adding 20 to 30 ounces of a strong decoction or infusion to the bath water and having the patient soak in it for at least ten minutes.

While some readers might think preparing their own herbal remedies using these instructions rather daunting, it really isn't all that difficult once one learns the basic concepts. The most important aspect to remember is to purchase quality herbal ingredients to work with. The remedy prepared will only be as good as the herb that was used. Choose a good source to purchase from and expect to pay a little more for good quality—and remember to always ask about sustainability issues such as where and how the plant was harvested. To learn more about how some of the rainforest plants featured in this book are combined into specific formulas for specific conditions, continue on to Chapter 4, where recipes are provided that utilize the preparation methods discussed in this chapter.

Curanderos set up shop at local markets to dispense herbal remedies.

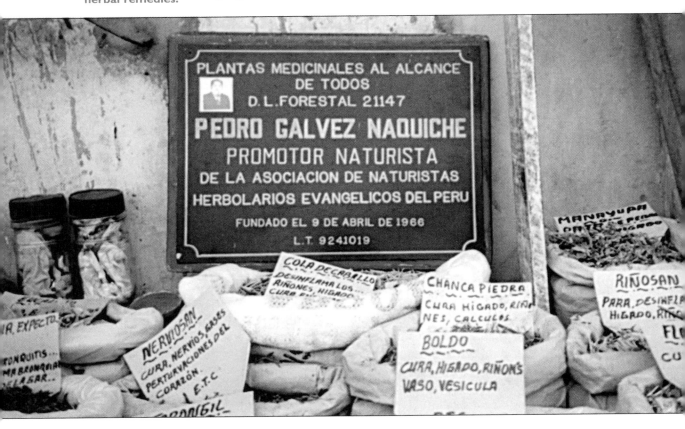

CHAPTER 4

RAINFOREST REMEDIES AND RECIPES

The following natural remedies are not complicated to prepare and can be adjusted easily if you want to prepare more or less than the amounts shown. The quantities shown are for dried plants. If you are lucky enough to be able to obtain freshly picked plants, then double the quantities given below. Either cut herbs or powdered herbs can be used. The amounts shown below are for powdered herbs, which are more widely available for these plants and more easily measured in a standard manner. If using cut-up leaves, barks, roots, etc., then generally double the amount shown below (a tablespoon of cut leaves can grind up to about a half-tablespoon or less of powdered herb, depending on how coarsely or finely cut they are). Before preparing and using any of the following recipes, please read about each herbal ingredient in Part Three. Some of the plants may be contraindicated for some people.

ALLERGY REMEDY

Combine 2 tablespoons each of nettle leaf, amor seco, and gervâo, and 1 tablespoon each of jatobá, guaco, picão preto, and carqueja into a glass jar, and shake well to disperse and mix the herbs together. When relief from seasonal allergies is needed, place a heaping teaspoon of the mixture into a coffee cup and pour 6–8 ounces of boiling water into the cup. Cover it with a saucer and let it steep for fifteen minutes, stirring once halfway through. Let the powder settle to the bottom of the cup and drink the infusion warm (leaving the sediment in the bottom). Repeat every six hours or so as needed to relieve allergy symptoms.

ARTHRITIS REMEDY

The following can be used for general arthritis pain and inflammation as and when needed. It's best prepared as a tincture. (See more instructions on preparing tinctures in Chapter 3, as needed.) The remedy can be stored for up to two years at room temperature.

Combine 2 tablespoons each of powdered chuchuhuasi, cat's claw, tayuya, iporuru, samambaia, and vassourinha, with 1 tablespoon each of nettle root, guaco, and manacá. Place powdered herb into a glass bottle or jar. Add 4 cups of 40-proof vodka (or 2 cups of 180-proof Everclear and 2 cups of distilled water). Shake well and seal or cork the container. Keep at room temperature and shake well every day for two weeks. At the end of two weeks, let the jar or bottle sit for three days without shaking. Line a tea strainer with a piece of cheesecloth and set over a large bowl. Carefully pour the tincture through the strainer, leaving most of the sediment in the bottom of the bottle. Pour the strained tincture back into a clean dark-colored bottle, seal, and store at room temperature away from direct sunlight. When you need relief from occasional arthritis pain and inflammation, take 1 or 2 teaspoons of the tincture directly by mouth or in a small amount of water or juice every six to eight hours as needed.

CALMING REMEDY

Combine ¼ cup each of damiana, passionflower, manacá, and mulungu and mix well. This combination can be prepared as a standard decoction or as a tincture following the instructions given in the previous chapter. Take one cup of the decoction as a sleeping aid or one-half cup to relieve stress. Dosages for the tincture are 1 teaspoon for stress and 2 teaspoons as a sleeping aid. This combination of plants is not pleasant tasting, so you may prefer to prepare the tincture, in which case you need only take a teaspoon and not a whole cup.

CANDIDA AND YEAST REMEDY

Combine 3 tablespoons jatobá, 2 tablespoons pau d'arco, 2 tablespoons anamu, and 1 tablespoon Brazilian peppertree powders (makes ½ cup). Prepare as a standard decoction following the instructions provided in the previous chapter. As the decoction is boiling, add 1 teaspoon of lemon juice to every 1 cup of water. For *Candida*, drink 1 cup of the decoction twice daily. The decoction can also be cooled to lukewarm and one cup used as a douche. For yeast infections, douche once daily for three consecutive days.

COLD AND FLU REMEDY

In a glass jar, combine 2 tablespoons each of powdered picão preto, fedegoso, mullaca, amor seco, mutamba, anamu, avenca, and guaco. Seal jar and shake well to mix (makes 1 cup). When needed for a cold or flu, shake jar well and then measure 2 level teaspoons of the mixture into a coffee cup. Pour 6–8 ounces of boiling water into the cup. Cover it with a saucer and let it steep fifteen minutes (stirring once halfway through). Let powder settle to the bottom and drink the tea warm or cold (leaving sediment in bottom of cup). Repeat every six hours.

This same remedy can be prepared as a tincture if preferred for longer-term storage. Follow the instructions for preparing tinctures in the previous chapter. Use 1 cup of the mixture of powdered plants with 4 cups alcohol/water. Dosages for the tincture are 1 teaspoon every six hours. For children, use 10 drops of the tincture for every 20 pounds of body weight every six hours.

INDIGESTION REMEDY

This remedy can be used to treat acidity in the stomach, gastroesophageal reflux (GERD), or high-acid indigestion. Place ½ teaspoon each of powdered carqueja, guacatonga, and espinheira santa in a coffee cup. Pour 6–8 ounces of boiling water into the cup, cover it with a saucer, and let it steep fifteen minutes (stirring once halfway through). Drink warm or cold, leaving the sediment in the bottom of the cup.

Alternatively, you can combine equal parts of all three plants (¼ or ½ cup of each) and stuff the well-mixed herbal powder into empty gelatin capsules (available at most health food stores in several sizes). Take 1–2 grams (2–4 capsules, depending on the size of the capsule) when needed for acid reflux or acid indigestion.

MENSTRUAL CRAMPS/PAIN REMEDY

Combine ½ cup of abuta with ¼ cup each of tayuya, manacá, and iporuru. Mix together in a large glass jar or bottle. Pour 2 cups of distilled water and 2½ cups of 180-proof alcohol (or 4½ cups of 40-proof vodka and no water) into the jar. Cap the jar and allow it to soak for two weeks, shaking the jar daily. At the end of two weeks, allow it to settle for three days without shaking, and then pour through a fine strainer or cheesecloth, leaving sediment in bottom of bottle. Place the strained tincture into a clean, preferably dark-colored glass jar or bottle with a lid. If kept sealed, in a cool (room temperature) dark place, this tincture will last for a year or longer. For menstrual pain and cramps, take 1 teaspoon of the tincture two to three times daily, or as needed. (Warning—this tincture tastes quite horrible!)

NATURAL COUGH SYRUP

In a ceramic pot with a lid, combine 4 tablespoons of guaco, 2 tablespoons of embauba, and 2 tablespoons amor seco. Add 8 cups of distilled water. Bring to a boil and place the lid on the pot. Reduce heat to medium and continue boiling until it is reduced to 4 cups (about thirty to forty-five minutes). Cool slightly and let powder settle to the bottom of the pot. Strain mixture through a cheesecloth-lined tea strainer into a clean pot, discarding sediment/powder. Add 1 cup of sugar and bring back to a boil. Boil, covered with a lid, for about twenty minutes, until it is syrupy. Remove from heat and add $\frac{1}{4}$ cup honey and 1 tablespoon lemon juice. Let cool. Pour into a glass jar or bottle and store in the refrigerator (will last several months). When needed for coughs or sore throats, take 1 tablespoon every four to six hours. Use 1-teaspoon dosages for children. (This one actually tastes pretty good!)

PAIN-RELIEVING MASSAGE OIL

Combine 1 cup of andiroba oil, $\frac{1}{2}$ cup copaiba oil, and $\frac{1}{2}$ cup of grapeseed oil together in a glass or plastic bottle and shake well to combine. Use as a regular massage oil, or rub lightly into painful or inflamed muscles, joints, sprains, and strains. If you live in the southern United States and can get your hands on some fresh scarlet bush leaves, infuse about $\frac{1}{2}$ cup of fresh, roughly chopped and bruised leaves in this combination of oil. Combine the oils and leaves in a glass Mason jar and put in a sunny window for a week to infuse them. Strain out the leaves and put in a clean bottle. This makes a wonderful topical pain-relief remedy!

PARASITE CLEANSE

Using ground powders, combine 5 tablespoons of amargo, 4 tablespoons of simarouba, 3 tablespoons of fedegoso, 2 tablespoons of epazote, and 2 tablespoons of boldo and mix well, making 1 cup. Use a heaping teaspoon per cup of water and prepare as a standard decoction. Take $\frac{1}{2}$ to 1 cup, depending on body weight, of the decoction twice daily for twenty-one consecutive days. This parasite cleanse remedy is generally used once annually (or twice annually if you are exposed to more parasites than the average American). This remedy is also a good one if you come down with amebic dysentery when traveling to Third World countries.

PROSTATE REMEDY

For prostate pain and inflammation, combine 2 tablespoons each of jatobá and nettle root with 1 tablespoon each of nettle leaf, cipó cabeludo, mutamba, and pau d'arco. Mix well and store in a glass jar. Prepare as needed as a standard decoction and drink 1 cup two to three times daily. This decoction can also be taken as 1 cup twice weekly to help prevent prostate problems and maintain a healthy prostate.

The above herbal remedies are just a few that are possible using the plants featured in this book. Don't be afraid to try your own combinations to prepare others. The tables of condensed information and condition-specific data in Part Two will help you select which plants to combine together for specific conditions. Just remember to read the information about each plant in Part Three to make sure there are no particular contraindications before using it in a remedy.

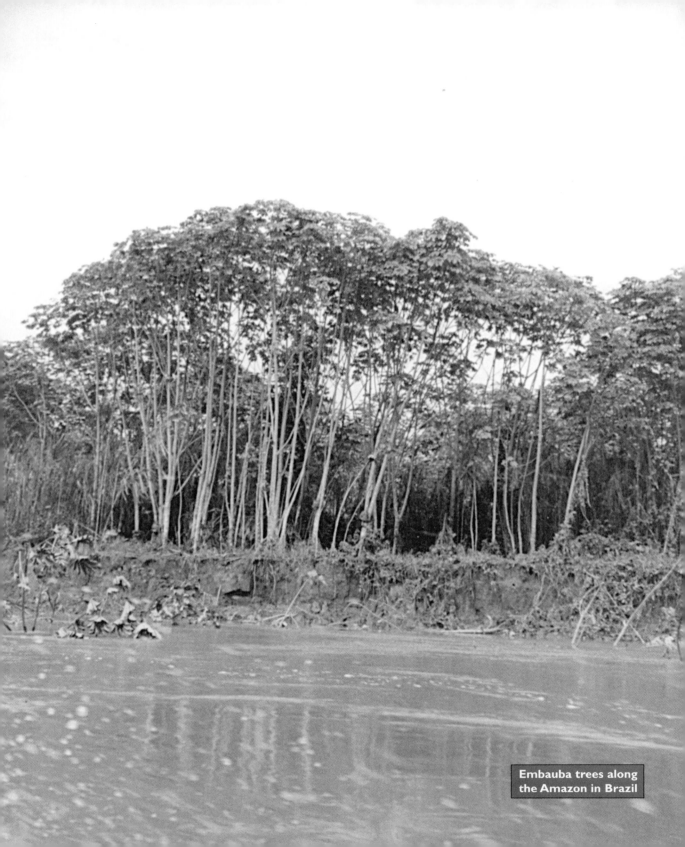

Embauba trees along
the Amazon in Brazil

PART TWO

QUICK GUIDES TO MEDICINAL PLANTS OF THE AMAZON

art Two provides information on seventy-three widely used medicinal plants of the Amazon rainforest. This material is presented in easily accessible table format for quick reference. Chapter 5 is a guide to the main properties and actions of common rainforest plants. Chapter 6 lists various diseases and disorders, and which medicinal plants are used in herbal therapy. Chapter 7 summarizes the specifics on each rainforest botanical. Together, these three chapters provide the reader with a guide to many of the most commonly used Amazonian plants, their properties and actions, and possible uses.

The tables and the summary provided in this section reorganize and cross reference much of the extensive information on each plant found in Part Three. Part Two can help readers identify which specific plants they should consider and research for their particular needs—be that a property (for example, an anti-inflammatory agent or a diuretic) or a way to treat a specific disease/disorder (for example, asthma or a yeast infection). However, since not all the plant information is completely summarized in these quick-reference guides, readers should always refer to the comprehensive information about each plant given in Part Three. Part Two should serve as an excellent starting point to an exploration of rainforest botanicals.

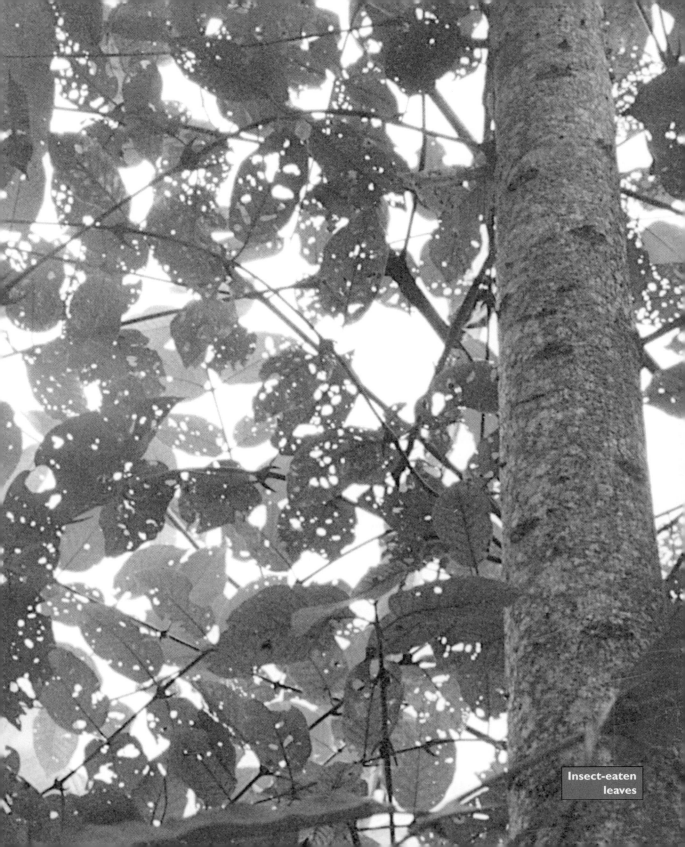

Insect-eaten
leaves

CHAPTER 5

PROPERTIES AND ACTIONS OF RAINFOREST PLANTS

This chapter presents valuable information, in an easy-to-use table, on the properties and actions attributed to the medicinal plants of the Amazon region. Table 5.1 defines the technical terms used to describe these properties, and lists those plants most commonly used for the particular property/action. This table also indicates those plants whose use for that action has been documented by research or by traditional medicinal use.

Scientists, herbalists, health practitioners, and researchers refer to the biological or therapeutic properties and actions of medicinal plants using general industry-standard words like anti-inflammatory, analgesic, antibacterial, and so on. Some words, such as *antibacterial* and *antiviral* are easy and self-explanatory. Other words, such as *vulnerary* or *vermifuge* may be much less familiar to nonprofessionals, and in most cases, simpler, more easily understood words have been used here. Some of the more technical terms may also have special nuances and meanings.

For example, the words *aperient, laxative, purgative,* and *cathartic* all refer to specific laxative-like actions the substances can have on bowel elimination, but there are differences in their exact meanings. A plant with an *aperient* action is used as a very mild or gentle "laxative" (generic term) to increase mucus and water in the intestine to aid in elimination, and may take a day or two to take effect. On the opposite end of the spectrum, a "laxative" that has a *purgative* or *cathartic* action promotes the immediate and complete evacuation of the bowel, oftentimes prior to liquefying, acts in a few hours or less, and can sometimes cause intestinal cramping because it stimulates the smooth muscles in the colon to move things along rather quickly. Therefore, just using the generic and well-known word "laxative" to describe these different properties and actions is not always helpful to the nonprofessional (especially one sitting in rush-hour traffic thinking they've taken a "laxative" instead of understanding it was really a purgative!).

In Table 5.1, column 1 lists the technical term for the property or action and corresponding lay term. A definition of the term or a cross reference to a simpler word for the particular property is provided in column 2. Rainforest plants having the specific property/action, as documented in this book and by hundreds of third-party documents, clinical studies, laboratory experiments, and/or herbal medicine books published in other countries, are then listed. Since many actions and properties can be attributed to the same plant (and many plants can have the same documented action), it can get confusing to the average person, and even to the professional, as to which plant to first turn for a particular action or property.

In an effort to simplify things, information about the uses of the different plants has been broken down in three ways. Column 3 lists the top five plants that practitioners and herbalists generally turn to first to achieve a particular action; these five plants are listed in order of preference. The table also differentiates whether the actions/properties have been documented through research or only through traditional use in herbal medicine. Those plants whose specific actions/properties have been documented through clinical research and/or laboratory studies are listed in column 4; these plants are listed alphabetically. Please remember that actions of the plants listed in this column may have been documented by a laboratory experiment, a test tube study, or preliminary animal research and not a human clinical study or medical trial. Finally, those plants whose actions/properties have been recorded just by their documented use in herbal medicine are listed in column 5; these plants are also listed alphabetically.

This information has been compiled and provided as a quick-reference guide to what has been actually documented on the plants. It is not intended to make specific medical claims for them. As always, it is best to refer to the text provided in Part Three, Medicinal Plants of the Rainforest, for more complete information on each plant's potential actions, properties, and uses, as well as on what actual research supports it. These documented actions may help explain why a specific plant is used in a particular way in herbal medicine systems. For example, a plant used in herbal medicine as a heart tonic or to lower high blood pressure might have been documented to have a hypotensive action in an animal study. Table 5.1 may also help the reader determine which plants he or she should read about in more detail; for example, someone with arthritis looking for plants with documented anti-inflammatory actions would look under anti-inflammatory and be guided to read, in Part Three, about the top five plants used for anti-inflammatory actions.

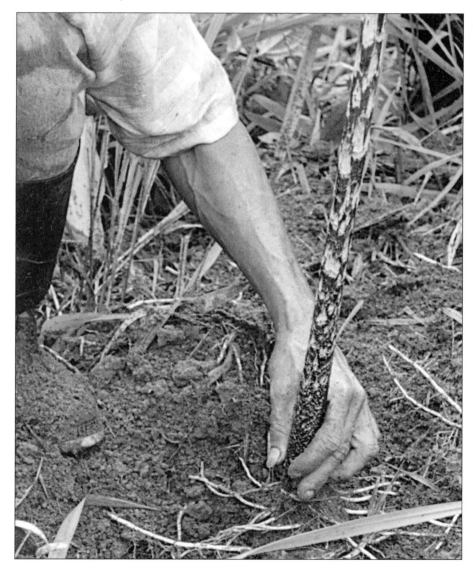

Harvesting jergón sacha root.

TABLE 5.1

Properties and Actions of Common Rainforest Plants

Technical Term (Lay Term)	Definition of Term
Abortifacient (Abortive)	A substance that causes or induces abortions.
ACE Inhibitor	A substance that inhibits angiotensin-converting enzyme, typically resulting in lowered blood pressure.
Adaptogen	A substance that restores or balances, in some unknown way, the normal functions of an organ or system.
Aldose Reductase Inhibitor	An agent that inhibits aldose reductase, an enzyme that converts glucose into a nerve toxin that results in nerve damage (e.g., diabetic neuropathy, macular degeneration).
Alterative	See **Adaptogen**.
Amebicide (Anti-amebic)	An agent used to kill amebas and treat amebic infections.
Analgesic (Pain-reliever)	A substance that relieves or reduces pain; also referred to as anodyne.
Anaphylactic	A substance that causes an allergic reaction.
Anesthetic	A substance that decreases or blocks nerve sensitivity to pain.
Antacid	A substance that reduces or neutralizes stomach acid.
Anti-allergy	See **Anti-anaphylactic**.
Anti-amebic	See **Amebicide**.
Anti-anaphylactic (Anti-allergy)	A substance that blocks or reduces an allergic reaction.
Antianxiolytic (Anti-anxiety)	An agent used to reduce or prevent anxiety.

Most Widely Used Herbs	Scientifically Validated Herbs	Traditionally Used
Not applicable	anamu, boldo, carqueja, chanca piedra, clavillia, pau d'arco	bitter melon, damiana, epazote, espinheira santa, fedegoso, gervâo, manacá, picão preto, scarlet bush, vassourinha
erva tostão, embauba, mutamba, abuta	abuta, embauba, erva tostão, mutamba	Not applicable
suma, cat's claw, erva tostão, samambaia, sarsaparilla	cat's claw, erva tostão, samambaia	damiana, guaraná, maca, manacá, muira puama, picão preto, sarsaparilla, suma, tayuya, velvet bean, yerba mate
chanca piedra, pedra hume caá, chuchuhuasi, annatto	annatto, chanca piedra, chuchuhuasi, pedra hume caá	Not applicable
simarouba, amargo, epazote, erva tostão, guava	amargo, epazote, erva tostão, graviola, guava, quinine, simarouba	bitter melon, carqueja, cashew, gervâo
internal—iporuru, tayuya, manacá, vassourinha, mulungu external—copaiba, andiroba, sangre de grado, kalanchoe, manacá	abuta, amargo, amor seco, anamu, andiroba, Brazilian peppertree, carqueja, catuaba, chanca piedra, chuchuhuasi, copaiba, embauba, erva tostão, gervâo, guacatonga, guaraná, guava, jurubeba, kalanchoe, macela, manacá, muira puama, nettle, passionflower, pau d'arco, scarlet bush, suma, tayuya, vassourinha, velvet bean	andiroba, boldo, cipó cabeludo, clavo huasca, epazote, espinheira santa, fedegoso, graviola, guaco, iporuru, juazeiro, mullaca, mulungu, quinine, sangre de grado, sarsaparilla, simarouba
Not applicable	balsam, Brazil nut, cashew, copaiba	Not applicable
sangre de grado, manacá, guaco, scarlet bush, Brazilian peppertree	Brazilian peppertree, chanca piedra, curare, sangre de grado, scarlet bush	copaiba, embauba, guacatonga, guaco, manacá
espinheira santa, guacatonga, carqueja, gervâo, jurubeba	carqueja, espinheira santa, gervâo, guacatonga, jurubeba	annatto, copaiba, epazote
amor seco, nettle, kalanchoe, gervâo, guaco	amor seco, gervâo, guaco, kalanchoe, nettle	erva tostão, pau d'arco, sangre de grado, suma, yerba mate
passionflower, mulungu, tayuya, manacá, damiana	mulungu, passionflower	anamu, catuaba, damiana, graviola, guava, manacá, muira puama, suma, tayuya, velvet bean

TABLE 5.1

Properties and Actions of Common Rainforest Plants

(continued)

Technical Term (Lay Term)	Definition of Term
Antibacterial	A substance that kills or inhibits bacteria.
Anticandidal (Anti-yeast)	An agent that inhibits or kills the yeast *Candida albicans*.
Anticarcinomic (Anticancerous)	A substance that kills or inhibits carcinomas (a cancer that arises in epithelium/tissue cells).
Anticoagulant (Blood thinner)	A substance that thins the blood and acts to inhibit blood platelets from sticking together and forming a clot.
Anticonvulsant	An agent that reduces or prevents convulsions.
Antidepressant	A substance used to treat depression.
Antidysenteric	An agent used to reduce or treat dysentery and diarrhea.
Antifungal	An agent that kills or inhibits the growth of fungi.
Antihelmintic	See **Vermifuge**.
Antihemorrhagic (Hemostatic, Styptic)	An agent that stops or prevents bleeding.

Most Widely Used Herbs	Scientifically Validated Herbs	Traditionally Used
internal—picão preto, mullaca, anamu, Brazilian peppertree, fedegoso external—copaiba, sangre de grado, mulateiro, anamu, andiroba	abuta, anamu, andiroba, annatto, avenca, balsam, bitter melon, Brazilian peppertree, cashew, catuaba, chanca piedra, clavillia, copaiba, embauba, erva tostão, fedegoso, graviola, guacatonga, guaco, guaraná, guava, jatobá, juazeiro, kalanchoe, macela, mulateiro, mullaca, mulungu, mutamba, pau d'arco, picão preto, sangre de grado, sarsaparilla, scarlet bush, simarouba, stevia, vassourinha	aveloz, cipó cabeludo, nettle, quinine
jatobá, pau d'arco, anamu, Brazilian peppertree, picão preto	anamu, avenca, Brazilian peppertree, clavillia, guaco, guava, jatobá, mulateiro, pau d'arco, picão preto, stevia	(See previous column.)
internal—graviola, mullaca, espinheira santa, vassourinha, guacatonga external—espinheira santa, sangre de grado, graviola, mullaca, copaiba	amargo, anamu, andiroba, bitter melon, Brazilian peppertree, cat's claw, chuchuhuasi, copaiba, epazote, espinheira santa, graviola, guacatonga, macela, mullaca, mutamba, pau d'arco, sangre de grado, simarouba, suma, vassourinha	aveloz, fedegoso, guaco, jergón sacha, samambaia, sarsaparilla
guaco, cipó cabeludo, boldo, mullaca, macela	cipó cabeludo, guaco, guaraná, macela, manacá, mullaca, picão preto	anamu, boldo, cat's claw, pau d'arco
erva tostão, amor seco, abuta, mulungu, nettle	abuta, amor seco, erva tostão, graviola, nettle	anamu, annatto, guava, jaborandi, kalanchoe, macela, mulungu, passionflower, tayuya
mulungu, tayuya, passionflower, muira puama, graviola	cat's claw, graviola, mulungu	Brazilian peppertree, damiana, muira puama, passionflower, tayuya, yerba mate
simarouba, sangre de grado, amargo, guava, cashew	amargo, cashew, gervâo, guava, pau d'arco, samambaia, sangre de grado, simarouba	cat's claw, chuchuhuasi, clavillia, scarlet bush
internal—jatobá, pau d'arco, anamu, fedegoso, picão preto external—jatobá, copaiba, sangre de grado, mulateiro, pau d'arco	abuta, anamu, Brazilian peppertree, clavillia, copaiba, embauba, fedegoso, graviola, guacatonga, guava, iporuru, jatobá, kalanchoe, mulateiro, mutamba, pau d'arco, picão preto, sangre de grado, sarsaparilla, scarlet bush, stevia, vassourinha	balsam, cashew, quinine
internal—abuta, sangre de grado, Brazilian peppertree, erva tostão, picão preto external—sangre de grado, juazeiro, nettle, mutamba, kalanchoe	abuta, annatto, sangre de grado	Brazilian peppertree, carqueja, cashew, embauba, fedegoso, guacatonga, jatobá, juazeiro, mullaca, mutamba, nettle, pedra hume caá, picão preto, simarouba

	Technical Term (Lay Term)	Definition of Term
TABLE 5.1 **Properties and Actions of Common Rainforest Plants** *(continued)*	**Antihepatotoxic** (Liver detoxifier)	A substance that protects the liver from toxins or clears toxins from the liver.
	Antihistamine	An agent used to counteract the effects of histamine production in allergic reactions.
	Anti-inflammatory	A substance used to reduce or prevent inflammation.
	Antileukemic	A substance that kills or inhibits the growth of leukemia cells.
	Antilithic	An agent that reduces or suppresses the formation of kidney stones and acts to dissolve those already present.
	Antimalarial	An agent used to treat malaria and/or kill the malaria-causing organism, *Plasmodium*.
	Antimicrobial	A substance that destroys or inhibits the growth of disease-causing bacteria, viruses, fungi, and other microorganisms. See also **Antibacterial, Anticandidal, Antifungal**, and **Antiviral**.
	Antimutagenic (Cellular protector)	An agent that can reduce, prevent, or reverse cells from mutating (for example, prevent healthy cells from mutating to cancer cells).
	Antioxidant	A substance that prevents oxidation and is thought to protect body cells from the damaging effects of oxidation (through free radical activity and lipid peroxidation).

Most Widely Used Herbs	Scientifically Validated Herbs	Traditionally Used
boldo, carqueja, erva tostão, chanca piedra, fedegoso	artichoke, boldo, carqueja, chanca piedra, erva tostão, fedegoso, macela, picão preto, sarsaparilla	amargo, cat's claw, epazote, mutamba
gervâo, guaco, nettle, amor seco, kalanchoe	abuta, amor seco, gervâo, guaco, kalanchoe, nettle	carqueja, erva tostão, iporuru, pau d'arco
internal—iporuru, guaco, amor seco, tayuya, cat's claw external—copaiba, andiroba, scarlet bush, guaco, kalanchoe	abuta, anamu, andiroba, boldo, carqueja, cashew, cat's claw, chuchuhuasi, copaiba, embauba, erva tostão, fedegoso, gervâo, guacatonga, guaco, iporuru, jatobá, juazeiro, jurubeba, kalanchoe, macela, manacá, mulungu, nettle, passionflower, pau d'arco, picão preto, samambaia, sangre de grado, sarsaparilla, scarlet bush, suma, tayuya, vassourinha, velvet bean, yerba mate	acerola, amargo, amor seco, annatto, bitter melon, chanca piedra, curare, epazote, espinheira santa, jaborandi, jergón sacha, mullaca, mutamba
mullaca, picão preto, vassourinha, simarouba, cipó cabeludo	bitter melon, cat's claw, cipó cabeludo, espinheira santa, mullaca, pau d'arco, picão preto, simarouba, suma, vassourinha	(See previous column.)
chanca piedra, boldo, cipó cabeludo, artichoke, erva tostão	chanca piedra	amargo, artichoke, avenca, boldo, cipó cabeludo, erva tostão, kalanchoe, velvet bean
quinine, simarouba, amargo, vassourinha, epazote	abuta, amargo, andiroba, chanca piedra, epazote, fedegoso, graviola, guava, pau d'arco, picão preto, quinine, simarouba, vassourinha	amor seco, anamu, annatto, damiana, bitter melon, carqueja, gervâo, guaco, jatobá, manacá, mullaca, mutamba, sarsaparilla, scarlet bush
cat's claw, chanca piedra, samambaia, fedegoso, boldo	boldo, cat's claw, chanca piedra, fedegoso, manacá, samambaia	guacatonga, simarouba
cat's claw, samambaia, gervâo, tayuya, fedegoso	abuta, acerola, anamu, annatto, artichoke, boldo, Brazil nut, camu-camu, cat's claw, chuchuhuasi, embauba, fedegoso, gervâo, guaraná, guava, macela, mulateiro, mutamba, samambaia, sangre de grado, tayuya, yerba mate	avenca, bitter melon, jatobá, pau d'arco, pedra hume caá, sarsaparilla, suma

Technical Term (Lay Term)	Definition of Term
Antiparasitic	A substance that kills parasites, either internally or externally.
Antiprotozoal	A substance that kills protozoa, a large family of single-cell microscopic organisms, many of which cause disease.
Antipyretic	See **Febrifuge**.
Antiseptic	A substance that destroys or inhibits germs and disease-causing organisms and is sufficiently nontoxic to cleanse wounds and prevent infections.
Antispasmodic (Muscle-relaxer)	A substance that relieves spasms or inhibits the contraction of smooth muscles.
Antitumorous	An agent that kills tumor cells and/or prevents the formation of tumors.
Antitussive	See **Cough Suppressant**.
Anti-ulcerogenic **Antiulcerous** (Anti-ulcer)	An agent used to protect against the formation of ulcers or as a treatment for ulcers.
Antivenin	An agent used against the venom of a snake, spider, or other venomous animal.

TABLE 5.1
Properties and Actions of Common Rainforest Plants
(continued)

Most Widely Used Herbs	Scientifically Validated Herbs	Traditionally Used
amargo, simarouba, epazote, boldo, fedegoso	amargo, andiroba, balsam, boldo, epazote, fedegoso, graviola, quinine, simarouba	annatto, bitter melon, clavillia, erva tostão, guava, jatobá, macela, mulateiro, nettle, pau d'arco, picão preto, scarlet bush, velvet bean
amargo, guaco, simarouba, bitter melon, anamu	amargo, anamu, bitter melon, epazote, erva tostão, graviola, guaco, guava, quinine, simarouba	boldo
mullaca, Brazilian peppertree, picão preto, annatto (leaf), guava (leaf)	balsam, Brazilian peppertree, copaiba, sangre de grado	abuta, andiroba, annatto, boldo, cashew, damiana, embauba, epazote, espinheira santa, fedegoso, guacatonga, guaraná, guava, mullaca, mulungu, nettle, picão preto, quinine, sarsaparilla
amor seco, abuta, vassourinha, manacá, mulungu	abuta, amargo, amor seco, annatto, boldo, Brazilian peppertree, chanca piedra, clavillia, curare, embauba, erva tostão, fedegoso, gervâo, graviola, guava, kalanchoe, macela, manacá, mullaca, mulungu, mutamba, passion-flower, quinine, vassourinha, velvet bean, yerba mate	anamu, chuchuhuasi, damiana, epazote, guaco, iporuru, picão preto
internal—graviola, mullaca, espinheira santa, vassourinha, guacatonga external—espinheira santa, sangre de grado, graviola, mullaca, copaiba	amargo, anamu, andiroba, bitter melon, Brazilian peppertree, cat's claw, chuchuhuasi, copaiba, epazote, espinheira santa, graviola, guacatonga, iporuru, kalanchoe, macela, mullaca, mutamba, pau d'arco, picão preto, sangre de grado, scarlet bush, simarouba, suma, vassourinha	aveloz, gervâo, jergón sacha, jurubeba, manacá
(internal peptic) gervâo, carqueja, espinheira santa, guacatonga, cat's claw (internal *H. pylori*) carqueja, guacatonga, bitter melon, balsam, pau d'arco (external) copaiba, gervâo, kalanchoe, juazeiro, picão preto	abuta, amargo, balsam, carqueja, cat's claw, chanca piedra, copaiba, espinheira santa, gervâo, guacatonga, jurubeba, kalanchoe, muira puama, picão preto	andiroba, bitter melon, epazote, guava, juazeiro, mutamba, pau d'arco, tayuya
jergón sacha, guaco, guacatonga, embauba, picão preto, tayuya	annatto, guacatonga, guaco, picão preto, velvet bean	abuta, amargo, anamu, curare, erva tostão, jergón sacha, manacá, pata de vaca, pau d'arco, tayuya, vassourinha

TABLE 5.1

Properties and Actions of Common Rainforest Plants

(continued)

Technical Term (Lay Term)	Definition of Term
Antiviral	A substance that destroys or inhibits the growth and viability of viruses.
Aperient	A substance that acts as a mild laxative by increasing fluids in the bowel.
Aphrodisiac	An agent that increases sexual activity and libido and/or improves sexual performance.
Appetite Stimulant	A substance used to increase or stimulate the appetite.
Appetite Suppressant	A substance that suppresses the appetite and/or eliminates the feelings of hunger.
Astringent	A substance that, by contracting blood vessels and certain body tissues (such as mucous membranes), reduces secretions and excretion of fluids and/or has a drying effect.
Bile Stimulant (Gallbladder)	A substance that increases the volume and flow of bile from the gallbladder; sometimes called choleretic.
Bile Stimulant (Liver)	A substance that increases the production and flow of bile in the liver; sometimes called chologogue.
Bitter	Having a sharp, acrid, and unpleasant taste that is thought to stimulate the flow of bile and other digestive juices to aid in digestion.

Most Widely Used Herbs	Scientifically Validated Herbs	Traditionally Used
internal—jergón sacha, mullaca, anamu, chanca piedra, bitter melon external—sangre de grado, bitter melon, carqueja, clavillia, vassourinha	amargo, anamu, bitter melon, Brazilian peppertree, carqueja, cat's claw, catuaba, chá de bugre, chanca piedra, clavillia, erva tostão, iporuru, kalanchoe, macela, mullaca, mutamba, pau d'arco, picão preto, sangre de grado, simarouba, stevia, vassourinha	andiroba, aveloz, avenca, copaiba, embauba, fedegoso, graviola, guacatonga, jergón sacha
carqueja, fedegoso, nettle, erva tostão, samambaia	fedegoso	amargo, annatto, Brazilian peppertree, carqueja, curare, damiana, erva tostão, guava, jurubeba, nettle, samambaia
(male) muira puama, catuaba, damiana, clavo huasca, velvet bean (female) clavo huasca, abuta, catuaba, suma, passionflower	damiana, muira puama, passionflower, suma, velvet bean	abuta, annatto, bitter melon, cashew, catuaba, chuchuhuasi, clavo huasca, guaraná, iporuru, maca, sarsaparilla
quinine, bitter melon, jatobá, amargo, boldo	amargo, quinine	amargo, avenca, bitter melon, boldo, chanca piedra, chuchuhuasi, clavo huasca, erva tostão, guaco, jatobá, muira puama, samambaia, suma
chá de bugre, guaraná, damiana, yerba mate	damiana, guaraná	chá de bugre, yerba mate
mutamba, pau d'arco, jatobá, Brazilian peppertree, guaraná	cashew, mulateiro	acerola, amargo, andiroba, annatto, artichoke, avenca, bitter melon, Brazilian peppertree, camu-camu, cat's claw, copaiba, damiana, embauba, espinheira santa, graviola, guacatonga, guaraná, guava, jatobá, juazeiro, macela, muira puama, mutamba, nettle, passionflower, pata de vaca, pau d'arco, pedra hume caá, picão preto, quinine, simarouba
artichoke, chanca piedra, boldo, erva tostão, macela	artichoke, boldo, chanca piedra, macela	abuta, amargo, balsam, erva tostão, jaborandi
boldo, artichoke, jurubeba, gervâo, jaborandi	artichoke, boldo, yerba mate	amargo, erva tostão, gervâo, jaborandi, jurubeba
amargo, quinine, carqueja, simarouba, artichoke	amargo, andiroba, artichoke, quinine	bitter melon, boldo, carqueja, damiana, macela, picão preto, simarouba, tayuya

Technical Term (Lay Term)	Definition of Term
Blood Cleanser	An agent used to cleanse or purify the blood; sometimes called a depurative.
Blood Thinner	See **Anticoagulant**.
Bronchodilator	An agent that dilates or relaxes bronchial muscles.
Cardiodepressant	An agent that decreases the contraction force of the heart and/or lowers heart rate.
Cardiotonic (Heart tonic)	A substance that strengthens, tones, or regulates heart functions without overt stimulation or depression.
Carminative	An agent used to prevent or expel gas from the stomach and intestines.
Cathartic	See **Purgative**.
Cellular Protector	See **Antimutagenic**.
Central Nervous System (CNS) Depressant	A substance that depresses the central nervous system.
Central Nervous System (CNS) Stimulant	A substance that stimulates the central nervous system.
Choleretic	See **Bile Stimulant** (Gallbladder).
Choliokinetic	A substance that increases the contractive power of the bile duct.
Chologogue	See **Bile Stimulant** (Liver).
Cicatrizant	See **Wound Healer**.

TABLE 5.1

Properties and Actions of Common Rainforest Plants

(continued)

Most Widely Used Herbs	Scientifically Validated Herbs	Traditionally Used
tayuya, sarsaparilla, samambaia, manacá, mullaca	sarsaparilla	amargo, amor seco, anamu, annatto, avenca, bitter melon, boldo, carqueja, cat's claw, chanca piedra, erva tostão, espinheira santa, fedegoso, guacatonga, guaco, guaraná, guava, jaborandi, jurubeba, manacá, mullaca, mutamba, nettle, pata de vaca, samambaia, tayuya, vassourinha, velvet bean, yerba mate
amor seco, guaco, embauba, gervâo, balsam	amor seco, gervâo, guaco	avenca, balsam, embauba, guaraná, manacá, velvet bean, yerba mate
graviola, mutamba, guava, nettle, jaborandi	graviola, guava, mutamba, nettle	jaborandi, manacá
embauba, Brazilian pepper-tree, erva tostão, picão preto, vassourinha	chá de bugre, embauba, guava, jurubeba, picão preto, quinine, stevia, vassourinha	abuta, acerola, annatto, artichoke, avenca, Brazilian peppertree, cat's claw, erva tostão, graviola, guaraná, juazeiro, macela, muira puama, mulungu, mutamba, passionflower, pau d'arco, pedra hume caá, yerba mate
jurubeba, epazote, bitter melon, carqueja, espinheira santa	copaiba	bitter melon, boldo, carqueja, chanca piedra, clavillia, clavo huasca, epazote, erva tostão, espinheira santa, guaraná, jatobá, jurubeba, kalanchoe, macela, picão preto, simarouba, suma, velvet bean
manacá, kalanchoe, passion-flower, mulungu, damiana	damiana, guava, kalanchoe, manacá, passionflower, vassourinha	embauba, gervâo, mulungu
muira puama, guaraná, catuaba, yerba mate, velvet bean	guaraná, muira puama	catuaba, velvet bean, yerba mate
artichoke, carqueja, jaborandi	artichoke	carqueja, jaborandi

TABLE 5.1

**Properties
and Actions
of Common
Rainforest
Plants**

(continued)

Technical Term (Lay Term)	Definition of Term
Contraceptive	An agent that prevents conception or interferes with fertility.
Cough Suppressant	A substance that suppresses coughing; also called antitussive.
COX Inhibitor	An agent that inhibits or interferes with the production of cyclooxygenase enzymes, which are linked to inflammatory processes and diseases.
Decongestant	A substance that relieves or reduces nasal or bronchial congestion.
Demulcent	See **Emollient**.
Detoxifier	A substance that promotes the removal of toxins from a system or organ.
Diaphoretic (Sweat promoter)	A substance that induces perspiration; also called sudorific.
Digestion Stimulant	An agent that stimulates or strengthens the activity of the stomach to improve the appetite and digestive processes; also called stomachic.
Disinfectant	An agent that destroys or inhibits the growth of harmful organisms.

Most Widely Used Herbs	Scientifically Validated Herbs	Traditionally Used
Not applicable	bitter melon, cat's claw, espinheira santa	amor seco, epazote, vassourinha
guaco, embauba, amor seco, passionflower, guava	guaco, guava, passionflower	abuta, amor seco, annatto, avenca, balsam, bitter melon, cashew, copaiba, damiana, embauba, espinheira santa, gervâo, iporuru, jatobá, jergón sacha, juazeiro, kalanchoe, macela, mutamba, picão preto, vassourinha, velvet bean
iporuru, picão preto, anamu	anamu, iporuru, picão preto	Not applicable
amor seco, nettle, embauba, jatobá, gervâo	nettle	abuta, amor seco, carqueja, cashew, cipó cabeludo, embauba, erva tostão, gervâo, jatobá, jurubeba, mutamba, picão preto, vassourinha
samambaia, chanca piedra, fedegoso, tayuya, nettle	artichoke, sarsaparilla	amor seco, avenca, bitter melon, boldo, cat's claw, chanca piedra, clavillia, erva tostão, espinheira santa, fedegoso, nettle, samambaia, tayuya, vassourinha
jaborandi, jatobá, mutamba, picão preto, guaco	jaborandi	abuta, anamu, avenca, carqueja, chá de bugre, chanca piedra, embauba, epazote, fedegoso, gervâo, guaco, jatobá, macela, manacá, mutamba, nettle, picão preto, samambaia, sarsaparilla, simarouba
jurubeba, artichoke, mutamba, carqueja, amargo	artichoke, boldo, carqueja, espinheira santa, jurubeba	abuta, amargo, amor seco, annatto, balsam, bitter melon, Brazilian peppertree, cashew, cat's claw, chanca piedra, chuchuhuasi, clavillia, clavo huasca, damiana, embauba, erva tostão, gervâo, graviola, guacatonga, guaraná, jatobá, juazeiro, muira puama, mutamba, nettle, quinine, sarsaparilla, simarouba, tayuya, yerba mate
mullaca, Brazilian peppertree, anamu, copaiba, espinheira santa	Brazilian peppertree	anamu, copaiba, espinheira santa, guacatonga, mullaca, mulungu, passionflower

Technical Term (Lay Term)	Definition of Term
Diuretic	A substance that increases urination.
Emetic	An agent that induces vomiting.
Emollient	An agent that has a protective and soothing action on the surfaces of the skin and membranes; also called demulcent.
Expectorant	An agent that increases bronchial mucous secretion by promoting liquefaction of the sticky mucus and expelling it from the body.
Febrifuge	An agent that reduces fever; also called antipyretic.
Galactagogue	See **Lactation Stimulant**.
Gastrotonic (Gastroprotective)	Substance that strengthens, tones, or regulates gastric functions (or protects from injury), without overt stimulation or depression.
Heart Tonic	See **Cardiotonic**.
Hemostatic	See **Antihemorrhagic**.
Hepatoprotective (Liver protector)	A substance that helps protect the liver from damage by toxins, other chemicals, or other disease processes.

TABLE 5.1

Properties and Actions of Common Rainforest Plants

(continued)

Most Widely Used Herbs	Scientifically Validated Herbs	Traditionally Used
erva tostão, amor seco, chanca piedra, cipó cabeludo, nettle	abuta, boldo, chanca piedra, embauba, erva tostão, jaborandi, nettle, passionflower, pata de vaca, sarsaparilla, scarlet bush, stevia, vassourinha	acerola, amor seco, anamu, annatto, artichoke, avenca, Brazilian pepper-tree, carqueja, cashew, cat's claw, chá de bugre, cipó cabeludo, clavillia, copaiba, curare, damiana, epazote, espinheira santa, fedegoso, gervâo, guaco, guaraná, jatobá, jergón sacha, juazeiro, jurubeba, manacá, mullaca, picão preto, samambaia, tayuya, velvet bean, yerba mate
Not applicable	aveloz, graviola	copaiba, jaborandi, yerba mate
andiroba, avenca, copaiba, samambaia, sarsaparilla	Not applicable	amor seco, andiroba, annatto, avenca, balsam, boldo, bitter melon, Brazil nut, copaiba, mulateiro, mutamba, nettle, picão preto, samambaia, sarsaparilla, vassourinha
embauba, guaco, samambaia, avenca, guava	guaco	abuta, amargo, anamu, andiroba, annatto, avenca, Brazilian peppertree, copaiba, damiana, embauba, guava, jatobá, juazeiro, mullaca, mutamba, samambaia, vassourinha
juazeiro, scarlet bush, manacá, vassourinha, kalanchoe	boldo, juazeiro, kalanchoe, manacá, nettle, scarlet bush, velvet bean	abuta, amargo, anamu, andiroba, annatto, avenca, bitter melon, Brazilian peppertree, carqueja, cashew, chanca piedra, chuchuhuasi, curare, fedegoso, gervâo, graviola, guaco, jurubeba, mullaca, mutamba, picão preto, quinine, samambaia, sarsaparilla, simarouba, vassourinha
jurubeba, picão preto, carqueja, cat's claw, guacatonga	annatto, artichoke, boldo, carqueja, cat's claw, chanca piedra, copaiba, gervâo, guacatonga, guava, jurubeba, macela, picão preto	abuta, amargo, avenca, bitter melon, epazote, muira puama
carqueja, erva tostão, chanca piedra, picão preto, boldo	annatto, artichoke, boldo, carqueja, chanca piedra, erva tostão, fedegoso, gervâo, jatobá, macela, picão preto	abuta, acerola, avenca, cat's claw, epazote, mutamba

	Technical Term (Lay Term)	Definition of Term
TABLE 5.1 **Properties and Actions of Common Rainforest Plants** *(continued)*	**Hepatotonic** (Liver tonic)	A substance that strengthens or tones the liver, sometimes employed to normalize liver enzymes and function.
	Hormonal (Female)	A substance that has a hormone-like effect similar to that of estrogen and/or a substance used to normalize female hormone levels.
	Hormonal (Male)	A substance that has a hormone-like effect similar to that of testosterone and/or a substance used to normalize male hormone levels.
	Hyperglycemic	A substance that raises blood sugar levels.
	Hypocholesterolemic (Cholesterol reducer)	A substance that lowers blood cholesterol levels.
	Hypoglycemic	An agent that lowers the concentration of glucose (sugar) in the blood.
	Hypotensive	A substance that lowers blood pressure.
	Hypothermal	See **Refrigerant**.
	Immune modulator	A substance that affects, modulates or selectively changes the functioning of the immune system (often used in auto-immune diseases).
	Immune stimulant	A substance that stimulates the activity of immune cells/function and/or increases the production of immune cells.
	Immune suppressant	A substance that suppresses the functioning of the immune system.
	Insecticide	A substance that kills insects.
	Insect Repellant	An agent that repels insects.
	Lactagogue	See **Lactation Stimulant**.

Most Widely Used Herbs	Scientifically Validated Herbs	Traditionally Used
carqueja, picão preto, gervâo, artichoke, chanca piedra	artichoke, chanca piedra, erva tostão, fedegoso, jurubeba, mulungu	abuta, acerola, amargo, anamu, avenca, boldo, carqueja, embauba, gervâo, juazeiro, macela, mullaca, pau d'arco, picão preto, vassourinha
abuta, damiana, Brazilian peppertree, suma, chuchuhuasi	abuta, cat's claw, damiana	Brazilian peppertree, chuchuhuasi, damiana, espinheira santa, maca, suma
muira puama, nettle, sarsaparilla, damiana, velvet bean	nettle, velvet bean	catuaba, chuchuhuasi, damiana, maca, muira puama, sarsaparilla, suma
Not applicable	annatto, guaraná	Not applicable
bitter melon, artichoke, suma, chanca piedra, velvet bean	artichoke, bitter melon, chanca piedra, guava, suma, velvet bean	acerola, annatto, avenca, carqueja, cat's claw, kalanchoe, muira puama, sarsaparilla, vassourinha, yerba mate
pata de vaca, pedra hume caá, chanca piedra, bitter melon, stevia	abuta, anamu, annatto, avenca, bitter melon, carqueja, chanca piedra, damiana, embauba, guava, macela, mullaca, mutamba, pata de vaca, pedra hume caá, stevia, vassourinha, velvet bean	amargo, cat's claw, iporuru, jatobá, mulateiro
graviola, abuta, chanca piedra, picão preto, erva tostão	abuta, Brazilian peppertree, carqueja, chanca piedra, embauba, erva tostão, fedegoso, graviola, guava, jurubeba, muira puama, mulungu, mutamba, nettle, passionflower, picão preto, stevia, vassourinha	annatto, artichoke, avenca, cashew, gervâo, guaraná, jaborandi, pedra hume caá, samambaia, velvet bean, yerba mate
cat's claw, samambaia	erva tostão, mullaca, nettle, picão preto, samambaia, sarsaparilla, suma, velvet bean	cat's claw, pau d'arco
cat's claw, anamu, mullaca, fedegoso, macela	anamu, bitter melon, cat's claw, chuchuhuasi, fedegoso, macela, mullaca, scarlet bush	chanca piedra, jergón sacha, maca, pau d'arco, simarouba, suma, yerba mate
Not applicable	aveloz, kalanchoe	Not applicable
amargo, graviola (seeds), andiroba, mulateiro, epazote	amargo, andiroba, epazote, graviola, kalanchoe, manacá, mulateiro, pau d'arco, quinine	annatto, bitter melon, Brazilian peppertree, fedegoso, macela, vassourinha
andiroba, annatto, mulateiro, amargo, vassourinha	andiroba	amargo, annatto, aveloz, mulateiro, vassourinha

TABLE 5.1

Properties and Actions of Common Rainforest Plants
(continued)

Technical Term (Lay Term)	Definition of Term
Lactation Stimulant	An agent that increases the production of breast milk and/or stimulates milk flow; also called a galactagogue or lactagogue.
Larvicidal	An agent that kills insect or parasite larva.
Laxative	A substance that stimulates evacuation of the bowels, causing looseness or relaxation of the intestinal muscles.
Molluscicidal	An agent that kills snails. (Typically used as a testing method to find agents to treat schistosomiasis.)
Muscle Relaxer	See **Antispasmodic**.
Nervine	A substance that has a normalizing or balancing effect on the nerves and/or central nervous system.
Neurasthenic	A substance used to treat nerve pain and/or weakness (neuralgia, sciatica, etc.).
Neuroprotective	A substance that protects brain cells from damage, helps repair damaged brain cells, and/or balances brain chemicals. In herbal medicine, neuroprotective plants are often used for memory disorders.
Pectoral	Pertaining to or used for the chest and respiratory tract.
Pediculicide	An agent that kills lice.
Piscicide	An agent that kills fish. (Also indicative that the substance possibly has other properties that make it toxic to parasites or bacteria.)

Most Widely Used Herbs	Scientifically Validated Herbs	Traditionally Used
nettle, erva tostão, gervâo, avenca, graviola (fruit juice)	None	avenca, bitter melon, epazote, erva tostão, gervâo, graviola, jaborandi, mulungu, nettle
amargo, gervâo, carqueja, boldo, bitter melon	amargo, bitter melon, carqueja, gervâo	balsam, boldo, jergón sacha, simarouba
guava, gervâo, tayuya, chanca piedra, amor seco	gervâo	amor seco, aveloz, bitter melon, boldo, chanca piedra, clavillia, embauba, epazote, espinheira santa, guaraná, guava, pau d'arco, simarouba, tayuya
graviola (seeds), bitter melon, macela, epazote, cashew	bitter melon, cashew, cipó cabeludo, epazote, jatobá, graviola, guacatonga, macela, pata de vaca	Not applicable
catuaba, damiana, tayuya, graviola, muira puama	damiana	amor seco, catuaba, cipó cabeludo, epazote, graviola, guaraná, guava, muira puama, quinine, sangre de grado, scarlet bush, suma, tayuya, yerba mate
sangre de grado, passionflower, mulungu, tayuya, manacá	passionflower, sangre de grado	catuaba, guaraná, guava, macela, manacá, muira puama, mulungu, quinine, suma, tayuya, velvet bean, yerba mate
samambaia, cat's claw, sarsaparilla, guaraná, velvet bean	cat's claw, graviola, guaraná, samambaia, sarsaparilla, velvet bean	catuaba, damiana, mulungu, simarouba, suma, yerba mate
avenca, samambaia, amor seco, embauba, balsam	None	abuta, amor seco, avenca, balsam, catuaba, chá de bugre, copaiba, embauba, epazote, gervâo, graviola, guaco, jatobá, kalanchoe, mutamba, picão preto, samambaia, sarsaparilla, vassourinha
amargo, andiroba, graviola (seed), balsam, fedegoso	amargo, balsam	andiroba, fedegoso, graviola, guacatonga, nettle
abuta, graviola, aveloz, chanca piedra, Brazilian peppertree, anamu	None	abuta, anamu, aveloz, Brazilian peppertree, cashew, graviola, guaraná, mulungu

<table>
<tr><td colspan="2">

TABLE 5.1

Properties and Actions of Common Rainforest Plants

(continued)

</td></tr>
</table>

Technical Term (Lay Term)	Definition of Term
Purgative	A substance used to cleanse or purge, especially causing the immediate evacuation of the bowel.
Refrigerant	A substance that lowers the temperature of the body or a part of the body, used to reduce the metabolic activity of tissues or to provide a local anesthetic effect; also sometimes known as hypothermal.
Sedative	A substance that soothes, calms, or tranquilizes, reducing or relieving stress, irritability, or excitement.
Sialogogue	A substance used to increase or promote the excretion of saliva.
Spasmolytic	See **Antispasmodic**.
Stimulant	A substance that promotes or increases the activity of a body system or function.
Stomachic	See **Digestive Stimulant**.
Styptic	See **Antihemorrhagic**.
Sudorific	See **Diaphoretic**.
Tonic	A substance that acts to restore, balance, tone, strengthen, or invigorate a body system without overt stimulation or depression.
Uterine Relaxant	An agent that relaxes the muscles in the uterus.
Uterine Stimulant	An agent that stimulates the uterus (and often employed during active childbirth).

Most Widely Used Herbs	Scientifically Validated Herbs	Traditionally Used
abuta, jatobá (fruit/seed), graviola (seed), manacá, aveloz	None	abuta, annatto (seeds), aveloz, bitter melon, cashew, clavillia, graviola (seeds), jatobá, manacá, yerba mate
scarlet bush, manacá, kalanchoe, mulateiro, mutamba	manacá, nettle, scarlet bush	annatto, avenca, bitter melon, carqueja, cashew, erva tostão, kalanchoe, mulateiro, mutamba, nettle, samambaia, sarsaparilla, vassourinha
manacá, mulungu, kalanchoe, passionflower, vassourinha	amargo, graviola, guava, kalanchoe, mulungu, passionflower, vassourinha	anamu, boldo, epazote, gervâo, macela, manacá, mullaca, nettle
jaborandi, espinheira santa, amargo, picão preto, Brazilian peppertree	jaborandi	amargo, Brazilian peppertree, espinheira santa, picão preto
guaraná, yerba mate, jatobá, chuchuhuasi, erva tostão	erva tostão, guaraná, yerba mate	abuta, artichoke, avenca, boldo, Brazilian peppertree, catuaba, chá de bugre, chuchuhuasi, copaiba, damiana, jatobá, maca, muira puama, picão preto, sarsaparilla, suma, yerba mate
cat's claw, suma, chuchuhuasi, catuaba, sarsaparilla	None	abuta, amargo, artichoke, avenca, bitter melon, Brazilian peppertree, carqueja, cashew, cat's claw, catuaba, chanca piedra, chuchuhuasi, clavillia, curare, damiana, espinheira santa, gervâo, jatobá, juazeiro, jurubeba, maca, muira puama, pata de vaca, quinine, samambaia, sarsaparilla, simarouba, tayuya, vassourinha
abuta, passionflower, boldo, chuchuhuasi, embauba	abuta, boldo	chanca piedra, chuchuhuasi, embauba, passionflower, pata de vaca
fedegoso, mutamba, picão preto, Brazilian peppertree, bitter melon	bitter melon, Brazilian peppertree, clavillia, fedegoso, graviola, mutamba, picão preto	avenca, carqueja, erva tostão, kalanchoe, nettle, velvet bean

TABLE 5.1

Properties and Actions of Common Rainforest Plants

(continued)

Technical Term (Lay Term)	Definition of Term
Vasoconstrictor	An agent that causes constriction of the blood vessels and decreases blood flow.
Vasodilator	A substance that causes a widening and/or relaxation of the blood vessels and therefore an increase in blood flow.
Vermifuge	A substance used to expel worms from the intestines.
Vulnerary	See **Wound Healer**.
Wound Healer	A substance used to heal wounds and promote tissue formation and the formation of a scab; also called vulnerary.

The Amazon River.

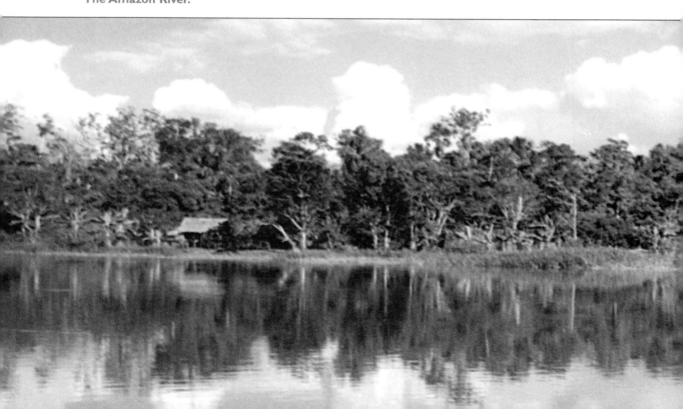

Most Widely Used Herbs	Scientifically Validated Herbs	Traditionally Used
fedegoso, guava, nettle, artichoke	fedegoso, guava	artichoke, nettle
graviola, boldo, gervâo, guaraná, yerba mate	boldo, catuaba, gervâo, graviola, guaraná, yerba mate	Brazilian peppertree, simarouba, stevia
amargo, epazote, simarouba, boldo, carqueja	amargo, bitter melon, boldo, carqueja, epazote, fedegoso, simarouba	anamu, andiroba, balsam, cat's claw, chanca piedra, clavillia, copaiba, erva tostão, gervâo, graviola, guaco, guava, jatobá, macela, mullaca, passionflower, pata de vaca, picão preto, scarlet bush, vassourinha, velvet bean
sangre de grado, copaiba, juazeiro, scarlet bush, Brazilian peppertree	balsam, Brazilian peppertree, copaiba, juazeiro, sangre de grado	acerola, amor seco, andiroba, annatto, avenca, bitter melon, cat's claw, clavillia, embauba, epazote, espinheira santa, gervâo, guacatonga, guaco, picão preto, sarsaparilla, scarlet bush, stevia, vassourinha

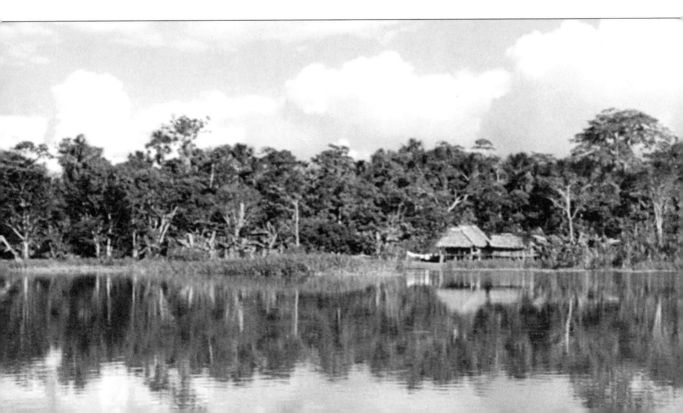

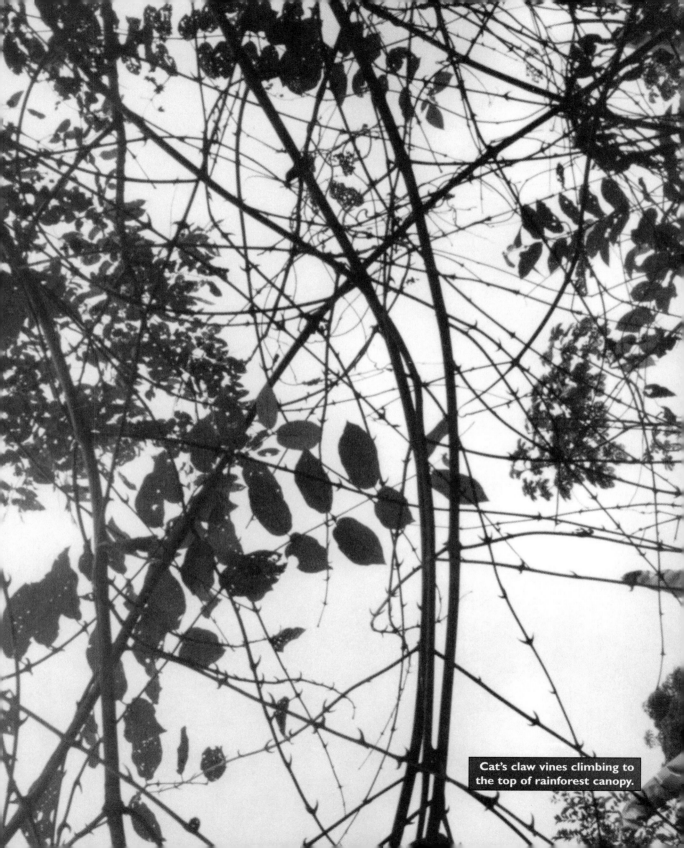

Cat's claw vines climbing to the top of rainforest canopy.

CHAPTER 6

HERBAL TREATMENT OF SPECIFIC DISEASES AND DISORDERS

The World Health Organization (WHO) estimates that up to 80 percent of the world's population still relies mainly on herbal medicine for primary health care, especially in developing nations and rainforest countries. People in tropical forests around the world have used the plants growing in their backyards as part of their healthcare systems for millennia. In fact, archaeologists have discovered the remains of plants used as medicine at archaeological dig sites in Latin and South America dating back to 8000 B.C. In the northwestern Amazon alone, at least 1,300 plant species are used to create *drogas do certão* or "wilderness drugs" for the primary health care needs in the region today. Many of these plant-based remedies have never been subjected to any type of scientific research.

Traditional uses of medicinal plants can be very important, especially to researchers and drug companies. If a plant has been used in a specific way for a specific purpose for many years and in many different geographical areas, there is probably a reason for it. It is this rapidly growing industry (called *ethnobotany*) that helps scientists target which plants to research first and what to study them for. Indigenous people originally discovered the medicinal uses of three-quarters of the plant-derived drugs in use today.

Let's face it, pharmaceutical drugs aren't getting any cheaper and most are out of the financial reach of a peasant or farmer in the Amazon who earns the equivalent of $50 monthly to support a family of seven. That doesn't mean he and his family can't afford to be sick, or aren't faced with many of the same illnesses and maladies as people in developed nations.

What it does mean is that plant-based medicines are often the most accessible and appropriate therapy for a wide diversity of health problems experienced by rural and rainforest inhabitants. Often, these populations cultivate and transplant wild medicinal plants in and around their homes and villages and use them to treat many common health problems they are faced with including fevers, fungal infections, respiratory problems, pain, gastrointestinal problems, and even as antidotes for poisonous snakebites. But that doesn't mean that many of these people wouldn't rather have a convenient aspirin or two to take occasionally for a simple headache, instead of going through the time-consuming steps of harvesting some leaves, bark, or roots out of the forest and boiling them into a tea remedy for headache. The sad fact is that even aspirin can be unavailable or too expensive for some forest dwellers.

Table 6.1 serves as a quick reference for matching a specific disorder or condition to the plants that have been used in the tropics, developing nations, and rainforests to treat it. Diseases not commonly found in developed nations but often common in developing nations, which lack adequate immunization programs, and tropical diseases, are included in the following table. The information has been provided as a summary of historical medicinal uses for the plants by disease and condition. It was compiled, cataloged, and condensed from more than 500 published sources of documentation listed in the References section of this book. The goal is to provide information and a starting point for categorizing and cross-referencing the extensive information provided in Part Three.

It is not intended to make any medical claim that the plants have been scientifically or clinically proven to cure or effectively treat the listed diseases or conditions in any way. It also is not meant to imply or suggest that the plants are more effective at treating the specific conditions than drugs or products available in the United States or other developed nations, but not available in the countries where these plants grow and where their history of medicinal use has been recorded. Sometimes it really is just easier and better to take an aspirin to relieve the occasional headache (if you have access to it and can afford it). Just because traditional herbal medicine and herbal remedies are often used in the Amazon and other remote areas to replace conventional medicine and drugs due to socioeconomic factors or simple unavailability, it is not advisable to use them here to replace or avoid proper medical care and drugs that could be beneficial. Again, conventional medicine and traditional medicine systems should ideally play complementary roles in health care—one should not substitute the other.

If you are looking for natural remedies for a serious medical disease or condition, please always seek the advice and help of qualified healthcare professionals. There are many healthcare professionals available these days with practical medical training as well as education and experience with medicinal plants, supplements, and nutrition and dietary recommendations. Find one. Books like this one, as well as the Internet, are good places to begin your research, especially when looking up and verifying both conventional and complementary products, therapies, treatments, and drugs. However, don't start and end there. Get qualified help and advice from experienced health professionals that can combine the best of both health systems, practices, products, and therapies into an effective and comprehensive treatment program. Please always remember that many medicinal plants (including those discussed in this book) have active biological properties and active chemicals that should be treated with care, respect, and knowledge. Some are not without side effects, and for most, there is little data on their suitability and contraindications in combination with the many pharmaceutical drugs that are commonly and routinely prescribed here in the United States.

TABLE 6.1 Specific Diseases/Disorders and Their Herbal Treatment

Condition	Plants Used in Herbal Medicine (in order of preference)
Abdominal Pain	jurubeba, carqueja, artichoke, erva tostão, kalanchoe, epazote, clavillia, abuta, bitter melon, fedegoso, chuchuhuasi
Abrasions	sangre de grado, andiroba, scarlet bush, mutamba, juazeiro, copaiba, fedegoso, balsam, kalanchoe See also **Wounds**
Abscesses	guaco, erva tostão, fedegoso, picão preto, sarsaparilla, epazote, graviola, cat's claw, samambaia, aveloz (topical), clavillia, balsam, jurubeba
Acid Reflux	See **Heartburn**
Acne	abuta, sarsaparilla, bitter melon, espinheira santa, damiana, fedegoso, tayuya, chuchuhuasi, artichoke, andiroba (external), clavillia, cat's claw
Adrenal Gland Disorders	chuchuhuasi, tayuya, erva tostão, espinheira santa, maca, catuaba, suma, muira puama, cat's claw, artichoke, passionflower
Aging (anti-)	samambaia, cat's claw, sarsaparilla, suma, yerba mate, andiroba (topical), annatto
AIDS and HIV	jergón sacha, mullaca, bitter melon, carqueja, amargo, chanca piedra, macela, clavillia, vassourinha, chá de bugre, catuaba, simarouba, cat's claw, pau d'arco

Condition	Plants Used in Herbal Medicine (in order of preference)
Allergies	amor seco, nettle, kalanchoe, gervâo, guaco, carqueja, jatobá, pau d'arco, picão preto, yerba mate, bitter melon, cat's claw, samambaia
Alopecia (hair loss)	nettle, mutamba, avenca, gervâo, catuaba, sarsaparilla, muira puama, chuchuhuasi, picão preto, guaraná (topical), quinine, jaborandi (topical), juazeiro (topical)
Alzheimer's Disease	samambaia, cat's claw, velvet bean, catuaba, sarsaparilla, guaraná, damiana, mulungu, simarouba, suma, yerba mate, anamu
Amebic Infections	simarouba, amargo, epazote, erva tostão, guava, graviola, quinine, bitter melon, carqueja, gervâo
Amenorrhea (absence of menstruation)	damiana, sarsaparilla, suma, espinheira santa, Brazilian peppertree, avenca, chuchuhuasi, vassourinha, macela, gervâo, epazote, maca, jergón sacha, tayuya, balsam, cat's claw
Amyloidosis	mullaca, vassourinha, simarouba, anamu, Brazilian peppertree, suma, graviola, cat's claw
Anal Warts	sangre de grado, vassourinha, bitter melon, clavillia, pau d'arco, macela, Brazilian peppertree, jergón sacha
Anemia	carqueja, jurubeba, amargo, chanca piedra, camu-camu, maca, erva tostão, vassourinha, fedegoso, acerola, artichoke, suma, nettle, espinheira santa, simarouba, pau d'arco, quinine
Angina	mulungu, abuta, Brazilian peppertree, embauba, picão preto, epazote, carqueja, cat's claw
Anorexia	amargo, samambaia, jatobá, jurubeba, boldo, damiana, sarsaparilla, clavo huasca, quinine, carqueja, simarouba, passionflower, yerba mate
Anxiety	mulungu, passionflower, tayuya, manacá, damiana, catuaba, damiana, graviola, guava, muira puama, velvet bean, suma, anamu, curare
Arrhythmia	Brazilian peppertree, quinine, guava, mulungu, abuta
Arteriosclerosis/ Atherosclerosis	macela, cat's claw, artichoke, yerba mate, acerola, guaco, guaraná, camu-camu, bitter melon, suma, vassourinha, sarsaparilla
Arthritis	amor seco, cat's claw, guaco, iporuru, tayuya, picão preto, chuchuhuasi, nettle, mulungu, scarlet bush, gervâo, kalanchoe, samambaia, anamu, manacá, pau d'arco, mullaca, sarsaparilla, vassourinha, graviola, cipó cabeludo, suma, copaiba (topical), andiroba (topical)
Arthritis, Rheumatoid	See **Autoimmune Disorders**
Asthma	amor seco, embauba, avenca, guaco, mutamba, samambaia, jatobá, mullaca, gervâo, abuta, macela, nettle, kalanchoe, chuchuhuasi, mulungu, bitter melon, espinheira santa, epazote, fedegoso, anamu, balsam, damiana
Athlete's Foot	jatobá, sangre de grado, copaiba, pau d'arco, Brazilian peppertree, fedegoso, anamu, mulateiro, scarlet bush, juazeiro
Autoimmune Disorders	mullaca, anamu, macela, fedegoso, cat's claw, samambaia, clavillia, Brazilian peppertree, erva tostão, picão preto, pau d'arco, velvet bean, nettle, suma, sarsaparilla

Condition	Plants Used in Herbal Medicine (in order of preference)
Back Injuries/Pain	tayuya, iporuru, cat's claw, guaco, amor seco, mulungu, manacá, picão preto, vassourinha, scarlet bush, gervâo, chuchuhuasi, sarsaparilla, cipó cabeludo, pau d'arco, copaiba (topical), kalanchoe (topical), andiroba (topical)
Bacterial Infections, General	picão preto, mullaca, anamu, mutamba, embauba, Brazilian peppertree, guava, fedegoso, sangre de grado, sarsaparilla, kalanchoe, macela, graviola, erva tostão, annatto, avenca, simarouba, vassourinha, guaco, bitter melon, cashew, clavillia, copaiba, juazeiro, mulateiro, scarlet bush, pau d'arco, chanca piedra, guacatonga, stevia, balsam
Bedsores	sangre de grado, copaiba, gervâo, anamu, annatto, scarlet bush
Benign Prostatic Hypertrophy (BPH)	nettle, mutamba, jatobá, vassourinha, cipó cabeludo, graviola, damiana, chanca piedra, pau d'arco
Bladder Disorders	jatobá, pau d'arco, abuta, anamu, chanca piedra, cipó cabeludo, erva tostão, fedegoso, annatto, clavillia, Brazilian peppertree, amor seco
Blennorrhagia (excessive mucus)	picão preto, erva tostão, jatobá, amor seco, chanca piedra, mutamba, embauba, vassourinha, amargo, cipó cabeludo, Brazilian peppertree, manacá, abuta, tayuya
Bloating	jurubeba, amargo, artichoke, simarouba, boldo, carqueja, bitter melon, gervâo, epazote, quinine, clavo huasca
Boils	anamu, guaco, mullaca, clavillia, mutamba, copaiba (topical), picão preto, fedegoso, mulateiro, pau d'arco, annatto (topical), scarlet bush (topical)
Bone Cancer	vassourinha, graviola See also **Cancer**
Bowel Disorders	cat's claw, boldo, macela, jurubeba, sangre de grado, simarouba, tayuya, anamu, mutamba, artichoke, bitter melon, carqueja, gervâo, guaco, cipó cabeludo, clavillia, epazote, annatto
Breathing Problems	embauba, amor seco, avenca, samambaia, guaco, mullaca, mutamba, guava, nettle, picão preto, gervâo, macela, jatobá, pau d'arco, abuta
Bronchitis	picão preto, embauba, guaco, samambaia, amor seco, avenca, jergón sacha, bitter melon, simarouba, gervâo, fedegoso, anamu, jatobá, mullaca, mutamba, Brazilian peppertree, macela, abuta, clavillia, epazote, juazeiro
Burns	scarlet bush, kalanchoe, sangre de grado, andiroba, mulateiro, juazeiro, sarsaparilla, nettle, mutamba, annatto
Bursitis	cat's claw, iporuru, chuchuhuasi, amor seco, tayuya, picão preto, guaco, gervâo, nettle, sarsaparilla
Cancer	graviola, espinheira santa, mullaca, mutamba, vassourinha, bitter melon, guacatonga, simarouba, cat's claw, anamu, pau d'arco, fedegoso, sangre de grado, suma, amargo, copaiba
Candida (yeast infections)	jatobá, pau d'arco, clavillia, anamu, fedegoso, Brazilian peppertree, graviola, sangre de grado, andiroba (topical), copaiba (topical), mulateiro (topical), guaco, guava

Condition	Plants Used in Herbal Medicine (in order of preference)
Carpal Tunnel Syndrome	manacá, mulungu, iporuru, tayuya, amor seco, pau d'arco, kalanchoe
Cartilage Disorders	tayuya, cat's claw, iporuru, maca, acerola, camu-camu
Cataract	bitter melon, jaborandi, annatto, erva tostão, fedegoso, gervâo, Brazilian peppertree, acerola, camu-camu, cat's claw
Catarrh	amor seco, jatobá, avenca, mutamba, balsam, nettle, guaco, cipó cabeludo, graviola, erva tostão, picão preto, chanca piedra
Cavities, Dental	stevia, juazeiro, anamu, cashew
Celiac Disease	cat's claw, macela, anamu, boldo, sangre de grado, jurubeba, simarouba, tayuya, gervâo
Cellulite	andiroba (topical), chá de bugre
Cellulitis	anamu, fedegoso, bitter melon, mullaca, clavillia, scarlet bush, sarsaparilla, Brazilian peppertree, picão preto, gervâo, simarouba, amor seco, cat's claw
Central Nervous System Disorders	manacá, kalanchoe, passionflower, mulungu, damiana, muira puama, guava, guaraná, catuaba, yerba mate, velvet bean, vassourinha
Cervical Dysplasia	abuta, graviola, andiroba, cat's claw, copaiba, anamu, fedegoso, erva tostão, bitter melon, clavillia, macela, jergón sacha, gervâo, chuchuhuasi, mullaca
Chagas Disease	epazote, guaco, mullaca, macela, anamu, pau d'arco, clavillia, embauba, copaiba, carqueja, andiroba
Chickenpox	mullaca, bitter melon, vassourinha, jergón sacha, macela, clavillia, chanca piedra, cat's claw, sangre de grado (topical), copaiba (topical)
Childbirth	abuta, anamu, avenca, bitter melon, embauba, scarlet bush, vassourinha, mutamba, sangre de grado, picão preto, gervâo
Cholecystitis	See **Gallbladder and Bile Duct Diseases**
Cholelithiasis	See **Gallstones**
Cholera	mutamba, guava, anamu, guaco, erva tostão, sangre de grado
Cholesterol, Elevated	artichoke, bitter melon, boldo, velvet bean, chanca piedra, guava, carqueja, yerba mate, suma, sarsaparilla, vassourinha, maca, cat's claw, annatto, acerola, andiroba
Chorea	guava, embauba, epazote
Chronic Fatigue Syndrome	cat's claw, mullaca, anamu, fedegoso, jergón sacha, chuchuhuasi, maca, pau d'arco, catuaba, clavillia, sarsaparilla, jatobá, guaraná, yerba mate, suma, macela, muira puama, mutamba, gervâo, erva tostão
Chronic Obstructive Pulmonary Disease (COPD)	embauba, abuta, amor seco, avenca, jatobá, samambaia, cat's claw, macela, epazote, gervâo, guaco, mullaca, mutamba
Cirrhosis	erva tostão, chanca piedra, carqueja, boldo, picão preto, artichoke, guaco, fedegoso, gervâo

Condition	Plants Used in Herbal Medicine (in order of preference)
Cold Sores	See **Herpes Simplex**
Colds and Flu	picão preto, fedegoso, mullaca, amor seco, mutamba, Brazilian peppertree, bitter melon, clavillia, gervâo, guava, simarouba, guaco, macela, jergón sacha, kalanchoe, anamu, avenca, pau d'arco, samambaia, balsam, acerola, camu-camu, cat's claw
Colic	guava, jurubeba, amor seco, passionflower, boldo, cashew, damiana
Colitis	cat's claw, boldo, simarouba, macela, picão preto, anamu, gervâo, tayuya, sangre de grado, cipó cabeludo, clavillia, jurubeba, amor seco
Colon Polyps	graviola, mutamba, sangre de grado, cat's claw, bitter melon, mullaca, vassourinha
Conjunctivitis	annatto (topical), picão preto, guava, vassourinha, Brazilian peppertree, epazote, sarsaparilla, fedegoso, clavillia, abuta
Constipation	jatobá, annatto, fedegoso, artichoke, graviola, boldo, clavillia, epazote
Convulsions	erva tostão, amor seco, abuta, mulungu, nettle, graviola, manacá, annatto, tayuya, anamu, guava, kalanchoe, macela, passionflower
Cough	guaco, embauba, amor seco, passionflower, guava, samambaia, avenca, mutamba, balsam, jatobá, picão preto, gervâo, jergón sacha, vassourinha, epazote, juazeiro, kalanchoe, macela, velvet bean
Crohn's Disease	cat's claw, sangre de grado, macela, boldo, mullaca, fedegoso, carqueja, anamu, Brazilian peppertree, clavillia, gervâo, guaco, cipó cabeludo, simarouba, tayuya, abuta, artichoke
Croup	avenca, embauba, jergón sacha, mutamba, guaco, balsam, epazote, guava, gervâo, samambaia
Cuts and Wounds	sangre de grado, scarlet bush, cat's claw, nettle, andiroba, juazeiro, copaiba, balsam, Brazilian peppertree, espinheira santa, sarsaparilla, guacatonga, guaco, picão preto
Cystic Fibrosis	amor seco, samambaia, nettle, embauba, gervâo, picão preto, abuta, erva tostão, amargo
Cystitis	See **Interstitial Cystitis**
Dandruff	copaiba, juazeiro, avenca, nettle, quinine, guaraná, balsam, brazil nut, artichoke
Degenerative Nerve Diseases	sangre de grado, samambaia, cat's claw, sarsaparilla, guaraná, velvet bean, passionflower, mulungu, tayuya, manacá, pau d'arco, yerba mate, picão preto
Dementia	See **Memory Disorders**
Dengue Fever	simarouba, amargo, jergón sacha, mullaca, anamu, chanca piedra, bitter melon, manacá, kalanchoe, guaco, scarlet bush, juazeiro, vassourinha
Depression	mulungu, tayuya, passionflower, muira puama, damiana, graviola, cat's claw, Brazilian peppertree, yerba mate
Dermatitis	Internal: samambaia, pau d'arco, cat's claw, sarsaparilla, boldo, fedegoso, tayuya, suma
	External: andiroba, copaiba, scarlet bush, sangre de grado, juazeiro, mutamba, guacatonga, mulateiro, balsam, annatto

Condition	Plants Used in Herbal Medicine (in order of preference)
Diabetes	pata de vaca, pedra hume caá, bitter melon, chanca piedra, stevia, annatto, chuchuhuasi, embauba, guava, macela, mullaca, mutamba, vassourinha, carqueja, anamu
Diabetic Kidney Problems	chanca piedra, erva tostão, sarsaparilla See also **Kidney Disorders, General**
Diabetic Macular Degeneration	chanca piedra, pedra hume caá, chuchuhuasi, annatto
Diabetic Neuropathy	sangre de grado, chanca piedra, pedra hume caá, chuchuhuasi, tayuya, annatto
Diaper Rash	andiroba, scarlet bush, copaiba, guava
Diarrhea	sangre de grado, amargo, simarouba, guava, bitter melon, Brazilian peppertree, carqueja, cashew, fedegoso, epazote, anamu
Digestive Disorders	artichoke, carqueja, jurubeba, espinheira santa, boldo, erva tostão, guacatonga, sangre de grado, amargo, quinine, cipó cabeludo, simarouba, annatto, bitter melon, cat's claw, gervâo, amor seco, picão preto
Diphtheria	mutamba, embauba, picão preto, mullaca, anamu, Brazilian peppertree, fedegoso, macela, avenca, guava, annatto, kalanchoe, erva tostão, simarouba, vassourinha, guaco, cashew, copaiba, jaborandi
Diverticulitis	cat's claw, boldo, abuta, sangre de grado, jurubeba, macela, tayuya, passionflower, gervâo, anamu
Dry Eye Syndrome	jaborandi
Dysentery	simarouba, amargo, guava, sangre de grado, epazote, erva tostão, Brazilian peppertree, cashew, mutamba, anamu, clavillia, fedegoso, gervâo
Dysmenorrhagia (painful menstruation)	abuta, erva tostão, vassourinha, amor seco, tayuya, iporuru, manacá, chuchuhuasi, passionflower, scarlet bush
Dyspepsia	See **Indigestion**
***E. coli* Infections**	anamu, guava, macela, bitter melon, mutamba, embauba, sangre de grado, jatobá, catuaba, kalanchoe, annatto
Ear Infections/Earaches	annatto (topical), gervâo (topical), clavillia, fedegoso, vassourinha, mullaca, guava (topical), boldo, kalanchoe (topical), picão preto, cashew
Eating Disorders	amargo, quinine, guava, sarsaparilla, damiana, simarouba, boldo, carqueja, jurubeba, artichoke
Eczema	sarsaparilla, andiroba, tayuya, samambaia, bitter melon, sangre de grado, copaiba, balsam, nettle, clavillia, cashew, guacatonga (topical), gervâo, guaco, vassourinha, pau d'arco, cat's claw, boldo, suma, fedegoso
Edema	chanca piedra, annatto, kalanchoe, chá de bugre, erva tostão, nettle, amor seco, anamu, guacatonga, Brazilian peppertree, jaborandi, curare, picão preto, jurubeba, carqueja

Condition	Plants Used in Herbal Medicine (in order of preference)
Elephantiasis	mutamba, pata de vaca, sarsaparilla, nettle, samambaia
Emphysema	jatobá, macela, anamu, embauba, manacá, samambaia, avenca, amor seco, epazote, gervâo, guaco, mullaca, mutamba
Encephalitis	simarouba, amargo, jergón sacha, mullaca, anamu, chanca piedra, bitter melon, manacá, kalanchoe, guaco, scarlet bush, juazeiro, vassourinha
Endocrine Disorders	maca, sarsaparilla, abuta, chuchuhuasi, damiana, suma, muira puama, catuaba, nettle
Endometriosis	abuta, graviola, tayuya, iporuru, gervâo, chuchuhuasi, erva tostão, cat's claw
Enteritis	See **Gastritis/Gastroenteritis**
Epilepsy	mulungu, manacá, amor seco, passionflower, catuaba, muira puama, graviola, tayuya
Epstein-Barr Virus	bitter melon, tayuya, cat's claw, suma, Brazilian peppertree, mullaca, jergón sacha, macela, chanca piedra, vassourinha, clavillia
Erectile Dysfunction	See **Impotence**
Erysipelas	vassourinha, gervâo, mutamba, jurubeba, fedegoso, scarlet bush, Brazilian peppertree, annatto, copaiba, fedegoso, anamu, erva tostão, kalanchoe, abuta, nettle
Eye Diseases	annatto, cashew, guava, jaborandi
Fatigue	jatobá, maca, guaraná, chuchuhuasi, yerba mate, suma, catuaba, muira puama, sarsaparilla
Fatty Liver	chanca piedra, artichoke, boldo, erva tostão, fedegoso, carqueja, picão preto, gervâo
Fever	juazeiro, scarlet bush, manacá, vassourinha, kalanchoe, velvet bean, nettle, boldo, quinine, amargo, curare, guaco, mutamba, simarouba
Fibroids	See **Uterine Fibroids**
Fibromyalgia	mullaca, anamu, macela, Brazilian peppertree, clavillia, manacá, chuchuhuasi, fedegoso, gervâo, tayuya, iporuru, muira puama, mulungu, amor seco, passionflower
Fistulas	guaco, erva tostão, fedegoso, picão preto, anamu, epazote, graviola, samambaia, clavillia
Flatulence	jurubeba, epazote, bitter melon, carqueja, espinheira santa, copaiba, boldo, chanca piedra, kalanchoe, macela, artichoke
Fractures	embauba, nettle, epazote, sangre de grado, clavillia, Brazilian peppertree, scarlet bush, kalanchoe
Fungal Infections	jatobá, pau d'arco, anamu, fedegoso, picão preto, copaiba, sangre de grado, mulateiro, Brazilian peppertree, clavillia, graviola, guava, kalanchoe, scarlet bush, embauba, guacatonga, vassourinha
Gallbladder and Bile Duct Diseases	artichoke, boldo, chanca piedra, erva tostão, amargo, carqueja, jurubeba, macela, abuta, avenca, balsam, bitter melon, fedegoso, gervâo
Gallstones	chanca piedra, boldo, carqueja, avenca, amargo, artichoke, cipó cabeludo, jurubeba, macela, erva tostão

Condition	Plants Used in Herbal Medicine (in order of preference)
Gastritis/ Gastroenteritis	jurubeba, carqueja, espinheira santa, guava, macela, boldo, epazote, picão preto, gervâo, guaco, sangre de grado, cat's claw, simarouba, amargo, pedra hume caá, tayuya, sarsaparilla
Gastrointestinal Bleeding	sangre de grado, Brazilian peppertree, abuta, carqueja, erva tostão, picão preto, cashew, mutamba, simarouba
Genital Warts	See **Human Papilloma Virus (HPV)**
Giardia Infections	guava, simarouba, anamu, mutamba
Glaucoma	jaborandi
Gonorrhea	mutamba, pau d'arco, picão preto, annatto, bitter melon, boldo, Brazilian peppertree, clavillia, embauba, chanca piedra, erva tostão, cat's claw, copaiba, curare, jaborandi
Gout	chanca piedra, carqueja, cipó cabeludo, tayuya, boldo, artichoke, epazote, manacá, guaco, sarsaparilla, jergón sacha, velvet bean, bitter melon, picão preto, yerba mate, chuchuhuasi, Brazilian peppertree, balsam
Gum Diseases	Brazilian peppertree, anamu, mulungu, macela, guava, samambaia, cat's claw, fedegoso, pau d'arco, gervâo, juazeiro, clavillia, cashew
Hair Loss	See **Alopecia**
Hangover	jurubeba
Hay Fever	See **Allergies**
Head Lice	amargo, andiroba, balsam, fedegoso, graviola (seeds), nettle
Headache	iporuru, tayuya, manacá, vassourinha, mulungu, pau d'arco, amor seco, scarlet bush, passionflower, kalanchoe, guaco, gervâo, guaraná, muira puama, chuchuhuasi, damiana, abuta, cat's claw
Heart Diseases, General	abuta, avenca, Brazilian peppertree, embauba, chá de bugre, cat's claw, guaraná, graviola, guava, mulungu, gervâo, artichoke, jurubeba, yerba mate, suma, vassourinha, sarsaparilla, chanca piedra, picão preto, stevia, quinine, boldo, bitter melon, samambaia, erva tostão
Heart Palpitations	mulungu, Brazilian peppertree, quinine, abuta, guava
Heart Valve Diseases	mullaca, Brazilian peppertree, anamu, clavillia, macela, fedegoso, tayuya, iporuru
Heartburn/Reflux	carqueja, espinheira santa, guacatonga, boldo, epazote, guaco, gervâo, picão preto, annatto, jergón sacha
Heat Stroke	scarlet bush, guaraná, manacá, kalanchoe, mulateiro, mutamba
Helicobacter pylori Stomach Ulcers	carqueja, pau d'arco, cashew, bitter melon (fruit), balsam, copaiba, guacatonga, guava
Hemochromatosis	damiana, mulungu, manacá
Hemorrhages	abuta, sangre de grado, Brazilian peppertree, erva tostão, mutamba, picão preto, annatto, pedra hume caá, scarlet bush, simarouba, kalanchoe, juazeiro
Hemorrhagic Fevers	embauba, guava, epazote, Brazilian peppertree, clavillia, mutamba, erva tostão, scarlet bush

Condition	Plants Used in Herbal Medicine (in order of preference)
Hemorrhoids	sangre de grado, Brazilian peppertree, copaiba, vassourinha, epazote, erva tostão, passionflower, picão preto, chuchuhuasi, artichoke, quinine, yerba mate, nettle
Hepatitis	chanca piedra, jergón sacha, mullaca, anamu, macela, sangre de grado, clavillia, fedegoso, bitter melon, vassourinha, mutamba, erva tostão, gervâo, carqueja, picão preto, mulungu
Hernia	jergón sacha, mulungu, fedegoso, pau d'arco, tayuya, iporuru
Herniated Disk	iporuru, tayuya, chuchuhuasi, amor seco, gervâo, guaco, picão preto, kalanchoe, sarsaparilla
Herpes Simplex (I & II)	jergón sacha, sangre de grado, mullaca, vassourinha, mutamba, simarouba, bitter melon, clavillia, pau d'arco, chá de bugre, macela, carqueja, chanca piedra, guacatonga, embauba, andiroba
Herpes Zoster (Shingles)	cat's claw, jergón sacha, mullaca, sangre de grado, pau d'arco, bitter melon, vassourinha, gervâo, clavillia, macela, passionflower
Hiatal Hernia	carqueja, guaco, guacatonga, espinheira santa, sangre de grado, tayuya, gervâo, picão preto, boldo, jergón sacha, epazote, annatto
High Blood Pressure	abuta, graviola, chanca piedra, picão preto, erva tostão, Brazilian peppertree, embauba, stevia, mulungu, mutamba, fedegoso, guava, carqueja, passionflower, vassourinha, jurubeba, nettle
HIV	See **AIDS and HIV**
Hives	nettle, kalanchoe, guaco, amor seco, pau d'arco, gervâo, picão preto, carqueja, sangre de grado (topical), andiroba (topical) See also **Allergies**
Hodgkin's Disease	bitter melon, graviola, pau d'arco, mullaca, vassourinha, anamu, mutamba, cat's claw, espinheira santa, simarouba, suma
Hot Flashes	manacá, scarlet bush, vassourinha, kalanchoe
Human Papilloma Virus (HPV)	andiroba, bitter melon, sangre de grado, jergón sacha, copaiba, vassourinha, clavillia, cat's claw, macela, mullaca, chanca piedra
Huntington's Disease	velvet bean, guava, embauba, epazote, mulungu, manacá, samambaia, cat's claw
Hypertension	See **High Blood Pressure**
Immune System Disorders	cat's claw, anamu, mullaca, fedegoso, samambaia, macela, suma, chuchuhuasi, sarsaparilla, bitter melon, acerola, camu-camu, erva tostão
Impetigo	sangre de grado, pau d'arco, anamu, mullaca, embauba, clavillia, fedegoso, copaiba (topical), andiroba (topical), annatto (topical), kalanchoe (topical)
Impotence	muira puama, velvet bean, catuaba, damiana, nettle, sarsaparilla, iporuru, suma, maca, macela, amor seco, mutamba, cashew
Indigestion	jurubeba, artichoke, amargo, espinheira santa, carqueja, boldo, damiana, gervâo, picão preto, guacatonga, bitter melon, passionflower, guaco, quinine, simarouba

Condition	Plants Used in Herbal Medicine (in order of preference)
Infectious Mononucleosis	picão preto, fedegoso, mullaca, Brazilian peppertree, mutamba, guaco, bitter melon, cat's claw, clavillia, anamu, jergón sacha, suma, macela
Infertility, Female	maca, abuta, suma, chuchuhuasi, iporuru
Infertility, Male	maca, velvet bean, catuaba, chuchuhuasi, muira puama, sarsaparilla
Inflammatory Conditions	iporuru, guaco, amor seco, tayuya, cat's claw, chuchuhuasi, guaco, copaiba, embauba, manacá, mulungu, erva tostão, scarlet bush, picão preto, samambaia, abuta, kalanchoe, gervâo, nettle, passionflower, pau d'arco, guacatonga, juazeiro, anamu, andiroba, boldo, carqueja, cashew, fedegoso, jurubeba, macela, sangre de grado, sarsaparilla, suma, vassourinha, velvet bean
Influenza	See **Colds and Flu**
Insect Bites and Stings	sangre de grado, guacatonga, guaco, scarlet bush, copaiba, kalanchoe, jergón sacha, embauba, vassourinha, amargo, mulateiro, picão preto, gervâo, abuta
Insect Repellant	andiroba, amargo, mulateiro, clavillia, simarouba, annatto, fedegoso, guaco, Brazilian peppertree, quinine, cashew, aveloz
Insomnia	manacá, mulungu, passionflower, catuaba, boldo, graviola, kalanchoe
Interstitial Cystitis	jatobá, copaiba, boldo, cipó cabeludo, pau d'arco, erva tostão, annatto, anamu, chanca piedra, Brazilian peppertree, abuta, samambaia, picão preto, sarsaparilla, pata de vaca, jurubeba, artichoke, mulungu, nettle
Intestinal Parasites	amargo, simarouba, epazote, boldo, fedegoso, carqueja, quinine, andiroba, balsam, graviola, bitter melon, gervâo, erva tostão
Irritable Bowel Syndrome	cat's claw, macela, sangre de grado, boldo, artichoke, jurubeba, simarouba, tayuya, anamu, abuta, fedegoso, gervâo, guaco, mullaca
Itching	andiroba, sangre de grado, nettle, kalanchoe, scarlet bush, artichoke, guaco, chanca piedra, guava, fedegoso, picão preto, gervâo, balsam, bitter melon, vassourinha, pau d'arco
Jaundice	chanca piedra, artichoke, erva tostão, boldo, fedegoso, carqueja, picão preto, avenca, abuta, vassourinha, scarlet bush, bitter melon, annatto, jurubeba, guava, curare
Jock Itch	See **Fungal Infections**
Kidney Disorders, General	chanca piedra, erva tostão, cipó cabeludo, vassourinha, mutamba, amor seco, nettle, amargo, jatobá, picão preto, samambaia, copaiba, abuta, carqueja, anamu, mullaca, sarsaparilla, damiana, cat's claw, annatto, fedegoso, gervâo, pata de vaca, curare
Kidney Failure and Dialysis	erva tostão, chanca piedra, samambaia, sarsaparilla, cat's claw
Kidney Stones	chanca piedra, amargo, abuta, boldo, cipó cabeludo, erva tostão, gervâo, kalanchoe, bitter melon, curare, avenca, pata de vaca
Laryngitis	guaco, sangre de grado, picão preto, avenca, guava, jatobá, amor seco, cat's claw, macela, balsam, epazote, jaborandi

Condition	Plants Used in Herbal Medicine (in order of preference)
Leishmaniasis	cashew, pau d'arco, chuchuhuasi, graviola, sarsaparilla, copaiba, kalanchoe
Leprosy	sarsaparilla, mutamba, guacatonga, bitter melon, fedegoso, vassourinha, andiroba, clavillia, tayuya, nettle, pata de vaca
Leukemia	mullaca, picão preto, vassourinha, simarouba, cipó cabeludo, anamu, suma, pau d'arco, cat's claw, bitter melon, espinheira santa, amargo, graviola
Lice	See **Head Lice**
Lipomas	espinheira santa, artichoke, embauba, andiroba (topical), sangre de grado (topical), vassourinha, erva tostão, picão preto, fedegoso, mullaca, cat's claw
Listeria Infections	anamu, pau d'arco, mullaca
Liver Disorders, General	erva tostão, picão preto, carqueja, fedegoso, boldo, chanca piedra, gervão, artichoke, amargo, macela, jurubeba, mulungu, guaco, annatto, avenca, epazote
Lupus	See **Autoimmune Disorders**
Lymphatic Diseases	manacá, sarsaparilla, kalanchoe, jergón sacha, cat's claw, suma, gervão, guaco, espinheira santa, graviola
Macular Degeneration	See **Diabetic Macular Degeneration**
Malaria	quinine, simarouba, amargo, vassourinha, epazote, fedegoso, graviola, guava, pau d'arco, picão preto, andiroba, chanca piedra, abuta, erva tostão
Measles	mullaca, amargo, sarsaparilla, clavillia, jergón sacha, macela, epazote, vassourinha, chanca piedra, sangre de grado (topical)
Memory Disorders	samambaia, catuaba, sarsaparilla, guaraná, suma, anamu, velvet bean, cat's claw, maca, muira puama, damiana, epazote
Men's Health, General	muira puama, sarsaparilla, catuaba, chuchuhuasi, mutamba, suma, cipó cabeludo, velvet bean, cat's claw
Menopause	abuta, espinheira santa, damiana, suma, sarsaparilla, chuchuhuasi, kalanchoe, mulungu, avenca, bitter melon, clavo huasca, maca, passionflower
Menorrhagia (excessive menstruation)	abuta, Brazilian peppertree, erva tostão, vassourinha, sarsaparilla, nettle, velvet bean, chanca piedra
Menstrual Cramps	abuta, manacá, amor seco, mulungu, iporuru, tayuya, passionflower, vassourinha, kalanchoe, scarlet bush
Metrorrhagia (bleeding between periods)	abuta, damiana, nettle, sarsaparilla, espinheira santa, suma, vassourinha, maca
Migraine	manacá, iporuru, passionflower, tayuya, pau d'arco, mulungu, guaraná, scarlet bush, vassourinha, kalanchoe
Molds	jatobá, Brazilian peppertree, anamu, pau d'arco, clavillia, fedegoso
Molluscum contagiosum	sangre de grado, bitter melon, clavillia, mullaca, macela, vassourinha, jergón sacha, copaiba

Condition	Plants Used in Herbal Medicine (in order of preference)
Morning Sickness	jurubeba
Mouth Ulcers	sangre de grado, guaco, Brazilian peppertree, pau d'arco, jatobá, clavillia, mutamba, copaiba (topical), fedegoso, anamu, bitter melon, mullaca, macela, jergón sacha, vassourinha, carqueja
Multiple Myeloma	graviola, mullaca, bitter melon, cat's claw, espinheira santa, guacatonga, vassourinha, mutamba, anamu, simarouba, amargo, suma
Multiple Sclerosis	jergón sacha, mullaca, macela, sangre de grado, tayuya, iporuru, manacá, pau d'arco, amor seco, mulungu, bitter melon, clavillia, vassourinha, gervâo
Mumps	clavillia, velvet bean, jergón sacha, cat's claw, bitter melon, macela, mullaca, vassourinha
Muscle Aches	scarlet bush (topical), copaiba (topical), amor seco, iporuru, cat's claw, tayuya, chuchuhuasi, kalanchoe, vassourinha, sarsaparilla, guaco, picão preto, gervâo, abuta
Muscle Cramps/ Spasms	amor seco, abuta, vassourinha, manacá, iporuru, mulungu, embauba, passionflower, graviola, macela, kalanchoe, erva tostão, fedegoso, gervâo, quinine, mutamba, mullaca, velvet bean, amargo, scarlet bush
Nausea and Vomiting	jurubeba, artichoke, gervâo, guava, fedegoso, carqueja, kalanchoe, macela, mullaca, boldo
Nephritis	chanca piedra, erva tostão, cipó cabeludo, sarsaparilla, mutamba, mullaca, guava, artichoke, abuta, picão preto, jatobá, damiana, jaborandi
Nervousness	See **Anxiety**
Neuralgia	manacá, sangre de grado, passionflower, mulungu, iporuru, tayuya, pau d'arco, macela, guaco, catuaba, gervâo, muira puama, guaraná, chuchuhuasi, cipó cabeludo, gervâo, quinine, abuta, nettle
Neurologic Diseases, General	mulungu, manacá, passionflower, velvet bean, damiana, muira puama, sarsaparilla, samambaia, sangre de grado, cat's claw, guaraná, catuaba, bitter melon
Neuromuscular Disorders	abuta, iporuru, tayuya, amor seco, passionflower, cat's claw, chuchuhuasi, picão preto, sarsaparilla, guaco, gervâo
Neuropathy	sangre de grado, chuchuhuasi, cat's claw, muira puama, annatto
Obesity	chá de bugre, guaraná, picão preto, yerba mate, carqueja, jurubeba, stevia
Osteoarthritis	cat's claw, tayuya, iporuru, chuchuhuasi, amor seco, picão preto, gervâo, sarsaparilla, guaco
Osteomyelitis	anamu, vassourinha, mullaca, simarouba, fedegoso, Brazilian peppertree, amor seco, picão preto, gervâo, bitter melon, macela, cat's claw See also **Bacterial Infections, General**
Otitis Media	See **Ear Infections/Earaches**
Pancreatitis	boldo, jergón sacha, artichoke, samambaia, picão preto, mullaca, mutamba, anamu, chanca piedra, nettle, epazote

Condition	Plants Used in Herbal Medicine (in order of preference)
Parasites, Skin	amargo, andiroba, balsam, mutamba, mulateiro, juazeiro, kalanchoe, epazote, bitter melon, guaco
Parkinson's Disease	velvet bean, embauba, mulungu, passionflower, manacá, pau d'arco, suma
Peptic Ulcers	gervâo, carqueja, espinheira santa, guacatonga, cat's claw, bitter melon, epazote, jurubeba, picão preto, copaiba, sangre de grado, boldo
Pertussis	See **Whooping Cough**
Pharyngitis	guaco, sangre de grado, picão preto, scarlet bush, avenca, guava, pau d'arco, amor seco, cat's claw, macela, balsam
Pinworms	See **Intestinal Parasites**
Pityriasis Rosea	See **Dermatitis**
Pleurisy	guaco, avenca, samambaia, copaiba, nettle, anamu, sarsaparilla, epazote, jaborandi See also **Bacterial Infections, General; Viral Infections**
Pneumonia, bacterial (Streptococcus & Klebsiella pneumoniae)	embauba, mutamba, picão preto, kalanchoe, avenca, guava, pau d'arco, erva tostão, macela, fedegoso, Brazilian peppertree, mullaca, cat's claw, guaco, simarouba, gervâo, samambaia
Pneumonia, fungal (Pneumocystis carinii)	embauba, jatobá, pau d'arco, kalanchoe, anamu, fedegoso, picão preto, guava, Brazilian peppertree, mutamba, copaiba, sarsaparilla, scarlet bush
Pneumonia, mycoplasmal (Mycoplasma pneumonia)	mullaca, macela, anamu, Brazilian peppertree, clavillia, fedegoso, embauba
Pneumonia, viral (several strains)	jergón sacha, vassourinha, mutamba, mullaca, anamu, macela, bitter melon, sangre de grado, pau d'arco, picão preto, embauba
Poison Ivy	sangre de grado (topical), andiroba (topical), gervâo, guaco, nettle, picão preto, pau d'arco
Premenstrual Syndrome (PMS)	damiana, manacá, mulungu, muira puama, suma, sarsaparilla, passionflower, guaraná
Prostatitis	jatobá, nettle, cipó cabeludo, mutamba, pau d'arco, Brazilian peppertree, chanca piedra, curare, artichoke, cat's claw
Psoriasis	samambaia, pau d'arco, fedegoso, sarsaparilla, cat's claw, suma, mullaca, boldo, bitter melon, cashew, jaborandi, andiroba (topical), copaiba (topical)
Respiratory Disorders, General	embauba, guaco, kalanchoe, avenca, vassourinha, samambaia, amor seco, Brazilian peppertree, jatobá, balsam, anamu, pau d'arco, picão preto, gervâo, mutamba, guava, espinheira santa, sarsaparilla, nettle, epazote, jergón sacha, juazeiro
Rheumatism	cat's claw, iporuru, chuchuhuasi, embauba, picão preto, tayuya, gervâo, vassourinha, mulungu, abuta, guaco, manacá, sarsaparilla, nettle, amor seco, samambaia, fedegoso, pau d'arco, scarlet bush, anamu, kalanchoe, suma, cipó cabeludo
Rheumatoid Arthritis	See **Autoimmune Disorders**

Condition	Plants Used in Herbal Medicine (in order of preference)
Rhinitis	See **Allergies**
Ringworm	jatobá, fedegoso, sangre de grado, copaiba, pau d'arco, anamu, balsam, Brazilian peppertree, clavillia, epazote, bitter melon, chanca piedra, velvet bean
Rosacea	mullaca, samambaia, pau d'arco, cat's claw, sarsaparilla, suma, pata de vaca, boldo, fedegoso
Salivary Gland Disorders	jaborandi, espinheira santa, amargo, picão preto, Brazilian peppertree
Salmonella Infections	simarouba, guava, embauba, bitter melon, erva tostão, macela, picão preto, abuta, guaraná
Sarcoidosis	samambaia, embauba, graviola See also **Autoimmune Disorders**
Scabies	amargo, bitter melon, andiroba, balsam, mutamba, fedegoso, pau d'arco, guava, scarlet bush, jergón sacha, mulateiro, copaiba, kalanchoe, amor seco
Scars	sangre de grado, andiroba, copaiba, samambaia, sarsaparilla
Schistosomiasis	pau d'arco, cipó cabeludo, macela, graviola (seeds), bitter melon, epazote, cashew, jatobá, guacatonga, pata de vaca, copaiba
Sciatica	tayuya, manacá, iporuru, mulungu, pau d'arco, quinine, kalanchoe, muira puama
Scleroderma	See **Autoimmune Disorders**
Sclerosis	picão preto, erva tostão, avenca, cat's claw, balsam
Scrofula	mullaca, anamu, clavillia, macela, fedegoso, Brazilian peppertree, amargo, sarsaparilla, samambaia, manacá, cashew, tayuya
Seborrhea	copaiba, juazeiro, guaraná, mulateiro, sarsaparilla, andiroba, tayuya, samambaia, bitter melon
Seizures	amor seco, mulungu, manacá, passionflower
Senility	See **Memory Disorders**
Sepsis	See **Bacterial Infections, General**
Sexual Dysfunction, Female	clavo huasca, catuaba, abuta, damiana, suma, chuchuhuasi, velvet bean, maca, sarsaparilla, vassourinha, simarouba
Sexual Dysfunction, Male	muira puama, catuaba, nettle, velvet bean, sarsaparilla, mutamba, iporuru, damiana, maca, amor seco, macela, cashew
Shingles	See **Herpes Zoster**
Sickle Cell Anemia	suma
Sinusitis	amor seco, nettle, kalanchoe, gervâo, guaco, carqueja, jatobá, pau d'arco, picão preto, yerba mate, bitter melon, cat's claw, samambaia
Skin Rash	See **Dermatitis**
Sleep Disorders	manacá, mulungu, kalanchoe, passionflower, vassourinha, graviola

Condition	Plants Used in Herbal Medicine (in order of preference)
Snakebite	jergón sacha, guaco, guacatonga, picão preto, tayuya, velvet bean, annatto, amargo, curare
Sore Throat	guaco, guava, sangre de grado, vassourinha, copaiba, picão preto, scarlet bush, samambaia, carqueja, fedegoso, cashew, abuta, pau d'arco, andiroba, juazeiro, kalanchoe, epazote, balsam
Spastic Colon	See **Irritable Bowel Syndrome**
Spleen Disorders	erva tostão, mulungu, carqueja, jurubeba, nettle, tayuya, avenca, artichoke, bitter melon, graviola, quinine
Sprains and Strains	tayuya, iporuru, embauba, manacá, abuta, amor seco, mulungu, cat's claw, chuchuhuasi, vassourinha, kalanchoe, cipó cabeludo, pau d'arco, amargo, gervâo, sarsaparilla, scarlet bush (topical), copaiba (topical), macela (topical)
Staphylococcus Infections	mutamba, mullaca, anamu, macela, copaiba, erva tostão, bitter melon, guava, avenca, Brazilian peppertree, pau d'arco, kalanchoe, mulungu, annatto, chanca piedra See also **Bacterial Infections, General**
Stomach Ulcers	See *Helicobacter pylori* **Stomach Ulcers; Peptic Ulcers**
Strep Throat	mutamba, mullaca, gervâo, copaiba, gervâo, bitter melon, pau d'arco, guaco, kalanchoe
Stress	manacá, catuaba, mulungu, passionflower, damiana, muira puama, kalanchoe
Stretch Marks	andiroba (topical), copaiba (topical), sangre de grado (topical), brazil nut (oil), samambaia
Sunburn	samambaia, cat's claw, gervâo, guaco
Sunstroke	See **Heat Stroke**
Syphilis	mutamba, sarsaparilla, manacá, clavillia, pau d'arco, boldo, Brazilian peppertree, samambaia, copaiba, cashew, vassourinha, guaco, scarlet bush, gervâo, abuta, damiana, tayuya, guacatonga, nettle, chanca piedra, velvet bean, pata de vaca, catuaba, jaborandi
Testicular Inflammation	abuta, curare
Tetanus	fedegoso, guaco, copaiba, andiroba, passionflower, annatto, curare, anamu, clavillia See also **Bacterial Infections, General**
Thrush	See *Candida;* **Fungal Infections**
Tick Bites	See **Insect Bites and Stings**
Tonsillitis	mutamba, picão preto, mullaca, carqueja, cashew, copaiba, guaco, anamu, Brazilian peppertree, fedegoso, gervâo, sangre de grado, clavillia
Trichomonas	guaco, anamu, epazote, simarouba, amargo, fedegoso
Tuberculosis	picão preto, anamu, fedegoso, Brazilian peppertree, amor seco, bitter melon, pau d'arco, sarsaparilla, kalanchoe, jatobá, manacá, copaiba, balsam, chanca piedra, velvet bean, acerola
Ulcerative Colitis	sangre de grado, cat's claw, macela, picão preto, boldo, sarsaparilla, fedegoso, guaco, pau d'arco, simarouba

Condition	Plants Used in Herbal Medicine (in order of preference)
Ulcers	See *Helicobacter pylori* **Stomach Ulcers; Peptic Ulcers**
Urinary Tract Infections	chanca piedra, anamu, jatobá, nettle, boldo, cipó cabeludo, copaiba, fedegoso, Brazilian peppertree, epazote, curare, vassourinha, amor seco, espinheira santa, picão preto, abuta, annatto, pau d'arco
Urticaria	See **Hives**
Uterine Diseases	abuta, amor seco, anamu, Brazilian peppertree, cipó cabeludo, clavillia, curare, fedegoso, guaco, jatobá, pau d'arco, sarsaparilla, picão preto
Uterine Fibroids	abuta, graviola, mutamba, cat's claw, chuchuhuasi, simarouba, Brazilian peppertree
Vaginal Diseases (Infection, vaginitis leucorrhea, etc.)	jatobá, pau d'arco, anamu, amor seco, clavillia, abuta, curare, annatto, Brazilian peppertree, guava, fedegoso, sangre de grado, cashew, picão preto, bitter melon, sarsaparilla
Varicose Veins	cat's claw, acerola, andiroba (topical), camu-camu
Vasculitis	gervâo, guaco, cat's claw
Viral Infections	jergón sacha, mullaca, sangre de grado, anamu, chanca piedra, macela, bitter melon, pau d'arco, vassourinha, mutamba, kalanchoe, amargo, clavillia, erva tostão, picão preto, simarouba, carqueja, catuaba, chá de bugre, iporuru, stevia, cat's claw, Brazilian peppertree
Vitiligo	See **Autoimmune Disorders**
Warts	aveloz (topical), sangre de grado (topical), copaiba (topical), bitter melon, embauba, clavillia, mullaca, vassourinha, pau d'arco, macela, jergón sacha, Brazilian peppertree, chanca piedra, sarsaparilla
Whooping Cough	jergón sacha, embauba, samambaia, kalanchoe, avenca, mulungu, guaco, guava, passionflower, mulungu See also **Bacterial Infections, General**
Women's Health, General	abuta, catuaba, clavo huasca, chuchuhuasi, damiana, suma, sarsaparilla, vassourinha, erva tostão, cat's claw
Wounds	See **Cuts and Wounds**
Yeast Infections	See *Candida*
Yellow Fever	amargo, jergón sacha, simarouba, mullaca, mutamba, gervâo, anamu, vassourinha, chanca piedra, bitter melon, manacá, kalanchoe, scarlet bush, juazeiro

CHAPTER 7

PLANT DATA
SUMMARY

This chapter provides a concise overview of the seventy-three rainforest plants detailed in the book. Table 7.1 highlights each botanical's main actions and uses, indicates which properties have been documented by research or traditional use, and lists any applicable cautions. Since this chapter provides only a summary, it is still important for the reader to read the comprehensive information given in Part Three. The summary can, however, guide the reader as to which plants he or she may be interested in exploring in greater detail.

TABLE 7.1	**Summary of Rainforest Plants**		
Plant	Main Preparation Method	Main Actions (in order)	Main Uses
Abuta vine wood (*Cissampelos pareira*)	decoction or capsules	antispasmodic, antihemorrhagic (reduces bleeding), muscle relaxant, uterine relaxant, hypotensive (lowers blood pressure)	• for menstrual problems (pain, cramps, excessive bleeding, fibroids, endometriosis) • as a female tonic (hormonal balancing, menopausal libido loss, hormonal acne, premenstrual syndrome, childbirth) • for heart problems (irregular heartbeat, high blood pressure, heart tonic) • as a general antispasmodic and muscle relaxer (asthma, stomach cramps, muscle pain/strains, irritable bowel syndrome [IBS], diverticulitis) • for kidney support (kidney stones, kidney/urinary infections and pain)
Acerola fruit (*Malpighia glabra*)	juice	antioxidant, nutritive, astringent, antifungal	• for its natural high vitamin C content • for colds/flu (for its vitamin C content) • for skin care/anti-aging (for its antioxidant and vitamin content) • as an overall health tonic (tones, balances, strengthens) • as a heart tonic (tones, balances, strengthens)
Amargo bark (*Quassia amara*)	infusion or capsules	antiparasitic, pediculicide (kills lice), digestive stimulant, bitter digestive aid, liver bile stimulant, antilithic (prevents kidney stones)	• for lice and skin parasites • for intestinal parasites and amebic infections • for malaria • for digestive problems (ulcers, dyspepsia, intestinal gas and bloating, sluggish digestion, anorexia) • as a liver/gallbladder aid to increase bile and eliminate toxins and stones
Amor Seco whole herb (*Desmodium adscendens*)	infusion or capsules	anti-asthmatic, antispasmodic, bronchodilator, muscle relaxer, antihistamine	• for asthma and allergies • for respiratory problems (bronchitis, chronic obstructive pulmonary disease [COPD], emphysema, excessive phlegm/mucus) • as a general antispasmodic, muscle relaxant, and pain-reliever for colic, stomach and bowel cramping, arthritis, muscle/joint aches, pain, injuries and spasms • for menstrual disorders (cramps, excessive bleeding, pain, vaginal discharge) • for convulsions (allergic reactions, epilepsy)

Properties/Actions Documented by Research	Other Properties/Actions Documented by Traditional Use	Cautions
antibacterial, antihistamine, anti-inflammatory, antioxidant, antispasmodic, diuretic, hypotensive (lowers blood pressure), muscle relaxant, uterine relaxant	analgesic (pain-reliever), antihemorrhagic (reduces bleeding), antiseptic, aphrodisiac, cardiotonic, diaphoretic (promotes sweating), expectorant, febrifuge (lowers fever), hepato-protective (liver protector), stimulant, tonic (tones, balances, strengthens)	It relaxes the uterus and is contraindicated in pregnancy. It may also potentiate medications used to treat hypertension.
antifungal, anti-inflammatory, antioxidant	astringent, cardiotonic	High dosages of vitamin C may cause diarrhea.
amebicide, analgesic (pain-reliever), anticancerous, antileukemic, anti-malarial, antiparasitic, antitumorous, antiulcerous, antiviral, bitter, gastroprotective, insecticide, larvicide, muscle relaxant, pediculicide (kills lice), sedative	antibacterial, antilithic (prevents kidney stones), antispasmodic, antivenin, carminative (expels gas), digestive stimulant, febrifuge (reduces fever), hepatoprotective (liver protector), hepatotonic (tones, balances, strengthens liver functions), hypoglycemic, liver and gallbladder bile stimulant, sialogogue (increases saliva), tonic (tones, balances, strengthens), vermifuge (expels worms)	It interferes with fertility. Large amounts might cause nausea and stomach irritation.
analgesic (pain-reliever), anti-anaphylactic (stops allergic reactions), anti-asthmatic, anticonvulsant, antihistamine, antispasmodic, bronchodilator, muscle relaxant, potassium maxi-K inhibitor	antidiuretic, antihemorrhagic (reduces bleeding), anti-inflammatory, blood cleanser, central nervous system (CNS) tonic (tones, balances, strengthens), contraceptive, cough suppressant, digestive stimulant, lactagogue (promotes milk flow), laxative, nervine (balancing/calming nerves), vermifuge (expels worms), wound healer	none

Plant	Main Preparation Method	Main Actions (in order)	Main Uses
Anamu whole herb (*Petiveria alliacea*)	capsules or infusion	anticancerous, antiviral, anticandidal, antibacterial, immune stimulant	• for cancer and leukemia • for immune disorders (to stimulate immune function and immune cell production) • for colds, flu, and viruses • for *Candida* and other yeast infections • for urinary tract infections
Andiroba seed oil (*Carapa guianensis*)	cold pressed oil	analgesic (pain-reliever), anti-inflammatory, insect repellant, antitumorous, wound healer	• for insect bites and stings • as an insect repellant • for psoriasis, dermatitis, heat rash, skin fungi, and other skin problems • for skin parasites • for skin cancer
Annatto leaves (*Bixa orellana*)	infusion	antimicrobial, diuretic, digestive stimulant, hepatoprotective (liver protector), hypocholesterolemic (lowers cholesterol)	• as a topical antiseptic for ear, eye, and skin infections • for digestive problems (heartburn, constipation, stomachache) • for prostate and urinary infections • for hypertension • for high cholesterol levels
Annatto seeds (*Bixa orellana*)	maceration or capsules	antioxidant, hepatoprotective (liver protector), insect repellant, diuretic, hypocholesterolemic (lowers cholesterol)	• to tone, balance, and strengthen liver function and for hepatitis and liver inflammation/pain • for high cholesterol • for skin care and skin anti-aging (for its antioxidant and ultraviolet ray [UV]-protective effect) • as a strong diuretic • for high blood pressure
Artichoke leaves (*Cynara scolymus*)	fluid extract or tincture	liver and gallbladder bile stimulant, hepatoprotective (liver protector), antihepatotoxic (liver detoxifier), hypocholesterolemic (lowers cholesterol)	• for gallstones and as a liver and gallbladder bile stimulant • for high cholesterol • for digestive disorders • for irritable bowel syndrome, Crohn's disease, and other bowel problems
Aveloz latex (*Euphorbia tirucalli*)	cold maceration or undiluted latex	tumor promoter, carcinogenic, immune suppressant, irritant, caustic	• for warts (topically applied)

Properties/Actions Documented by Research	Other Properties/Actions Documented by Traditional Use	Cautions
abortive, analgesic (pain-reliever), antibacterial, anticancerous, anticandidal, antifungal, anti-inflammatory, antileukemic, antiprotozoal, antitumorous, antiviral, COX inhibitor (linked to inflammation), hypoglycemic, immune stimulant, uterine stimulant	anti-anxiety, antioxidant, anti-rheumatic, antispasmodic, diaphoretic (promotes sweating), diuretic, febrifuge (reduces fever), insecticide, menstrual stimulant, sedative, vermifuge (expels worms)	It has abortive and hypoglycemic effects.
analgesic (pain-reliever), antibacterial, anticancerous, anti-inflammatory, antimalarial, antiparasitic, antitumorous, insect repellant	antiseptic, balsamic, emollient, febrifuge (reduces fever), vermifuge (expels worms), wound healer	none
aldose reductase inhibitor (linked to diabetic complications), antibacterial, antihemorrhagic (reduces bleeding), antivenin	antacid, anti-inflammatory, antiseptic, aperient (mild laxative), aphrodisiac, astringent, digestive stimulant, diuretic, febrifuge (reduces fever), hypocholesterolemic (lowers cholesterol), hypotensive (lowers blood pressure), wound healer	It may potentiate medications used to treat hypertension.
antioxidant, hepatoprotective (liver protector), hyperglycemic, also used as a food-coloring agent	expectorant, hypocholesterolemic (lowers cholesterol), hypotensive (lowers blood pressure), insect repellant, wound healer	It might raise blood sugar levels and may potentiate medications used to treat hypertension.
antihepatotoxic (clears toxins in liver), antioxidant, liver and gallbladder bile stimulator, hepatoprotective (liver protector), hepatotonic (tones, balances, strengthens the liver), hypocholesterolemic (lowers cholesterol)	astringent, blood cleanser, cardiotonic (tones, balances, strengthens the heart), detoxifier, digestive stimulant, diuretic, hypotensive (lowers blood pressure), stimulant, tonic (tones, balances, strengthens)	none
antimicrobial, carcinogenic, caustic, emetic (induces vomiting), immune suppressant, irritant, tumor promoter	laxative	It is not recommended for internal use. It may trigger latent Epstein-Barr infection and promote tumor growth.

Plant	Main Preparation Method	Main Actions (in order)	Main Uses
Avenca leaves and root (*Adiantum capillus-veneris*)	infusion or tincture	cough suppressant, decongestant, expectorant, menstrual stimulant, antimicrobial	• for respiratory problems (coughs, bronchitis, colds, flu, pneumonia, excessive mucus/phlegm) • for hair loss • for gallstones • for menstrual disorders (interruption or absence of menstrual cycle) • as a blood cleanser and liver detoxifier
Balsam resin (*Myroxylon balsamum*)	filtered resin diluted in warm water	emollient (soothes membranes), cough suppressant, antiseptic, anti-inflammatory, antiparasitic	• for coughs and lung congestion • for skin rashes and wounds • for head lice • for skin parasites and ringworm • for colds, flu, and strep throat
Bitter melon fruit and fruit seed (*Momordica charantia*)	fruit juice	hypoglycemic, hypocholesterolemic (lowers cholesterol), antibacterial, carminative (expels gas), bitter	• for diabetes • for high cholesterol and triglyceride levels • for *H. pylori* ulcers • as a bitter digestive aid for intestinal gas, bloating, stomachache, and sluggish digestion • for intestinal parasites
Bitter melon leaves/stem (*Momordica charantia*)	decoction or capsules	anticancerous, antiviral, antibacterial, digestive stimulant, hypoglycemic	• for cancer • for viral infections (HIV, herpes, Epstein-Barr, hepatitis, influenza, and measles) • for bacterial infections (*Staphylococcus, Streptococcus,* and *Salmonella*) • as a bitter digestive aid (for dyspepsia and sluggish digestion) • for diabetes
Boldo leaves (*Peumus boldus*)	infusion or tincture	liver and gallbladder bile stimulant, digestive stimulant, hepatoprotective (liver protector), vermifuge (expels worms)	• for gallstones and as a gallbladder stimulant (to stimulate bile) • to tone, balance, and strengthen liver function (increases liver bile and detoxifies the liver) • for upper digestive tract disorders (ulcers, sluggish digestion, lack of bile, dyspepsia) • for bowel disorders (colitis, leaky gut, constipation, spastic colon, irritable bowel syndrome [IBS]) • for intestinal worms and liver flukes

Properties/Actions Documented by Research	Other Properties/Actions Documented by Traditional Use	Cautions
antibacterial, anticandidal, anti-fertility, antiviral, contraceptive, hypoglycemic	antioxidant, astringent, liver bile stimulator, blood cleanser, cardiotonic (tones, balances, strengthens the heart), cough suppressant, decongestant, detoxifier, diaphoretic (promotes sweating), diuretic, expectorant, hepatoprotective (liver protector), hypocholesterolemic (lowers cholesterol), hypoglycemic, hypotensive (lowers blood pressure), menstrual stimulant, stimulant, tonic (tones, balances, strengthens), wound healer	It has been documented in animals to have contraceptive and anti-fertility effects. It may lower blood sugar levels.
antibacterial, antiparasitic, antiseptic	antifungal, anti-inflammatory, cough suppressant, expectorant	Some people are allergic or sensitive to the resin and develop rashes or hives.
abortive, antimicrobial, contraceptive, hypocholesterolemic (lowers cholesterol), hypoglycemic	antifungal, antiparasitic, antivenin, bitter, cardiotonic (tones, balances, strengthens the heart), digestive stimulant, emetic (causes vomiting), menstrual stimulator, purgative (strong laxative), vermifuge (expels worms)	It lowers blood sugar levels and has abortive and contraceptive effects.
antibacterial, anticancerous, anti-fertility, antileukemic, antiprotozoal, antitumorous, antiviral, hypoglycemic, immune stimulant	antifungal, anti-inflammatory, antimalarial, antiparasitic, antiseptic, bitter, carminative (expels gas), digestive stimulant, febrifuge (reduces fever), hypotensive (lowers blood pressure), lactagogue (promotes milk flow), menstrual stimulator, purgative, vermifuge (expels worms), wound healer	It may lower blood sugar levels.
abortive, anti-inflammatory, anti-oxidant, antiparasitic, antispasmodic, digestive stimulant, diuretic, febrifuge (reduces fever), gastroprotective, hepatoprotective (liver protector), hepatotonic (tones, balances, strengthens the liver), hypocholester-olemic (lowers cholesterol), hypoglycemic, liver and gallbladder bile stimulant, muscle relaxant, platelet aggregation inhibitor, uterine relaxant, vasorelaxant (relaxes blood vessels), vermifuge (expels worms)	analgesic (pain-reliever), antihepatotoxic (liver detoxifier), blood cleanser, cardiotonic (tones, balances, strengthens the heart), carminative (expels gas), hepatotonic (tones, balances, strengthens the liver), laxative, stimulant	It has abortive and blood-thinning effects and may cause birth defects. Don't use while pregnant. Don't exceed recommended dosages.

Plant	Main Preparation Method	Main Actions (in order)	Main Uses
Brazil nut (*Bertholletia excelsia*)	eaten as a food	nutritive, antioxidant, emollient	• as a nutritive • as an antioxidant (for its selenium content) • as an emollient (oil is used for the skin and hair)
Brazilian Peppertree bark or fruit (*Schinus molle*)	tincture or decoction	antibacterial, anticandidal, antifungal, antihemorrhagic (reduces bleeding), cardiotonic (tones, balances, strengthens the heart)	• as a broad-spectrum antimicrobial and antiseptic against bacterial, viral, and fungal infections • for *Candida* and yeast infections • to tone, balance, and strengthen heart function and as a heart regulator for arrhythmia and mild hypertension • to stop bleeding and heal wounds internally and externally • for Mycoplasmal infections
Camu-Camu fruit (*Myrciaria dubia*)	fruit juice	antioxidant, nutritive, astringent	• for its natural high vitamin C content • for colds/flu (for its vitamin C content) • for skin care/anti-aging (for its antioxidant, mineral, and vitamin content)
Carqueja whole herb (*Baccharis genistelloides*)	tincture or capsules	antacid, antiulcerous, digestive stimulant, hepatotonic (tones, balances, strengthens the liver), detoxifier	• for digestive disorders (ulcers, gastro-enteritis, acid reflux, and ileocecal valve disorders) and to slow digestion • to tone, balance, and strengthen liver function (also to eliminate liver flukes, increase liver bile, and to remove toxins from the liver) • for gallbladder disorders (stones, pain, lack of bile, sluggish action, toxin build-up) • as a detoxifier (blood, liver, gallbladder, pancreas) • for viral infections (stomach viruses, HIV, herpes simplex)
Cashew leaves or bark (*Anacardium occidentalis*)	decoction	antiseptic, antidysenteric, antibacterial, antiulcerous, astringent	• for diarrhea, dysentery, and colic • as an internal and external antiseptic against bacterial infections • for stomach ulcers (all kinds) • for ear and eye infections • to stop bleeding and heal wounds

Properties/Actions Documented by Research	Other Properties/Actions Documented by Traditional Use	Cautions
antioxidant	emollient, wound healer	Brazil nuts can cause an allergic reaction in some people.
analgesic (pain-reliever), antibacterial, anticancerous, anticandidal, antifungal, anti-inflammatory, antispasmodic, antitumorous, antiviral, hypotensive (lowers blood pressure), wound healer	antidepressant, antihemorrhagic (reduces bleeding), antiseptic, aperient (mild laxative), astringent, cardiotonic (tones, balances, strengthens the heart), digestive stimulant, diuretic, menstrual stimulant, stimulant, tonic	It has a mild hypotensive effect (lowers blood pressure).
antioxidant (vitamin C)	nutritive	none
abortive, analgesic (pain-reliever), antacid, antihepatotoxic (liver detoxifier), anti-inflammatory, antiulcerous, antiviral, digestive stimulant, gastrotonic (tones, balances, strengthens the gastric system), hepatoprotective (liver protector), hepatotonic (tones, balances, strengthens the liver), hypoglycemic, hypotensive (lowers blood pressure), insect repellant, uterine stimulant	antidiabetic, aperient (mild laxative), bitter digestive aid, blood cleanser, carminative (expels gas), diaphoretic (promotes sweating), diuretic, febrifuge (reduces fever), tonic (tones, balances, strengthens), vermifuge (expels worms)	It has hypotensive (lowers blood pressure) and hypoglycemic actions. It should not be used during pregnancy.
antibacterial, antidiabetic, anti-inflammatory, antiulcerous, astringent	antidiabetic, antidysenteric, cough suppressant, decongestant, digestive stimulant, diuretic, febrifuge (reduces fever), hypotensive (lowers blood pressure), purgative (strong laxative), refrigerant (reduces body temperature), tonic (tones, balances, strengthens), wound healer	none

Plant	Main Preparation Method	Main Actions (in order)	Main Uses
Cat's Claw vine bark (*Uncaria tomentosa*)	decoction, fluid extract, or capsules	immune stimulant, anti-inflammatory, antimutagenic (cellular protector), anticancerous, antiulcerous	• as an immune stimulant and an adjunctive therapy for cancer (to reduce side effects of chemotherapy and protect cells) • as a bowel cleanser and anti-inflammatory for Crohn's disease, colitis, diverticulitis, irritable bowel syndrome (IBS), and other bowel problems • as an anti-inflammatory for arthritis (all kinds) and muscle pains/strains/injuries • as a general daily tonic (to tone, balance, and strengthen all body functions) • for stomach ulcers and ulcerative colitis and as an ulcer preventative/stomach and bowel protector
Catuaba bark (*Erythroxlyum catuaba*)	tincture or decoction	aphrodisiac, nervine (balances/calms nerves), anti-anxiety, central nervous system tonic (tones, balances, strengthens the nervous system), antiviral	• as an aphrodisiac and libido stimulant for males and females • to tone, balance, and calm the central nervous system (and for nerve pain, exhaustion, overstimulation) • for nervousness, emotional stress, and insomnia (related to overactive neuro-transmitters) • as a general tonic (tones, balances, strengthens overall body functions) • for poor memory, Alzheimer's disease, and dementia
Chá de bugre leaves (*Cordia salicifolia*)	infusion	appetite suppressant, diuretic, stimulant, cardiotonic (tones, balances, strengthens the heart), antiviral	• for weight loss (as an appetite suppressant) • as a mild diuretic • for cellulite • to tone, balance, and strengthen heart function • for herpes simplex

Properties/Actions Documented by Research	Other Properties/Actions Documented by Traditional Use	Cautions
anticancerous, antidepressant, anti-inflammatory, antileukemic, antimutagenic (cellular protector), antioxidant, antitumorous, anti-ulcerous, antiviral, contraceptive, immune stimulant	analgesic (pain-reliever), anticoagulant (blood thinner), antidysenteric, blood cleanser, detoxifier, diuretic, gastrotonic (tones, balances, strengthens the gastric system), hypocholesterolemic (lowers cholesterol), tonic (tones, balances, strengthens overall body functions), wound healer	Do not use before or after an organ or bone marrow transplant since it boosts immune function. May also have a mild blood thinning effect.
analgesic (pain-reliever), antibacterial, antiviral, vasodilator, vasorelaxant	anti-anxiety, aphrodisiac, cardiotonic (tones, balances, strengthens the heart), central nervous system tonic (tones, balances, strengthens), nervine (balances/calms nerves), tonic (tones, balances, strengthens)	none
anticancerous, antiviral, cardiotonic (tones, balances, strengthens the heart)	appetite suppressant, cough suppressant, diuretic, febrifuge (reduces fever), stimulant, wound healer	It contains naturally occurring caffeine.

Plant	Main Preparation Method	Main Actions (in order)	Main Uses
Chanca Piedra whole herb (*Phyllanthus niruri*)	infusion or fluid extract	antilithic (prevents and eliminates kidney stones), hepatoprotective (liver protector), diuretic, anti-hepatotoxic (liver detoxifier), antiviral	• for kidney stones and gallstones (active stones and as a preventative) • to tone, balance, strengthen, detoxify, and protect the liver (and to balance liver enzymes) • for viruses, including hepatitis A, B, and C, herpes, and HIV • to tone, balance, strengthen, detoxify, and protect the kidneys and to reduce uric acid and increase urination • for hypertension and high cholesterol levels
Chuchuhuasi bark (*Maytenus krukovii*)	tincture	muscle relaxant, anti-inflammatory, analgesic (pain reliever), menstrual stimulant, tonic (tones, balances, strengthens overall body functions)	• as an analgesic, a muscle relaxant, and an anti-inflammatory for arthritis, rheumatism, and back pain • as an aphrodisiac for loss of libido (male and female) • to cool and balance adrenal function • to tone, balance, and strengthen female hormonal systems and for menstrual disorders, libido loss, menstrual pain, and cramps • as a general tonic (tones, balances, strengthens overall body functions) and mild immune stimulant
Cipó Cabeludo vine/leaf (*Mikania hirsutissima*)	infusion or fluid extract	analgesic (pain-reliever), antibacterial, decongestant, antilithic (prevents or eliminates kidney stones), antileukemic	• for prostatitis, benign prostatic hypertrophy (BPH), and prostate pain • for urinary tract disorders (infections, cystitis, nephritis, urethritis, kidney stones) • as a pain-reliever for neuralgia, arthritis, and general muscle pain • as a decongestant to remove excessive mucus in the bowel, urinary tract, and lungs • for leukemia

Properties/Actions Documented by Research	Other Properties/Actions Documented by Traditional Use	Cautions
analgesic (pain-reliever), antibacterial, antihepatotoxic (liver detoxifier), antilithic (prevents and eliminates kidney stones), antimalarial, anti-mutagenic (cellular protector), antispasmodic, antiulcerous, antiviral, contraceptive, diuretic, gastrotonic (tones, balances, strengthens the gastric system), hepatoprotective (liver protector), hepatotonic (tones, balances, strengthens the liver), hypo-cholesterolemic (lowers cholesterol), hypoglycemic, hypotensive (lowers blood pressure), uterine relaxant	anti-inflammatory, blood cleanser, carminative, detoxifier, diaphoretic (promotes sweating), febrifuge (reduces fever), laxative, menstrual stimulant, tonic (tones, balances, strengthens overall body systems), vermifuge (expels worms)	It may increase the effect of diabetic, high blood pressure, and diuretic drugs. Don't use during pregnancy.
aldose reductase inhibitor (linked to diabetic complications), analgesic (pain-reliever), anticancerous, anti-inflammatory, antioxidant, antitumorous, immune stimulant, protein kinase C inhibitor (linked to inflammation processes)	adrenal tonic (tones, balances, strengthens the adrenals), antidysenteric, antispasmodic, aphrodisiac, digestive stimulant, febrifuge (reduces fever), menstrual stimulant, tonic (tones, balances, strengthens overall body functions)	none
antibacterial, anticoagulant, antileukemic, molluscicidal (kills snails)	analgesic (pain-reliever), antilithic (prevents or eliminates kidney stones), anti-rheumatic, blood cleanser, decongestant, diuretic, nervine (balances/calms nerves)	Contains coumarin and might thin the blood and/or increase the effect of coumadin drugs.

Plant	Main Preparation Method	Main Actions (in order)	Main Uses
Clavillia whole herb (*Mirabilis jalapa*)	infusion or capsules	antiviral, antibacterial, anticandidal, antifungal, antispamodic	• as a broad-spectrum antimicrobial for bacterial, fungal, and viral infections • for *Candida* and yeast infections • as a bowel cleanser and laxative • for skin problems (eczema, dermatitis, acne, rashes, liver spots, skin fungi, ringworm) • for vaginal discharge, infections, and sexually transmitted diseases
Clavo Huasca vine bark (*Tynanthus panurensis*)	tincture	aphrodisiac, analgesic (pain reliever), digestive stimulant, febrifuge (reduces fever), stimulant	• as an aphrodisiac for pre-menopausal women • for muscle pain and aches • as a digestive aid to calm the stomach, increase appetite, and expel intestinal gas • as a male aphrodisiac; for erectile function • as a general tonic (tones, balances, strengthens overall body functions)
Copaiba resin (*Copaifera officinalis*)	cold-filtered resin	anti-inflammatory, analgesic (pain-reliever), anticancerous, antimicrobial, wound healer	• as a topical analgesic (pain-reliever) and anti-inflammatory for wounds, rashes, dermatitis, bug bites, boils, and psoriasis • as an antiseptic, disinfectant, and antimicrobial agent for internal and external bacterial infections • for nail and skin fungi • for skin cancer • for stomach ulcers and stomach cancer
Curare root (*Chondrodendron tomentosum*)	decoction	antibacterial, antiseptic, wound healer, anti-inflammatory, febrifuge (reduces fever)	• for prostatitis • for urinary tract infections • to tone, balance, and strengthen the kidneys (also as a diuretic and for kidney stones) • for vaginal discharge and sexually transmitted diseases • for testicular inflammation
Damiana leaf (*Turnera aphrodisiaca*)	infusion or capsules	aphrodisiac, antidepressant, central nervous system depressant, anti-anxiety, tonic (tones, balances, strengthens overall body functions)	• as a male and female sexual stimulant used to treat erectile dysfunction and anorgasmia • to tone, balance, and strengthen the central nervous system and for emotional stress, depression, and anxiety • for general hormonal balancing • for nervous stomach, colic, and dyspepsia • for mood disorders (obsessive compulsive disorder, hypochondria, neurosis, paranoia, etc.)

Properties/Actions Documented by Research	Other Properties/Actions Documented by Traditional Use	Cautions
abortive, antibacterial, anticandidal, antifungal, antispasmodic, antiviral, uterine stimulant	antidysenteric, antiparasitic, carminative (expels gas), detoxifier, digestive stimulant, diuretic, purgative (strong laxative), tonic (tones, balances, strengthens overall body functions), vermifuge (expels worms), wound healer	Do not use during pregnancy.
none	analgesic (pain-reliever), anti-rheumatic, aphrodisiac, carminative (expels gas), digestive stimulant, muscle relaxant, tonic (tones, balances, strengthens overall body functions)	none
analgesic (pain-reliever), anti-bacterial, anticancerous, antifungal, anti-inflammatory, antitumorous, antiulcerous, gastroprotective (protects the gastric tract), wound healer	anesthetic, antacid, antiseptic, antiviral, astringent, carminative (expels gas), cough suppressant, disinfectant, diuretic, emetic (causes vomiting), emollient, expectorant, laxative, stimulant	It may cause a measles-like rash in those allergic to the resin.
none	antibacterial, anti-inflammatory, antiseptic, antilithic (to prevent or eliminate kidney stones), diuretic, febrifuge (reduces fever), menstrual stimulant, wound healer	Do not use while pregnant.
aphrodisiac, central nervous system depressant	anti-anxiety, antidepressant, antiseptic, antispasmodic, aperient (mild laxative), astringent, bitter digestive stimulant, cough suppressant, diuretic, expectorant, hormonal, nervine (balances/calms nerves), tonic (tones, balances, strengthens overall body functions)	It may reduce the absorption of iron.

Plant	Main Preparation Method	Main Actions (in order)	Main Uses
Embauba leaf (*Cecropia peltata*)	infusion	cough suppressant, anti-asthmatic, decongestant, antispasmodic, cardiotonic (tones, balances, strengthens the heart)	• for asthma • for upper respiratory problems (coughs, bronchitis, COPD, emphysema, pulmonary sarcoidosis) • for upper respiratory bacterial and viral infections • for high blood pressure • for Parkinson's disease
Epazote whole herb (*Chenopodium ambrosioides*)	decoction or capsules	antiparasitic, vermifuge (expels worms), insecticidal, digestive stimulant, hepatoprotective (liver protector)	• for intestinal worms and parasites • for skin parasites, lice, and ringworm • to tone, balance, and strengthen the liver (and for liver flukes and parasites) • to tone, balance, and strengthen the stomach and bowel (and for acid reflux, intestinal gas, cramping, chronic constipation, hemorrhoids, etc.) • for coughs, asthma, bronchitis, and other upper respiratory problems
Erva tostão root and leaf (*Boerhaavia diffusa*)	decoction or capsules	hepatotonic (tones, balances, strengthens the liver), antilithic (prevents or eliminates kidney stones), hepatoprotective (liver protector), diuretic, menstrual stimulant	• for liver disorders (jaundice, hepatitis, cirrhosis, anemia, flukes, detoxification, chemical injury, etc.) • for gallbladder disorders (stones, sluggish function, low bile production, emptying, and detoxification) • for kidney and urinary tract disorders (stones, nephritis, urethritis, infections, renal insufficiency/injury, etc.) • for menstrual disorders (pain, cramps, excessive bleeding, uterine spasms, water retention) • to tone, balance, and strengthen the adrenals (and for adrenal exhaustion and excess cortisol production)

Properties/Actions Documented by Research	Other Properties/Actions Documented by Traditional Use	Cautions
ACE inhibitor (typically lowers blood pressure), analgesic (pain reliever), antibacterial, antifungal, anti-inflammatory, antioxidant, antispasmodic, cardiotonic (tones, balances, strengthens the heart), diuretic, hypoglycemic, hypotensive (lowers blood pressure)	anti-asthmatic, antihemorrhagic (reduces bleeding), antiseptic, antivenin, antiviral, astringent, cough suppressant, central nervous system depressant, decongestant, diaphoretic (promotes sweating), digestive stimulant, expectorant, hepatotonic (tones, balances, strengthens the liver), laxative, menstrual stimulant, wound healer	It may increase the effect of diabetic and high blood pressure drugs.
amebicide, antibacterial, anticancerous, antimalarial, antiparasitic, antitumorous, ascaricide (kills Ascaris parasitic worms), insecticidal, molluscicidal (kills snails), vermifuge (expels worms)	analgesic (pain-reliever), antacid, antihepatotoxic (liver detoxifier), anti-inflammatory, antimicrobial, antiseptic, antispasmodic, antiulcer, carminative, contraceptive, diaphoretic (promotes sweating), digestive stimulant, diuretic, gastrototonic (tones, balances, strengthens), hepatoprotective (liver protector), lactagogue (promotes milk flow), laxative, menstrual stimulant, nervine (balances/ calms nerves), sedative, tonic (tones, balances, strengthens overall body functions), wound healer	It should not be used during pregnancy or while breastfeeding. Don't use essential oil internally.
ACE inhibitor (typically lowers blood pressure), analgesic (pain reliever), antiamebic, antibacterial, anticonvulsant, antihemorrhagic (reduces bleeding), anti-inflammatory, antispasmodic, antiviral, liver and gallbladder bile stimulant, diuretic, hepatoprotective (liver protector), hepatotonic (tones, balances, strengthens the liver), hypotensive (lowers blood pressure), immune modulator (selectively lowers overactive immune cells)	antihistamine, antilithic (prevents or eliminates kidney stones), aperient (mild laxative), blood cleanser, cardiotonic (tones, balances, strengthens the heart), carminative (expels gas), detoxifier, digestive stimulant, kidney tonic (tones, balances, strengthens the kidneys), lactagogue (promotes milk flow), menstrual stimulant, uterine stimulant, vermifuge (expels worms)	It is contraindicated in some heart diseases; it has hypotensive (lowers blood pressure), cardiac depressant, and ACE-inhibitor effects.

Plant	Main Preparation Method	Main Actions (in order)	Main Uses
Espinheira Santa leaf (*Maytenus ilicifolia*)	decoction or capsules	anticancerous, antacid, antiulcerous, menstrual stimulant, detoxifier	• for cancer (melanoma, carcinoma, adenocarcinoma, lymphoma, leukemia) • for stomach disorders (ulcers, acid reflux, gastritis, dyspepsia, indigestion, and to tone, balance, and strengthen the gastric tract) • as a menstrual stimulant and for estrogen hormonal balancing during menopause • for adrenal exhaustion and to support adrenal function • for detoxification (skin, blood, kidney, stomach, adrenals)
Fedegoso whole herb (*Cassia occidentalis*)	infusion	antimicrobial, antihepatotoxic (liver detoxifier), hepatotonic (tones, balances, strengthens the liver), antiparasitic, immune stimulant	• as a broad-spectrum internal and external antimicrobial to treat bacterial and fungal infections • for liver disorders (jaundice, hepatitis, cirrhosis, anemia, detoxification, injury/failure, bile stimulant, etc.) • for intestinal worms, internal parasites, skin parasites • as an immune stimulant • as a cellular protector and a preventative to cell damage (immune, liver, kidney, cancer preventative)
Gervâo whole herb (*Stachytarpheta jamaicensis*)	infusion	antihistamine, bronchodilator, anti-inflammatory, antacid, antiparasitic	• for allergies and respiratory conditions (cold, flu, asthma, bronchitis, etc.) • for digestive problems (indigestion, acid reflux, ulcers, constipation, dyspepsia, slow digestion) • as a general pain-reliever and anti-inflammatory for various internal/external painful inflammatory disorders • to tone, balance, strengthen, protect, and detoxify the liver (and as a liver bile stimulant and for chronic liver conditions) • for intestinal worms and internal/external parasites

Properties/Actions Documented by Research	Other Properties/Actions Documented by Traditional Use	Cautions
antacid, anticancerous, antileukemic, antitumorous, antiulcerous, contraceptive, estrogenic	analgesic (pain-reliever), anti-asthmatic, anti-fertility, anti-inflammatory, antiseptic, astringent, blood cleanser, carminative (expels gas), detoxifier, diuretic, gastrototonic (tones, balances, strengthens the gastric tract), laxative, menstrual stimulant, sialogogue (increases saliva), tonic (tones, balances, strengthens overall body functions)	Do not use with estrogen-positive cancers. It may have estrogen-like actions.
antibacterial, antifungal, anti-hepatotoxic (liver detoxifier), anti-inflammatory, antimalarial, antimutagenic (cellular protector), antioxidant, antiparasitic, antispasmodic, aperient (mild laxative), hepatoprotective (liver protector), hepatotonic (tones, balances, strengthens the liver), hypotensive (lowers blood pressure), immune stimulant, insecticidal, muscle relaxant, weak uterine stimulant, vasoconstrictor	analgesic (pain-reliever), anticancerous, antihemorrhagic (reduces bleeding), antiseptic, antiviral, astringent, bile stimulant, blood cleanser, cardiotonic (tones, balances, strengthens the heart), contraceptive, detoxifier, diaphoretic (promotes sweating), digestive stimulant, diuretic, febrifuge (reduces fever), menstrual stimulant, tonic (tones, balances, strengthens overall body functions), vermifuge (expels worms)	It may speed the clearance of some drugs in the liver (thereby reducing their effect). It is mildly hypotensive (lowers blood pressure).
analgesic (pain-reliever), antacid, anti-anaphylactic (reduces allergic reactions), antidysenteric, antihistamine, anti-inflammatory, antioxidant, antispasmodic, antiulcerous, bronchodilator, gastrototonic (tones, balances, strengthens the gastric tract), hepatoprotective (liver protector), larvicidal, laxative, neurasthenic (reduces nerve pain), vasodilator	abortive, amebicide, antiparasitic, antitumorous, bile stimulant (liver), blood cleanser, cough suppressant, central nervous system depressant, decongestant, diaphoretic (promotes sweating), digestive stimulant, diuretic, expectorant, febrifuge (reduces fever), gastroprotective (protects the gastric tract), hepatotonic (tones, balances, strengthens the liver), hypotensive (lowers blood pressure), lactagogue (promotes milk flow), menstrual stimulant, nervine (balances/calms nerves), refrigerant (lowers body temperature), sedative, tonic (tones, balances, strengthens overall body functions), vermifuge (expels worms), wound healer	Avoid use when pregnant, or if you are allergic to aspirin or have a heart condition.

Plant	Main Preparation Method	Main Actions (in order)	Main Uses
Graviola leaf/stem/bark (*Annona muricata*)	infusion or capsules	anticancerous, antitumorous, antimicrobial, antiparasitic, hypotensive (lowers blood pressure)	• for cancer (all types) • as a broad-spectrum internal and external antimicrobial to treat bacterial and fungal infections • for internal parasites and worms • for high blood pressure • for depression, stress, and nervous disorders
Guacatonga leaf (*Casearia sylvestris*)	infusion or capsules	anticancerous, antitumorous, antiulcerous, antivenin, anti-inflammatory	• for cancer (sarcoma, carcinoma, and adenocarcinoma) • for stomach disorders (ulcers, acid reflux, indigestion, dyspepsia, stomachache) • as an antivenin for snake, spider, and bee bites and stings • as a topical analgesic (pain-reliever) and anti-inflammatory for skin diseases, rashes, and wounds • as a blood purifier and general detoxifier
Guaco leaf (*Mikania cordifolia, M. glomerata*)	fluid extract, syrup, or decoction	cough suppressant, bronchodilator, expectorant, antimicrobial, anti-inflammatory	• for upper respiratory problems (coughs, bronchitis, colds/flu, asthma, allergies, etc.) • for various internal and external bacterial and protozoal infections • for *Candida* and yeast infections • for snakebite and insect bites and stings • as an analgesic (pain-reliever) and anti-inflammatory for arthritis, rheumatism, intestinal inflammation, and ulcers
Guaraná seed (*Paullina cupana*)	infusion or capsules	stimulant, antioxidant, memory enhancer, nervine (balances/calms nerves), cardiotonic (tones, balances, strengthens the heart)	• as a caffeine stimulant for energy • as a weight loss aid (suppresses appetite and increases fat burning) • for headaches and migraines • to tone, balance, and strengthen the heart, as a blood cleanser, and to reduce/prevent sticky blood and blood clots • as a refrigerant (lowers body temperature) to prevent overheating and heat stroke

Properties/Actions Documented by Research	Other Properties/Actions Documented by Traditional Use	Cautions
antibacterial, anticancerous, anticonvulsant, antidepressant, antifungal, antimalarial, antimutagenic (cellular protector), antiparasitic, antispasmodic, antitumorous, cardiodepressant, emetic (causes vomiting), hypotensive (lowers blood pressure), insecticidal, sedative, uterine stimulant, vasodilator	antiviral, cardiotonic (tones, balances, strengthens the heart), decongestant, digestive stimulant, febrifuge (reduces fever), nervine (balances/calms nerves), pediculicide (kills lice), vermifuge (expels worms)	It has cardiodepressant, vasodilator, and hypotensive (lowers blood pressure) actions. Large dosages can cause nausea and vomiting. Avoid combining with ATP-enhancers like CoQ_{10}.
analgesic (pain-reliever), antacid, antibacterial, anticancerous, antifungal, anti-inflammatory, antitumorous, antiulcerous, antivenin, gastroprotective (protects the gastric tract)	anesthetic, antihemorrhagic (reduces bleeding), antimutagenic (cellular protector), antiseptic, antiviral, astringent, blood cleanser, detoxifier, digestive stimulant, wound healer	none
anti-anaphylactic (reduces allergic reactions), antibacterial, anticandidal, anticoagulant (blood thinner), antihistamine, anti-inflammatory, antiprotozoal, antivenin, bronchodilator, cough suppressant, expectorant	analgesic (pain-reliever), anesthetic, anti-asthmatic, anticancerous, antispasmodic, blood cleanser, diaphoretic (promotes sweating), febrifuge (reduces fever), vermifuge (expels worms), wound healer	It contains up to 10 percent coumarin (coumadin), which has a blood-thinning effect.
analgesic (pain-reliever), antibacterial, antioxidant, hyperglycemic, memory enhancer, nervine (balances/calms nerves), neurasthenic (reduces nerve pain), platelet aggregation inhibitor (to prevent clogged arteries), stimulant, vasodilator	anticoagulant (blood thinner), antiseptic, aphrodisiac, appetite suppressant, astringent, blood cleanser, cardiotonic (tones, balances, strengthens the heart), carminative (expels gas), central nervous system stimulant, digestive stimulant, diuretic, hypotensive (lowers blood pressure), laxative, menstrual stimulant, thermogenic (increases fat burning)	Avoid if allergic or sensitive to caffeine.

Plant	Main Preparation Method	Main Actions (in order)	Main Uses
Guava leaf (*Psidium guajava*)	decoction	antidysenteric, antiseptic, antibacterial, antispasmodic, cardiotonic (tones, balances, strengthens the heart)	• for dysentery (bacterial and amebic), diarrhea, colic, and infantile rotavirus enteritis • as a broad-spectrum antimicrobial for internal and external bacterial, fungal, candidal, and amebic infections • to tone, balance, protect, and strengthen the heart (and for arrhythmia and some heart diseases) • as a cough suppressant, analgesic (pain reliever), and febrifuge (reduces fever) for colds, flu, sore throat, etc. • as a topical remedy for ear and eye infections
Iporuru leaf and bark (*Alchornea castaneifolia*)	infusion	anti-inflammatory, analgesic (pain-reliever), antiviral, antifungal, fertility aid	• for arthritis and rheumatism • as an internal and external anti-inflammatory and pain-reliever for muscle and joint injuries • for fungal and viral infections • for erectile dysfunction and female fertility
Jaborandi leaf (*Pilocarpus jaborandi*)	infusion	diaphoretic (promotes sweating), sialagogue (increases saliva), anti-glaucomic, diuretic, febrifuge (reduces fever)	• for glaucoma • for detoxification through copious sweating • for dry mouth disorders • for hair loss (applied topically) • for colds, flu, and pneumonia
Jatobá bark (*Hymenaea courbaril*)	tincture or decoction	anticandidal, antifungal, antibacterial, stimulant, cough suppressant	• for *Candida* and yeast infections • for fungal infections (athlete's foot, nail fungus, etc.) • for prostatitis • for cystitis and urinary tract infections • as a natural stimulant and energy tonic (tones, balances, strengthens overall body functions)
Jergón sacha root (*Dracontium loretense*)	cold maceration, capsules, or tincture	antiviral, antivenin, cough suppressant, protease inhibitor (typically used for viral infections), anti-inflammatory	• for snakebite • for viral infections (HIV, hepatitis, whooping cough, influenza, parvovirus, and others) • for upper respiratory problems (cough, bronchitis, asthma, etc.) • for spider, bee, scorpion, and other venomous insect bites • as a topical wound healer

Properties/Actions Documented by Research	Other Properties/Actions Documented by Traditional Use	Cautions
amebicide, analgesic (pain-reliever), antibacterial, anticandidal, anti-dysenteric, antifungal, antimalarial, antioxidant, antispasmodic, antiulcerous, cardiodepressant, cardiotonic (tones, balances, strengthens the heart), central nervous system depressant, cough suppressant, gastrototonic (tones, balances, strengthens the gastric tract), hypotensive (lowers blood pressure), sedative, vasoconstrictor	anti-anxiety, anticonvulsant, antiseptic, astringent, blood cleanser, digestive stimulant, menstrual stimulant, nervine (balances/calms nerves), vermifuge (expels worms)	It has a cardiac depressant effect and is contra-indicated in some heart conditions.
antifungal, anti-inflammatory, antitumorous, antiviral, COX inhibitor (typically reduces inflammation)	analgesic (pain-reliever), anti-arthritic, antihistamine, anti-rheumatic, antispasmodic, aphrodisiac, cough suppressant, fertility aid, hypoglycemic, wound healer	none
diaphoretic (promotes sweating), digestive stimulant, diuretic, sialagogue (increases saliva)	anticonvulsant, anti-inflammatory, cardiac depressant, hypotensive (lowers blood pressure), lactagogue (promotes milk flow), spasmogenic (induces spasms)	Use under practitioner supervision only. See contraindications in main plant section.
antibacterial, anticandidal, antifungal, anti-inflammatory, hepatoprotective (liver protector), molluscicidal (kills snails)	antidysenteric, antispasmodic, astringent, carminative (expels gas), cough suppressant, digestive stimulant, diuretic, purgative (strong laxative), stimulant, tonic (tones, balances, strengthens overall body functions), vermifuge (expels worms), wound healer	It has a natural stimulant effect; take before 6 pm to avoid insomnia.
none	anticancerous, anti-inflammatory, antivenin, antiviral, cough suppressant, diuretic, immune stimulant, larvicidal	none

Plant	Main Preparation Method	Main Actions (in order)	Main Uses
Juazeiro bark (***Ziziphus joazeiro***)	decoction, maceration, or tincture	analgesic (pain-reliever), antibacterial, anti-inflammatory, febrifuge (reduces fever), astringent	• as a topical wound-healer • as a mouthwash for cavities, gingivitis, and tooth extractions • for fevers (all kinds) • as a topical hair remedy for dandruff, hair loss, and seborrhea • for upper respiratory bacterial infections, coughs, and bronchitis
Jurubeba leaf (***Solanum paniculatum***)	infusion or fluid extract	gastroprotective (protects the gastric tract), digestive stimulant, antiulcerous, carminative (expels gas)	• to speed digestion and stimulate digestive function • to provide relief from sour stomach, gas, bloating, and general dyspepsia • for stomach ulcers • to tone, balance, strengthen, and protect the liver • to tone, balance, and strengthen the heart
Kalanchoe leaf (***Kalanchoe pinnata***)	infusion or fresh leaf juice	immunomodulator (selectively changes some immune functions), central nervous system depressant, analgesic (pain-reliever), antimicrobial, anti-inflammatory	• applied externally and taken internally for all types of pain and inflammation • applied externally and taken internally for various bacterial, viral, and fungal infections • for leishmaniasis • for earaches (leaf juice dropped into ear) • for upper respiratory infections, flu, and fever
Maca root (***Lepidum meyenii***)	eaten fresh/dried, or in capsules	tonic (tones, balances, strengthens overall body functions), nutritive, fertility enhancer, endocrine function support, anti-fatigue	• as a natural source of nutrients (amino acids, minerals, etc.) • to support endocrine function • to reduce fertility problems (both male and female) • to support erectile function • as an aphrodisiac

Properties/Actions Documented by Research	Other Properties/Actions Documented by Traditional Use	Cautions
analgesic (pain-reliever), antibacterial, anti-inflammatory, febrifuge (reduces fever), wound healer	antiulcerous, astringent, cardiotonic (tones, balances, strengthens the heart), cavity prevention, cough suppressant, digestive stimulant, diuretic, hepatotonic (tones, balances, strengthens the liver)	none
analgesic (pain-reliever), antacid, antiulcerous, cardiotonic (tones, balances, strengthens the heart), digestive stimulant, gastroprotective (protects the gastric tract), gastro-totonic (tones, balances, strengthens the gastric tract), hepatotonic (tones, balances, strengthens the liver), hypotensive (lowers blood pressure)	anti-inflammatory, antilithic (prevents or eliminates kidney stones), antitumorous, aperient (mild laxative), bile stimulant (liver), blood cleanser, carminative (expels gas), decongestant, diuretic, febrifuge (reduces fever), nervine (balances/calms nerves), tonic (tones, balances, strengthens overall body functions)	It might reduce fertility in men. It has a mild hypotensive (lowers blood pressure) and stimulant effect on the heart and should be used with caution if you have a heart condition.
analgesic (pain-reliever), anti-allergic, anti-anaphylactic (reduces allergic reactions), antibacterial, antifungal, antihistamine, anti-inflammatory, antitumorous, antiulcerous, antiviral, central nervous system depressant, febrifuge (reduces fever) gastro-protective (protects the gastric tract), immune modulator (modulates some overactive immune cells), immunosuppressive (suppresses some immune cells), insecticidal, muscle relaxant, sedative	anticonvulsant, antilithic (prevents or eliminates kidney stones), carminative (expels gas), cough suppressant, diuretic, hypocholesterolemic (lowers cholesterol), menstrual stimulant, refrigerant (lowers body temperature), tonic (tones, balances, strengthens overall body functions), uterine stimulant, vasoconstrictor, wound healer	Avoid long-term use because of its immune suppressant effects.
aphrodisiac, fertility enhancer, increases sperm count/motility	hormonal, immunostimulant, stimulant, tonic (tones, balances, strengthens overall body functions)	Large amounts may cause intestinal gas.

Plant	Main Preparation Method	Main Actions (in order)	Main Uses
Macela whole herb (*Achyrocline satureoides*)	infusion or tincture	analgesic (pain-reliever), anti-bacterial, anti-inflammatory, antiviral, bile stimulant	• applied externally for pain and inflammation • for respiratory problems (asthma, bronchitis, flu, and upper respiratory bacterial and viral infections) • for arteriosclerosis • for viral infections (hepatitis, HIV, herpes, etc.) • for gallbladder and liver disorders
Manacá root (*Brunfelsia uniflora*)	tincture or decoction	sedative, analgesic (pain reliever), central nervous system depressant, anti-inflammatory, blood cleanser	• for arthritis and rheumatism (internal and external) and general painful and inflammatory conditions • to cleanse and stimulate the lymphatic system (and for swollen lymph glands) • to relieve menstrual pain and cramps • for colds, flu, and fevers • for sexually transmitted diseases
Muira puama root and bark (*Ptychopetalum olacoides*)	tincture	aphrodisiac, tonic (balances, strengthens overall body functions), neurasthenic (reduces nerve pain), antidepressant, central nervous system tonic (tones, balances, strengthens the central nervous system)	• for erectile dysfunction and impotency • as a male aphrodisiac and libido promoter • as a tonic (tones, balances, strengthens) for males • for hair loss and balding • central nervous system tonic (tones, balances, strengthens) and antidepressant
Mulateiro bark (*Calycophyllum spruceanum*)	decoction	antifungal, anticandidal, astringent, insecticidal, wound healer	• for fungal infections of the skin (athlete's foot, nail fungus, etc.) • for skin parasites • for *Candida* and yeast infections • as a skin aid for wrinkles, scars, freckles, and age spots • for diabetes

Properties/Actions Documented by Research	Other Properties/Actions Documented by Traditional Use	Cautions
analgesic (pain-reliever), antibacterial, anticoagulant (blood thinner), anti-inflammatory, antioxidant, antispasmodic, antitumorous, antiviral, bile stimulant, gastrototonic (tones, balances, strengthens the gastric tract), hepatoprotective (liver protector), hepatotonic (tones, balances, strengthens the liver), hypoglycemic, immunostimulant, molluscicidal (kills snails)	anticonvulsant, antiseptic, astringent, bitter digestive aid, cardiotonic (tones, balances, strengthens the heart), carminative (expels gas), cough suppressant, diaphoretic (promotes sweating), digestive stimulant, menstrual stimulant, muscle relaxant, neurasthenic (reduces nerve pain), sedative, vermifuge (expels worms)	It has a sedative effect and might increase the effects of other sedatives. People with diabetes should use with caution as it has a mild hypoglycemic effect.
analgesic (pain-reliever), anticoagulant (blood thinner), anti-inflammatory, antimutagenic (cellular protector), antispasmodic, central nervous system depressant, febrifuge (reduces fever), insecticide, refrigerant (lowers body temperature)	abortive, anesthetic, antitumorous, antivenin, blood cleanser, diaphoretic (promotes sweating), laxative, lymphatic stimulant, menstrual stimulant, sedative	Use with caution in combination with MAO inhibitors, sedatives, and blood thinners. Avoid if allergic to aspirin/salicylates. Do not exceed recommended dosages.
adaptogen, analgesic (pain-reliever), anti-fatigue, antiulcerous, aphrodisiac, central nervous system tonic (tones, balances, strengthens), hypotensive (lowers blood pressure), nervine (balances/calms nerves), neurasthenic (reduces nerve pain)	antidepressant, anti-rheumatic, anti-stress, astringent, cardiotonic (tones, balances, strengthens the heart), digestive stimulant, gastrototonic (tones, balances, strengthens the gastric tract), hypocholesterolemic (lowers cholesterol), stimulant, tonic (tones, balances, strengthens overall body functions)	none
antibacterial, anticandidal, antifungal, antioxidant, insecticidal, insect repellant	antidiabetic, antiparasitic, astringent, emollient, wound healer	none

Plant	Main Preparation Method	Main Actions (in order)	Main Uses
Mullaca whole herb (*Physalis angulata*)	infusion or capsules	antibacterial, antimycoplasmal, anticancerous, immuno-modulator, antiviral	• for bacterial and viral infections of all kinds • for cancer and leukemia • for Mycoplasma and mycobacteria infections • for skin diseases (dermatitis, psoriasis, skin infections, rosacea, scleroderma, etc.) • for viral infections of all kinds
Mulungu bark and root (*Erythrina mulungu*)	tincture or decoction	antidepressant, anti-anxiety, sedative, nervine (balances/calms nerves), hepatotonic (tones, balances, strengthens the liver)	• for mental disorders (depression, anxiety, stress, hysteria, panic disorders, compulsive disorders, etc.) • as a sedative for insomnia, restlessness, and sleep disorders • for liver disorders (hepatitis, obstructions, high liver enzyme levels, sclerosis, etc.) • for high blood pressure and heart palpitations • for drug and nicotine withdrawal
Mutamba bark (*Guazuma ulmifolia*)	decoction or capsules	antibacterial, antiviral, antifungal, antioxidant, hypotensive (lowers blood pressure)	• as a topical hair remedy for hair loss and baldness • as a digestive aid for stomachache, diarrhea, dysentery, and stomach inflammation • as an external skin remedy for wounds, rashes, skin parasites, dermatitis, fungal infections, and leprosy • for viral and bacterial infections (including syphilis, gonorrhea, upper respiratory viruses, and kidney infections) • as an astringent to stop bleeding
Nettle leaf and stem (*Urtica dioica*)	infusion or capsules	anti-allergy, anti-anaphylactic, anti-inflammatory, decongestant, diuretic	• for seasonal allergies, rhinitis, and sinusitis • for prostatitis • for arthritis, rheumatism, and other inflammatory conditions • for high blood pressure • for kidney and urinary tract infections and inflammation

Properties/Actions Documented by Research	Other Properties/Actions Documented by Traditional Use	Cautions
antibacterial, anticancerous, anticoagulant (blood thinner), antileukemic, antimycobacterial, antispasmodic, antitumorous, antiviral, hypoglycemic, hypotensive (lowers blood pressure), immunomodulator (modulates some overactive immune cells), immunostimulant	analgesic (pain-reliever), anti-asthmatic, antihemorrhagic (reduces bleeding), anti-inflammatory, antiseptic, blood cleanser, disinfectant, diuretic, expectorant, febrifuge (reduces fever), hepatotonic (tones, balances, strengthens the liver), sedative, vermifuge (expels worms)	It may thin the blood and lower blood pressure.
anti-anxiety, antibacterial, antidepressant, anti-inflammatory, antimycobacterial, anti-spasmodic, hepatotonic (tones, balances, strengthens the liver), hypotensive (lowers blood pressure), sedative	analgesic (pain-reliever), anticonvulsant, antiseptic, cardiotonic (tones, balances, strengthens the heart), central nervous system depressant, hypnotic, lactagogue (promotes milk flow), nervine (balances/calms nerves), neurasthenic (reduces nerve pain)	It may lower blood pressure and may cause drowsiness.
ACE inhibitor (typically lowers blood pressure), antibacterial, anticancerous, antifungal, antioxidant, antispasmodic, antitumorous, antiviral, cardiac depressant, cardiotonic (tones, balances, strengthens the heart), hypoglycemic, hypotensive (lowers blood pressure), muscle relaxant, uterine stimulant	antihemorrhagic (reduces bleeding), anti-inflammatory, antiulcerous, astringent, blood cleanser, cough suppressant, decongestant, diaphoretic (promotes sweating), digestive stimulant, emollient, febrifuge (reduces fever), hepatoprotective (liver protector), hepatotonic (tones, balances, strengthens the liver), wound healer	Use with caution and under a doctor's supervision if you have a heart condition.
analgesic (pain-reliever), anti-allergy, anti-anaphylatic, anticonvulsant, antihistamine, anti-inflammatory, decongestant, diuretic, hypotensive (lowers blood pressure), immuno-modulator (selectively modulates overactive immune cells)	anti-asthmatic, antibacterial, antidiabetic, antihemorrhagic (reduces bleeding), anti-rheumatic, astringent, blood cleanser, diaphoretic (promotes sweating), febrifuge (reduces fever), laxative, menstrual stimulant, wound healer	It may lower blood pressure and heart rate. Avoid chronic use due to its diuretic effects.

Plant	Main Preparation Method	Main Actions (in order)	Main Uses
Nettle root (Urtica dioica)	infusion or capsules	anti-androgenic, blood cleanser, hormonal regulator, diuretic, hair growth promoter	• for benign prostatic hyperplasia (BPH) • as a diuretic for kidney disorders, hypertension, and diabetes • for male pattern baldness and hair loss • for high blood pressure • as a blood cleanser and general detoxification aid
Passionflower leaf (Passiflora incarnata)	infusion	antidepressant, analgesic (pain-reliever), antispasmodic, sedative, central nervous system depressant	• for mood disorders (depression, anxiety, stress) • for insomnia and sleep disorders • for headaches, migraines, and general pain • for stomach problems (colic, nervous stomach, indigestion, etc.) • to relieve menstrual cramps and premenstrual syndrome (PMS)
Pata de Vaca leaf (Bauhinia forficata)	infusion	antidiabetic, hypoglycemic, diuretic, tonic (tones, balances, strengthens overall body functions), astringent	• for diabetes • for kidney and urinary disorders (including polyuria, cystitis, and kidney stones) • as a blood cleanser and to build blood cells • applied topically for elephantiasis • for skin disorders (rashes, dermatitis, skin ulcers, etc.)
Pau d'Arco bark (Tabebuia impetiginosa)	decoction or tincture	anticandidal, antifungal, antiviral, antibacterial, anticancerous	• for *Candida*, yeast, and other fungal infections (taken internally and used as a douche or topically) • for leukemia and cancer • for colds, flu, and other upper-respiratory bacterial and viral infections • for sexually transmitted diseases (syphilis, gonorrhea, etc.) • for psoriasis and dermatitis
Pedra Hume Caá leaf (Myrcia salicifolia)	infusion or capsules	antidiabetic, hypoglycemic, aldose reductase inhibitor (prevents diabetic complications), astringent, hypotensive (lowers blood pressure)	• for diabetes • as a preventative to diabetic neuropathy and macular degeneration • for hypertension and as a heart tonic (tones, balances, strengthens the heart) • for enteritis, diarrhea, and dysentery • as an astringent to stop bleeding and hemorrhages

Properties/Actions Documented by Research	Other Properties/Actions Documented by Traditional Use	Cautions
analgesic (pain-reliever), anti-androgenic, cardiodepressant, diuretic, febrifuge (reduces fever), hormonal regulator, hypotensive (lowers blood pressure), refrigerant (lowers body temperature), sedative	anticonvulsant, anti-inflammatory, blood cleanser, cardiotonic (tones, balances, strengthens the heart), emollient, hepatotonic (tones, balances, strengthens the liver), laxative, menstrual stimulant, neurasthenic (reduces nerve pain)	It may lower blood pressure and heart rate. Avoid chronic use due to its diuretic effects.
analgesic (pain-reliever), anti-anxiety, anti-inflammatory, antispasmodic, aphrodisiac, central nervous system depressant, cough suppressant, diuretic, hypotensive (lowers blood pressure), sedative	anticonvulsant, antidepressant, astringent, cardiotonic (tones, balances, strengthens the heart), disinfectant, nervine (balances/calms nerves), neurasthenic (reduces nerve pain), tranquilizer, vermifuge (expels worms)	It may cause drowsiness or have a tranquilizing effect.
diuretic, hypoglycemic	antidiabetic, antivenin, astringent, blood cleanser, tonic (tones, balances, strengthens overall body functions), uterine relaxant, vermifuge (expels worms)	Diabetics should use under a doctor's supervision as insulin medications may need adjusting.
analgesic (pain-reliever), antibacterial, anticancerous, anticandidal, antifungal, anti-inflammatory, antileukemic, antimalarial, antiparasitic, anti-tumorous, antiviral, insecticidal	anti-allergy, anticoagulant (blood thinner), antidysenteric, antioxidant, anti-rheumatic, antiulcerous, antivenin, astringent, cardiotonic (tones, balances, strengthens the heart), hepatotonic (tones, balances, strengthens the liver), immunostimulant, laxative	In excessive amounts, it may cause gastrointestinal upset or nausea.
aldose reductase inhibitor, alpha-glucosidase inhibitor, antidiabetic, appetite suppressant, hypoglycemic	antihemorrhagic (reduces bleeding), antioxidant, astringent, cardiotonic (tones, balances, strengthens the heart), gastrototonic (tones, balances, strengthens the gastric tract), hypotensive (lowers blood pressure)	It may lower blood sugar levels. It is contraindicated in hypoglycemia. Diabetics should monitor their glucose levels closely.

Plant	Main Preparation Method	Main Actions (in order)	Main Uses
Picão Preto whole herb (*Bidens pilosa*)	decoction or capsules	antimicrobial, anti-inflammatory, hepatoprotective (liver protector), antiulcerous, antidiabetic	• as a broad-spectrum antimicrobial for various internal and external infections (caused by virus, bacteria, yeast, fungi) • to tone, balance, strengthen, protect, and detoxify the liver • for arthritis, rheumatism, and other inflammatory conditions • for diabetes • for stomach ulcers and digestive disorders
Quinine bark (*Cinchona sp*)	decoction	antimalarial, bitter digestive aid, antiparasitic, antispasmodic, febrifuge (reduces fever)	• for malaria • as a bitter digestive aid to stimulate digestive juices • for nocturnal leg cramps • for intestinal parasites and protozoa • for arrhythmia and other heart conditions
Samambaia root and leaf (*Polypodium decumanum*)	infusion or capsules	immunomodulator (selectively modulates overactive immune cells), antipsoriatic, neuro-protective (protects brain cells), cough suppressant, anti-inflammatory	• for psoriasis and other skin conditions • for Alzheimer's disease, dementia, and memory problems • for coughs, bronchitis, chest colds, and other upper respiratory problems • for autoimmune disorders • as a general tonic (tones, balances, strengthens overall body functions), cellular protector, and anti-aging aid

Properties/Actions Documented by Research	Other Properties/Actions Documented by Traditional Use	Cautions
antibacterial, anticandidal, anti-coagulant (blood thinner), antifungal, antihepatotoxic (liver detoxifier), anti-inflammatory, antileukemic, antimalarial, antitumorous, anti-ulcerous, antivenin, antiviral, cardio-tonic (tones, balances, strengthens the heart), COX inhibitor (reduces inflammation), gastro-protective (protects gastric tract), hepatoprotective (liver protector), hepatotonic (tones, balances, strengthens the liver), hypoglycemic, hypotensive (lowers blood pressure), immunomodulator (selectively modulates overactive immune cells), uterine stimulant	abortive, antidiabetic, antihemorrhagic (reduces bleeding), antiparasitic, antiseptic, antispasmodic, astringent, bitter, carminative, cough suppressant, diaphoretic (promotes sweating), diuretic, emollient, febrifuge (reduces fever), menstrual stimulant, stimulant, vermifuge (expels worms), wound healer	It may potentiate the effects of antidiabetic, blood thinning, and high blood pressure drugs.
anti-arrhythmic, antimalarial, antiparasitic, antiprotozoal, antispasmodic, bitter digestive aid, cardiotonic (tones, balances, strengthens the heart)	amebicide, analgesic (pain-reliever), antibacterial, antifungal, antiseptic, astringent, digestive stimulant, febrifuge (reduces fever), insecticide, nervine (balances/calms nerves), neurasthenic (reduces nerve pain)	It contains quinine alkaloids that are toxic in large doses. Do not exceed recommended dosages. See other contraindications in main plant section.
antidysenteric, anti-inflammatory, antimutagenic (cellular protector), antioxidant, antipsoriatic, immuno-modulator, neuroprotective (protects brain cells)	anticancerous, aperient (mild laxative), blood cleanser, cough suppressant, detoxifier, diaphoretic (promotes sweating), expectorant, febrifuge (reduces fever), hypotensive (lowers blood pressure), tonic (tones, balances, strengthens overall body functions)	Do not use in combination with digitalis and some heart drugs.

Plant	Main Preparation Method	Main Actions (in order)	Main Uses
Sangre de Grado resin (**Croton lechleri**)	undiluted resin is taken internally (in small amount of juice/water) or applied topically	wound healer, antifungal, antiseptic, antiviral, anti-hemorrhagic (reduces bleeding)	• to stop bleeding and to seal and heal wounds, burns, cuts, tooth extractions • for herpes virus ulcers (taken internally and applied topically) • for skin fungi, rashes, and dermatitis • for insect bites, poison ivy, and other itchy or allergic skin reactions • for stomach ulcers, ulcerative colitis, dysentery, and diarrhea
Sarsaparilla root (**Smilax officinalis**)	capsules or decoction	blood cleanser, immuno-modulator (selectively reduces overactive immune cells), antimutagenic (cellular protector), detoxifier, tonic (tones, balances, strengthens overall body functions)	• for psoriasis, dermatitis, leprosy, and other skin disorders • as a blood purifier and general detoxification aid • as a general tonic (tones, balances, strengthens), stimulant, and hormonal regulator • for arthritis, rheumatism, and autoimmune disorders which cause inflammation • for syphilis and other sexually transmitted diseases
Scarlet Bush leaf and stem (**Hamelia patens**)	decoction or tincture	analgesic, anti-inflammatory, antiseptic, febrifuge (reduces fever), refrigerant (reduces body temperature)	• as a topical anti-inflammatory and analgesic (pain-reliever) remedy for skin problems (rashes, bites, stings, etc.) and for bruises, strains, muscle aches, sprains, etc. • as a topical astringent, antiseptic, and antimicrobial remedy for wounds, cuts, burns, skin fungi, etc. • for fevers and to lower body temperature (to prevent sunstroke, overheating) • taken internally for inflammation (rheumatism, arthritis, etc.) • taken internally for pain (headaches, menstrual cramps, post-partum pain, etc.)

Properties/Actions Documented by Research	Other Properties/Actions Documented by Traditional Use	Cautions
anesthetic, anti-allergic, antibacterial, antidysenteric, antifungal, antihemorrhagic (reduces bleeding), anti-inflammatory, antileukemic, antioxidant, antiseptic, antitumorous, antiviral, neurasthenic (reduces nerve pain), wound healer	analgesic (pain-reliever), anticancerous, anti-itch, antiulcerous, astringent, blood cleanser	The red resin stains clothes/fabric permanently.
antibacterial, antifungal, anti-inflammatory, antimutagenic (cellular protector), blood cleanser, detoxifier, diuretic, hepatoprotective (liver protector), immunomodulator (selectively reduces overactive immune cells), neuroprotective (protects brain cells)	absorption aid, analgesic (pain-reliever), anticancerous, antioxidant, anti-rheumatic, antiseptic, aphrodisiac, diaphoretic (promotes sweating), digestive stimulant, febrifuge (reduces fever), stimulant, tonic (tones, balances, strengthens), wound healer	Excessive dosages can cause gastrointestinal irritation.
analgesic (pain-reliever), anesthetic, antibacterial, antifungal, anti-inflammatory, antitumorous, diuretic, immunostimulant, nervine (balances/calms nerves), refrigerant (lowers body temperature)	antidysenteric, antihemorrhagic (reduces bleeding), antiparasitic, astringent, febrifuge (reduces fever), vermifuge (expels worms), wound healer	none

Plant	Main Preparation Method	Main Actions (in order)	Main Uses
Simarouba bark (*Simarouba amara*)	decoction or tincture	antidysenteric, amebicide, antiparasitic, antiviral, antihemorrhagic (reduces bleeding)	• for dysentery (amebic and bacterial) and diarrhea • for intestinal worms and internal parasites • for malaria • as an astringent to stop bleeding internally (stomach ulcers, hemorrhages, etc.) and externally for wounds • for viral infections
Stevia leaf (*Stevia rebaudiana*)	infusion or dry powder extract	sweetener, hypoglycemic, hypotensive (lowers blood pressure), cardiotonic (tones, balances, strengthens the heart), antimicrobial	• as a natural sweetener • for diabetes • for high blood pressure • for cavity prevention • as a weight loss aid
Suma root (*Pfaffia paniculata*)	decoction or capsules	adaptogen, tonic (tones, balances, strengthens), aphrodisiac, steroidal, immunostimulant	• as a general tonic (tones, balances, strengthens) for balancing, energizing, rejuvenating, and muscle growth • for hormonal disorders (menopause, PMS, etc.) • for chronic fatigue and general tiredness • for sexual disorders (impotency, frigidity, low libido, etc.) • for sickle cell anemia
Tayuya root (*Cayaponia tayuya*)	infusion or capsules	analgesic (pain-reliever), nervine (balances/calms nerves), neurasthenic (reduces nerve pain), anti-inflammatory, detoxifier	• to relieve pain of all types (arthritis, migraines and headaches, stomachaches, menstrual pain, etc.) • for central nervous system disorders (sciatica, neuralgia, multiple sclerosis, epilepsy, nerve injuries, etc.) • as a general detoxifier and blood cleanser • for acne, eczema, dermatitis, and other skin problems • for emotional fatigue and depression

Properties/Actions Documented by Research	Other Properties/Actions Documented by Traditional Use	Cautions
amebicide, antibacterial, anti-cancerous, antidysenteric, antileukemic, antimalarial, antimutagenic (cellular protector), antiparasitic, antitumorous, antiviral, vermifuge (expels worms)	analgesic (pain-reliever), antihemorrhagic (reduces bleeding), astringent, bitter, carminative, diaphoretic (promotes sweating), digestive stimulant, febrifuge (reduces fever), menstrual stimulant, tonic (tones, balances, strengthens overall body functions)	Large dosages might cause nausea and vomiting.
antibacterial, anticandidal, antifungal, antiviral, cardiotonic (tones, balances, strengthens the heart), diuretic, hypoglycemic, hypotensive (reduces blood pressure), sweetener	tonic (tones, strengthens, balances overall body functions), vasodilator, wound healer	none
analgesic (pain-reliever), anti-cancerous, anti-inflammatory, antileukemic, antitumorous, aphrodisiac, cellular protector, hypocholesterolemic (lowers cholesterol), immunomodulator (selectively modulates overactive immune cells), steroidal	adaptogen, anti-allergy, antioxidant, cardiotonic (tones, balances, strengthens the heart), carminative (expels gas), estrogenic, immunostimulant, nervine (balances/calms nerves), stimulant, tonic (tones, balances, strengthens overall body functions)	It may have estrogen-like effects. Do not use with estrogen-positive cancers.
analgesic (pain-reliever), anti-inflammatory, antioxidant	anticonvulsant, antidepressant, anti-rheumatic, antisyphilitic, antiulcerous, antivenin, bitter, blood cleanser, detoxifier, digestive stimulant, diuretic, laxative, nervine (balances/calms nerves), neurasthenic (reduces nerve pain), sedative, tonic (tones, balances, strengthens overall body functions)	none

Plant	Main Preparation Method	Main Actions (in order)	Main Uses
Vassourinha whole herb (*Scoparia dulcis*)	infusion or capsules	anti-inflammatory, antimicrobial, analgesic (pain-reliever), antispasmodic, anticancerous	• for menstrual problems (pain, cramps, premenstrual syndrome [PMS], to promote and normalize menstruation) • for upper-respiratory bacterial and viral infections • to relieve pain of all types (arthritis, migraines and headaches, stomachaches, muscle pain, etc.) • to tone, balance, and strengthen heart function (and for mild hypertension) • for sexually transmitted diseases and urinary tract infections
Velvet Bean seed (*Mucuna pruriens*)	capsules or standardized extract	anti-Parkinson's, androgenic, aphrodisiac, hypoglycemic, anabolic	• for Parkinson's disease (contains natural L-dopa) • for impotency and erectile dysfunction • as an aphrodisiac and to increase testosterone • as a muscle builder and anabolic/androgenic aid to stimulate growth hormone • as a weight-loss aid
Yerba Mate leaf (*Ilex paraguariensis*)	infusion	stimulant, tonic (tones, balances, strengthens overall body functions), thermogenic (increases fat-burning), nervine (balances/calms nerves), anti-allergy	• as a stimulant (for its caffeine content) • as an overall tonic (tones, balances, strengthens the body) and digestive aid • for obesity and as part of weight loss regimens • as a general nervine (balances/calms nerves) for nerve pain, nervous fatigue, and depression • for allergies and sinusitis

Properties/Actions Documented by Research	Other Properties/Actions Documented by Traditional Use	Cautions
analgesic (pain-reliever), antibacterial, anticancerous, antifungal, anti-inflammatory, antileukemic, antispasmodic, antitumorous, antiviral, cardiotonic (tones, balances, strengthens heart function), central nervous system depressant, diuretic, hypoglycemic, hypotensive (lowers blood pressure), sedative	abortive, antimalarial, antivenin, contraceptive, cough suppressant, decongestant, detoxifier, emollient, expectorant, febrifuge (reduces fever), hepatotonic (tones, balances, strengthens the liver), insecticide, menstrual stimulant, refrigerant (lowers body temperature), tonic (tones, balances, strengthens overall body functions), vermifuge (expels worms), wound healer	Use with caution in combination with barbiturates and antidepressants. It has hypoglycemic effects.
anabolic, analgesic (pain-reliever), androgenic, anti-inflammatory, anti-Parkinson's, antispasmodic, antivenin, aphrodisiac, febrifuge (reduces fever), hormonal, hypocholesterolemic (lowers cholesterol), hypoglycemic, immunomodulator, nervine (balances/calms nerves), neurasthenic (reduces nerve pain)	antilithic (prevents or eliminates kidney stones), antiparasitic, blood cleanser, carminative (expels gas), central nervous system stimulant, cough suppressant, diuretic, hypotensive (lowers blood pressure), menstrual stimulant, uterine stimulant, vermifuge (expels worms)	It contains L-dopa and has androgenic and hypoglycemic activity. See further cautions in next chapter.
anti-inflammatory, antioxidant, antispasmodic, bile stimulant, stimulant, thermogenic (increases fat burning), vasodilator	anti-allergy, antidepressant, appetite suppressant, blood cleanser, cardiotonic (tones, balances, strengthens the heart), central nervous system stimulant, digestive stimulant, hypotensive (lowers blood pressure), nervine (balances/calms nerves), neurasthenic (reduces nerve pain), neuroprotective (protects brain cells), purgative (strong laxative)	It contains natural caffeine. Don't use if allergic to caffeine or zanthines.

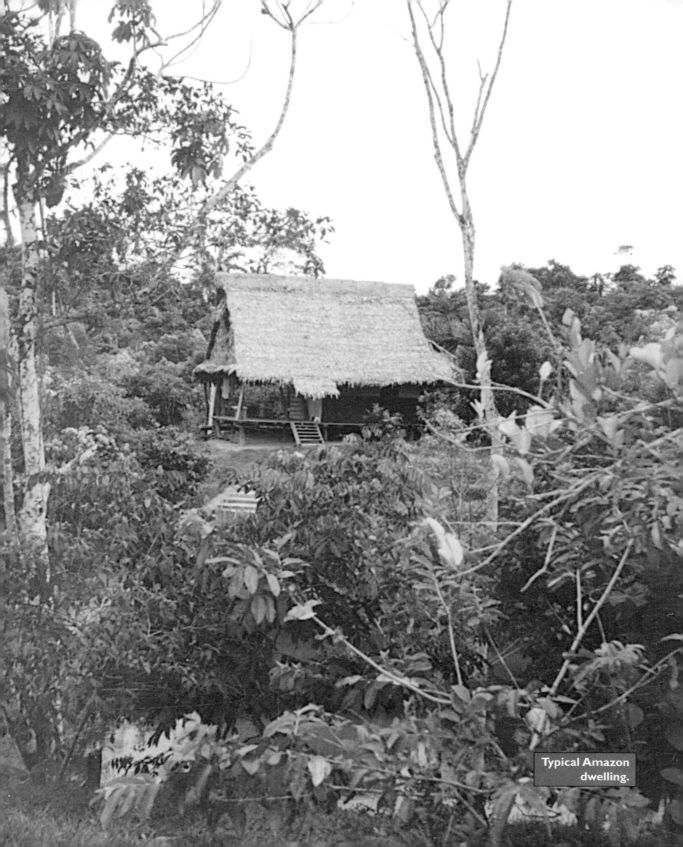

Typical Amazon dwelling.

PART THREE

MEDICINAL PLANTS OF THE AMAZON

Part Three is a valuable resource to more than seventy medicinal plants found in the Amazon rainforest. Each plant is listed alphabetically and includes extensive information. This material is the result of years of research, focusing on both scientific studies and traditional uses.

For quick reference, each entry is introduced by such important facts as the plant's family, genus, species, other common names, parts used, main actions, and standard dosages. Illustrations of each plant are also included.

For each plant, traditional uses by indigenous tribes and in herbal medicine systems worldwide are detailed. Specifics regarding plant chemicals are invaluable for professionals and anyone interested in learning more about the plants' possible biological activities. (Such data is not often so readily accessible!) Clinical research and scientific studies are summarized which help explain and validate the traditional uses of the plants by indigenous peoples. Practical uses, methods of preparation, contraindications, possible drug interactions, and documented uses according to region are also provided. Whether you absorb this entire section, or only focus on plants with specific properties, Part Three offers a wealth of essential information that will teach you what you need to know about each plant and how to use it effectively and safely.

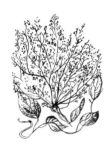

ABUTA
HERBAL PROPERTIES AND ACTIONS

Main Actions	Other Actions	Standard Dosage
• stops bleeding	• kills bacteria	Vine Wood
• balances menstruation	• prevents convulsions	**Decoction:** 1 cup two or three times daily
• relieves pain	• fights free radicals	
• reduces spasms	• prevents ulcers	**Tincture:** 2–3 ml two or three times daily
• relaxes muscles	• reduces mucus	
• stops inflammation	• reduces fever	**Tablets/Capsules:** 1–2 g two or three times daily
• increases urination	• protects liver	
• lowers blood pressure	• balances hormones	

Family: Menispermaceae

Genus: *Cissampelos*

Species: *pareira*

Common Names: abuta, abutua, barbasco, imchich masha, butua, false pareira, pareira, aristoloche lobee, bejuco de raton, feuille coeur, liane patte cheval, gasing-gasing

Parts Used: whole vine, seed, bark, leaf, root

Abuta is a woody, climbing rainforest vine with leaves up to 30 cm long. It produces inedible, dark, grape-sized berries. It belongs to the genus *Cissampelos*, of which thirty to forty species are represented in the tropics. Abuta vine is blackish-brown and tough; when freshly cut it has a waxy luster. Abuta is found throughout the Amazon in Peru, Brazil, Ecuador, and Colombia, and it is cultivated by many to beautify their gardens.

The common name of this plant has caused some confusion in herbal commerce today. In Brazil, this plant is well known as *abutua*, and in Peru it is known as *abuta* or *barbasco*. References to abuta in herbal commerce today may apply to either *Cissampelos pareira* or to a completely different plant, *Abuta grandiflora*. Another tropical vine, *Abuta grandiflora*, also has the common name of abuta in South America, but this is a very different plant with different chemicals and uses in herbal medicine. This plant is referred to in Peru as *chiric sanago* as well as *abuta* (hence the confusion).

TRIBAL AND HERBAL MEDICINE USES

Abuta (*Cissampelos pareira*) is commonly referred to as the *midwives' herb* throughout South America because of its long history of use for all types of women's ailments. The vine or root of abuta is used in tropical countries to prevent a threatened miscarriage and to stop uterine hemorrhages after childbirth. Midwives in the Amazon still carry abuta with them for menstrual cramps and pre- and post-natal pain, excessive menstrual bleeding, and uterine hemorrhaging. Abuta is also believed to aid poor digestion, drowsiness after meals, and constipation.

Virtually all parts of the plant have been used by indigenous peoples throughout the South American rainforest for thousands of years for other ailments, and are still in use today. Members of the Palikur tribe in Guyana use a poultice of abuta leaves as a topical pain-reliever, and the Wayãpi Indians use a decoction of the leaf and stem as an oral analgesic. Ecuadorian Ketchwa tribes use the leaf decoction for eye infections and snakebite. The Créoles in Guyana soak the leaves, bark, and roots in rum and use it as an aphrodisiac. Indigenous tribes in Peru use the seeds of abuta for snakebite, fevers, sexually transmitted diseases, and as a diuretic and expectorant. Amazonian herbal healers (called *curanderos*) toast the seeds of abuta and then brew them into a tea to treat internal hemorrhages and external bleeding. They also brew a leaf tea for rheumatism and a vine wood-and-bark tea to treat irregular heartbeat and excessive menstrual bleeding.

Abuta is called the "midwives' herb" as it is used for many women's ailments.

In Brazil, abuta is widely employed in herbal medicine today as a diuretic and as a tonic (a general overall balancer), as well as to reduce fever and relieve pain. It is often employed for menstrual cramps, difficult menstruation, excessive bleeding and uterine hemorrhages, fibroid tumors, pre- and post-natal pain, colic, constipation, poor digestion, and dyspepsia. In Mexico, abuta has a long history of use for muscle inflammation, snakebite, rheumatism, diarrhea, dysentery, and menstrual problems.

In North American herbal medicine, abuta is used for many of the same conditions as in South America as well as for inflammation of the testicles and minor kidney problems.

PLANT CHEMICALS

Cissampelos plants, including abuta, contain a group of plant chemicals called isoquinoline alkaloids. Since the late 1960s, these chemicals have received a great deal of attention and research.[1,2] Out of thirty-eight alkaloids thus far discovered in abuta, the one called tetrandrine is the most well documented. Clinical research over the years has found tetrandrine to have pain-relieving, anti-inflammatory, and fever-reducing properties.[3] More than one hundred recent clinical studies also describe this chemical's promising actions against leukemia and some other cancer cells, and research is ongoing. However, the therapeutic dosages of tetrandrine used in these animal studies are much higher than one can reasonably obtain from natural abuta root or vine. (The average-weight person would need to take about 2 lbs. of abuta root each day to obtain the therapeutic dosage of tetrandrine used in the animal studies.) Other recently published studies examined tetrandrine's possible cardioactive and blood pressure-reducing (hypotensive) effects through numerous pathways and mechanisms of action at much smaller dosages.

Abuta contains cardioactive plant chemicals that lower blood pressure.

Another well-known alkaloid chemical, berberine, has been documented to have hypotensive, antifungal, and antimicrobial actions. This chemical has been used for the treatment of irregular heartbeat, cancer, *Candida*, diarrhea, and irritable bowel syndrome.[4] Another alkaloid called cissampeline is sold as a skeletal muscle relaxant drug in Ecuador.[5]

The main chemicals in abuta are alkaloids, arachidic acid, bebeerine, berberine, bulbocapnine, cissamine, cissampareine, corytuberine, curine, 4-methylcurine, cyclanoline, cycleanine, dicentrine, dehydrodicentrine, dimethyltetrandrinium, essential oil, grandirubrine, hayatine, hayatinine, insularine, isochondodendrine, isomerubrine, laudanosine, linoleic acid, magnoflorine, menismine, norimeluteine, nor-ruffscine, nuciferine, pareirine, pareirubrine alkaloids, pareitropone, quercitol, stearic acid, and tetrandrine.

BIOLOGICAL ACTIVITIES AND CLINICAL RESEARCH

In 1962, researchers reported abuta demonstrated anti-inflammatory, smooth muscle relaxant, antispasmodic, and uterine relaxant actions in various laboratory animals.[6] Subsequent studies with animals confirmed the plant's antispasmodic [7] and anti-inflammatory actions.[8] These documented effects are quite similar to abuta's traditional uses for menstrual disorders (including cramping and pain). In other animal studies, a root extract was reported to have a diuretic effect, a finding that confirms another of abuta's traditional medicine uses.[9]

Clinical research documenting muscle relaxant, antispasmodic, and uterine relaxant effects help explain abuta's long history of use for menstrual difficulties.

Other *in vivo* research on extracts of abuta indicated that the leaf has antiulcerous actions[10] and that the root has a very mild hypoglycemic action[11] at high dosages. Studies have also shown that the abuta root has other possible therapeutic uses: it demonstrated anticonvulsant actions in mice;[12] and, in dogs, it was shown to significantly lower blood pressure.[6,7] In addition, test-tube (*in vitro*) studies over the years have reported that abuta has antioxidant properties;[13] antibacterial actions against *Staphylococcus, Pseudomonas, Salmonella*, and *Klebsiella*;[10,14] and antimalarial effects.[15,16] One of these *in vitro* studies also reported that a root extract demonstrated a toxic effect against colon cancer cells.[16]

CURRENT PRACTICAL USES

Abuta is still used in the Amazon and outlying areas for the same purposes for which it has been used traditionally for centuries—as a childbirth aid and for general women's ailments. South and North American natural health practitioners commonly rely on abuta as an excellent natural remedy for menstrual difficulties, including cramping and pain, premenstrual syndrome (PMS), excessive bleeding, and fibroid tumors. Its ability to curb excessive menstrual bleeding very quickly can be quite remarkable. It is often employed in overall female balancing formulas, in kidney formulas (for its diuretic and smooth-muscle relaxant effects), and, in combination with other plants, in heart tonics and hypertension remedies.

Toxicity studies with animals confirm the safety of the plant; rats given 10 g of abuta per kg of body weight evidenced no toxic effects.[17]

Traditional Preparation

In South America, a standard decoction is generally prepared with the vine wood and taken two or three times daily in 1-cup doses. (It tastes quite horrible, however!) The natural remedy in North American herbal medicine systems for menstrual difficulties is generally 1–2 g of the powdered vine in tablets or capsules two or three times daily, or 2–3 ml of a standard tincture twice daily, or as needed.

Contraindications   Abuta has been documented to lower blood pressure in two animal studies; therefore, abuta is probably contraindicated for people with low blood pressure. An alkaloid in abuta, tetrandrine, has been documented to have various actions on heart function in animals and humans. Those with a heart condition or taking heart medications should consult with their doctor before using this plant.

Abuta has demonstrated to be a uterine relaxant and has been traditionally employed as a childbirth aid. A pregnant woman should use it only under the supervision of a qualified healthcare practitioner.

Drug Interactions   Abuta may potentiate prescription heart medications.

Worldwide Ethnomedical Uses

Region	Uses
Amazonia	for childbirth, colic, fever, muscle spasms and pain, nervous children, pinta, snakebite
Argentina	for diarrhea, menstrual disorders, respiratory tract infections, urinary tract infections
Brazil	for abortions, anemia, asthma, bladder problems, colic, congestion, constipation, contusions, cramps, cystitis, digestive problems, detoxification (by inducing sweating), dysentery, dyspepsia, drowsiness, edema, excessive phlegm and mucus, fever, gallbladder problems (to stimulate bile), hepatitis, inflammation, kidney stones, menstrual disorders, muscle aches, pains and spasms, testicular inflammation, threatened miscarriage, pre-and post-natal pain, rheumatism, snakebite, stomach problems, urinary tract disorders, uterine hemorrhages, water retention
Guatemala	for cramps, erysipelas, fever, menstrual disorders, rheumatism, snakebite, water retention, and to increase perspiration
Mexico	for bladder problems, dermatitis, diarrhea, dysentery, edema, excessive phlegm and mucus, fever, insect bites, jaundice, menstrual disorders, muscle inflammation, nephritis, pain, pimples, rheumatism, snakebite, urogenital problems, vaginal discharge, water retention, and as a female balancing aid
Nicaragua	for bites, fever, skin rash, sores, stings, sexually transmitted diseases
United States	for hemorrhages and excessive bleeding, constipation, kidney stones, menstrual disorders, muscle spasms, premenstrual syndrome (PMS), testicular inflammation, urinary tract irritation, water retention
Venezuela	for bladder problems, kidney stones, snakebite, and as a diuretic
Elsewhere	for abortions, anemia, arrow poisoning, asthma, boil, childbirth, constipation, cough, cystitis, diabetes, diarrhea, dyspepsia, excessive phlegm and mucus, edema, eye problems, fetal growth problems, fever, hemorrhages, hypertension, indigestion, itch, kidney stones, malaria, menstrual disorders, pain, post-menstrual hemorrhages, rheumatism, snakebite, sores, sterility, threatened miscarriage, urogenital inflammation, uterine hemorrhage, sexually transmitted diseases, water retention, wounds and as a female balancing aid

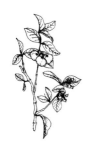

ACEROLA		
HERBAL PROPERTIES AND ACTIONS		
Main Actions	**Other Actions**	**Standard Dosage**
• is nutritious	• kills fungi	Fruit
• fights free radicals	• dries secretions	**Fresh Juice:** 1 cup two or three times daily
	• increases urination	**Tablets/Capsules:** 1–2 g twice daily or follow the label directions based on vitamin C content

Family: Malpighiaceae

Genus: *Malpighia*

Species: *glabra, punicifolia*

Common Names: acerola, Antilles cherry, Barbados cherry, cereso, cerezo, escobillo, health tree

Parts Used: fruit, leaves

Acerola (*Malpighia glabra*) is a small tree or shrub that grows up to 5 m high in the dry, deciduous forest. It produces an abundance of bright red fruit 1–2 cm in diameter, with several small seeds that look similar to the European cherry. For this reason, acerola is also known as the Antilles, Barbados, Puerto Rican, or West Indian cherry tree. The mature fruits are juicy and soft with a pleasant, tart flavor. Acerola can be found growing wild and under cultivation on the sandy soils throughout northeastern Brazil. It is native to northern South America, Central America, and Jamaica. Its cousin, *M. punicifolia,* is present as far north as Florida and Texas.

TRIBAL AND HERBAL MEDICINE USES

Acerola juice is as common and popular in Brazil as orange juice is in North America. As a natural remedy in Brazil, a handful of fresh fruit is eaten for fever and dysentery. It is also used there as an anti-inflammatory, astringent, stimulant for the liver and renal systems, diuretic, and to support heart function as well as to heal wounds. It is employed as a nutritive aid for anemia, diabetes, high cholesterol levels, liver problems, rheumatism, tuberculosis, and during convalescence.

In North America, the use of acerola is mostly based on its high content of vitamin C, which has long been thought in conventional and alternative health practices as a powerful antioxidant.

PLANT CHEMICALS

Until the plant camu-camu appeared on the scene, acerola was considered the richest known source of natural vitamin C. Oranges provide 500 to 4,000 parts per million (ppm) of vitamin C, or ascorbic acid, whereas acerola has been found in tests to provide ascorbic acid in a range of 16,000 to 172,000 ppm[1,2] Acerola can contain up to 4.5 percent vitamin C, compared to 0.05 percent in a peeled orange. The vitamin C content of acerola varies depending on ripeness, season, climate, and locality.[3] As the fruit begins to ripen, it loses a great deal of its vitamin content; for this reason, most commercially-produced acerola is harvested while still green.

Acerola also provides twice as much magnesium, pantothenic acid, and potassium as oranges. It also contains vitamin A (4,300 to 12,500 IU/100 g, compared to approximately 11,000 IU for raw carrots) and thiamine, riboflavin, and niacin in concentrations comparable to those in other fruits.

Acerola contains 4–5 times more vitamin C than oranges.

Thus far, 150 other constituents have been identified in acerola.[4] In addition to ascorbic acid and the other vitamins mentioned above, acerola contains 3-methyl-3-butenol, dehydroascorbic acid, calcium, dextrose, diketogulonic acid, fructose, furfural, hexadecanoic acid, iron, limonene, l-malic acid, phosphorus, protein, and sucrose.

BIOLOGICAL ACTIVITIES AND CLINICAL RESEARCH

Acerola has not been the subject of much clinical research since it is mainly consumed as a food, rather than used as an herbal remedy. In one *in vitro* study, the leaves, bark, and fruit of acerola were reported to have antifungal properties.[5] New findings show that acerola may potentiate the benefits and actions of other supplements (the cholesterol-lowering actions of soy and alfalfa, in one study).[6]

Recent research in cosmetology indicates that vitamin C is a powerful antioxidant and free radical scavenger for the skin, and acerola extracts are now appearing in skin care products that fight cellular aging. In addition to its vitamin content, acerola contains mineral salts that have shown to aid in the remineralization of tired and stressed skin, and its mucilage and proteins have skin-hydrating properties and promote capillary conditioning.

CURRENT PRACTICAL USES

In North America, acerola is used for its high content of vitamin C. Dried acerola fruit extracts can now be found in tablet form and as an ingredient in many over-the-counter multivitamin products in the United States as a natural form of vitamin C.

Traditional Preparation

In South America, acerola juice is freely consumed like most other fruit juices. Consumers in the United States should take acerola supplements based on the vitamin C content provided in the products available in the marketplace. The adult recommended dietary allowance (RDA) for vitamin C is 60–75 mg daily. Therapeutic dosages of vitamin C for colds and flu, general illnesses, and debility are 1–5 g daily.

Contraindications

A study published in 2002 reported that acerola caused allergic reactivity similar to that of the well-known allergen latex. Those who may be allergic to latex may also be allergic to acerola in supplement form or to its addition in various fruit juices.[7]

Large dosages of vitamin C can cause diarrhea.

Drug Interactions   None reported.

Worldwide Ethnomedical Uses

Region	Uses
Brazil	for anemia, diabetes, dysentery, fever, heart function, high cholesterol levels, inflammation, liver problems, rheumatism, tuberculosis, water retention, wounds, and as a drying/astringent agent
Guatemala	for diarrhea
Mexico	for fever and as an astringent
Venezuela	for bowel inflammation, breast disorders, dysentery
Elsewhere	for diarrhea, dysentery, hepatitis, liver disorders, and as an astringent

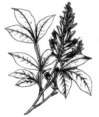

Family: Simaroubaceae

Genus: *Quassia*

Species: *amara*

Common Names:
amargo, bitter ash, bitterholz, bitterwood, bois amer, bois de quassia, crucete, quassia, cuassia, fliegenholz, guabo, hombre grande, jamaica bark, kashshing, maraubá, marupá,

AMARGO
HERBAL PROPERTIES AND ACTIONS

Main Actions
- kills parasites
- kills lice
- expels worms
- kills insects
- kills larva
- treats malaria
- prevents ulcers
- stimulates digestion
- increases bile
- reduces fever

Other Actions
- reduces inflammation
- kills cancer cells
- kills leukemia cells
- prevents tumors
- kills viruses
- dries secretions
- cleanses blood
- mildly laxative
- sedates
- increases saliva

Standard Dosage
Wood, Bark

Infusion: 1 cup two or three times daily

Tablets/Capsules: 1–2 g two or three times daily

Cold Maceration: 1 cup two or three times daily

Amargo is a small tropical tree, growing only 2–6 m in height. It is indigenous to Brazil, Peru, Venezuela, Suriname, Colombia, Argentina, and Guyana. It has beautiful red flowers and fruits that turn red as they mature. Known botanically as *Quassia amara*, it is marketed and used interchangeably with another tree

palo muneco, pau amarelo, quassia amarga, quassiawood, ruda, simaruba, simaruba-baum, quassiaholz, quassia de cayenne, quassie, quina, simaba, Suriname wood

Parts Used: wood, leaves

TRIBAL AND HERBAL MEDICINE USES

Amargo is widely used for all kinds of parasites, worms, and lice, both internally and externally.

species, *Picrasma excelsa*. Sharing the common name of *quassia* (and many of *Quassia amara's* constituents and uses), *P. excelsa* is much taller (up to 25 m in height) and occurs farther north in the tropics of Jamaica, the Caribbean, the Lesser Antilles, and northern Venezuela. In herbal medicine in the United States and Europe, very little distinction is made between the two species of trees; they are used identically and just called *quassia*. The name *amargo* means "bitter" in Spanish and describes its very bitter taste.

In the Amazon rainforest, amargo is used much in the same manner as quinine bark: for malaria and fevers and as a bitter digestive aid. It grows at lower elevations (where quinine does not) and contains many of the same antimalarial phytochemicals (plant chemicals) as quinine. In addition, it is used as an insecticide and tonic, and for hepatitis. Brazilian Indians use the leaves in a bath for measles, as well as in a mouthwash used after tooth extractions. Indians in Suriname use the bark for fever and parasites. Throughout South America, amargo is a tribal remedy for debility, digestion problems, fever, liver problems, parasites, malaria, snakebite, and back spasms.

In current Brazilian herbal medicine systems, amargo is considered a tonic, digestion stimulant, blood cleanser, insecticide, and mild laxative. It is recommended for diarrhea, intestinal worms, dysentery, dyspepsia, excessive mucus, expelling worms, intestinal gas, stomachache, anemia, and liver and gastrointestinal disorders. In Peru, amargo is employed as a bitter digestive aid to stimulate gastric and other digestive secretions as well as for fevers, tuberculosis, kidney stones, and gallstones. In Mexico, the wood is used for liver and gallbladder diseases and for intestinal parasites. In Nicaragua, amargo is used to expel worms and intestinal parasites, as well as for malaria and anemia. Throughout South America, the bitter principals of amargo are used to stimulate the appetite and secretion of digestive juices, as well as to expel worms and intestinal parasites.

In herbal medicine in the United States and Europe, amargo is employed as a bitter tonic for stomach, gallbladder, and other digestive problems (by increasing the flow of bile, digestive juices, and saliva); as a laxative, amebicide, and insecticide; and to expel intestinal worms. In Europe, it is often found in various herbal drugs that promote gallbladder, liver, and other digestive functions. In Britain, a water extract of the wood is used topically against scabies, fleas, lice, and other skin parasites. U.S. herbalist David Hoffman recommends it as an excellent remedy for dyspeptic conditions, to stimulate production of saliva and digestive juices, and to increase the appetite (as well as for lice infestations and threadworms). He also notes, "It may safely be used in all cases of lack of appetite such as anorexia nervosa and digestive sluggishness."

PLANT
CHEMICALS

Chemicals in amargo
make it fifty times more
bitter than quinine!

Amargo bark contains many active constituents including bitter principles reported to be fifty times more bitter than quinine.[2] While amargo contains many of the same types of antimalarial chemicals as quinine bark, it also contains another chemical called quassin. The large amount of quassin in the bark and wood gives amargo a bitterness rating of 40,000.[3] The bark also contains the phytochemicals quassimarin and similakalactone D. Quassimarin has demonstrated antileukemic and antitumorous properties in various studies,[4–6] and similakalactone D has been documented to have antimalarial,[7,8] antiviral,[9] antitumor,[8] and anticancer activities.[10] Other quassinoids have demonstrated antiamebic actions *in vivo* and *in vitro*.

BIOLOGICAL
ACTIVITIES
AND CLINICAL
RESEARCH

Human studies reveal
amargo is 99 percent
effective for head lice.

Several early clinical studies performed on amargo verified its traditional use as a natural insecticide, documenting it as an effective treatment for head lice infestation in humans.[11–14] One of these studies reported a 99 percent effectiveness in 454 patients who had only two topical treatments one week apart.[12] In a 1991 double-blind placebo trial on 148 children with head lice, those treated with an amargo bark extract reported fewer new cases, demonstrating a preventative activity against lice.[13] In addition, an amargo water extract has been reported to work quite well against aphids in the garden,[14] and researchers in India have discovered larvicidal activity against several types of insects, including mosquitoes.[15] Since amargo has long been used for malaria in South America, researchers studied this biological effect as well. One study showed strong *in vivo* antimalarial activity in mice.[16]

Amargo was reported to have antiviral activity when scientists at Texas Christian University demonstrated in 1996 that a water extract was active *in vitro* against cells infected with HIV.[17] A 1978 *in vivo* study reported that amargo wood and/or sap extracts (as well as the isolated chemical quassimarin) inhibited the growth of leukemia in mice.[5] In 2002, an extract of the amargo wood was shown to have antiulcerous actions in mice, inhibiting the formation of gastric ulcers (induced by stress and various chemical means).[18] Prior to this study, a U.S. patent was awarded on the quassinoid phytochemicals in amargo, finding them to have "remarkable antiulcer effects with low toxicities."[19] In another *in vivo* study, amargo was reported to have pain-relieving, muscle-relaxant, and sedative effects in rats and mice.[20]

CURRENT
PRACTICAL USES

In South America, amargo is still heavily relied on as a natural remedy for parasites of all kinds. It is slowly catching on here in North American herbal medicine practices as a remedy for parasites and head lice, but it is predominately used here as a bitter digestive aid and remedy for digestive disorders. Amargo wood is listed by the U.S. Food and Drug Administration (FDA) as generally regarded as safe (GRAS). The wood and its main bitter chemical, quassin, also are approved as food additives—and are employed in beverages and baked goods for their bitter taste. Toxicity studies performed on rats and mice reported no toxicity in oral dosages up to 5 g per kg of body weight.[18]

Traditional Preparation

The traditional remedy as a digestive aid is $\frac{1}{2}$ teaspoon of wood powder infused in 1 cup of boiling water. This is taken ten to fifteen minutes before or with meals. Alternatively, 1 g in tablets or capsules can be taken two or three times daily on an empty stomach for an internal parasite cleanse. Another remedy calls for 2 teaspoons of wood powder or chips to be soaked in 1 cup of cold water overnight (a cold maceration). This is drunk for internal parasites, gallstones, and digestive disorders. This maceration can also be used topically for skin/hair parasites or as a bug spray, especially for aphids on plants and fleas on the dog. For head lice or fleas, prepare a cold maceration (allowing it to macerate/soak for twenty-four hours). Strain and pour through the hair or apply directly to the skin. It can be washed off in an hour (or simply left on the dog). For lice, repeat every three days for three applications, and for fleas, apply once monthly. Also, a small handful of amargo wood chips can be placed in backyard ponds/fountains (or a few chips in bird baths) to kill mosquito larvae without harming fish or birds.

Contraindications

Amargo should not be used during pregnancy. Amargo has been documented to have an anti-fertility effect in studies with male rats.[21] Men undergoing fertility treatment or wishing to have children probably should avoid using amargo.

Large amounts of amargo can irritate the mucous membrane of the stomach and can lead to nausea and vomiting. Do not exceed recommended dosages.

Drug Interactions

None reported. However, amargo may interfere with male fertility drugs.

Worldwide Ethnomedical Uses

Region	Uses
Brazil	for anemia, anorexia, colic, debility, dental pain, diarrhea, digestion disorders, dysentery, dyspepsia, fever, flatulence, gallbladder problems, gallstones, gastrointestinal disorders, gonorrhea, kidney stones, liver problems, malaria, measles, urinary insufficiency, vaginal discharge, and as a bitter digestive stimulant
Costa Rica	for diabetes, diarrhea, fever, worms
Europe	for bile insufficiency, digestive disorders, fleas, gallstones, liver disease, parasites, scabies, threadworms, and as a bitter digestive stimulant
Guatemala	for constipation, diabetes, high blood pressure, nervousness
Mexico	for digestive disorders, gallbladder problems, intestinal parasites, liver disorders, worms, and as a digestive stimulant

Nicaragua	for anemia, bug bites, intestinal parasites, malaria, stings, worms, and as an astringent
Panama	for hyperglycemia, fever, liver disorders, malaria, snakebite
Peru	for cleansing blood, digestive disorders, edema, fever, gallstones, hepatitis, intestinal parasites, kidney stones, stimulating digestion, tuberculosis, worms, and as an insecticide
South America	for anorexia, cleansing blood, debility, digestive disorders, carcinoma, cirrhosis, constipation, fever, fleas, hyperglycemia, indigestion, leukemia, lice, liver disorders, malaria, parasites, scabies, snakebite, spasms, stimulating digestion, worms, and as an aphidicide and insecticide
Turkey	for diarrhea, digestive difficulty, dysentery, fever, malaria, urinary insufficiency, and as an astringent and tonic
United States	for alcoholism, anorexia, bowel cleansing, convalescence, debility, digestive disorders, fever, gallbladder problems, increasing saliva, intestinal parasites, lice, liver support, spasms, stimulating bile production, stimulating digestion, worms
Venezuela	for constipation, dysentery, fever, worms, and as a tonic
Elsewhere	for amebic infections, bacterial infections, cancer, carcinoma, fever, liver disorders, malaria, snakebite, stimulating digestion, tumors, worms, and as an insecticide and tonic

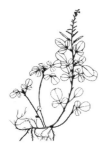

Family: Fabaceae

Genus: *Desmodium*

Species: *adscendens*

Common Names:
amor seco, amor-do-campo, strong back, pega pega, margarita, beggar-lice, burbur, manayupa, hard man, hard stick, mundubirana, barba de boi, mundurana, owono-bocon, dipinda dimukuyi, dusa karnira, tick-clover, tick-trefoil

Parts Used: aerial parts, leaves

AMOR SECO
HERBAL PROPERTIES AND ACTIONS

Main Actions
- reduces pain
- blocks allergies
- reduces asthma
- reduces convulsions
- blocks histamine
- reduces inflammation
- reduces spasms
- dilates bronchials
- relaxes muscles

Other Actions
- cleanses blood
- detoxifies
- increases urination
- mildly laxative
- heals wounds

Standard Dosage
Leaves, Whole herb
Infusion: 1–3 cups daily
Tincture: 4–6 ml daily
Capsules/Tablets: 4–5 g daily

Amor seco is a weedy, perennial herb that grows to 50 cm tall and produces numerous light-purple flowers and green fruits in small, beanlike pods. It is indigenous to many tropical countries and grows in open forests, pastures, along roadsides, and like many weeds—just about anywhere the soil is disturbed. In Brazil, the plant is known as *amor seco* or *amor-do-campo*; Peruvians call the plant *manayupa*. The *Desmodium* genus is a large one, with about 400 species of perennial and annual herbs growing in temperate and tropical regions in the Western hemisphere, Australia, and South Africa. In the South American tropics, *Desmodium axillare,* a closely related plant, is used interchangeably in herbal medicine systems.

TRIBAL AND HERBAL MEDICINE USES

Today, tribes in the Amazon rainforest use amor seco medicinally much as they have for centuries. A tea of the plant is given for nervousness, and it is used in baths to treat vaginal infections. Some tribes believe the plant has magic powers, and it is taken by lovers to rekindle a waning romance. Rio Pastaza natives in the Amazon brew a leaf tea and wash the breasts of mothers with it to promote milk flow. Additional indigenous tribal uses include a leaf decoction for consumption, an application of pounded leaves and lime juice for wounds, and a leaf infusion for convulsions and venereal sores. A survey, in which more than 8,000 natives in various parts of Brazil were interviewed, showed that a decoction of the dried roots of amor seco is a popular tribal remedy for malaria.[1] The indigenous Garifuna tribe in Nicaragua uses a leaf decoction of amor seco internally for diarrhea and sexually transmitted diseases, and to aid digestion.

Amor seco is also quite popular in herbal medicine throughout South and Central America. In Peruvian herbal medicine today, a leaf tea is used as a blood cleanser; to detoxify the body from environmental toxins and chemicals; as a urinary tract cleanser; and to treat ovarian and uterine problems such as inflammation and irritation, vaginal discharges, and hemorrhages. In Belize (where the plant is called "strong back"), the entire plant is soaked in rum for twenty-four hours, and then $\frac{1}{4}$ cup is taken three times daily for seven to ten days for backaches. Alternatively, an entire plant is boiled in 3 cups of water for ten minutes, and 1 cup of warm tea is taken before meals for three to five days for relief of backache, muscle pains, kidney ailments, and impotence. In Brazilian herbal medicine, the dried leaves are used for the treatment of asthma, vaginal discharge, body aches and pains, ovarian inflammation, excessive urination, excessive mucus, and diarrhea. In Ghana, a leaf decoction is a popular remedy for bronchial asthma, constipation, dysentery, and colic, and is also used to dress wounds.

PLANT CHEMICALS

Amor seco is known to be rich in flavonoids, alkaloids, and chemicals known as soyasaponins. A novel soyasaponin in amor seco is dehydrosoyasaponin. It is considered a highly active chemical with therapeutic actions for asthma. Amor seco also contains a chemical called astragalin, which is a well known antibacterial chemical found in the popular medicinal plant astragalus. Amor seco's traditional uses for infections, sexually transmitted diseases, and wounds are probably related to this particular chemical in the plant.

Main chemicals found in amor seco include astragalin, beta-phenylethylamines, cosmosiin, cyanidin-3-o-sophoroside, dehydrosoyasaponins, hordenine, pelargonidin-3-o-rhamnoside, salsoline, soyasaponins, tectorigenin, tetrahydroisoquinolines, and tyramine.

BIOLOGICAL ACTIVITIES AND CLINICAL RESEARCH

Herbalists in Ghana have long used amor seco leaves to treat bronchial asthma. The treatment was so successful that it attracted attention from the scientific community. In 1977, a clinical observational study on humans showed that 1 to 2 teaspoons of dried amor seco leaf powder daily (in three dosages) produced improvement and remission in most asthma patients treated.[2,3] In an effort to understand the anti-asthmatic properties of this effective natural remedy, scientists conducted various animal studies to determine how it worked. In ten different studies, researchers found that amor seco interfered with the production of many of the chemicals normally produced during an asthma attack: chemicals called spasmogens that cause contractions in the lung; histamine that triggers the allergic response; and chemicals called leukotrienes that are known to stimulate bronchoconstriction and increase mucus production in the airway—all key features of asthma.[4–14] Many substances and allergens can cause a life-threatening allergic reaction called anaphylactic shock, or anaphylaxis. Several of these animal studies reported that amor seco had an anti-anaphylactic action against many known substances that trigger such reactions.

Human and animal studies indicate that amor seco is beneficial for asthma.

Bronchoconstriction (the tendency of airways to constrict or become too narrow, thereby making it hard to breath) in response to various stimuli and allergens is a universal feature of asthma and anaphylactic reactions. Some researchers noted that amor seco has a muscle-relaxing effect in lung tissues (bronchodilator) and inhibited contractions and constriction induced by a variety of substances.[8,15] Amor seco has also been shown to activate the chemical process known as potassium maxi-K channels.[16] Maxi-K channels play an important role in regulating the tone of airway smooth muscle and the release of constrictive substances in the lungs. One of amor seco's chemicals, dehydrosoyasaponin I, was cited as being "the most potent known potassium (maxi-K) channel opener."[16] This effect is also thought to contribute to amor seco's therapeutic activity in asthma.

Amor seco's documented anti-allergic activity acts to inhibit not only contraction of smooth muscle in the airways of the upper respiratory tract but also muscle contraction at multiple other sites throughout the body.[6] These documented antispasmodic and muscle relaxant actions help explain why amor seco has been traditionally used for backaches and muscle spasms. Amor seco has also recently been documented in animal studies to have pain-relieving actions as well as anticonvulsant actions.[17]

CURRENT PRACTICAL USES

Natural health practitioners and herbalists in South America today use this herbal remedy mainly for asthma and allergies and for muscle spasms and back pain. With some newer published research linking arthritis and rheumatism to various allergic reactions (and some of the same allergy-induced chemical processes found in asthma), the indigenous use of amor seco for back pain and arthritis may become the subject of future research. Amor seco is easy to administer and is highly effective at low dosages. In addition, its lack of side effects or toxicity places it in the first line of defense in the herbalist's medicine chest of natural remedies.

Traditional Preparation	Generally, 1–3 cups of amor seco leaf tea (standard infusion) daily, 4–6 ml of a standard tincture, or 4–5 g of powdered leaves in capsules daily are used for most conditions.
Contraindications	None known.
Drug Interactions	None reported.

Worldwide Ethnomedical Uses

Region	Uses
Africa	for asthma, bronchitis, central nervous system disorders, colic, ringworms, wounds
Amazonia	for backache, convulsions, headache, inflammation, muscle spasms, nervousness, pain, stimulating breast milk, and as a contraceptive
Belize	for aches (back, joint, muscle), headache, kidney disorders
Brazil	for body aches, cough, diarrhea, excessive mucus, excessive urination, inflammation, malaria, ovarian inflammation, spasms, vaginal discharge
Ghana	for anaphylaxis, asthma, colic, constipation, dysentery, wounds
Nicaragua	for diarrhea, digestive disorders, sexually transmitted diseases
Peru	for detoxifying blood, hemorrhage, inflammation, nervousness, ovarian problems, urinary problems, vaginitis
Trinidad	for detoxifying blood, malnutrition, sexually transmitted diseases, urinary disorders
United States	for asthma, backache, headache, impotency, joint aches, kidney, muscle pain, muscle spasms
Elsewhere	for asthma, constipation, convulsion, cough, fractures, scabies, sores, stimulating milk flow, tuberculosis, sexually transmitted diseases, worms, wounds

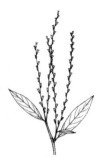

Family: Phytolaccaceae

Genus: *Petiveria*

Species: *alliacea*

Common Names:
anamu, apacin, apacina, apazote de zorro, aposin, ave, aveterinaryte, calauchin, chasser vermine, congo root, douvant-douvant, emeruaiuma, garlic weed, guinea henweed, guine, guinea, guinea hen leaf, gully root, huevo de gato, kojo root, mapurite, mucura-caa, mucura, mucuracáa, ocano, payche, pipi, tipi, verbena hedionda, verveine puante, zorrillo

Part Used: whole herb

TRIBAL AND HERBAL MEDICINE USES

ANAMU
HERBAL PROPERTIES AND ACTIONS

Main Actions	Other Actions	Standard Dosage
• reduces pain	• reduces spasms	Whole Herb
• kills bacteria	• reduces anxiety	**Infusion:** $1/4$ to $1/2$ cup two
• kills cancer cells	• reduces fever	or three times daily
• kills fungi	• lowers blood sugar	**Tablets/Capsules:** 1–3 g
• reduces inflammation	• kills insects	daily
• kills leukemia cells	• promotes menstruation	
• reduces free radicals	• sedates	
• prevents tumors	• increases perspiration	
• kills viruses	• expels worms	
• kills *Candida*		
• increases urination		
• enhances immunity		

Anamu is an herbaceous perennial that grows up to 1 m in height. It is indigenous to the Amazon rainforest and tropical areas of Central and South America, the Caribbean, and Africa. It produces dark green leathery leaves that lie close to the ground and tall spikes lined with small white flowers that float airily above the leaves. It is sometimes called "garlic weed," as the plant, and especially the roots, have a strong garlic odor. It is called *mucura* in the Peruvian Amazon, *anamu* or *tipi* in Brazil, and *guine* in other parts of Latin America.

In the Amazon rainforest, anamu is used as part of an herbal bath against witchcraft by the Indians and local jungle herbal healers called *curanderos*. The Ka'apor Indians call it *mikur-ka'a* (which means opossum herb) and use it for both medicine and magic. The Caribs in Guatemala crush the root and inhale it for sinusitis, and the Ese'Ejas Indians in the Peruvian Amazon prepare a leaf infusion for colds and flu. The Garifuna indigenous people in Nicaragua also employ a leaf infusion or decoction for colds, coughs, and aches and pains, as well as for magic rituals. The root is thought to be more powerful than the leaves. It is considered a pain-reliever and is often used in the rainforest in topical remedies for the skin. Other indigenous Indian groups beat the leaves into a paste and use it externally for headache, rheumatic pain, and other types of pain. This same jungle remedy is also used as an insecticide.

Anamu has a long history in herbal medicine in all of the tropical countries where it grows. In Brazilian herbal medicine, it is considered an antispasmodic, diuretic, menstrual promoter, stimulant, and sweat promoter. Herbalists and natural health practitioners there use anamu for edema, arthritis, malaria, rheumatism, and poor memory, and as a topical analgesic and anti-inflammatory for skin afflictions. Throughout Central America, women use anamu to relieve birthing pains and facilitate easy childbirth, as well as to induce abortions. In Guatemalan herbal medicine, the plant is called *apacín* and a leaf decoction is taken internally for digestive ailments and sluggish digestion, flatulence, and fever. A leaf decoction is also used externally as an analgesic for muscular pain and for skin diseases. Anamu is commonly used in big cities and towns in South and Central America as a natural remedy to treat colds, coughs, influenza, respiratory and pulmonary infections, and cancer, and to support the immune system. In Cuba, herbalists decoct the whole plant and use it to treat cancer and diabetes, and as an anti-inflammatory and abortive.

PLANT CHEMICALS

Many biologically active compounds have been discovered in anamu, including flavonoids, triterpenes, steroids, and sulfur compounds. Anamu contains a specific sulfur compound named dibenzyl trisulfide. In a plant-screening program at the University of Illinois at Chicago that evaluated more than 1,400 plant extracts as novel therapies for the prevention and treatment of cancer, anamu was one of thirty-four plants identified with active properties against cancer. The researchers reported that dibenzyl trisulfide was one of two of the active compounds in anamu with anticancerous actions.[1] Anamu also contains the phytochemicals astilbin, benzaldehyde, and coumarin, all of which have been documented with antitumorous and/or anticancerous properties as well.[2–4]

Anamu contains chemicals with tested anticancerous actions.

Main chemicals found in anamu include allantoin, astilbin, barbinervic acid, benzylhydroxytrisulfide, coumarin, daucosterol, dibenzyl sulfide, engeletin, friedelinol, ilexgenin A, leridal, leridol, lignoceric acid, linoleic acid, myricitrin, nonadecanoic acid, oleic acid, palmitic acid, petiveral, pinitol, proline, sitosterol, stearic acid, and trithiolaniacine.

BIOLOGICAL ACTIVITIES AND CLINICAL RESEARCH

The research published on anamu (and the plant chemicals described above) reveals that the herb has a broad range of therapeutic properties, including antileukemic, antitumorous, and anticancerous activities against several types of cancer cells. In an *in vitro* study by Italian researchers in 1990, water extracts and ethanol extracts of anamu retarded the growth of leukemia cells and several other strains of cancerous tumor cells.[5] Three years later, the researchers followed up with another study, which showed that the same extracts had a cytotoxic effect, actually killing some of these cancer cells, rather than just retarding their growth. This study indicated that whole herb water extracts of anamu were toxic to leukemia and lymphoma cancer cells but only inhibited the growth of breast cancer cells.[6] More recently, a study published in 2002 documented an *in vitro* toxic effect against a liver cancer cell line;[7] another *in vitro* study in 2001 reported that anamu retarded the growth of brain cancer cells.[8] A German study documenting anamu's activity against brain cancer cells related its actions to the sulfur compounds found in the plant.

Human and animal research confirms anamu is a natural immune stimulant.

In addition to its documented anticancerous properties, anamu has also been found in both *in vivo* and *in vitro* studies to be an immunostimulant. In a 1993 study with mice, a water extract stimulated immune cell production (lymphocytes and Interleukin II).[9] In the same year, another study with mice demonstrated that an anamu extract increased natural killer cell activity by 100 percent and stimulated the production of even more types of immune cells (Interferon, Interleukin II, and Interleukin 4). Additional research from 1997 to 2001 further substantiated anamu's immunostimulant actions in humans and animals.[11–13]

Anamu's traditional use as a remedy for arthritis and rheumatism has been validated by clinical research confirming its pain-relieving and anti-inflammatory properties. One research group in Sweden reported that anamu possesses cyclooxygenase-1 (COX-1) inhibitory actions.[14] COX-1 inhibitors are a new (and highly profitable) class of arthritis drugs being sold today by pharmaceutical companies. Another research group in Brazil documented significant anti-inflammatory effects in rats using various models,[15–17] and researchers in 2002 noted a significant pain-relieving effect in rats.[18] The pain-relieving and anti-inflammatory effects were even verified when an ethanol extract was applied topically in rats, again validating traditional use.[19]

Many clinical reports and studies document that anamu shows broad-spectrum antimicrobial properties against numerous strains of bacteria, viruses, fungi, and yeast. In a 2002 study, anamu extracts inhibited the replication of the bovine diarrhea virus; this is a test model for hepatitis C virus.[20] A Cuban research group documented anamu's antimicrobial properties *in vitro* against numerous pathogens, including *Escherichia coli, Staphylococcus, Pseudomonas,* and *Shigella* and, interestingly enough, their crude water extracts performed better than any of the alcohol extracts.[21] A German group documented good activity against several gram-positive and gram-negative bacteria, *Mycobacterium tuberculosis,* several strains of fungi, and *Candida*.[22] Anamu's antifungal properties were documented by one research group in 1991,[23] and again by a separate research group in 2001.[24] Its antimicrobial activity was further demonstrated by researchers from Guatemala and Austria who, in separate studies in 1998, confirmed its activity *in vitro* and *in vivo* studies against several strains of protozoa, bacteria, and fungi.[25,26]

While anamu has not been used widely employed for diabetes, it has been clinically documented to have hypoglycemic actions. Researchers in 1990 demonstrated the *in vivo* hypoglycemic effect of anamu, showing that anamu decreased blood sugar levels by more than 60 percent one hour after administration to mice. This finding reflects herbal medicine practice in Cuba where anamu has been used as an herbal aid for diabetes for many years.[27]

CURRENT PRACTICAL USES

With the many documented properties and actions of this tropical plant, it is no wonder that anamu has enjoyed such a long history of use in herbal medicine. Continuing research on this plant's attributes is quantifying and qualifying the richness of indigenous herbal traditions. Today, in South America, anamu is being used for its immune stimulant and anticancerous properties as a support aid for cancer and leukemia patients. This use is catching on here in the United States, and anamu is now available in capsules and tablets under several labels. It is also being employed in various formulas for its antimicrobial actions against bacteria, viruses, yeast, and fungi, as well as in other formulas supporting immune function.

In the first published study on toxicity in 1992, researchers noted that, at high dosages, anamu extract delayed cell proliferation *in vitro*. When they tested the extract in mice, they noted that it caused a change in bone marrow cells; however, they were using 100 to 400 times the traditional dosage given to humans.[28] In two independent studies published later by other researchers, oral doses of leaf and root extracts did not cause any toxicity in rats and mice at up to 5 g per kg of body weight.[15,29] Methanol extracts of the plant did, however, cause uterine contractions in an early study;[30] such contractions can lead to abortion, one of anamu's well documented uses in traditional herbal medicine.

Traditional Preparation

The traditional remedy calls for a decoction or infusion prepared with 30 g of dried anamu whole herb in a liter of water; $1/4$ cup to $1/2$ dosages are taken one to three times daily or used topically, depending on the condition treated. Since most of the chemicals are water soluble, powdered whole herb in tablets or capsules (1–3 grams) daily can be substituted, if desired.

Contraindications

Methanol extracts of anamu cause uterine contractions, which can lead to abortion. As such, anamu is contraindicated for pregnant women.

Anamu contains a low concentration of coumarin, which has a blood-thinning effect. People with blood disorders such as hemophilia and people on blood-thinning medications should not use this plant without the supervision and advice of a qualified healthcare practitioner.

This plant has been shown to have hypoglycemic effects in mice. People with hypoglycemia and diabetes should not use this plant unless they are under the care of a healthcare practitioner to monitor their blood sugar levels.

Drug Interactions   None published. However, due to anamu's natural coumarin content, it is conceivable that it may potentiate the effects of coumadin (Warfarin®).

Worldwide Ethnomedical Uses

Region	Uses
Argentina	for colds, diarrhea, fever, headache, menstrual problems, respiratory tract infections, rheumatism, swellings, toothache, urinary infections, urinary insufficiency
Brazil	for abortions, asthma, arthritis, cancer, diabetes, fever, headache, inflammation, increasing perspiration, intestinal parasites, malaria, menstrual disorders, osteoarthritis, pain, rheumatism, spasms, toothache, urinary insufficiency, sexually transmitted diseases, worms, and as an insecticide and sedative
Colombia	for cavity prevention, childbirth, snakebite
Cuba	for abortions, cancer, diabetes, inflammation
Guatemala	for abscesses, blood disorders, boils, dermatitis, diarrhea, erysipelas, fever, headache, menstrual problems, pimples, ringworm, sinusitis, skin disease, skin eruptions, skin fungus, stomach cramps
Latin America	for abortions, absence of menses, cleansing blood, hysteria, increasing perspiration, nerves, reducing phlegm, spasms, urinary insufficiency
Mexico	for abortions, boils, catarrh, childbirth, cleansing blood, colds, delayed menses, epilepsy, fever, headache, heat rash, hives, hysteria, increasing perspiration, influenza, nerves, paralysis, pimples, rabies, repelling insects, rheumatism, reducing phlegm, spasms, toothache, tumor, urinary insufficiency, sexually transmitted diseases, worms
Nicaragua	for aches, colds, coughs, heart problems, kidney disorders, liver support, pains, pulmonary disorders, respiratory disorders, snakebite
Paraguay	for abortions, digestive diseases, fever, flu, menstrual disorders, pain (muscular), sinusitis, skin disease, toothache, and as an insecticide
Peru	for colds, flu
Puerto Rico	for abortions, cholera, childbirth, fever, menstrual problems
Trinidad	for abortions, cleansing blood, cystitis, flu, head cold, irritations, menstrual disorders, thinning blood, sexually transmitted diseases
Venezuela	for abortions, cavities, cleansing blood, intestinal parasites, menstrual difficulties, root canal problems, spasms, worms
Elsewhere	for abortions, asthma, cancer, childbirth, colds, coughs, fever, headache, increasing perspiration, inflammation, intestinal parasites, lung disorders, menstrual problems, nervousness, pain, reducing phlegm, rheumatism, snakebite, spasms, toothache, urinary insufficiency, sexually transmitted diseases, worms; and as an aphrodisiac, insecticide, and sedative

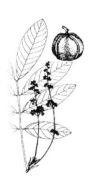

ANDIROBA		
HERBAL PROPERTIES AND ACTIONS		
Main Actions	**Other Actions**	**Standard Dosage**
• heals wounds	• soothes skin	Seed Oil
• reduces pain	• reduces fever	**External:** Applied topically to the skin as needed.
• reduces inflammation	• prevents tumors	
• kills bacteria		**Internal:** 2 ml two to three times daily
• kills parasites		
• expels worms		
• repels insects		
• kills insects		

Family: Meliaceae

Genus: *Carapa*

Species: *guianensis, procera*

Common Names: andiroba, andiroba-saruba, bastard mahogany, Brazilian mahogany, iandirova, carapa, carapá, cedro macho, crabwood, figueroa, krapa, nandiroba, requia, tangare, y-andiroba

Parts Used: seed oil, bark, leaves

Andiroba is a tall rainforest tree that grows up to 40 m high. It is in the same family as mahogany, and it has been called Brazilian mahogany or bastard mahogany due to their similarity. It can be found growing wild throughout the Amazon rainforest, usually on rich soils, in swamps, and in the alluvial flats, marshes, and uplands of the Amazon Basin. It can also be found wild or under cultivation in Brazil in the Islands region, Tocantins, Rio Solimoes, and near the seaside. It is one of the large-leafed trees of the rainforest and can be identified by its large and distinctively textured leaves.

Andiroba wood is soft, yet durable, and much sought by sawmills. It has, in the past, been shipped to the United States for use in the furniture industry and for other uses. Its durability and impalatability to insects have guaranteed commercial demand for the wood, and as a result, the species has been devastated in all areas near major towns in Amazonia. It could, however, be cultivated easily in the Amazon or other regions of Brazil.

The andiroba tree produces a brown, woody, four-cornered nut, some 3–4 inches across that resembles a chestnut. The nut contains several oil-rich kernels or seeds that average about 63 percent oil, which is pale yellow in color. Andiroba oil is a sustainable rainforest product that has a long history of use in South America as well as commercial value. A single tree will produce, on average, about 200 kg of nuts annually. Approximately 6 kg of nuts are required to produce 1 kg (about a liter) of andiroba oil, using the traditional extraction method. This traditional method is efficient, if somewhat primitive. The seeds are collected from rivers, where they float after being shed by trees or from the forest floor. They are then boiled in a large pot of water, left for some two weeks until they have rotted, and then squeezed (in a primitive press known as a *tip-iti*) to extract the oil. One consequence of this extraction method is that crude andiroba oil is frequently associated with a red coloring that is derived from the skin of the seeds. Because the oil becomes rancid very quickly, it must be used quickly. Local usage is mostly limited to immediate use or to the manufacture of soap or candles.

TRIBAL AND HERBAL MEDICINE USES

The indigenous peoples in the Amazon have used andiroba in many ways for centuries, and virtually all parts of the tree, as well as the seed oil, are utilized. The Munduruku Indians traditionally used the oil for the mummification of human heads taken as war trophies. The Wayãpi, Palikur, and Creole Indian tribes have used andiroba oil to remove ticks from their scalps, for other skin parasites, and even in the process of tanning animal hides. The indigenous tribes of Northwest Amazonia brew the bark, and sometimes the leaves, into a tea for fevers and intestinal worms; they also apply this tea externally for ulcers, skin parasites, and other skin problems. Indians have also used the oil as a solvent for extracting the plant pigments and colorants with which they paint their skin. Several Indian tribes in the Amazon combine andiroba oil with the reddish-orange pigment extracted from annatto seeds. They rub the oily bright orange paste all over their bodies, and even into their hair, to protect themselves from biting insects and to repel rainwater (to which they are constantly exposed in the rainforest).

Indians in the Amazon use andiroba oil as an effective insect repellant and to kill skin parasites.

Andiroba oil burns well and is used as a natural lamp fuel in the rainforest. In the early 1800s, the street lamps of Belém, Brazil were fueled with andiroba oil. Not only does it burn cleanly with little smoke but it also repels mosquitoes, flies, and other pests. Traditional forest dwellers and river people in Brazil called *caboclos* make a medicinal soap using crude andiroba oil, wood ash, and cocoa skin residue. This soap is especially recommended for the treatment of skin diseases and as an insect repellent. They also apply andiroba oil directly on joints to relieve arthritis pain and mix it with hot water and human milk and drop it into the ear for ear infections. To aid digestion, the bark is soaked in water for a day and 1 cup is taken before meals.

Many of these uses continue today in the Brazilian herbal medicine systems. Andiroba oil is used by Brazilian city dwellers either in pure form or mixed with other oils or natural products. They apply it externally to wounds and bruises, use it as a massage oil and natural insect repellant, and employ it topically for many skin diseases and conditions, including psoriasis. A common natural remedy in Brazil is prepared by soaking ¼ of a *cabacinha* (the fruit of *Luffa operculata*) in 250 ml of hot andiroba oil for several hours. This warm maceration is rubbed into the skin to relieve arthritis and rheumatism and to cauterize wounds. A teaspoon of this preparation is also gargled for sore throats and taken internally for coughs. Andiroba is also still widely used as an insect repellent and for treating insect bites for both people and animals.

The oil is commercially manufactured into anti-inflammatory, antibacterial, anti-arthritic, and insect repellant soaps as well as turned into candles that are sold as natural insect repellents. The oil is also used in Brazil as a furniture polish that is thought to protect wooden furniture from termites and other wood-chewing insects.

PLANT CHEMICALS

Andiroba oil is a rich source of essential fatty acids including oleic, palmitic, stearic, and linoleic acids. It yields up to 65 percent unsaturated fatty acids and can contain up to 9 percent linoleic acid. (Linoleic acid has been shown in various studies over the years to lower cholesterol levels, reduce blood pressure, and provide anti-cancer benefits.)

All parts of the andiroba tree (including the oil) tastes very bitter. This bitterness is attributed to a group of terpene chemicals called *meliacins*, which are very similar to the bitter antimalarial chemicals found in other tropical plants. One of these *meliacins*, named *gedunin*, has recently been documented with antiparasitic properties and an antimalarial effect equal to that of quinine.[1,2]

Chemical analysis of andiroba oil, bark, and leaves has also identified the presence of another group of chemicals called limonoids. The anti-inflammatory and insect-repellent properties of andiroba oil are attributed to the presence of these limonoids, including a novel one which has been named andirobin. Another limonoid called *epoxyazadiradione* is found in andiroba oil; it has been documented with *in vitro* anti-tumor effects (neuroblastoma and osteosarcoma cancer cell lines were tested).[3]

Main chemicals found in andiroba include andirobin, arachidic acid, acetoxy-gedunins, epoxyazadiradiones, deacetoxygedunins, hydroxylgedunins, gedunins, hexadecenoic acid, linoleic acid, linolenic acid, oleic acid, palmitic acid, palmitoleic acid, and stearic acid.

BIOLOGICAL ACTIVITIES AND CLINICAL RESEARCH

Tests of crude andiroba oil by Brazilian scientists have produced evidence of its anti-inflammatory and pain-relieving properties.[4] The bark has also demonstrated *in vitro* antibacterial activity in another clinical study.[5] Thus far, at least three chemicals found in andiroba have been found to have antiparasitic and/or insecticidal actions.[6,7] A branch of the Brazilian government has been examining andiroba's insect-repellant properties[8] and will be producing an insect-repellent product utilizing andiroba oil. It will be provided to the military and other government workers who are exposed to mosquitoes and other biting bugs in the forests of Brazil. In 1999, a U.S. patent was filed detailing that andiroba oil, when applied topically, prevented the formation of cellulite through a chemical enzyme-blocking action. (Unfortunately, they reported it didn't have the ability to get rid of existing cellulite.)[9]

Research confirms andiroba's traditional uses as an insect repellant as well as for pain and inflammation.

Some of the more recent research has focused on andiroba's anticancerous actions. In 2002, researchers reported that the seed oil could prevent and even reverse cervical dysplasia.[10] Cervical dysplasia is a precancerous condition that can oftentimes develop into cervical cancer. In addition, the leaf, bark, seeds, and flowers have shown some activity against sarcoma cancer cells *in vitro*,[5] and the crude oil passed a preliminary screening test to predict anti-tumor activity.[4]

CURRENT PRACTICAL USES

Andiroba oil is well known in Brazil and widely employed to heal many skin conditions and as a natural insect repellant. In the last several years, several andiroba oil products sold in capsules have appeared in Brazilian stores and pharmacies and are recommended for cancer and internal healing. North American practitioners and consumers are just beginning to learn of andiroba's powerful healing properties. Andiroba oil can be applied topically several times daily to rashes, muscle/joint aches and injuries, wounds, insect bites, boils, and ulcers. It can also be used by itself or combined with other oils as a healing and anti-inflammatory massage oil as well as placed in the ears for ear infections. It's also a great natural remedy for ear mites in dogs and cats: just place several drops in the affected ears daily for a week.

Traditional Preparation

For skin conditions, insect bites, and sore muscles and joints, liberally apply the oil topically several times daily. For ear infections, place two drops of the oil inside the ears. For internal use, 2 ml in a small glass of warm water is taken two or three times daily. This can also be used as a gargle for sore throats.

Contraindications

None reported.

Drug Interactions

None reported.

Worldwide Ethnomedical Uses

Region	Uses
Amazonia	for arthritis, colds, chiggers, digestion, feet (tired), fever, flu, insect bites, itch, leprosy, lice, malaria, mites, parasites, repelling/killing insects, skin problems, tetanus, ulcers, worms
Brazil	for acne, bruises, arthritis, cancer, constipation, cough, cuts, dermatitis, diabetes, diarrhea, ear infections, fevers, hepatitis, herpes, inflammation, bites, malaria, muscle aches, pain, parasites, psoriasis, repelling insects, rheumatism, skin diseases, skin rashes, skin ulcers, sores, splenitis, throat problems, worms
Guatemala	as an insect repellent
Guyana	for inflammation, muscle pain, repelling/killing insects, rheumatism, skin rash, skin problems, ticks, wounds
Nicaragua	for diarrhea, skin problems, and as an astringent
Panama	for arthritis

Peru	for dermatitis, fever, herpes, skin sores, worms
Trinidad	for colds, fever, flu, killing insects, muscle pain, sore feet, and as a massage oil
Venezuela	for itch, leprosy, malaria, parasites, skin problems
Elsewhere	for arthritis, herpes, repelling/killing insects, skin disorders, tetanus

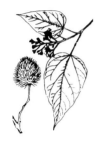

Family: Bixaceae

Genus: *Bixa*

Species: *orellana*

Common Names:
achiote, achiotec, achiotl,
achote, annatto, urucu,
beninoki, bija, eroya,
jafara, kasujmba-kelling,
kham thai, onoto,
orleanstrauch, orucu-
axiote, rocou, roucou,
ruku, roucouyer, unane,
uruku, urucum, urucu-üva

Parts Used: bark, seeds,
leaves, roots, shoots

ANNATTO
HERBAL PROPERTIES AND ACTIONS

Main Actions
- reduces acid
- kills bacteria
- fights free radicals
- kills parasites
- kills germs
- increases urination
- stimulates digestion
- lowers blood pressure
- mildly laxative
- protects liver

Other Actions
- reduces inflammation
- stops coughing
- dries secretions/oils
- cleanses blood
- soothes membranes
- reduces phlegm
- reduces fever
- raises blood sugar
- heals wounds

Standard Dosage
Seed and Leaves

Leaf Decoction: $1/2$ cup two
or three times daily

Seed Powder: 5–10 mg
twice daily

TRIBAL AND HERBAL MEDICINE USES

Annatto is a profusely fruiting shrub or small tree that grows 5–10 m in height. Approximately fifty seeds grow inside prickly reddish-orange heart-shaped pods at the ends of the branches. The trees are literally covered by these brightly colored pods, and one small annatto tree can produce up to 270 kg of seeds. The seeds are covered with a reddish aril, which is the source of an orange-yellow dye. Annatto is known as *achiote* in Peru and as *urucum* in Brazil. It grows throughout South and Central America and the Caribbean, and can be found in some parts of Mexico as well.

Traditionally, the crushed seeds are soaked in water that is allowed to evaporate. A brightly colored paste is produced, which is added to soups, cheeses, and other foods to give them a bright yellow or orange color. Annatto seed paste produced in South America is exported to North America and Europe, where it is used as a food coloring for margarine, cheese, microwave popcorn, and other yellow or orange foodstuffs. Many times, this natural food coloring replaces the very expensive saffron in recipes and dishes around the world. Annatto paste is also used as a natural dye for cloth and wool and is sometimes employed in the paint, varnish, lacquer, cosmetic, and soap industries.

Although mostly only the seed paste or seed oil is used today, the rainforest tribes have used the entire plant as medicine for centuries.

Throughout the rainforest, indigenous tribes have used annatto seeds as body paint and as a fabric dye. It has been traced back to the ancient Mayan Indians, who employed it as a principal coloring agent in foods, for body paints, and as a coloring for arts, crafts, and murals. Although mostly only the seed paste or seed oil is used commercially today, the rainforest tribes have used the entire plant as medicine for centuries. A tea made with the young shoots is used by the Piura tribe as an aphrodisiac and astringent, and to treat skin problems, fevers, dysentery, and hepatitis. The leaves are used to treat skin problems, liver disease, and hepatitis. The plant has also been considered good for the digestive system. The Cojedes tribe uses an infusion of the flowers to stimulate the bowels and aid in elimination as well as to avoid phlegm in newborn babies. Traditional healers in Colombia have also used annatto as an antivenin for snakebites. The seeds are believed to be an expectorant, while the roots are thought to be a digestive aid and cough suppressant.

Today in Brazilian herbal medicine, a leaf decoction of annatto is used to treat heartburn and stomach distress caused by spicy foods, and as a mild diuretic and mild laxative. It is also used for fevers and malaria, and, topically, to treat burns. Annatto is a common remedy in Peruvian herbal medicine today, and the dried leaves are called *achiotec*. Eight to ten dried leaves are boiled for ten minutes in 1 liter of water for this popular Peruvian remedy. One cup is drunk warm or cold three times daily after meals to treat prostate disorders and internal inflammation, arterial hypertension, high cholesterol, cystitis, obesity, renal insufficiency, and to eliminate uric acid. This decoction is also recommended as a vaginal antiseptic and wound healer, as a wash for skin infections, and for liver and stomach disorders. *Curanderos* (herbal healers) in the Peruvian Amazon squeeze the juice from the fresh leaves and place it in the eye for inflammation and eye infections, and they use the juice of twelve fruits taken twice daily for five days to "cure" epilepsy.

PLANT CHEMICALS

Bixin, extracted and used as a food colorant, has been shown to protect against ultraviolet rays and to have antioxidant and liver protective properties.

Analysis of annatto seeds indicates that they contain 40 percent to 45 percent cellulose, 3.5 percent to 5.5 percent sucrose, 0.3 percent to 0.9 percent essential oil, 3 percent fixed oil, 4.5 percent to 5.5 percent pigments, and 13 percent to 16 percent protein, as well as alpha- and beta-carotenoids and other constituents.[1] Annatto oil is extracted from the seeds and is the main source of pigments named *bixin* and *norbixin,* which are classified as carotenoids. Bixin, extracted and used as a food colorant, has been shown to protect against ultraviolet rays and to have antioxidant and liver protective properties in clinical research.[2–7]

In addition to bixin and norbixin, annatto contains bixaghanene, bixein, bixol, crocetin, ellagic acid, ishwarane, isobixin, phenylalanine, salicylic acid, threonine, tomentosic acid, and tryptophan.

BIOLOGICAL ACTIVITIES AND CLINICAL RESEARCH

Much has been done in the laboratory validating annatto's traditional uses and finding new ones. A water extract of the root has demonstrated hypotensive activity in rats, as Peruvian herbal systems have practiced.[8] The same extract demonstrated smooth muscle-relaxant activity in guinea pigs and lowered gastric secretions in rats,[8] which help to explain its use as a digestive aid and for stomach disorders. Annatto seed extracts have been documented to raise blood glucose levels in some species of animals and to lower them in others.[9–11] Annatto leaves were reported in yet another study to possess aldose reductase inhibition actions, a process implicated in the advancement of diabetic neuropathy.[12] A 2000 study confirmed the effectiveness of a leaf-and-bark extract at neutralizing hemorrhages in mice injected with snake venom,[13] a practice used in Colombia for many years. Annatto demonstrated antigonorrheal activity in a 1995 study,[14] and in other research, flower and leaf extracts demonstrated *in vitro* antibacterial activity against several bacteria, including *E. coli* and *Staphylococcus*.[15] This supports its use in traditional medicine systems for gonorrhea and other types of infections.

CURRENT PRACTICAL USES

Although not widely available in the United States, standard decoctions of annatto leaves are taken by the half-cupful two or three times daily for prostate and urinary difficulties, as well as for high cholesterol and hypertension. Ground annatto seed powder is also used in small dosages of 10–20 mg daily for high cholesterol and hypertension. Higher dosages can cause a marked increase in urination. It has been noted that some individuals are highly sensitive to annatto seed and this diuretic effect can be caused at much lower doses, even by just eating a bag of popcorn in which annatto was used as a coloring or flavoring ingredient.

Annatto's history of use as a food coloring is well established worldwide, and current trends show that it is being used increasingly in body care products. Annatto oil is an emollient, and its high carotenoid content provides beneficial antioxidant properties.[16] In body care products, annatto oil provides antioxidant benefits while adding a rich, sunny color to creams, lotions, and shampoos.

Traditional Preparation

In South America, a standard leaf decoction is prepared. One-half cup amounts are taken two or three times daily with meals for various conditions. Ground annatto seed powder is also used in small dosages (of 5–20 mg daily).

Contraindications

The seed extract was reported to elevate blood sugar levels in dogs, and it is therefore contraindicated for people with diabetes. A 1991 study documents an allergic reaction of one patient to bixin, the dye chemical in annatto seeds, stating it's "a potential rare cause of anaphylaxis."[17]

Drug Interactions   None reported.

Worldwide Ethnomedical Uses

Region	Uses
Argentina	for diarrhea, fevers, heart support
Brazil	for burns, constipation, fevers, heartburn, hepatitis, malaria, stomachache, urinary insufficiency
Colombia	as an antivenin, aphrodisiac
Cuba	as an aphrodisiac
Guatemala	for gonorrhea
Haiti	for fever and as a douche and insect repellent
Mexico	for burns, constipation, digestion, dysentery, epilepsy, erysipelas, fever, gonorrhea, headache, inflammation, malaria, sexually transmitted diseases, sore throat, tumors, urinary insufficiency, vaginitis, wounds; and as an aphrodisiac, astringent, and insect repellent
Paraguay	as an insecticide and insect repellent
Peru	for conjunctivitis, cystitis, dysentery, epilepsy, fevers, high cholesterol, digestion, hypertension, obesity, prostatitis, renal problems, urinary problems, urogenital infections, wounds, and as an antiseptic, aphrodisiac, astringent, and dye
Trinidad	for diabetes, dysentery, flu, jaundice, renal insufficiency, sexually transmitted diseases, skin disease
Elsewhere	for blood cleansing, cancer, diabetes, dysentery, fever, kidney problems, parasites, skin disorders, to stop bleeding, and as an aphrodisiac, astringent, dye, and cosmetic

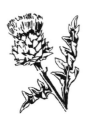

Family: Asteraceae

Genus: *Cynara*

Species: *scolymus*

Common Names:
globe artichoke,
alcachofra, alcachofera,
artichaut, tyosen-azami

Parts Used: leaves, flowers

ARTICHOKE
HERBAL PROPERTIES AND ACTIONS

Main Actions
- reduces cholesterol
- lowers blood pressure
- stimulates bile
- supports liver
- supports gallbladder
- enhances digestion
- fights free radicals
- detoxifies

Other Actions
- dries secretions
- supports heart
- cleanses blood
- increases urination

Standard Dosage
Leaves
Infusion: 1–3 cups daily
Liquid Extract: 2–3 ml with each meal
Tablets/Capsules: 2–3 g three times daily
Standardized Extracts: follow label directions

Alcachofra is the Brazilian name for the globe artichoke. A member of the milk thistle family, it grows to a height of about 2 m and produces a large, violet-green flower head. The flower petals and fleshy flower bottoms are eaten as a vegetable throughout the world, which has led to its commercial cultivation in many parts of South and North America (chiefly California) as well as in Europe. The artichoke was used as a food and medicine by the ancient Egyptians, Greeks, and Romans; in Rome, the artichoke was an important menu item at feasts. It wasn't until the fifteenth century, however, that it made its appearance throughout Europe.

TRIBAL AND HERBAL MEDICINE USES

Artichoke has been used in traditional medicine for centuries as a specific liver and gallbladder remedy. In Brazilian herbal medicine systems, leaf preparations are used for liver and gallbladder problems, diabetes, high cholesterol, hypertension, anemia, diarrhea (and elimination in general), fevers, ulcers, and gout. In Europe, it is also used for liver and gallbladder disorders; in several countries, standardized herbal drugs are manufactured and sold as prescription drugs for high cholesterol and digestive and liver disorders. Other uses around the world include treatment for dyspepsia and chronic albuminuria.

In France, a patent has been filed that describes an artichoke extract for treating liver disease, high cholesterol levels, and kidney insufficiency. In all herbal medicine systems where it is employed, artichoke is used to increase bile production in the liver, increase the flow of bile from the gallbladder, and to increase the contractive power of the bile duct. These bile actions are beneficial in many digestive, gallbladder, and liver disorders. Artichoke is also often used to mobilize fatty stores in the liver and detoxify it, and as a natural aid to lower cholesterol.

PLANT CHEMICALS

Artichoke has plant chemicals in it that help lower cholesterol and protect the liver.

The artichoke is popular for its pleasant bitter taste, which is attributed mostly to a plant chemical called *cynarin* found in the green parts of the plant. Cynarin is considered one of artichoke's main biologically active chemicals. It occurs in the highest concentration in the leaves of the plant, which is why leaf extracts are most commonly employed in herbal medicine. Other documented "active" chemicals include flavonoids, sesquiterpene lactones, polyphenols, and caffeoylquinic acids.

In the 1970s, European scientists first documented cynarin's ability to lower cholesterol in humans.[1–4] Over the years, other researchers have continued to document artichoke's or cynarin's effect in this area. One study, published in 2000, was a double-blind, randomized, placebo-controlled study that used an artichoke leaf extract that was standardized to its cynarin content.[5] For six weeks, 143 patients with high cholesterol were given the extract; at the end of the test, results showed a decrease of 10–15 percent in total cholesterol, low density lipoprotein (LDL), and ratio of LDL to high-density lipoprotein (HDL) cholesterol. Scientists now report that the cholesterol-lowering effect of artichoke can be attributed to chemicals other than just cynarin,[6] including several newly discovered ones.[7]

The liver detoxifying and protective properties of artichoke first came to the attention of researchers in 1966 (in a study that supported its effect on liver regeneration in rats).[8] A 1987 study that focused on the effects of rat liver cells subjected to harmful chemical agents found both cynarin and caffeic acids (both in artichoke) to have significant protective effects.[9]

Artichoke's main plant chemicals are caffeic acid, caffeoylquinic acids, caryophyllene, chlorogenic acid, cyanidol glucosides, cynaragenin, cynarapicrin, cynaratriol, cynarin, cynarolide, decanal, eugenol, ferulic acid, flavonoids, folacin, glyceric acid, glycolic acid, heteroside-B, inulin, isoamerboin, lauric acid, linoleic acid, linolenic acid, luteolin glucosides, myristic acid, neochlorogenic acid, oleic acid, palmitic acid, phenylacetaldehyde, pseudotaraxasterol, scolymoside, silymarin, sitosterol, stearic acid, stigmasterol, and taraxasterol.

BIOLOGICAL ACTIVITIES AND CLINICAL RESEARCH

Investigations are still being conducted on artichoke's beneficial effects on liver and gallbladder functions. A 2002 finding noted that an artichoke leaf extract reversed damage done by harmful chemicals in rat liver cells and, in doing so, enhanced bile production.[10–12]

A portion of artichoke's liver-protective properties is thought to be attributed to its documented antioxidant actions.[13–14] A 2002 study focused on the antioxidant effects of artichoke extract in cultured blood vessel cells and reported that the extract demonstrated "marked protective properties against oxidative stress induced by inflammatory mediators."[15] Artichoke's antioxidant properties were also confirmed in an earlier (2000) study that focused on human white blood cells under various induced oxidative stresses.[16]

Clinical studies confirm artichoke's traditional uses to support liver and gallbladder functions.

A 1999 clinical investigation focused on gallbladder function. It "showed the efficacy and safety of artichoke extracts (*Cynara scolymus* L.) in the treatment of hepatobiliary dysfunction and digestive complaints, such as sensation of fullness, loss of appetite, nausea and abdominal pain."[17] A 2000 study took this notion a step further. It was known that artichoke extract was indicated for dyspepsia, a digestive disorder involving the esophagus, duodenum, and upper gastrointestinal tract, but there are many symptom overlaps between dyspepsia and irritable bowel syndrome (IBS).[18] A subgroup of patients with IBS was distilled from the dyspepsia study group and was monitored for six weeks after the original study had ended. Of the IBS patients, 96 percent rated artichoke leaf extract as better than or at least equal to previous therapies administered for their IBS symptoms.

CURRENT PRACTICAL USES

The history of artichoke is a perfect example of science finally catching up to the longstanding traditional uses of a medicinal plant. While scientists still argue today over which specific chemical or group of chemicals is responsible for each documented beneficial action, the traditional uses for high cholesterol, as well as for liver, gallbladder, and digestive disorders, are being validated. While many Europeans still have to see their doctors for an artichoke extract prescription, concentrated natural leaf extracts and standardized extracts are widely available in the United States at health food stores. With the growing American trend to find more natural and healthy alternatives, these products will probably gain in popularity as consumers learn more of the most recent research studies. However, the most effective method to control cholesterol is with a sensible diet. Unfortunately, there are no magic bullets.

Traditional Preparation

Traditionally, 1 to 3 cups of a standard leaf infusion are taken daily after meals; 3–4 ml of a concentrated 4:1 liquid extract, or 3–5 g daily of dried herb in capsules or tablets can be substituted, if desired. With standardized extract products, follow the instructions on the product label.

Contraindications

None reported for internal use. Dermatitis, following contact with the fresh plant and leaves, has been reported.

Artichoke has been documented in traditional uses to be hypoglycemic; however, no clinical studies have been published to confirm this action. Diabetics and people with hypoglycemia should use this plant product with caution and monitor their blood sugar levels closely in anticipation of these possible effects.

Drug Interactions

Artichoke extracts have been documented to lower blood cholesterol in human and animal studies and, as such, may potentiate the effects of cholesterol-lowering and statin drugs.

Worldwide Ethnomedical Uses

Region	Uses
Brazil	for acne, anemia, arthritis, arteriosclerosis, asthma, bile insufficiency, blood cleansing, bronchitis, diabetes, diarrhea, dyspepsia, digestive disorders, dandruff, fever, flatulence, gallbladder disorders, gallstones, gout, heart function, hemorrhage, hemorrhoids, high cholesterol, hypertension, hyperglycemia, inflammation, kidney insufficiency, liver disorders, nephritis, obesity, prostatitis, rheumatism, seborriasis, ulcers, urethritis, urinary disorders, and as an astringent and vasoconstrictor
Dominican Republic	for bile insufficiency, digestive problems, gallbladder disorders
Europe	for bile insufficiency, cancer, detoxification, dyspepsia, gallbladder disorders, high cholesterol, hyperglycemia, jaundice, liver disorders, nausea
Haiti	for edema, hypertension, kidney disorders, liver problems, urinary insufficiency
Mexico	for cystitis, gallstones, hypertension, liver disorders
Elsewhere	for diabetes, edema, rheumatism, urinary insufficiency

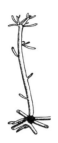

AVELOZ
HERBAL PROPERTIES AND ACTIONS

Main Actions	Other Actions	Standard Dosage
• promotes tumors	• moderately laxative	Latex
• causes cancer		Not recommended
• suppresses immune system		
• causes vomiting		
• irritates membranes		
• activates viruses		

Family: Euphorbiaceae

Genus: *Euphorbia*

Species: *tirucalli, insulana*

Common Names: aveloz, milkbush, pencil tree, kayu patah tulang, kayu urip, mentulang, paching tawa, tikel balung, tulang-tulang, cega-olho, coral-verde, labirinto, cassoneira, arvore-do-lapis, cassoneira, garrancho, Indian tree spurge, fingertree, milkhedge, petroleum-plant, rubber euphorbia, euphorbe antivenerien, almeidinha, consuelda

Parts Used: latex, branches, roots

TRIBAL AND HERBAL MEDICINE USES

Aveloz is a succulent cactus-like plant growing to a height of about 10 m. Introduced from Africa as a garden plant, it is now naturalized in tropical areas and rainforests in the Amazon, Madagascar, and South Africa. In Africa, it is a common garden plant and its thick rapid growth promotes its use as a natural barrier fence. The main trunk and branches are woody and brown, but the younger branches are green and cylindrical, looking like many pencils and earning the plant its common name—pencil tree. Leaves are minute and are shed early, and the function of the leaves is taken over by the green branches. All parts of the plant ooze a caustic milky white sap when damaged, like many other Euphorbia species.

Aveloz is called "petroleum plant" because it produces a hydrocarbon substance very much like gasoline. This plant is being studied by Petrobas, the national petroleum company in Brazil. It is thought that the hydrocarbon produced by the plant could be used directly in existing gasoline refineries; estimates of ten to fifty barrels of oil per acre of cultivated aveloz with cost estimates of $3–10 per barrel have been postulated.[1]

In Africa, aveloz is regarded as an insect repellant. The root is used for snakebite; the latex is used for skin tumors and syphilis ulcers; the seeds and latex are used for intestinal parasites; and decoctions of the wood are used for bacterial infections. In Malaysia, the stems are pounded and applied to swellings, and in the Dutch Indies, the pounded stems are used as a poultice to extract thorns. A root infusion is used for aching bones and a poultice of the root or leaves is used for nose ulcers and hemorrhoids. A wood decoction is used for leprosy and paralysis of the hands and feet after childbirth. In India, the latex is used for asthma, cough, earache, neuralgia, rheumatism, toothache, and warts. A decoction of the branches or root is used for colic and gastric problems. In Brazil, the latex is used externally to remove warts and tumors and to treat rheumatism. The latex is diluted in water and used internally for snakebite, as well as benign and cancerous tumors. In Peru, the plant is used much like in India, for abscesses, asthma, cancer, colic, cough, earache, neuralgia, rheumatism, stomachache, and toothache.

PLANT CHEMICALS

The chemistry of the plant does not validate any of the herbal medicine uses. In fact, the plant contains many harmful chemicals that make it unsuitable for many of the traditional uses, especially those for cancer. The latex of aveloz is a rich source of terpenes, including phorbol esters and ingenol esters.[2] These phorbol esters are highly irritating and have been clinically documented to actually promote tumors.[3–5] One particular phorbol in aveloz, 4-deoxyphorbol ester, has been clinically documented to enhance Epstein-Barr virus (EBV) infection, cause DNA damage to immune cells, and cause a suppression of the immune system in general.[6–8]

Chemicals in aveloz may activate dormant Epstein-Barr viruses and suppress the immune system.

In addition to this one chemical, an extract of aveloz was also shown to reduce the ability of certain immune cells (T-cells) to kill EBV.[6,8] EBV is a member of the herpes virus family. It is one of the most common human viruses—as many as 95 percent of adults in the United States have been infected at some point in their lives.[9] After the initial infection, EBV establishes a lifelong dormant infection in the immune system (inside of B-cells). EBV infection can lead to mononucleosis, and some EBV carriers will develop cancer, either Burkitt's lymphoma or nasopharyngeal carcinoma.[9]

Aveloz contains 4-deoxyphorbol ester, beta-sitosterol, caoutchouc, casuariin, corilagin, cycloeuphordenol, cyclotirucanenol, ellagic acids, euphorbins, euphol, euphorone, euphorcinol, gallic acids, glucosides, hentriacontane, hentriacontanol, ingenol, isoeuphoral, kamepferol, pedunculagin, phenols, phorbol esters, proteases, putranjivain A–B, sapogenin acetates, succinic-acid, taraxasterol, taraxerin, tirucallol, and tirucallin A–B.

BIOLOGICAL ACTIVITIES AND CLINICAL RESEARCH

The studies on aveloz, its chemicals, and EBV were conducted by several research groups who were trying to understand why EBV and Burkitt's lymphoma were endemic in areas where aveloz was widely used as a local remedy (usually for parasites) and/or as a common-living fence in Africa.[2–8] Their research concluded that exposure to the latex of aveloz directly activates latent EBV infections, and exposure to this plant is now considered a causative factor in the development of Burkitt's lymphoma.[6–11] Burkitt's lymphoma is a non-Hodgkin's malignant lymphoma associated with EBV, and in clinical research, treatment of a Burkitt's lymphoma cell line with the latex of aveloz found the latex to reactivate latent EBV and promote tumor growth in general.[10–13]

Research indicates that taking aveloz internally (for any reason) has no clinical merit or benefit, especially for cancer.

CURRENT PRACTICAL USES

Since the 1970s, aveloz has been promoted as a "cure" for cancer when the latex is taken internally or used externally. While the plant has a folk use for certain types of cancer, it has been more widely used for external tumors. The latex is caustic and irritating and has been traditionally used to "burn off" warts and possibly skin tumors. Taking the latex of aveloz internally (for any reason) has no clinical merit or benefit, especially for cancer.

Aveloz is confirmed to suppress the immune system.[8] Suppression of the immune system makes the body less resistant to infections and some cancers, and it is therefore not recommended for cancer patients. Even more important, the latex has also been documented to promote tumor growth and/or to trigger certain cancers. Again, this certainly is not beneficial, indicated, or prudent for cancer patients. Unfortunately, aveloz sap still continues to be touted as a cancer cure in Brazil and now in the United States without any merit or scientific basis. As one group of researchers stated, "cancer management with *Euphorbia tirucalli* presents no scientific basis, at least up to the moment, since the phorbol esters have already presented tumor-promoting activity."[2]

Aveloz is not recommended as a natural remedy for any reason due to its toxicity and its immune suppression and tumor-promoting properties. It is hoped that the time will come where aveloz will go into our cars as a natural gasoline, rather than into desperate cancer patients who will try anything in their search for a cure.

Traditional Preparation

None recommended.

Contraindications

The latex is considered a poison and has caused deaths in Africa. Contact of the latex with the eyes can cause blindness. The caustic latex can also cause skin burns, ulcerations, and dermatitis. Taking pure latex internally is known to induce hemorrhages and stomach ulcers. Used internally, even in small quantities and in diluted form, the latex can cause digestive disturbances such as nausea, vomiting, and diarrhea. In addition, internal use of the latex may cause burning and ulceration of the mouth and throat.

Drug Interactions

None reported.

Worldwide Ethnomedical Uses

Region	Uses
Africa	for parasites, sexual impotence, snakebite, syphilis, tumors
Asia	for broken bones, hemorrhoids, pain, swellings, ulceration

Brazil	for abscess, asthma, bacterial infections, cancer, constipation, fungal infections, rheumatism, scorpion bite, snakebite, spasms, syphilis, tumor, viruses, warts, and as an expectorant and irritant
Dutch Indies	for bone aches, hemorrhoids, leprosy, nose ulcers, paralysis, thorns
India	for abscess, asthma, colic, constipation, cough, earache, gastralgia, neuralgia, rheumatism, syphilis, toothache, warts
Peru	for abscesses, asthma, cancer, colic, cough, earache, neuralgia, rheumatism, stomachache, toothache
Elsewhere	for dermatosis, paralysis, pain, poisoning

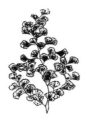

Family: Adiantaceae

Genus: *Adiantum*

Species: *capillus-veneris*

Common Names:
avenca, maidenhair fern, adianto, alambrillo, barun, cabello de venus, capilera, capille e jenere, celantillo, centaurea, cilantrillo, culandrillo, culantrillo de pozo, culantrillo, fern karn dam, frauenhaar, hansraj, helecho culantrillo, herba capillorum veneris, ladies' hair, venus hair fern

Parts Used: leaves, rhizome

AVENCA
HERBAL PROPERTIES AND ACTIONS

Main Actions
- suppresses coughs
- reduces phlegm
- kills viruses
- kills bacteria
- detoxifies
- fights free radicals
- supports heart
- cleanses blood
- increases urination
- lowers blood sugar
- stimulates menstruation

Other Actions
- dries secretions
- protects liver
- reduces cholesterol
- reduces blood pressure
- stimulates
- supports gallbladder
- heals wounds

Standard Dosage
Leaves or rhizome
Infusion: 1/2 cup twice daily
Tincture: 1–3 ml twice daily
Capsules/Tablets: 2 g twice daily

Avenca is a small, slow-growing evergreen fern found throughout the world in moist forests. It reaches 35 cm tall, growing in stands from its creeping rhizome, and bears leaves up to 50 cm long. It can be found in the rainforests of the Amazon as well as in the more temperate, moist forests of Southern Europe and the United States (where it is commonly referred to as *maidenhair fern*). It is called *culantrillo* in Peru and *avenca* in Brazil. These days avenca can be found in many plant stores and nurseries, where it is sold as an ornamental landscape fern for shade gardens.

TRIBAL AND HERBAL MEDICINE USES

In the Peruvian Amazon, local people prepare the fronds of the plant as an infusion or syrup and use it as a diuretic, as an expectorant and to calm coughs, to promote perspiration and menstruation, and to treat urinary disorders, colds, rheumatism, heartburn, gallstones, alopecia (hair loss), and sour stomach. In the highlands of the Peruvian Andes, local shamans and healers decoct the rhizome and use it for alopecia, gallstones, and jaundice. In the Brazilian Amazon, it is recommended as a good expectorant and used for bronchitis, coughs, and other respiratory problems.

Avenca's history of use
in herbal medicine for
respiratory problems
dates back to 23 A.D.

Avenca has long held a place in herbal medicine systems worldwide. In European herbal medicine, its documented use predates the era of Dioscorides and Pliny (23–79 A.D.). According to the well-known British herbalist Nicholas Culpepper (1787 ed.), "This and all other Maiden Hair Ferns is a good remedy for coughs, asthmas, pleurisy, etc., and on account of its being a gentle diuretic also in jaundice, gravel and other impurities of the kidneys." In France, the fronds and rhizomes were once made into a syrup called "Sirop de Capillaire," which was a favorite medicine for upper respiratory problems such as coughs and excessive mucus. The plant is also used widely throughout the world for dandruff, hair loss, and menstrual difficulties.

In Brazilian herbal medicine today, the frond and leaf are employed for hair loss, coughs, bronchitis, laryngitis and throat dryness, and to improve appetite and digestion, stimulate renal function, regulate menstruation, and facilitate childbirth. In Peruvian herbal medicine, the frond and rhizome are used for hair loss, gallstones, hepatic calculi, hydrophobia, asthma, coughs, catarrh, and to regulate menstruation. In India, the entire plant is used for its cooling effects, for diabetes, colds, bronchial disease, and for its menstrual-promoting properties. Externally it is used for boils, eczema, and wounds.

PLANT CHEMICALS

Chemical analysis of avenca reveals an array of compounds including triterpenes, flavonoids, phenylpropanoids, and carotenoids. Interestingly, despite its ancient use, there has been no specific research on avenca to isolate and test its chemicals for biological activities.

Adiantone, adiantoxide, astragalin, beta-sitosterol, caffeic acids, caffeylgalactose, caffeylglucose, campesterol, carotenes, coumaric acids, coumarylglucoses, diplopterol, epoxyfilicane, fernadiene, fernene, filicanes, hopanone, hydroxy-adiantone, hydroxy-cinnamic acid, isoadiantone, isoquercetin, kaempferols, lutein, mutatoxanthin, naringin, neoxanthin, nicotiflorin, oleananes, populnin, procyanidin, prodelphinidin, quercetins, querciturone, quinic acid, rhodoxanthin, rutin, shikimic acid, violaxanthin, and zeaxanthin are chemicals found in avenca.

BIOLOGICAL ACTIVITIES AND CLINICAL RESEARCH

The plant has demonstrated little toxicity. However, in animal studies, it has been shown to have an anti-fertility effect. In the 1980s, two separate researchers in India found that a pet ether extract of the plant had an anti-implantation effect in rats, preventing conception.[1,2]

In 1989, scientists in Iraq demonstrated avenca's antimicrobial properties.[3] A methanol extract of the aerial parts was reported to have *in vitro* antimicrobial actions against *Bacillus, E. coli, Staphylococcus, Proteus, Pseudomonas,* and *Candida*. French scientists demonstrated that an ethanol extract of the rhizome evidenced antiviral properties *in vitro* against *Vesicular stomatitis* virus.[4] Other early (1967) research showed that a water extract of the entire plant had hypoglycemic activity when given to mice (10 mg/kg) orally.[5] Much later (in 1993), Belgian scientists confirmed that avenca leaves had *in vivo* hypoglycemic properties in mice. In one study, a water extract of the aerial parts was given to mice (25 mg/kg) orally and found to reduce glucose-induced hyperglycemia.[6] An ethanol extract, however, showed no activity. They reconfirmed these findings in 1995 by demonstrating that a water extract reduced glucose-induced hyperglycemia.[7]

CURRENT PRACTICAL USES

Despite the plant's ancient history of use for respiratory disorders, no clinical research has been done to validate these traditional uses. In spite of the lack of scientific research done on avenca, herbalists and healthcare practitioners throughout the world continue to use the plant based on its traditional uses (for literally thousands of years): for respiratory disorders and hair loss, and to regulate menstruation.

Traditional Preparation

One-half cup leaf infusion can be taken twice daily or 1–3 ml of a 4:1 root tincture used twice daily. If desired, 1–2 g of powdered leaf or root in tablets or capsules twice daily can be substituted.

Contraindications

Avenca has been documented to lower blood sugar levels in animal studies. People with diabetes and people with hypoglycemia should use this plant with caution and monitor their blood sugar levels accordingly.

Avenca has a long history of use in herbal medicine systems to stimulate the uterus and promote menstruation; it is contraindicated in pregnancy.

The plant has shown to have an anti-implantation effect in animal studies and may prevent conception. Couples seeking fertility treatment or pregnancy should not take avenca.

Due to its effect on fertility and menstruation, avenca may have estrogen-like effects and should probably be avoided by women with estrogen-positive cancers.

Drug Interactions

Avenca may potentiate insulin and antidiabetic drugs.

Worldwide Ethnomedical Uses

Region	Uses
Amazonia	for blood cleansing, coughs, excessive mucus, menstrual problems, respiratory problems, urinary disorders, urinary insufficiency, and to increase perspiration
Brazil	for asthma, bronchitis, childbirth, cough, digestion, excessive mucus, flu, hair loss, kidney problems, laryngitis, menstrual disorders, respiratory problems, rheumatism, throat (sore), urinary insufficiency, and to stimulate the appetite
Egypt	for asthma, chest colds, cough, edema, flu, hepatitis, snakebite, spider bite, splenitis, urinary insufficiency, and to increase perspiration
England	for asthma, cough, hair loss, jaundice, kidney stones, menstrual disorders, pleurisy, shortness of breath, swellings, urinary insufficiency, yellow jaundice
Europe	for alcoholism, bronchitis, bronchial diseases, cough, dandruff, detoxification, diabetes, excessive mucus, flu, hair loss, menstrual problems, and to sooth mucous membranes
India	for boils, bronchial diseases, colds, diabetes, eczema, fever, menstrual problems, skin diseases, wounds
Iraq	for bronchitis, colds, cough, excessive mucus, flu, menstrual disorders, respiratory difficulty, reducing secretions, urinary insufficiency, and to increase perspiration
Mexico	for birth control, bladder problems, blood cleansing, constipation, hair loss, kidney stones, liver function, menstrual disorders, respiratory distress
Peru	for asthma, colds, cough, congestion, excessive mucus, flu, gallstones, hair loss, heartburn, hydrophobia, liver problems, menstrual disorders, respiratory problems, sore throat, stomach problems, urinary insufficiency, and to increase perspiration
United States	for chills, coughs, excessive mucus, fever, flu, lung problems, menstrual disorders, menstrual pain, respiratory ailments, sclerosis (spleen), sores, urinary insufficiency, and to sooth membranes and increase perspiration

Rain clouds gathering over the rainforest.

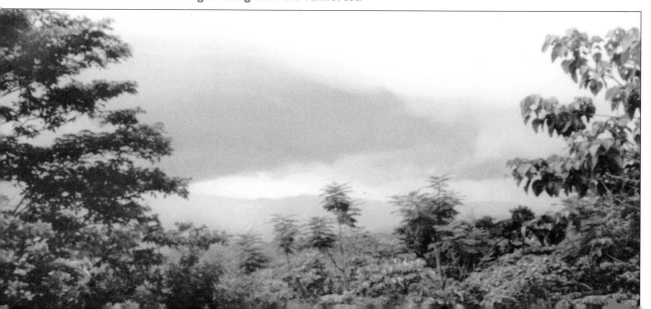

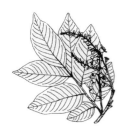

BALSAM OF PERU / BALSAM OF TOLU
HERBAL PROPERTIES AND ACTIONS

Main Actions	Other Actions	Standard Dosage
• kills bacteria	• reduces inflammation	Gum or Oil
• kills fungi	• reduces phlegm	**Internal:** 5–8 drops twice daily
• kills parasites	• suppresses coughs	
• kills germs		**External:** Apply to affected area.

Family: Fabaceae

Genus: *Myroxylon*

Species: *balsamum*, *pereirae*

Common Names: Balsam of Peru, Balsam of tolu, Peru balsam, tolu balsam, bálsamo, baume de tolu, pau de balsamo, tache, estoraque, cabreúva veremelha, nabal, chirraca, sádalo

Parts Used: resin, bark

Balsam of tolu (*Myroxylon balsamum*), a tall tree native to northern South America, is found predominantly in Colombia, Peru, Venezuela, and some areas of Argentina, Brazil, Paraguay, and Bolivia. A closely related species called balsam of Peru (*M. pereirae*) is native to Central America farther north. Balsam of Peru was named such because it was originally assembled and shipped to Europe from the ports of Callao and Lima, Peru, but the species is not indigenous to Peru.

Both trees grow up to 35 m in height and produce white flowers and winged seedpods. Balsam trees are tapped like rubber trees to collect their resinlike gums that are used commercially and sold as "balsam." A tree must be at least twenty years old before it can be tapped for its gum, and one tree produces only about 3 kg of gum annually. Today, El Salvador is the main exporter of balsam of Peru (exporting approximately 50 metric tons annually), and Colombia and Venezuela are the main producers of balsam of tolu. The gum has a vanilla-like smell and taste and is used as a food additive and flavoring in cough syrups, soft drinks, confectioneries, and chewing gums.

TRIBAL AND HERBAL MEDICINE USES

The indigenous tribes of Mexico and Central America use the leaves and fruit of *M. pereirae* for asthma, colds and flu, rheumatism, and external wounds. The Choco Indians use the powdered bark as an underarm deodorant. The sap of *M. balsamum* has documented indigenous uses for colds and lung ailments, and Amazon rainforest tribes have employed it for abscesses, asthma, bronchitis, catarrh, headache, rheumatism, sores, sprains, tuberculosis, sexually transmitted diseases, and wounds.

Balsam has been officially listed as an herbal drug in the *U.S. Pharmacopoeia* since the early 1800s to treat bronchitis and other respiratory problems.

The indigenous use of balsam of Peru led to its export to Europe in the seventeenth century, where it was first documented in the *German Pharmacopeia*. It was used as an antibacterial, antifungal, and antiparasitic agent in cases of scabies, ringworm, lice, superficial ulcerations, wounds, bedsores, diaper rash, and chilblains. In Britain, balsam is used topically for scabies, prurigo (chronic inflammation of the skin), pruritus, and acute eczema, as well as taken internally for asthma and bronchitis and to generally lessen mucous secretions.

Balsam of Peru has been in the *U.S. Pharmacopeia* since 1820, with documented uses for bronchitis, laryngitis, dysmenorrhea, diarrhea, dysentery, and leucorrhea. Today, it is used extensively in topical preparations for the treatment of wounds, ulcers, and scabies. It can be found in hair tonics, antidandruff preparations, and feminine hygiene sprays and as a natural fragrance in soaps, detergents, creams, lotions, and perfumes. Balsam of tolu was also included in the *U.S. Pharmacopeia* in 1820 with similar uses as balsam of Peru. Additionally, it is a cough suppressant and respiratory aid used in cough lozenges and syrups, for sore throats, and as a vapor inhalant for respiratory ailments. The internal dosage is reported to be to 1 g taken three times daily.

PLANT CHEMICALS

Balsam contains 50 percent to 64 percent volatile oil and 20 percent to 28 percent resin. The volatile oil contains benzoic and cinnamic acid esters. The benzoic and cinnamic acids are believed to be the main active constituents of the resin. The oil contains about 60 percent cinnamein, a volatile oil that is extracted by steam distillation and used commercially in the perfume, cosmetic, and soap industries.

Many chemicals are found in balsam of Peru: alpha-bourbonene, alpha-cadinene, alpha-calacorene, alpha-copaene, alpha-curcumene, alpha-muurolene, alpha-pinene, benzaldehyde, benzoic, benzoic-acids, benzyl-alcohol, benzyl-benzoate, benzyl-cinnamate benzyl-ferulate, benzyl-isoferulate, beta-bourbonene, beta-elemene, cadalene, calamenene, caryophyllene, cinnamaldehyde, cinnamein, cinnamic-acids, cinnamyl-benzoate, cinnamyl-cinnamate, cis-ocimene, coumarin, d-cadinene, dammaradienone, delta-cadinene, dihydromandelic-acid, eugenol, farnesol, ferulic-acid, gamma-muurolene, hydroxyhopanone, l-cadinol, methyl-cinnamate, nerolidol, oleanolic-acid, p-cymene, peruresinotannol, peruviol, resin, styrene, sumaresinolic-acid, tannin, toluresinotannol-cinnamate, vanillin, and wax.

BIOLOGICAL ACTIVITIES AND CLINICAL RESEARCH

Although having beneficial properties, research shows that balsam can cause allergic skin rashes in some people when used topically.

Balsam of Peru and balsam of tolu have been documented to have antiseptic, antiparasitic, and antibacterial properties as well as to promote the growth of epithelial (tissue) cells.[1-3] The plants have been reported to inhibit *Mycobacterium tuberculosis*[3] as well as the common ulcer-causing bacteria *H. pylori*[4] in test-tube studies.

At least six clinical studies published in recent years indicate that balsam can cause allergic reactions in sensitive individuals. Allergic reactions reported are generally skin rashes and dermatitis when the balsam comes into contact with the skin—even in small amounts found in soaps, perfumes, and other common body care products. These allergic reactions are attributed to the gum's benzoic acids, to which some people are highly sensitive.

CURRENT PRACTICAL USES Balsam of Peru and balsam of tolu are widely available now in the U.S. natural products market. The resinous gum, or the essential oil distilled from the gum, is sold in small bottles and used topically, in aromatherapy, and taken internally in small amounts. Generally, its topical use is recommended for skin rashes, eczema, and skin parasites. In aromatherapy, it is considered warming, opening, and comforting and is used in various nervous tension and stress formulas. It is taken internally (5–10 drops) for upper respiratory problems and excessive mucus.

Traditional Preparation For topical use, mix 1 part balsam gum or oil with 3 parts of a carrier oil—for example, mix 1 teaspoon of balsam with 3 teaspoons of almond or grape seed oil—and apply it topically to wounds, rashes, or skin parasites twice daily. For internal use, place 5 drops of the essential oil in a small glass of warm water and take twice daily for excessive mucus and upper respiratory problems.

Contraindications Balsam has been reported to cause allergic skin reactions. Discontinue use if a skin rash develops.

Drug Interactions None known.

Worldwide Ethnomedical Uses

Region	Uses
Amazonia	for abscesses, asthma, bronchitis, flu, headache, rheumatism, sexually transmitted diseases, sores, sprains, tuberculosis, wounds
Caledonia	for bronchitis, cough, skin sores, wounds; also used in perfumes
Dominican Republic	for excessive mucus, digestion, sores, wounds
Europe	for bacterial infections, cancer, chilblains, fungal infections, lice, parasites, scabies, skin rash, skin problems, ulcers, wounds
Mexico	for asthma, bronchitis, colic, flu, freckles, gout, itch, menstrual problems, osteomyelitis, parasites, rheumatism, ringworm, scabies, sexually transmitted diseases, sores, spasm, stomachache, tumor, urinary insufficiency, worms
South Africa	for bronchitis, colds, coughs; used as an antiseptic, expectorant, and in perfumes
United States	for bronchitis, coughs, dandruff, diarrhea, dysmenorrhea, dysentery, hair support, leucorrhea, laryngitis, respiratory ailments, scabies, sore throat, wounds, ulcers, and as a natural fragrance in skin care products
Elsewhere	for asthma, bacterial infections, coughs, digestion, flu, headache, inflammation, respiratory problems, rheumatism, sclerosis, sexually transmitted diseases, topical cleanser, tuberculosis, umbilicus, and in deodorants

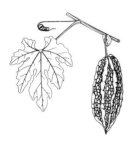

BITTER MELON
HERBAL PROPERTIES AND ACTIONS

Main Actions	Other Actions	Standard Dosage
• kills bacteria	• reduces inflammation	Leaves, Fruit
• kills viruses	• fights free radicals	**Decoction:** 1 cup one or two times daily
• kills cancer cells	• enhances libido	
• kills leukemia cells	• cleanses blood	**Tincture:** 1–3 ml twice daily
• prevents tumors	• dries secretions	**Tablets/Capsules:** 1 g twice daily
• prevents ulcers	• detoxifies	
• treats diabetes	• expels worms	
• reduces blood sugar	• balances hormones	
• reduces blood pressure	• enhances immunity	
• stimulates digestion	• kills insects	
• lowers body temperature	• mildly laxative	
	• promotes milk flow	

Family: Cucurbitaceae

Genus: *Momordica*

Species: *charantia*

Common Names: bitter melon, papailla, melao de sao caetano, bittergourd, balsam apple, balsam pear, karela, k'u kua kurela, kor-kuey, ku gua, pava-aki, salsamino, sorci, sorossi, sorossie, sorossies, pare, peria laut, peria

Parts Used: whole plant, fruit, seed

Bitter melon grows in tropical areas, including parts of the Amazon, east Africa, Asia, and the Caribbean, and is cultivated throughout South America as a food and medicine. It's a slender, climbing annual vine with long-stalked leaves and yellow, solitary male and female flowers borne in the leaf axils. The fruit looks like a warty gourd, usually oblong and resembling a small cucumber. The young fruit is emerald green, turning to orange-yellow when ripe. At maturity, the fruit splits into three irregular valves that curl backwards and release numerous reddish-brown or white seeds encased in scarlet arils. The Latin name *Momordica* means "to bite," referring to the jagged edges of the leaves, which appear as if they have been bitten. All parts of the plant, including the fruit, taste very bitter.

TRIBAL AND HERBAL MEDICINE USES

In the Amazon, local people and indigenous tribes grow bitter melon in their gardens for food and medicine. They add the fruit and/or leaves to beans and soup for a bitter or sour flavor; parboiling it first with a dash of salt may remove some of the bitter taste. Medicinally, the plant has a long history of use by the indigenous peoples of the Amazon. A leaf tea is used for diabetes, to expel intestinal gas, to promote menstruation, and as an antiviral for measles, hepatitis, and feverish conditions. It is used topically for sores, wounds, and infections, and internally and externally for worms and parasites.

In Brazilian herbal medicine, bitter melon is used for tumors, wounds, rheumatism, malaria, vaginal discharge, inflammation, menstrual problems, diabetes, colic, fevers, and worms. It is also used to induce abortions and as an aphrodisiac. It is prepared into a topical remedy for the skin to treat vaginitis, hemorrhoids, scabies, itchy rashes, eczema, leprosy, and other skin problems. In Mexico, the entire plant is used for diabetes and dysentery; the root is a reputed aphrodisiac. In Peruvian herbal medicine, the leaf or aerial parts of the plant are used to treat measles, malaria, and all types of inflammation. In Nicaragua, the leaf is commonly used for stomach pain, diabetes, fevers, colds, coughs, headaches, malaria, skin complaints, menstrual disorders, aches and pains, hypertension, infections, and as an aid in childbirth.

PLANT CHEMICALS

Bitter melon contains an array of biologically active plant chemicals including triterpenes, proteins, and steroids. One chemical has clinically demonstrated the ability to inhibit the enzyme guanylate cyclase, which is thought to be linked to the cause of psoriasis and also necessary for the growth of leukemia and cancer cells.[1–7] In addition, a protein found in bitter melon, momordin, has clinically demonstrated anticancerous activity against Hodgkin's lymphoma in animals.[8] Other proteins in the plant, alpha- and beta-momorcharin and cucurbitacin B, have been tested for possible anticancerous effects. A chemical analog of these bitter melon proteins has been developed, patented, and named "MAP-30"; its developers reported that it was able to inhibit prostate tumor growth.[9] Two of these proteins—alpha- and beta-momorcharin—have also been reported to inhibit HIV virus in test tube studies.[10–12] In one study, HIV-infected cells treated with alpha- and beta-momorcharin showed a nearly complete loss of viral antigen while healthy cells were largely unaffected.[12] The inventor of MAP-30 filed another patent which stated it was "useful for treating tumors and HIV infections."[13] Another clinical study showed that MAP-30's antiviral activity was also relative to the herpes virus *in vitro*.[14]

Anticancerous, antiviral, and hypoglycemic chemicals are present in bitter melon, which may explain many of its traditional uses.

In numerous studies, at least three different groups of constituents found in all parts of bitter melon have clinically demonstrated hypoglycemic (blood sugar-lowering) properties or other actions of potential benefit against diabetes mellitus.[15–24] These chemicals that lower blood sugar include a mixture of steroidal saponins known as charantins, insulin-like peptides, and alkaloids. The hypoglycemic effect is more pronounced in the fruit of bitter melon where these chemicals are found in greater abundance.

Alkaloids, charantin, charine, cryptoxanthin, cucurbitins, cucurbitacins, cucurbitanes, cycloartenols, diosgenin, elaeostearic acids, erythrodiol, galacturonic acids, gentisic acid, goyaglycosides, goyasaponins, guanylate cyclase inhibitors, gypsogenin, hydroxytryptamines, karounidiols, lanosterol, lauric acid, linoleic acid, linolenic acid, momorcharasides, momorcharins, momordenol, momordicilin, momordicins, momordicinin, momordicosides, momordin, multiflorenol, myristic acid, nerolidol, oleanolic acid, oleic acid, oxalic acid, pentadecans, peptides, petroselinic acid, polypeptides, proteins, ribosome-inactivating proteins, rosmarinic acid, rubixanthin, spinasterol, steroidal glycosides, stigmasta-diols, stigmasterol, taraxerol, trehalose, trypsin inhibitors, uracil, vacine, v-insulin, verbascoside, vicine, zeatin, zeatin riboside, zeaxanthin, and zeinoxanthin are all found in bitter melon.

BIOLOGICAL ACTIVITIES AND CLINICAL RESEARCH

More than 100 studies with animals and humans indicate bitter melon can lower blood sugar and cholesterol levels.

To date, close to 100 *in vivo* studies have demonstrated the blood sugar-lowering effect of this bitter fruit. The fruit has also shown the ability to enhance cells' uptake of glucose,[25] to promote insulin release, and to potentiate the effect of insulin.[26,27] In other *in vivo* studies, bitter melon fruit and/or seed has been shown to reduce total cholesterol. In one study, elevated cholesterol and triglyceride levels in diabetic rats were returned to normal after ten weeks of treatment.[29]

Several *in vivo* studies have demonstrated the antitumorous activity of the entire plant of bitter melon. In one study, a water extract blocked the growth of rat prostate carcinoma;[6] another study reported that a hot water extract of the entire plant inhibited the development of mammary tumors in mice.[30] Numerous *in vitro* studies have also demonstrated the anticancerous and antileukemic activity of bitter melon against numerous cell lines, including liver cancer, human leukemia, melanoma, and solid sarcomas.[3,31–33]

Bitter melon, like several of its isolated plant chemicals, also has been documented with *in vitro* antiviral activity against numerous viruses, including Epstein-Barr, herpes, and HIV viruses.[34] In an *in vivo* study, a leaf extract increased resistance to viral infections and had an immune-stimulant effect in humans and animals, increasing interferon production and natural killer cell activity.[35]

In addition to these properties, leaf extracts of bitter melon have demonstrated broad-spectrum antimicrobial activity. Various extracts of the leaves have demonstrated *in vitro* antibacterial activities against *E. coli, Staphylococcus, Pseudomonas, Salmonella, Streptobacillus,* and *Streptococcus;*[36–39] an extract of the entire plant was shown to have antiprotozoal activity against *Entamoeba histolytica.*[40] The fruit and fruit juice have demonstrated the same type of antibacterial properties and, in another study, a fruit extract demonstrated activity against the stomach ulcer-causing bacteria *Helicobacter pylori.*[41]

Many *in vivo* clinical studies have demonstrated the relatively low toxicity of all parts of the bitter melon plant when ingested orally. However, toxicity and even death in laboratory animals has been reported when extracts are injected intravenously.[42] Other studies have shown extracts of the fruit and leaf (ingested orally) to be safe during pregnancy.[43,44] The seeds, however, have demonstrated the ability to induce abortions in rats and mice, and the root has been documented as a uterine stimulant in animals.[45-48] The fruit and leaf of bitter melon have demonstrated an *in vivo* anti-fertility effect in female animals;[49,50] and in male animals, to affect the production of sperm negatively.[51]

CURRENT PRACTICAL USES

Over the years, scientists have verified many of the traditional uses of this plant, which continues to be an important natural remedy in herbal medicine systems. Bitter melon capsules and tinctures are becoming more widely available in the United States and are employed by natural health practitioners for diabetes, viruses, colds and flu, cancer and tumors, high cholesterol, and psoriasis. Concentrated fruit and seed extracts can be found in capsules and tablets, as well as whole herb/vine powders and extracts in capsules and tinctures.

Traditional Preparation

Traditionally, ½ to 1 cup of a standard leaf or whole herb decoction is taken one or two times daily, or 1–3 ml of a 4:1 tincture is taken twice daily. Powdered leaf in tablets or capsules—1 to 2 g daily—can be substituted, if desired. The traditional South American remedy for diabetes is to juice 1–2 fresh bitter melon fruits and drink twice daily. For seed or fruit extracts in capsules or tinctures, follow the label instructions.

Contraindications

Bitter melon traditionally has been used as an abortive and has weak uterine stimulant activity; therefore, it is contraindicated during pregnancy.

This plant has been documented to reduce fertility in both males and females and should therefore not be used by those undergoing fertility treatment or seeking pregnancy.

The active chemicals in bitter melon can be transferred through breast milk; therefore, it is contraindicated in women who are breastfeeding.

All parts of bitter melon (especially the fruit and seed) have demonstrated in numerous *in vivo* studies that they lower blood sugar levels. As such, it is contraindicated in persons with hypoglycemia. Diabetics should check with their physicians before using this plant, and use with caution while monitoring their blood sugar levels regularly, as the dosage of insulin medications may need adjusting.

Although all parts of the plant have demonstrated active antibacterial activity, none has shown activity against fungi or yeast. Long-term use of this plant may result in the killing of friendly bacteria with resulting opportunistic overgrowth of yeast (*Candida*). Cycling off the use of the plant (every twenty-one to thirty days for one week) may be warranted, and adding probiotics to the diet may be beneficial if this plant is used for longer than thirty days.

Drug Interactions

Bitter melon may potentiate insulin and antidiabetic drugs and cholesterol-lowering drugs.

Worldwide Ethnomedical Uses

Region	Uses
Brazil	for abortions, burns, colic, constipation, dermatosis, diabetes, diarrhea, eczema, fever, flu, hemorrhoids, hepatitis, hives, itch, impotency, leprosy, leukemia, libido, liver inflammation, malaria, menstrual problems, pain, rheumatism, scabies, skin problems, tumor, vaginal discharge, vaginitis, worms, wounds
China	for breast cancer, diabetes, fever, halitosis, impotency, renal insufficiency, kidney problems
Cuba	for anemia, colitis, diabetes, fever, hyperglycemia, intestinal parasites, kidney stones, liver problems, menstrual problems, sterility (female), worms
Haiti	for anemia, constipation, dermatosis, eye infections, fever, liver diseases, skin problems, rhinitis, and as an appetite stimulant and insecticide
India	for abortions, birth control, constipation, diabetes, eczema, fat loss, food, fever, gout, hemorrhoids, hydrophobia, hyperglycemia, increasing milk flow, intestinal parasites, jaundice, kidney stones, leprosy, liver disorders, menstrual disorders, pneumonia, psoriasis, rheumatism, scabies, skin problems, snakebite, vaginal discharge
Malaysia	for abdominal pain, asthma, burns, Celiac disease, dermatosis, diarrhea, headache, intestinal parasites, stomachache, worms
Mexico	for bowel function, burns, diabetes, dysentery, impotency, libido, scabies, sores, worms
Nicaragua	for aches, anemia, childbirth, colds, constipation, cough, diabetes, fever, headache, hypertension, infections, lung disorders, malaria, pain, pregnancy, rashes, skin problems
Panama	for colds, diabetes, fever, flu, gallbladder problems, hives, hypertension, itch, malaria, menstrual problems, and as an insecticide
Peru	for colic, constipation, contusions, diabetes, diarrhea, fever, hepatitis, inflammation, intestinal parasites, lung problems, malaria, measles, menstrual problems, skin sores, pus, wounds
Trinidad	for diabetes, dysentery, fever, hypertension, malaria, rheumatism, worms

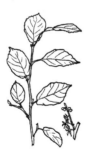

Family: Monimiaceae

Genus: *Peumus*

Species: *boldus*

BOLDO

HERBAL PROPERTIES AND ACTIONS

Main Actions
- stimulates digestion
- protects liver
- detoxifies liver
- stimulates bile
- supports gallbladder
- cleanses blood
- expels worms
- kills parasites
- increases urination

Other Actions
- supports heart
- stimulates
- reduces gas
- moderately laxative
- reduces inflammation
- reduces spasms
- relieves pain

Standard Dosage

Leaves

Infusion: $\frac{1}{2}$ cup one or two times daily

Tincture: 2–4 ml twice daily

Capsules/Tablets: 1–2 g twice daily

Common Names:
boldo, boldu, boldus,
boldoa, boldina, baldina,
molina

Part Used: leaves

Boldo is a slow-growing, shrubby evergreen tree that grows 6–8 m in height and produces small, berry-like fruit. The plant's scented flowers are either male or female, and only one sex is found on any one plant; as such, male and female plants must be grown together for the plants to reproduce. Boldo is found in the Andean regions of Chile and Peru, and also is indigenous to parts of Morocco. It is cultivated in Italy, Brazil, and North Africa to meet the demand for its medicinal leaves in European and Canadian markets, where it is widely used.

TRIBAL AND HERBAL MEDICINE USES

Indigenous uses of boldo have been widely documented. Legend has it that the medicinal uses of the plant were discovered by chance: a Chilean shepherd noticed that his sheep were healthier and had fewer liver problems, when they grazed on native boldo plants growing in his fields. Since this discovery, the plant has been used by the indigenous peoples of Chile for liver, bowel, and gallbladder troubles. It is also widely used in Chilean folk medicine to expel intestinal worms, for insomnia, rheumatism, cystitis, colds, hepatitis, constipation, flatulence, poor digestion, gallstones, earaches, and it is considered a general tonic. For many years, the fruit has been eaten as a spice, the wood has been used for charcoal, and the bark has been used in tanning hides. In parts of Peru, boldo leaves are used by indigenous tribes against liver diseases, to treat gallstones, and as a diuretic.

Boldo's uses in other traditional medicine systems are well documented. Worldwide, the plant is used in homeopathy and herbal medicine in the treatment of digestive disorders, as a laxative, a diuretic, for liver problems, and to increase the production of bile in the gallbladder. The leaves are used against intestinal worms, and botanist Dr. James Duke reports its traditional use for urogenital inflammations, gonorrhea, syphilis, gout, jaundice, dyspepsia, rheumatism, head colds, and earaches. In Brazilian herbal medicine systems, boldo is used for a variety of disorders including hepatitis, liver congestion, constipation, flatulence, dizziness, stomach and intestinal cramps and pain, gallstones, insomnia, rheumatism, and a lack of appetite. Throughout the rest of South America, boldo is used for gonorrhea, as well as for liver, gallbladder, and digestive complaints.

Boldo is the subject of a German therapeutic monograph that allows the use (as an herbal drug) for mild gastrointestinal spasms and dyspeptic disorders. In Germany, it is employed for liver and gallbladder complaints, gastric disorders, and to stimulate gastric secretions (especially bile production and secretion in the gallbladder and liver). It is also used for loss of appetite and as an antispasmodic. It is used for similar purposes in other countries throughout Europe.

In American herbal medicine systems, boldo is used to stimulate the secretion of saliva, bile flow and liver activity; it's chiefly valued as a remedy for gall-stones, liver problems, and gallbladder pain.

PLANT CHEMICALS

Boldo has many biologically active chemicals. At least seventeen alkaloids have been documented thus far, several of which are believed to be boldo's main active constituents.[1–5] Much of the biological activity of the plant has been attributed to a single alkaloid called *boldine.*

In various studies over the years boldine has shown to protect the liver,[6,7] to stimulate the production of bile in the liver,[4] as well as to stimulate digestion, increase the secretion of gastric juices, and stimulate the production of bile and its secretion from the gallbladder.[8–10] In other laboratory tests, boldine has demonstrated diuretic, fever reducing, and anti-inflammatory properties as well as the ability to reduce excess uric acid.[11–13] In animal studies, boldine exhibited anti-inflammatory and antispasmodic activities,[14,15] as well as the ability to protect against colon damage and inflammation in induced colitis and colon inflammation in animals.[16] Other research on boldine indicates that it has a strong cellular protective and antioxidant effect in the blood[17] and can normalize sticky blood (inhibits platelet aggregation).[18,19] In 2002, boldine was reported to have an effect on the cardiovascular system as well. Researchers found that it increased coronary blood flow, depressed cardiac force and heart rate, and had a vasorelaxant effect.[20]

One of boldo's main chemicals is responsible for the plant's ability to benefit the liver, gallbladder, and many digestive functions.

Most of these studies validate the plant's traditional uses for many types of digestive and elimination problems, gallbladder problems, and liver disorders. With so many studies on this important active alkaloid, it is understandable that most boldo herbal drugs sold in Europe are standardized for boldine content.

In addition to boldine, boldo contains ascaridole, benzaldehyde, boldin, boldoglucin, bornyl-acetate, 1,8-cineol, coclaurine, coumarin, cuminaldehyde, 2-decanone, 6(a)-7 dehydroboldine, diethylphthalate, eugenol, farnesol, fenchone, gamma terpinene, 2-heptanone, isoboldine, kaempferols, laurolitsine, laurotetainine, norboldine, norisocorydine, pachycarpine, P-cymene, P-cymol, pro-nuciferine, 2-octanone, reticuline, rhamnosides, sabinene, sinoacutine, terpinoline, thymol, trans verbenol, 2-tridecanone, and 2-undecanone.

BIOLOGICAL ACTIVITIES AND CLINICAL RESEARCH

Researchers verified indigenous uses of boldo leaves in the 1950s and 1960s and showed that leaf extracts had diuretic, digestion stimulation, and bile-producing properties in animal studies.[21,22] Although these properties are attributed largely to the plant chemical boldine, one study with rats indicated that an alcohol extract of boldo leaves was more active than boldine alone.[8] An ethanol extract of the leaf administered to mice was shown to have a liver protective effect, preventing liver damage from chemical exposure.[11] A recent human study demonstrated that boldo relaxes smooth muscle tissue and prolongs intestinal transit (which again validates its traditional uses for digestive functions).[23] The antioxidant property of boldo leaves has also been documented,[24] and animal studies confirm that boldo leaf has an anti-inflammatory effect.[11] A U.S. monograph reports that boldo can increase urine output by 50 percent, which validates the plant's traditional use as a diuretic.[25]

Clinical research confirms most of boldo's traditional uses.

Toxicity studies show that boldo should not be consumed regularly or in high dosages, and it should be respected for its very active qualities. The essential oil of the plant contains a compound called asaridole. Asaridole has antiparasitic and worm-expelling properties,[26] but it is also a documented liver toxin. Therefore, distilled essential oil products of boldo should only be used externally. In addition, boldine has been reported to have toxic effects in high dosages. In large quantities (higher than it occurs in traditional dosages of the natural leaf), it causes cramps, convulsions, and muscle paralysis, eventually leading to respiratory paralysis.[27] It also has demonstrated a uterine relaxant effect in rats.[28] In a 2000 study with rats, an extract of dry boldo leaves and the chemical boldine showed abortive actions and lowered the blood levels of bilirubin, cholesterol, glucose, alanine aminotransferase (ALT), aspartate aminotransferase (AST), and urea. These researchers reported, however, that the long-term administration of regular dosages of the leaf extract and boldine did not cause any toxic effect over a period of ninety days.[29]

CURRENT PRACTICAL USES

Centuries ago, boldo was a little-known plant growing in farmers' pastures in Chile. Today, huge fields of boldo are cultivated around the world to supply the market demand for a specific herbal remedy or herbal drug for gallstones and gallbladder inflammation and for many types of liver, stomach, and digestive conditions. However, persons with gallstones should seek the help and advice of a qualified and trained healthcare practitioner before self-medicating with boldo. It has such a pronounced effect on the gallbladder that it can cause the gallbladder to dump stones and grit rapidly, possibly causing a blockage in the bile ducts below the gallbladder and/or damaging the pancreas. It is best used in small quantities and with other plants to avoid these problems.

Many digestive disorders are due to a lack of bile and digestive juices, which results in sluggish digestion (causing bloating and an uncomfortable feeling of fullness after a meal, intestinal gas, fermentation and belching, and poor absorption of nutrients in the stomach and bowel). Boldo is one of the best natural remedies for these types of digestive problems because it stimulates the production and secretion of bile and other digestive juices in the stomach, gallbladder, and liver, thereby maximizing and speeding digestive processes in general. It also is one of the first natural remedies natural health practitioners use to assist in detoxifying the liver and to prevent liver damage from toxins and drugs that are known to have a toxic effect on the liver. However, consumers should not exceed the recommended dosages for boldo: it is a very powerful and active plant that should be treated with respect.

There are several boldo products available in capsules, tablets, and liquid extracts in the U.S. market, including extracts providing a standardized amount of boldine. These standardized extracts are sold as herbal drugs in Europe by prescription only; however, they are sold as over-the-counter herbal supplements in the United States.

Traditional Preparation   As a digestive aid or liver detoxifier, use ½ cup of a leaf infusion one or two times daily with meals or 2–4 ml of a 4:1 tincture twice daily. Or, if desired, take 1–2 g of powdered leaf in tablets or capsules twice daily. For standardized extracts, follow the label instructions.

Contraindications   Boldo has demonstrated abortive properties and caused fetal birth defects in animal studies and therefore should not be used during pregnancy or while breastfeeding.

Chemicals in boldo may thin the blood. Those taking blood-thinning medications (such as Warfarin®) or those with disorders that have a tendency towards thin blood (such as thrombocytopenia or hemophilia) should not take boldo unless under the supervision of a qualified healthcare practitioner.

Boldo has diuretic effects and is contraindicated for long-term, chronic use. Do not exceed the recommended dosages.

Drug Interactions   Boldo may potentiate the effects of blood-thinning medications such as Warfarin®.

One *in vivo* clinical study suggests that boldo and/or boldine can decrease metabolic activation and/or metabolism of toxins, drugs, and chemicals in the liver.[30] As such, boldo may decrease the effect or reduce the half-life of certain drugs that should be metabolized in the liver.

Worldwide Ethnomedical Uses

Region	Uses
Asia	for digestive problems, dyspepsia, hangover, intestinal gas, liver disorders
Brazil	for anorexia, bile insufficiency, cholecystitis, constipation, debilitation, digestive disorders, dizziness, dyspnea, gallstones, gastritis, gonorrhea, hepatitis, insomnia, intestinal gas, liver congestion, liver disorders, liver support, rheumatism, stomach problems, stomach pain, urinary insufficiency, weakness, and to stimulate digestion

Chile	for anorexia, bile insufficiency, bowel problems, high cholesterol, colds, cough, constipation, cystitis, diarrhea, dyspepsia, earache, edema, fluid retention, gallbladder problems, gallstones, gastric sluggishness, hypothyroidism, inflammation, intestinal gas, intestinal cramps, intestinal parasites, jaundice, liver disorders, liver support, liver protection, obesity, rheumatism, sores, stomachache, stomach cramps, urinary insufficiency, worms, and as an antioxidant, antiseptic, digestive stimulant, and sedative
Europe	for bile insufficiency, digestion problems, dyspepsia, gallbladder pain, gallstones, gastrointestinal spasms, gonorrhea, gout, liver disorders, spasms, urinary insufficiency, and as an appetite stimulant and digestive stimulant
Latin America	for anorexia, bile insufficiency, bowel problems, colds, constipation, cystitis, digestion problems, dyspepsia, earache, gallbladder problems, gallstones, gonorrhea, gout, hepatitis, intestinal gas, intestinal parasites, jaundice, kidney stones, liver disorders, liver support, malaria, pain, parasites, rheumatism, spasms, stomach pain, syphilis, urogenital inflammation, urethritis, urinary insufficiency, worms, and as an antiseptic, digestive stimulant, and general tonic
Mexico	for bile disorders, digestive disorders, gallbladder problems, gallstones, liver disorders, liver support, pain, rheumatism, and as a digestive stimulant
Turkey	for liver support, rheumatism, urinary insufficiency, worms and used as an antiseptic, digestive stimulant, sedative, and tonic
United States	for bile stimulation, cystitis, digestive problems, elimination problems, gallbladder disorders, gallstones, gastrointestinal spasms, gout, hepatitis, inflammation, kidney disorders, liver disorders, pain, uric acid elimination, urinary infections, urinary insufficiency, urinary antiseptic, and used as an antiseptic (urinary), digestive stimulant, sedative, and tonic

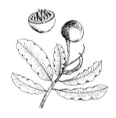

BRAZIL NUT

HERBAL PROPERTIES AND ACTIONS

Main Actions	Other Actions	Standard Dosage
• fights free radicals	• none	Nut, Nut oil
• is nutritious		
• is soothing		

Family: *Lecythidaceae*

Genus: *Bertholletia*

Species: *excelsia*

Common Names: Brazil nut, castania, castanheiro do para, para-nut, creamnut, castana-de-para, castana-de-Brazil

Parts Used: nut, seed oil

The Brazil nut tree is enormous, frequently attaining the height of 40 to 50 m or more, and it can reach ages of 500–800 years old. The tree is called *castanheiro do para* in Brazil and is found throughout the Amazon rainforest in Brazil, Peru, Colombia, Venezuela, and Ecuador. The fruit is a large, round woody capsule or pod, about the size of a large grapefruit and weighing up to 2.2 kg. The fruit pods grow at the ends of thick branches, then ripen and fall from the tree from January to June, usually with a loud crashing sound as they fall 150 feet through the canopy like cannon balls. Inside each fruit pod, wedged in like orange segments, are twelve to twenty-five Brazil nuts, each within its own individual shell. Mature Brazil nut trees can produce approximately 300 or more of these fruit pods annually.

Today, the monetary value of exporting Brazil nuts from the Amazon (which began in the 1600s with Dutch traders) is second only to that of rubber. The United States alone imports more than 9 metric tons of Brazil nuts annually. Virtually all Brazil nut production comes from wild forest trees and wild harvesting. The trees grow very slowly, taking as long as ten to thirty years before producing nuts, and they require a specific species of bee to pollinate the flowers. Both of these factors make the trees unsuitable and unprofitable for plantation cultivation.

The Brazil nut tree is a good example of the intricate ecosystem of the Amazon, where plants and animals are inexplicably intertwined. Not only is the pollination of this tree so specialized, requiring one particular insect species to produce the fruit, but only one species of animal is capable of chewing through the extremely tough fruit pod to disburse the seeds for new tree growth. The agouti, a rather large rat (up to 10 pounds!) with extremely sharp front teeth, is solely responsible for reseeding the forest with Brazil nuts and ensuring the next generation of trees. In the Amazon rainforest, the tree, bee, and agouti are all dependent on one another for survival.

TRIBAL AND HERBAL MEDICINE USES

The Brazil nut is a three-sided nut with white meat or flesh that consists of 70 percent fat and 17 percent protein. For centuries, the indigenous tribes of the rainforest have relied on Brazil nuts as an important and significant staple in their diet—so important that the nuts have even been used as a trade commodity, much like money. Indigenous tribes eat the nuts raw or grate them and mix them into gruels. In the Brazilian Amazon, the nuts are grated with the thorny stilt roots of *Socratea* palms into a white mush known as *leite de castanha* and then stirred into manioc flour. This food is a valuable source of calories, fat, and protein for much of the Amazon's rural and tribal peoples.

With such a high oil content, fresh Brazil nuts will even burn like miniature candles when lit. The oil is extracted from the nuts and used by indigenous and rural people for cooking oil, lamps, soap, and livestock feed. The empty seedpods, often called "monkey's pots," are used to carry around small smoky fires to discourage attacks of black flies, as cups to collect rubber latex from tapped trees, and as drinking cups. The husks of these seedpods have also been used in Brazilian folk medicine to brew into tea to treat stomachaches, and the tree bark is brewed into tea to treat liver ailments.

PLANT CHEMICALS

Brazil nut oil contains mainly palmitic, oleic, and linoleic and alpha linolenic acids and small amounts of myristic and stearic acids and phytosterols. In addition to protein and fat, Brazil nuts provide the highest natural source of selenium. One single Brazil nut exceeds the U.S. Recommended Daily Allowance of

One single Brazil nut exceeds the U.S. Recommended Daily Allowance of selenium.

selenium. The proteins found in Brazil nuts are very high in sulfur-containing amino acids like cysteine (8 percent) and methionine (18 percent) and are also extremely rich in glutamine, glutamic acid, and arginine.[1–5] The presence of these amino acids (chiefly methionine) enhances the absorption of selenium and other minerals in the nut.

In addition to the chemicals discussed above, Brazil nuts contain antimony, cerium, cesium, europium, fatty acids, lanthanum, lutetium, samarium, scandium, selenoprotein, tantalum, tungsten, and ytterbium.

BIOLOGICAL ACTIVITIES AND CLINICAL RESEARCH

Since the Brazil nut has long been a common food, rather than an herbal remedy, it hasn't been the subject of any clinical research. Anyone using it "therapeutically" employs the nuts for their high content of natural selenium. Selenium is an essential trace mineral in the human body with antioxidant, anti-cancer, and cancer-preventative properties (especially, it seems, for prostate cancer).[6–8]

CURRENT PRACTICAL USES

Brazil nuts and their oil are mainly used as a food in the United States. Brazil nut oil is clear yellowish oil with a pleasant, sweet smell and taste. It makes a wonderful light oil for salad dressings: try combining it with raspberry vinegar for tasty vinaigrette. In addition, Brazil nut oil is often used in soaps, shampoos, and hair conditioning/repair products in South America, and this use is beginning to catch on in the United States as well. It is a wonderful hair conditioner, bringing shine, silkiness, and softness to hair and renewing dry, lifeless hair and split ends. Brazil nut oil in skin creams helps lubricate and moisturize the skin, provides antioxidant benefits with its high selenium content, helps prevents dryness, and leaves skin soft, smooth, and hydrated.

Traditional Preparation

A Brazil nut a day is a great way to get the daily recommended amount of natural selenium.

Contraindications

Brazil nuts, like many other nuts, can cause allergic reactions in some sensitive individuals. If you are allergic to other nuts, like peanuts, you might be allergic to Brazil nuts as well.

Drug Interactions

None known.

Worldwide Ethnomedical Uses

Region	Uses
Amazonia	for liver problems, stomachache, and used as a food, emollient, soap, and insect repellant
Venezuela	used as a food and insect repellant

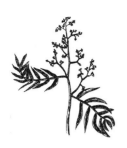

Family: Anacardiaceae

Genus: *Schinus*

Species: *molle,*
terebinthifolius, aroeira

Common Names:
Brazilian peppertree,
Peruvian peppertree,
California peppertree,
aroeira, aroeira salsa,
escobilla, Peruvian mastic
tree, mastic-tree,
aguaribay, American
pepper, anacahuita,
castilla, false pepper,
gualeguay, Jesuit's balsam,
molle del Peru, mulli,
pepper tree, pimentero,
pimientillo, pirul

Parts Used: fruit, bark,
leaf

BRAZILIAN PEPPERTREE
HERBAL PROPERTIES AND ACTIONS

Main Actions	Other Actions	Standard Dosage
• kills bacteria	• relieves pain	Leaf, Bark
• kills fungi	• kills cancer cells	**Bark decoction:** ½ cup twice daily
• kills *Candida* yeast	• relieves depression	
• reduces inflammation	• reduces spasms	**Leaf infusion:** ½ cup twice daily
• dries secretions	• kills viruses	
• regulates heartbeat	• stimulates digestion	**Tincture:** 2–3 ml twice daily
• lowers blood pressure	• increases urination	
• mildly laxative	• stimulates menstruation	
• stimulates uterus	• reduces phlegm	
• heals wounds	• kills insects	

Brazilian peppertree is a shrubby tree with narrow, spiky leaves. It grows 4 to 10 m tall, with a trunk 25 to 35 cm in diameter. It produces an abundance of small flowers formed in panicles that bear a great many small, flesh-colored, berry-like fruits in December and January. It is indigenous to South and Central America and can also be found in semitropical and tropical regions of the United States and Africa. In both North and South America, three different trees—*Schinus molle, Schinus aroeira,* and *Schinus terebinthifolius*—are all interchangeably called "peppertrees."

All parts of the tree have high oil and essential oil contents that produce a spicy, aromatic scent. The leaves of the Brazilian peppertree have such high oil content that leaf pieces jerk and twist when placed in hot water as the oil is released. The berries, which have a peppery flavor, are used in syrups, vinegar, and beverages in Peru; are added to Chilean wines; and are dried and ground up for a pepper substitute in the tropics. The dried berries have also been used as an adulterant of black pepper in some countries.

TRIBAL AND HERBAL MEDICINE USES

Virtually all parts of this tropical tree, including its leaves, bark, fruit, seeds, resin, and oleoresin (or balsam) have been used medicinally by indigenous peoples throughout the tropics. The plant has a very long history of use and appears in religious artifacts and on idols among some of the ancient Chilean Amerindians.

Throughout South and Central America, Brazilian peppertree is reported to be an astringent, antibacterial, diuretic, digestive stimulant, tonic, antiviral, and wound healer. In Peru, the sap is used as a mild laxative and a diuretic, and the entire plant is used externally for fractures and as a topical antiseptic. The oleoresin is used externally as a wound healer, to stop bleeding, and for toothaches, and it is taken internally for rheumatism and as a purgative. In South Africa, a leaf tea is used to treat colds, and a leaf decoction is inhaled for colds, hypertension, depression, and irregular heartbeat. In the Brazilian Amazon, a bark tea is used as a laxative, and a bark-and-leaf tea is used as a stimulant and antidepressant. In Argentina, a decoction is made with the dried leaves and is taken for menstrual disorders and is also used for respiratory and urinary tract infections and disorders.

In Brazilian herbal medicine today, Brazilian peppertree is employed for heart problems (hypertension and irregular heartbeat), infections of all sorts, menstrual disorders with excessive bleeding, tumors, and general inflammation.

Brazilian peppertree is still employed in herbal medicine today in many countries. It is used for many conditions in the tropics, including menstrual disorders, bronchitis, gingivitis, gonorrhea, gout, eye infections, rheumatism, sores, swellings, tuberculosis, ulcers, urethritis, urogenital disorders, sexually transmitted diseases, warts, and wounds. In Brazilian herbal medicine today, the dried bark and/or leaves are employed for heart problems (hypertension and irregular heartbeat), infections of all sorts, menstrual disorders with excessive bleeding, tumors, and general inflammation. A liquid extract or tincture prepared with the bark is used internally as a stimulant, tonic, and astringent, and externally for rheumatism, gout, and syphilis.

PLANT CHEMICALS

Phytochemical analysis of Brazilian peppertree reveals that the plant contains tannins, alkaloids, flavonoids, steroidal saponins, sterols, terpenes, and a large amount of essential oil.[1–3] The essential oil present in the leaves, bark, and fruit is a rich source of chemicals (over fifty constituents identified thus far, including biologically active triterpenes and sesquiterpenes). Some of these chemicals scientists have not seen before, and many of the plant's documented biological activities are attributed to its essential oil. The fruit can contain up to 5 percent essential oil, and the leaves can contain up to 2 percent essential oil.[1,2]

The list of chemicals found in the Brazilian peppertree is long: amyrin, behenic acid, bergamont, bicyclogermacrene, bourbonene, cadinene, cadinol, calacorene, calamenediol, calamenene, camphene, car-3-ene, carvacrol, caryophyllene, cerotic acid, copaene, croweacin, cubebene, cyanidins, cymene, elemene, elemol, elemonic acid, eudesmol, fisetin, gallic acid, geraniol butyrate, germacrene, germacrone, guaiene, gurjunene, heptacosanoic acid, humulene, laccase, lanosta, limonene, linalool, linoleic acid, malvalic acid, masticadienoic acid, masticadienonalic acid, masticadienonic acid, muurolene, muurolol, myrcene, nerol hexanoate, octacosanoic acid, oleic acid, paeonidin, palmitic acid, pentacosanoic acid, phellandrene, phellandrene, phenol, pinene, piperine, piperitol, protocatechuic acid, quercetin, quercitrin, raffinose, sabinene, sitosterol, spathulene, terpinene, terpineol, terpinolene, and tricosanoic acid.

BIOLOGICAL ACTIVITIES AND CLINICAL RESEARCH

In laboratory tests, the essential oil (as well as leaf and bark extracts) has demonstrated potent antimicrobial properties. Brazilian peppertree has displayed good-to-very strong *in vitro* antifungal actions against numerous fungi, as well as *Candida*.[4–7] One research group indicated that the antifungal action of the essential oil was more effective than the antifungal drug Multifungin®.[6] The essential oil and leaves have clinically demonstrated *in vitro* antibacterial activity against numerous bacterial strains (which probably explains why it is an herbal remedy for so many infectious conditions in its native countries).[5–10] In 1996, a U.S. patent was awarded for an essential oil preparation of Brazilian peppertree as a topical bactericidal medicine used against *Pseudomonas* and *Staphylococcus* for humans and animals, and as an ear, nose, and/or throat preparation against bacteria.[11] Another patent was awarded in 1997 for a similar preparation used as a topical antibacterial wound cleanser.[12] In much earlier *in vitro* tests, a leaf extract of Brazilian peppertree demonstrated antiviral actions against several plant viruses.[13] In addition to these documented antimicrobial properties, Brazilian peppertree passed an anti-cancer plant screening program in 1976 by demonstrating antitumorous actions.[14] In 2002, researchers in Argentina documented that it was toxic *in vitro* against a human liver cancer cell line.[15]

Brazilian peppertree is effective against numerous bacteria, fungi, and yeast.

Over the years, several research groups have conducted animal studies on Brazilian peppertree that have further substantiated some of its many traditional uses in herbal medicine. A fruit extract and a leaf extract were shown to lower blood pressure in dogs and rats,[16,17] as well as to stimulate uterine activity in guinea pigs and rabbits.[17,18] Leaf extracts have clinically demonstrated pain-relieving activity in mice[19] and antispasmodic properties in rats and guinea pigs (including uterine antispasmodic actions).[16,20] In 1974, the anti-inflammatory effect of Brazilian peppertree was documented; the herb was used to treat 100 patients with chronic cervicitis and vaginitis effectively.[21] In 1995 and 1996, other researchers documented the anti-inflammatory properties of this plant once again.[22–24]

CURRENT PRACTICAL USES

A monograph published in 1976 on Brazilian peppertree's essential oil indicated no toxicity in animals and humans ingesting or applying the essential oil topically.[25] Today, herbalists and natural health practitioners in both North and South America use Brazilian peppertree mostly for colds, flu, and other upper respiratory infections; as a remedy for hypertension and for irregular heartbeat; for fungal infections and *Candida;* and as a female balancing aid for numerous menstrual disorders, including menstrual cramps and excessive bleeding.

Traditional Preparation	The leaves are best prepared as an infusion, and the bark is best prepared as a decoction or an alcohol tincture. Generally, ½ cup of a bark decoction twice daily is used for colds, flu, sore throats and other upper respiratory infections; 2–3 ml of a 4:1 tincture taken two or three times daily can be substituted, if desired. This traditional remedy is also used as a heart tonic and for irregular heartbeat. A leaf decoction twice daily or as needed is generally used for menstrual disorders.
Contraindications	This plant was shown to stimulate the uterus in animal studies and therefore should not be used in pregnancy.
Drug Interactions	None reported. However, this plant has exhibited hypotensive actions in animal studies; in light of such, it is conceivable that the use of this plant may potentiate high blood pressure medications.

Worldwide Ethnomedical Uses

Region	Uses
Argentina	for diarrhea, menstrual disorders, respiratory tract infections, inflammation, urinary tract infections, wounds
Brazil	for bronchitis, constipation, cough, cystitis, depression, diarrhea, eye diseases, fever, flu, gonorrhea, heart problems, hemorrhage, inflammation, menstrual disorders, respiratory tract infections, rheumatism, spasms, tumors, urethritis, urinary tract disorders, and as an astringent, stimulant, and tonic
Colombia	for diarrhea, lung diseases, rheumatism
Mexico	for asthma, bronchitis, cataract, colic, conjunctivitis, constipation, cough, digestive disorders, flu, foot fungus, gonorrhea, gum diseases, mouth sores, rheumatism, sexually transmitted diseases, sores (skin), stomachache, toothache, tuberculosis, tumors, ulcers, urogenital diseases, warts, wounds, and as an astringent
Paraguay	for gonorrhea, menstrual disorders, sores, urethritis, urinary insufficiency, wounds
Peru	for constipation, fevers, fractures, rheumatism, toothache, tumors, urinary insufficiency, warts, wounds, and as an antiseptic
South Africa	for arrhythmia, colds, cough, depression, gout, hypertension, inflammation, pain, rheumatism
Turkey	for constipation, coughs, excessive mucus, gonorrhea, urinary insufficiency, and as a digestive stimulant and tonic
Uruguay	for menstrual disorders, rheumatism, wounds, and as an antiseptic
Elsewhere	for bronchitis, constipation, coughs, excessive mucus, edema, eye diseases, gingivitis, gout, hypertension, menstrual disorders, rheumatism, sexually transmitted diseases, sores, swelling, urinary insufficiency, urogenital inflammation, viruses, and to stimulate digestion

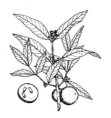

CAMU-CAMU

HERBAL PROPERTIES AND ACTIONS

Main Actions	Other Actions	Standard Dosage
• is nutritious • fights free radicals	• dries secretions	Fruit **Fresh Juice:** 1 cup two or three times daily **Tablets/Capsules:** 1–2 g twice daily or follow the label directions based on vitamin C content

Family: Myrtaceae

Genus: *Myrciaria*

Species: *dubia*

Common Names: camu-camu, rumberry

Part Used: fruit

Camu-camu is a low-growing shrub found throughout the Amazon rainforest, mainly in swampy or flooded areas. It grows to a height of about 2–3 m and has large, feathery leaves. It produces round, light orange-colored fruits about the size of lemons, which contain a significant amount of vitamin C. Its high vitamin C content has created a demand for camu-camu fruit in the natural products market. Some groups are now beginning to study cultivation methods for this important new rainforest resource, which is still harvested wild throughout the Amazon region. Ethnobotanist Mark Plotkin notes in his book, *Tales of a Shaman's Apprentice,* that "a forest stand of camu-camu is worth twice the amount to be gained from cutting down the forest and replacing it with cattle," and he believes that camu-camu cultivation holds real economic promise for local economies. Usually, camu-camu fruit is wild-harvested in canoes because the fruits mature at high water or during flooding seasons in the Amazon rainforest.

TRIBAL AND HERBAL MEDICINE USES

Camu-camu has never been documented as a traditional herbal remedy for any condition in the Amazon region. In fact, it was not widely eaten as a fruit by the indigenous people, due to its sour, acidic taste. In recent years, camu-camu has become popular in Iquitos, Peru, where it is made into drinks and ice creams.

PLANT CHEMICALS

Camu-camu fruit has the highest recorded amount of natural vitamin C known on the planet. Oranges provide 500–4,000 ppm vitamin C, or ascorbic acid; acerola has tested in the range of 16,000–172,000 ppm. Camu-camu provides up to 500,000 ppm, or about 2 g of vitamin C per 100 g of fruit.[1] In comparison to oranges, camu-camu provides thirty times more vitamin C, ten times more iron, three times more niacin, twice as much riboflavin, and 50 percent more phosphorus.[1] Camu-camu is also a significant source of potassium, providing 711 mg per kg of fruit.[2] It also has a full complement of minerals and amino acids that can aid in the absorption of vitamin C. Alpha-pinene and d-limonene (compounds known as terpenes) predominate as the volatile compounds in this fruit.[3]

Camu-camu provides thirty times more vitamin C than oranges.

As with any vitamin C-rich fruit, however, the time between harvesting and consumption is crucial; the fruit may lose up to a quarter of its vitamin C content in less than a month (even if frozen).[4] Even with this loss, camu-camu still has a dramatic edge over its next challenger, acerola, for vitamin C content.

In addition to the chemicals mentioned above, camu-camu contains beta-carotene, calcium, leucine, protein, serine, thiamin, and valine.

BIOLOGICAL ACTIVITIES AND CLINICAL RESEARCH

There has been no research conducted or published on any medicinal or therapeutic properties of camu-camu. However, there are a few herbal supplement companies in the United States marketing camu-camu extracts in powders and pills and alluding to claims of its benefits—from curing viral infections, colds, flu, cold sores, and autoimmune disorders to even weight loss. The fact is there just isn't any research to back up these claims. There is some research suggesting high dosages of vitamin C offer a benefit for various illnesses and conditions, yet even some of those studies are controversial. And, remember, this research is on vitamin C, not on camu-camu specifically.

Make no mistake—camu-camu is a great source of natural vitamin C. In addition, it comes with many other naturally occurring vitamins, minerals, and amino acids that may well help with the absorption and efficient uptake of vitamin C. This is thought to be superior to just taking an ascorbic acid tablet alone. Don't believe some of the more far-reaching and far-fetched marketing claims that are in the marketplace today, however. The only studied and verified health benefit today regarding camu-camu is based upon its vitamin C content—and not other "mysterious" chemicals that surround it.

CURRENT PRACTICAL USES

In the North American nutritional market, suggested daily servings are based upon the vitamin C content in the product sold, which can vary. Adjust the serving size or dosage based upon the amount of vitamin C the product contains.

Traditional Preparation

None documented.

Contraindications

None reported. Side effects for high or excessive dosages of vitamin C include gastrointestinal disturbances and diarrhea.

Drug Interactions

None reported.

Worldwide Ethnomedical Uses

Region	Uses
United States	Nutritive

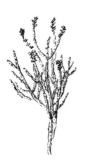

Family: Asteraceae

Genus: *Baccharis*

Species: *genistelloides*

Common Names: carqueja, bacanta, bacárida, cacaia-amarga, cacalia amara, cacália-amarga, cacália-amargosa, cacliadoce, carqueja amara, carqueja-amargosa, carqueja-do-mato, carquejilla, carquejinha, chinchimani, chirca melosa, condamina, cuchi-cuchi, quimsa-kuchu, quina-de-condamiana, quinsu-cucho, tiririca-de-balaio, tres-espigas, vassoura

Parts Used: entire plant, aerial parts

CARQUEJA
HERBAL PROPERTIES AND ACTIONS

Main Actions
- protects liver
- detoxifies liver
- aids digestion
- reduces acid
- treats ulcers
- relieves pain
- expels worms
- mildly laxative
- reduces inflammation
- lowers blood sugar
- cleanses blood
- tones gastric tract

Other Actions
- induces abortions
- kills viruses
- increases urination
- reduces fever
- promotes sweating

Standard Dosage
Aerial parts

Infusion: 1/2 cup two or three times daily

Tincture: 2–4 ml two or three times daily

Capsules/Tablets: 2 g twice daily

Carqueja is a perennial green herb that grows to a height of 1–2 m and produces yellowish-white flowers at the top of the plant. The bright green, flat, winged stalks have a fleshy, succulent consistency and the "wings" take the place of leaves. The *Baccharis* genus is composed of more than 400 species native to tropical and subtropical America. Carqueja is known by several botanical names in Brazil, including *Baccharis genistelloides*, *B. triptera*, and *B. trimera*; however, all refer to the same plant. The herb is found throughout the Amazon rainforest in Peru, Brazil, and Colombia, as well as in tropical parts of Argentina, Paraguay, and Uruguay. Other common species called *carqueja* in Brazil include *Baccharis trinervis* and *B. gaudichaudiana*, which look similar (but smaller in height and with smaller wings) and are sometimes used as substitutes for *B. genistelloides*. Another well-known species in the family (but very different from carqueja) is a small shrub, *B. cordifolia*, which is toxic to grazing animals.

TRIBAL AND HERBAL MEDICINE USES

Indigenous peoples of the rainforest have used carqueja for centuries to cure common ailments. Its uses in herbal medicine were first recorded in Brazil in 1931 by Pio Correa, who wrote about an infusion of carqueja being used for sterility in women and impotency in men. Correa described carqueja as having the therapeutic properties of a tonic, bitter, fever reducer, and digestive aid, with cited uses for dyspepsia, gastroenteritis, liver diseases, and diarrhea. Carqueja has long been used in Brazilian medicine to treat liver diseases, to strengthen stomach and intestinal function, and to help purge obstructions of the liver and gallbladder. Almost every book published in Brazil on herbal medicine includes carqueja, since it has shown to be so effective for liver and digestive disorders, as well as being a good blood cleanser and fever reducer. Other popular uses for carqueja in Brazilian herbal medicine today are to treat malaria, diabetes, stomach ulcers, sore throat and tonsillitis, angina, anemia, diarrhea, indigestion, urinary inflammation, kidney disorders, intestinal worms, leprosy, and poor blood circulation. In Peruvian herbal medicine today, carqueja is used for liver ailments, gallstones, diabetes, allergies, gout, intestinal gas and bloating, and sexually transmitted diseases.

PLANT CHEMICALS

Carqueja is a rich source of flavonoids. Certain flavonoids, such as silymarin in milk thistle, have shown liver-protective properties and are used for many liver conditions in herbal medicine systems. Carqueja is rather like the South American version of milk thistle. It contains up to 20 percent flavonoids, including quercetin, luteolin, nepetin, apigenin, and hispidulin. The flavonoids are considered carqueja's main active constituents. Several novel plant chemicals called clerodane diterpenoids have been identified in carqueja and, in 1994, scientists showed that these chemicals had maximum effects against worms.[1] This could possibly explain carqueja's long history of use as an agent to expel intestinal worms.

Carqueja contains many chemicals: 3,5-dicaffeoylquinic acid, alpha-phellandrene, alpha-terpinene, alpha-ylangene, beta-caryophyllene, beta-phellandrene, beta-pinene, calacorene, camphene, carquejol, cirsimaritin, clerodane diterpenoids, elemol, eriodictyol, essential oils, eudesmol, eugenol, eupatorin, eupatrin, farnesene, farnesol, flavonoids, genkwanin, germacrene D, glycosides, hispidium, hispidulin, ledol, limonene, linalool, luteolin, muurolene, myrcene, neptin, nerolidol, palustrol, pentadecanol, quercetin, resins, sabinene, saponins, spatholenol, spathulenol, squalene, terpinolene, viridiflorene, and viridiflorol.

BIOLOGICAL ACTIVITIES AND CLINICAL RESEARCH

Carqueja's liver protective properties were confirmed in a clinical study when a crude flavonoid fraction of carqueja, as well as a crude leaf/stem extract, dose-dependently increased the survival rate to 100 percent in mice administered lethal dosages of phalloidin—a liver toxin (as compared to only a 24 percent survival rate in the control group).[2] While these scientists indicated that the single flavonoid hispidulin evidenced the highest liver-protective effect of the flavonoids tested (it increased survival to 80 percent), the crude extract and the whole flavonoid fraction provided a stronger liver detoxifying and protective effect than the single flavonoid. This led to the conclusion that other constituents in the crude extract, besides the flavonoids, had liver-protective effects and/or there were interactions between the flavonoids and other plant chemicals that potentiated the flavonoids' effects.

Animal research confirms carqueja's antacid, anti-ulcer, and liver protective benefits.

Other traditional uses of carqueja have been studied and validated by research. Its antacid, anti-ulcer, and hypotensive properties were documented in two Brazilian animal studies in 1992.[3-4] Its anti-ulcer and pain-relieving properties were reported in a 1991 clinical study that showed that carqueja reduced gastric secretions and had an analgesic effect in rats with *H. pylori* ulcers. That study concluded that carqueja "may relieve gastrointestinal disorders by reducing acid secretion and gastrointestinal hyperactivity."[5] A later study, in 2000, confirmed its antiulcerogenic effect when a water extract of carqueja administered to rats protected them from alcohol-induced ulcers.[6] Other researchers documented carqueja's pain-relieving effects.[7] This same research group in Spain also reported a strong anti-inflammatory effect—a 70 percent to 90 percent inhibition—when mice were treated with the carqueja extract prior to being treated with various chemicals that induced inflammation. [7]

Carqueja has also long been used in South America as a natural aid for diabetes, and several studies confirm its blood sugar-lowering effect in mice, rats, and humans (in both normal and diabetic subjects).[8-10]

Finally, carqueja's traditional use for colds, flu, and stomach viruses has also been verified by research. Some of the more recent research has focused on its antiviral properties. In a clinical study published in 1999, researchers in Spain reported that a water extract of carqueja showed *in vitro* antiviral actions against Herpes simplex I and *Vesicular stomatitis* viruses at low dosages.[11] Researchers in Texas had already reported in 1996 that a water extract of carqueja provided an *in vitro* inhibition of HIV virus replication in T-cells.[12] In subsequent research, they have attributed this anti-HIV effect to a single chemical found in the water extract of carqueja—3,5-dicaffeoylquinic acid—and reported that this plant chemical is a potent inhibitor of HIV at dosages as low as only 1 mcg/ml.[13]

CURRENT PRACTICAL USES

Carqueja is one of the more widely known and used medicinal plants in Brazil and other parts of South America. It is as popular in Brazil as a natural herbal liver and digestive aid as milk thistle is in the United States and Europe. Many of its traditional uses have been verified by research, and it appears in the official pharmacopoeias of several South American countries as a specific liver and digestive aid. Carqueja is considered safe and nontoxic. Toxicity studies with rats indicated no toxic effects when various leaf/stem extracts were given at up to 2 g/kg in body weight.[6]

Herbalists and natural health practitioners in the United States are just learning of the many effective uses of carqueja. They document that it helps strengthen digestive, ileocecal valve, stomach, and liver functions; fortifies, cleanses and detoxifies the blood and the liver; expels intestinal worms; is helpful for poor digestion, liver disorders, anemia, or loss of blood; and removes obstructions in the gallbladder and liver.

| Traditional Preparation | Traditionally, 2 g in capsules or tablets or 2–4 ml of a standard tincture are taken with each meal as a digestive aid or liver remedy. Alternatively, a standard infusion is prepared with 5 g (about a teaspoon) of dried herb to 4–6 ounces water and infused for ten minutes. This traditional remedy is usually taken two or three times daily with meals as a digestive aid. For topical use (pain and inflammation), 60 g of herb (about 2 ounces) is decocted in 1 liter of water and applied to the affected area. |

Traditional
Preparation
Traditionally, 2 g in capsules or tablets or 2–4 ml of a standard tincture are taken with each meal as a digestive aid or liver remedy. Alternatively, a standard infusion is prepared with 5 g (about a teaspoon) of dried herb to 4–6 ounces water and infused for ten minutes. This traditional remedy is usually taken two or three times daily with meals as a digestive aid. For topical use (pain and inflammation), 60 g of herb (about 2 ounces) is decocted in 1 liter of water and applied to the affected area.

Contraindications
Carqueja should not be used during pregnancy, as it has demonstrated uterine stimulant and abortive effects in rats.[10]

The use of this plant is contraindicated in persons with low blood pressure due to its documented hypotensive effects. Persons with any heart condition or taking heart medications should check with their physician prior to using this plant.

Carqueja has been documented to lower blood glucose levels in human and animal studies. As such, it is contraindicated in persons with hypoglycemia, and people with diabetes should check with their doctor prior to using this plant, and use with caution while monitoring their blood sugar levels accordingly.

Drug Interactions
Carqueja may potentiate the effects of antihypertensive drugs and insulin and antidiabetic drugs.

Carqueja may speed the clearance of some drugs metabolized in the liver, thereby reducing the pharmacological effect and/or side effects of drugs that are metabolized in the liver.

Worldwide Ethnomedical Uses

Region	Uses
Bolivia	for abortions, digestion, gastrointestinal problems, ulcers
Brazil	for abortions, acid stomach, anemia, angina, anorexia, bile disorders, blood purification, bronchitis, Chagas disease, circulation, colds, constipation, detoxification, diabetes, diarrhea, digestion disorders, dyspepsia, edema, fevers, flu, gallstones, gallbladder disorders, gastritis, gastroenteritis, gout, heartburn, high cholesterol, hypertension, ileocecal disorders, impotence, indigestion, intestinal disorders, intestinal parasites, kidney stones, leprosy, liver detoxification, liver disorders, liver protection, malaria, nausea, obesity, rheumatism, sexually transmitted diseases, sore throat, spleen disorders, stomach problems, sterility, tonsillitis, ulcers (gastric), ulcers (skin), urinary insufficiency, urinary tract disorders, worms
Colombia	for stopping bleeding, promoting menstruation, ulcers, wounds
Paraguay	for diabetes, high cholesterol, infertility
Peru	for bloating, bronchopulmonary disorders, diabetes, digestive disorders, dislocations, flu, gallstones, gastritis, gastrointestinal disorders, gout, intestinal gas, liver diseases, malaria, rheumatic pain, promoting menstruation, sexually transmitted diseases, stomachache, urinary disorders, uterine problems

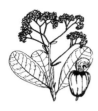

CASHEW
HERBAL PROPERTIES AND ACTIONS

Main Actions	Other Actions	Standard Dosage
• kills bacteria	• reduces inflammation	Leaf, Bark
• stops diarrhea	• suppresses coughs	**Decoction:** $^1/_2$ cup 2–3
• kills germs	• increases libido	times daily
• dries secretions	• aids digestion	
• increases urination	• reduces fever	
	• lowers blood sugar	
	• reduces blood pressure	
	• lowers body temperature	

Family: Anacardiaceae

Genus: *Anacardium*

Species: *occidentale*

Common Names: cajueiro, cashew, cashu, casho, acajuiba, caju, acajou, acaju, acajaiba, alcayoiba, anacarde, anacardier, anacardo, cacajuil, cajou, gajus, jocote maranon, maranon, merey, noix d'acajou, pomme cajou, pomme, jambu, jambu golok, jambu mete, jambu monyet, jambu terong

Parts Used: fruit, leaves, bark, nut/seed

Cashew is a multipurpose tree of the Amazon that grows up to 15 m high. It has a thick and tortuous trunk with branches so winding that they frequently reach the ground. Cashew trees are often found growing wild on the drier, sandy soils in the central plains of Brazil, and are cultivated in many parts of the Amazon rainforest.

The cashew tree produces many resources and products. The bark and leaves of the tree are used medicinally, and the cashew nut has international appeal and market value as a food. Even the shell oil around the nut is used medicinally and has industrial applications in the plastics and resin industries for its phenol content. Then, there is the pseudo-fruit—a swollen peduncle that grows behind the real fruit that yields the cashew nut. The pseudo-fruit, a large pulpy and juicy part, has a fine sweet flavor and is commonly referred to as the "cashew fruit" or the "cashew apple." Fresh or frozen cashew fruit concentrate is as common a juice product in South American food stores as orange juice is in the United States. It is very perishable, however; therefore, no fresh cashew fruit is exported into the United States or Europe from South America.

The cashew nut is defined botanically as the fruit. It grows externally in its own kidney-shaped hard shell at the end of this pseudo-fruit, or peduncle. The nut kernel inside is covered with an inner shell, and between the two shells is a thick, caustic, and toxic oil called cardol. Cashew nuts must be cleaned to remove the cardol, and then roasted or boiled to remove the toxins before they can be eaten.

TRIBAL AND HERBAL MEDICINE USES

Native to the northeast coast of Brazil, cashew was domesticated long before the arrival of Europeans at the end of the fifteenth century. It was "discovered" by European traders and explorers and first recorded in 1578. It was taken from Brazil to India and East Africa, where it soon became naturalized. In sixteenth-century Brazil, cashew fruits and their juice were taken by Europeans to treat fever, sweeten breath, and "conserve the stomach."

The cashew tree and its nuts and fruit have been used for centuries by the indigenous tribes of the rainforest, and it is a common cultivated plant in their gardens. The Tikuna tribe in northwest Amazonia considers the fruit juice medicinal against influenza, and they brew a tea of leaves and bark to treat diarrhea. The Wayãpi tribe in Guyana uses a bark tea as a diarrhea remedy and colic remedy for infants. Tribes in Suriname use the toxic seed oil as an external worm medicine to kill botfly larvae under the skin. In Brazil, a bark tea is used as a douche for vaginal discharge and as an astringent to stop bleeding after a tooth extraction. A wine made from the fruit is used for dysentery in other parts of the Amazon rainforest. The fruit juice and a bark tea are very common diarrhea remedies throughout the Amazon today, used by *curanderos* and local people alike.

In Peruvian herbal medicine today, cashew leaf tea (called *casho*) is employed as a common diarrhea remedy; a bark tea is used as an antiseptic vaginal douche; and the seeds are used for skin infections. In Brazilian herbal medicine, the fruit is taken for syphilis and as a diuretic, stimulant, and aphrodisiac. A leaf tea is prepared as a mouthwash and gargle for mouth ulcers, tonsillitis, and throat problems and is used for washing wounds. An infusion and/or maceration of the bark is used to treat diabetes, weakness, muscular debility, urinary disorders, and asthma. The leaves and/or the bark is also used in Brazil for eczema, psoriasis, scrofula, dyspepsia, genital problems, and sexually transmitted diseases, as well as for impotence, bronchitis, cough, intestinal colic, leishmaniasis, and syphilis-related skin disorders. North American practitioners use cashew for diabetes, coughs, bronchitis, tonsillitis, intestinal colic, and diarrhea, and as a general tonic.

> Cashew fruit juice and a tea made from the tree bark are very common diarrhea remedies throughout the Amazon today, used by herbal healers and local people alike.

PLANT CHEMICALS

In addition to being delicious, cashew fruit is a rich source of vitamins, minerals, and other essential nutrients. It has up to five times more vitamin C than oranges and contains a high amount of mineral salts. Volatile compounds present in the fruit include esters, terpenes, and carboxylic acids.[1] The bark and leaves of cashew are a rich source of tannins, a group of plant chemicals with documented biological activity. These tannins, in a 1985 rat study, demonstrated anti-inflammatory and astringent effects,[2] which may be why cashew is effective in treating diarrhea. Anacardic acids are found in cashew, with their highest concentration in the nutshells. Several clinical studies have shown that these chemicals curb the darkening effect of aging by inhibiting tyrosinase activity, and that they are toxic to certain cancer cells.[3–7]

The main chemicals found in cashew are alanine, alpha-catechin, alpha-linolenic acid, anacardic acids, anacardol, antimony, arabinose, caprylic acid, cardanol, cardol, europium, folacin, gadoleic acid, gallic acid, gingkol, glucuronic acid, glutamic acid, hafnium, hexanal, histidine, hydroxybenzoic acid, isoleucine, kaempferols, L-epicatechin, lauric acid, leucine, leucocyanidin, leucopelargonidine, limonene, linoleic acid, methylglucuronic acid, myristic acid, naringenin, oleic acid, oxalic acid, palmitic acid, palmitoleic acid, phenylalanine, phytosterols, proline, quercetin-glycoside, salicylic acid, samarium, scandium, serine, squalene, stearic acid, tannin, and trans-hex-2-enal tryptophan.

BIOLOGICAL ACTIVITIES AND CLINICAL RESEARCH

Cashew's antimicrobial properties were first documented in a 1982 *in vitro* study.[8] In 1999, another study was published indicating it had good *in vitro* antibacterial activity against *E. coli* and *Pseudomonas*.[9] A 2001 study reported that a bark extract exhibited *in vitro* antimicrobial activity against thirteen of fifteen microorganisms tested.[10] In 1999, researchers reported that cashew fruit exhibited antibacterial activity against *Helicobacter pylori* bacteria, which is now considered to cause acute gastritis and stomach ulcers.[11] Its effectiveness against leishmanial ulcers also was documented in two clinical studies.[12,13] Finally, two studies (one in mice and the other in rats) in 1989 and 1998 document the protective quality of a leaf extract against lab-induced diabetes.[14,15] Although the extract did not act as hypoglycemic as some others, it did stabilize blood glucose levels near pretest levels.

Cashew has demonstrated broad spectrum antibacterial actions in many laboratory tests.

CURRENT PRACTICAL USES

The different products produced from this tree offer a wide range of applications. The fruit is used to make highly nutritive snacks and juices, and fruit extracts are now being used in body-care products. Because of its high amount of vitamin C and mineral salts, cashew fruit is used as a catalyst in the treatment of premature aging of the skin and to re-mineralize the skin. It is also an effective scalp conditioner and tonic and is often used in shampoos, lotions, and scalp creams for the conditioning activity of its proteins and mucilage. Cashew leaf or bark tea is still widely used throughout the tropics as an effective diarrhea and colic remedy, considered gentle enough for children. Unfortunately, there are not many cashew products available in the U.S. market, besides of course, cashew nuts.

Traditional Preparation

The natural rainforest remedy for diarrhea and dysentery is $\frac{1}{2}$ cup of a standard decoction of leaves and twigs, taken two or three times daily.

Contraindications

Skin contact with various parts of the fresh plant (leaves, bark, fruit, fruit oil) may cause dermatitis and produce an allergic response. Cashew nuts and fruits have also been documented to cause food allergy reactions.

Drug Interactions

None reported.

Worldwide Ethnomedical Uses

Region	Uses
Africa	for malaria
Brazil	for asthma, bronchitis, corns, cough, diabetes, dyspepsia, eczema, fever, genital disorders, impotence, intestinal colic, leishmaniasis, libido stimulation, muscular debility, pain, psoriasis, scrofula, sexually transmitted diseases, syphilis, throat (sore), tonsillitis, ulcers (mouth), urinary disorders, urinary insufficiency, warts, wounds, and as a gargle and mouthwash
Haiti	for cavities, diabetes, stomatitis, toothache, warts
Malaysia	for constipation, dermatosis, diarrhea, flu, nausea, thrush
Mexico	for diabetes, diarrhea, freckles, leprosy, skin, swelling, syphilis, ulcer, warts
Panama	for asthma, colds, congestion, diabetes, diarrhea, hypertension, inflammation
Peru	for diarrhea, flu, infection, skin infections, and as an antiseptic and douche
Trinidad	for asthma, cough, diarrhea, dysentery, dyspepsia, stomachache
Turkey	for diarrhea, fever, poisoning, warts
Venezuela	for dysentery, leprosy, sore throat, and as a gargle
Elsewhere	for asthma, colds, colic, congestion, corns, cough, debility, diabetes, diarrhea, dysentery, scurvy, skin problems, tumor, urinary insufficiency, warts

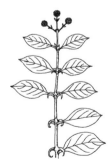

CAT'S CLAW
HERBAL PROPERTIES AND ACTIONS

Main Actions
- stimulates immune system
- reduces inflammation
- protects cells
- fights free radicals
- cleanses bowel
- kills cancer cells
- kills leukemia cells
- tones and balances

Other Actions
- relieves pain
- kills viruses
- detoxifies
- cleanses blood
- increases urination
- reduces blood pressure
- reduces cholesterol
- decreases depression

Standard Dosage

Inner Vine Bark

Decoction: 1 cup twice daily

Capsules/Tablets: 1–2 g two or three times daily

Fluid Extracts: 2–4 ml twice daily

Tinctures: 2–4 ml twice daily

Standardized Extracts: follow the label instructions

Family: Rubiaceae

Genus: *Uncaria*

Species: *tomentosa*, *guianensis*

Common Names: cat's claw, uña de gato, paraguayo, garabato, garbato casha, samento, toro, tambor huasca, uña huasca, una de gavilan, hawk's claw, saventaro

Parts Used: bark, root, leaves

TRIBAL AND HERBAL MEDICINE USES

Cat's claw has been used medicinally by the Aguaruna, Asháninka, Cashibo, Conibo, and Shipibo Indian tribes of Peru for at least 2,000 years.

Cat's claw (*U. tomentosa*) is a large, woody vine that derives its name from hook-like thorns that grow along the vine and resemble the claws of a cat. Two closely related species of *Uncaria* are used almost interchangeably in the rainforests: *U. tomentosa* and *U. guianensis*. Both species can reach over 30 m high into the canopy. *U. tomentosa* has small, yellowish-white flowers, whereas *U. guianensis* has reddish-orange flowers and thorns that are more curved. Cat's claw is indigenous to the Amazon rainforest and other tropical areas of South and Central America, including Peru, Colombia, Ecuador, Guyana, Trinidad, Venezuela, Suriname, Costa Rica, Guatemala, and Panama.

There are other species of plants with a common name of cat's claw (or *uña de gato*) in Mexico and Latin America; however, they are entirely different plants, not belonging to the *Uncaria* genus, or even the Rubiaceae family. Several of the Mexican *uña de gato* varieties have toxic properties.

Both South American *Uncaria* species are used by the indigenous peoples of the Amazon rainforest in very similar ways and have long histories of use. Cat's claw (*U. tomentosa*) has been used medicinally by the Aguaruna, Asháninka, Cashibo, Conibo, and Shipibo tribes of Peru for at least 2,000 years. The Asháninka Indian tribe in central Peru has the longest recorded history of use of the plant. They are also the largest commercial source of cat's claw from Peru today. The Asháninka use cat's claw to treat asthma, inflammations of the urinary tract, arthritis, rheumatism, and bone pain; to recover from childbirth; as a kidney cleanser; to cure deep wounds; to control inflammation and gastric ulcers; and for cancer. Indigenous tribes in Piura region of Peru use cat's claw to treat tumors, inflammations, rheumatism, and gastric ulcers. Other Peruvian indigenous tribes use cat's claw to treat diabetes, urinary tract cancer in women, hemorrhages, menstrual irregularity, cirrhosis, fevers, abscesses, gastritis, rheumatism, tumors, and inflammations as well as for internal cleansing and to "normalize the body." Reportedly, cat's claw has also been used as a contraceptive by several different tribes of Peru (but only in very large dosages). Fernando Cabieses, MD, a noted authority on Peruvian medicinal plants, explains that the Asháninka boil 5 to 6 kg (about 12 lbs.) of the root in water until it is reduced to little more than 1 cup. This decoction is then taken (1 cup daily) during the period of menstruation for three consecutive months; this supposedly causes sterility for three to four years.[1]

Cat's claw has been used in Peru and Europe since the early 1990s as an adjunctive treatment for cancer and AIDS, as well as for other diseases that target the immune system.[2–4] In herbal medicine today, cat's claw is employed around the world for many different conditions, including immune disorders, gastritis, ulcers, cancer, arthritis, rheumatism, rheumatic disorders, neuralgias, chronic inflammation of all kinds, and such viral diseases as herpes zoster (shingles). Brent Davis, DC, has written several articles on cat's claw and refers to it as the "opener of the way" for its ability to cleanse the entire intestinal tract and its effectiveness in treating stomach and bowel disorders (such as Crohn's disease, leaky bowel syndrome, ulcers, gastritis, diverticulitis, and other inflammatory conditions of the bowel, stomach, and intestines). Julian Whitaker, MD, reports using cat's claw for its immune-stimulating effects, for cancer, to help prevent strokes and heart attacks, to reduce blood clots, and for diverticulitis and irritable bowel syndrome.

PLANT CHEMICALS

Alkaloid chemicals in cat's claw are the subject of four U.S. patents indicating they increase immune function by up to 50 percent in relatively small amounts.

Cat's claw has several groups of plant chemicals that account for much of the plant's actions and uses. First and most studied is a group of oxidole alkaloids that has been documented with immune-stimulant and antileukemic properties. Another group of chemicals called quinovic acid glycosides have documented anti-inflammatory and antiviral actions. Antioxidant chemicals (tannins, catechins, and procyanidins) as well as plant sterols (beta-sitosterol, stigmasterol, and campesterol) account for the plant's anti-inflammatory properties. A class of compounds known as carboxyl alkyl esters found in cat's claw has been documented with immunostimulant, anti-inflammatory, anticancerous, and cell-repairing properties.

Cat's claw contains ajmalicine, akuammigine, campesterol, catechin, carboxyl alkyl esters, chlorogenic acid, cinchonain, corynantheine, corynoxeine, daucosterol, epicatechin, harman, hirsuteine, hirsutine, iso-pteropodine, loganic acid, lyaloside, mitraphylline, oleanolic acid, palmitoleic acid, procyanidins, pteropodine quinovic acid glycosides, rhynchophylline, rutin, sitosterols, speciophylline, stigmasterol, strictosidines, uncarine A through F, and vaccenic acid.

BIOLOGICAL ACTIVITIES AND CLINICAL RESEARCH

Clinical research confirms that cat's claw vine-bark extracts boost immune function, which have been used since the 1980s in Europe for immune-related conditions.

With so many documented traditional uses of this important rainforest plant, it is not surprising that it came to the attention of Western researchers and scientists. Studies began in the early 1970s when Klaus Keplinger, a journalist and self-taught ethnologist from Innsbruck, Austria, organized the first definitive work on cat's claw. Keplinger's work in the 1970s and 1980s led to several extracts of cat's claw being sold in Austria and Germany as herbal drugs,[2–4] as well as the filing of four U.S. patents describing extraction procedures for the immune-stimulating oxindole alkaloids.[5–8] These novel oxindole alkaloids fueled worldwide interest in the medicinal properties of this valuable vine of the rainforest. Other independent researchers in Spain, France, Japan, Germany, and Peru followed Keplinger, many of them confirming his research on the immuno-stimulating alkaloids in the vine and root. Many of these studies published from the late 1970s to early 1990s indicated that the whole oxindole alkaloid fraction, whole vine bark and/or root bark extracts, or six individually-tested oxindole alkaloids, when used in relatively small amounts, increased immune function by up to 50 percent.[9–16] These study results were substantiated by Canadian researchers at the University of Ottawa (1999) and by Peruvian researchers (1998), both working with whole vine extract.[17,18]

Proprietary extracts of cat's claw have been manufactured since 1999. Clinical studies, funded by the manufacturers of these extracts, have been published showing that these cat's claw products continue to provide the same immune-stimulating benefits as has been documented for almost twenty years.[19–22]

But then facts concerning cat's claw's benefits became confusing, as often happens with market-driven research. A manufacturer of a cat's claw extract funded a test tube study about these immune-stimulating alkaloids. The research indicated that, supposedly, two different types (chemotypes) of cat's claw vines are growing in the rainforest, and/or that cat's claw produces "good alkaloids" and "bad alkaloids." It has coined the "good ones" pentacyclic (POA) alkaloids and the "bad ones" tetracyclic (TOA) alkaloids; both are oxindole alkaloids. The research and marketing attempt to suggest that one set of "bad alkaloids" counteracts the immune benefits of the "good alkaloids."

This research has not been confirmed by independent researchers—that is, those who are not selling cat's claw or being paid by companies selling cat's claw. This research has also not been confirmed in humans or animals. This market-driven research would seek to discount or disprove all the definitive, independent research done over the last three decades in Japan, Peru, Germany, Spain, and the United States (including the four U.S. patents filed by these same researchers). Much of the previous independent research was performed on whole oxindole extracts and whole root or vine extracts (some in humans and animals). This research documented the presence of both types of alkaloids, both of which showed immune-stimulant actions. Indeed, some of the "new research" refuted the marketer's original (and independently confirmed) findings! As for the possibility of a new chemotype: a plant doesn't change its chemical constituency in five years. Again, two species of cat's claw exist—*U. tomentosa* and *U. guianensis;* they have a similar chemical makeup but a different ratio of oxindole alkaloids. Admittedly *U. tomentosa* has declined in the Peruvian rainforest because of overharvesting in the last five to eight years. The lower growing and easier-to-find *U. guianensis* variety is a common "adulterant" in many large lots of cat's claw bulk material being exported out of South America today.

In addition to its immune-stimulating activity, *in vitro* anticancerous properties have been documented for these alkaloids and other constituents in cat's claw. Five of the oxindole alkaloids have been clinically documented with *in*

Unsubstantiated product-sponsored research has confused consumers about the long-established and well-researched immune-stimulating effects of cat's claw's oxindole alkaloids.

Recent research has reported that cat's claw may provide an anticancerous action (especially against breast cancer cells) and may be beneficial in reducing chemotherapy side effects.

vitro antileukemic properties,[25] and various root and bark extracts have demonstrated antitumorous and anticancerous properties.[2,26–30] Italian researchers reported in a 2001 *in vitro* study that cat's claw directly inhibited the growth of a human breast cancer cell line by 90 percent,[31] while another research group reported that it inhibited the binding of estrogens in human breast cancer cells *in vitro*.[32] Swedish researchers documented it inhibited the growth of lymphoma and leukemia cells *in vitro* in 1998.[33] Early reports on Keplinger's observatory trials with cancer patients—taking cat's claw in conjunction with such traditional cancer therapies as chemotherapy and radiation—reported fewer side effects to the traditional therapies (such as hair loss, weight loss, nausea, secondary infections, and skin problems).[2] Subsequent researchers have shown how these effects might be possible—they have reported that cat's claw can aid in DNA cellular repair and prevent cells from mutating; it also can help prevent the loss of white blood cells and immune cell damage caused by many chemotherapy drugs (a common side effect called leukopenia).[19–21]

Another significant area of study has focused on cat's claw's anti-inflammatory properties. While plant sterols and antioxidant chemicals found in cat's claw account for some of these properties, new and novel plant chemicals called *quinovic acid glycosides* were documented to be the most potent anti-inflammatory constituents of the plant.[34] This study and subsequent ones indicated that cat's claw (and, especially, its glycosides) could inhibit inflammation from 46 percent up to 89 percent in various *in vivo* and *in vitro* tests.[35–41] The results of these studies validated its long history of indigenous use for arthritis and rheumatism, as well as for other types of inflammatory stomach and bowel disorders. It was also clinically shown to be effective against stomach ulcers in an *in vivo* rat study.[42]

Other research validates cat's claw's long history of indigenous use for arthritis and rheumatism, as well as for other types of inflammatory stomach and bowel disorders.

Research in Argentina reports that cat's claw is an effective antioxidant;[43] other researchers in 2000 concluded that it is an antioxidant as well as a remarkably potent inhibitor of tumor necrosis factor (TNF) alpha production. TNF represents a model for tumor growth driven by an inflammatory cytokine chemical.[44] Other researchers in the United States reported in 2002 that the anti-inflammatory actions of cat's claw are not attributable to immune-stimulating alkaloids, but rather to another group of chemicals called *carboxyl alkyl esters*.[45] This would explain why a product comprised of mostly alkaloids showed only modest benefit to arthritis patients—in a study by another group that was incidentally selling a special alkaloid preparation of cat's claw.[46] The same group of anti-inflammatory glycoside chemicals also demonstrated *in vitro* antiviral properties in another earlier study.[47]

In addition to the immunostimulant alkaloids, cat's claw contains the alkaloids rhynchophylline, hirsutine, and mitraphylline, which have demonstrated

Cat's claw most recently has shown possible applications for heart function, Alzheimer's disease, and mild depression.

the ability to lower blood pressure and dilate blood vessels.[48,49] Rhyncho-phylline has shown to prevent blood clots in blood vessels, dilate peripheral blood vessels, lower the heart rate, and lower blood levels of cholesterol.[49,50] Some of the newer research indicates that cat's claw might be helpful to people with Alzheimer's disease; this could be attributable to the antioxidant effects already confirmed or, possibly, to the dilation of peripheral blood vessels in the brain by alkaloids such as rhynchophylline.[51,52]

Another research group recently reported that cat's claw's immune-stimu-lating alkaloids pteropodine and isopteropodine might have other properties and applications. They reported that these two chemicals have shown to have a positive modulating effect on brain neurotransmitters called *5-HT(2) receptors*.[53] These receptor sites are targets for drugs used in treating a variety of conditions, including depression, anxiety, eating disorders, chronic pain conditions, and obesity.[54]

CURRENT PRACTICAL USES

Cat's claw has grown quite popular in the natural products industry and is mostly taken today to boost immune function, as an overall tonic and preventative to stay healthy, for arthritis and inflammation, for bowel and colon problems, and as a complementary therapy for cancer. The most common forms used today are cat's claw capsules and tablets, both of which have become widely available in most health food stores at reasonable prices. There are also newer (and more expensive) proprietary extracts of cat's claw in tablets and capsules, some backed by research—albeit paid-for research.

A good-quality, natural cat's claw vine-bark with naturally occurring chemicals is the best value, money wise. It contains all the chemicals that nature provides in the proper ratio (including immune-stimulating alkaloids, anti-inflammatory glycosides, and antioxidant chemicals), without chemical intervention. Some invasive extraction and manufacturing techniques may only extract one particular type of chemical, or change the complex ratio of naturally occurring chemicals in the plant—which ignores the efficiency and synergy of the plant. Scientists do not fully know how all these complex chemicals work together in harmony. In fact, scientists are still discovering new and novel active chemicals in this plant, even after over twenty years of research on cat's claw. As the market demand has increased for this rainforest plant over the last five years, more companies have gone into the business of harvesting it, and the quality of the bulk materials coming in from South America can be sometimes questionable. Oftentimes, a combination of *U. tomentosa* and *U. guianensis* is harvested and sold as "cat's claw" (as, presently, the *guianensis* species is found more easily). Pick a good quality and trusted label and manufacturer for the best results and the best value.

Traditional Preparation

For general immune and prevention benefits, practitioners usually recommend 1 g daily of vine powder in tablets or capsules. Therapeutic dosages of cat's claw are reported to be as high as 20 g daily and average 2–3 g two or three times daily. Generally, as a natural aid for arthritis, bowel, and digestive problems, taking 3–5 g daily is recommended, if a good product is obtained. Alternatively, a standard vine bark decoction can be used in much the same way indigenous people of the Amazon use it. The dosage for a standard decoction for general health and maintenance is $\frac{1}{2}$–1 cup of a decoction once daily and up to 1 cup three times daily in times of special needs. Adding lemon juice or vinegar to the decoction when boiling will help extract more alkaloids and fewer tannins from the bark. Use about $\frac{1}{2}$ teaspoon of lemon juice or vinegar per cup of water. For standardized and/or proprietary extract products, follow the label instructions.

Contraindications

Cat's claw has been clinically documented with immune-stimulant effects and is contraindicated before or following any organ or bone marrow transplant or skin graft.

Cat's claw has been documented with anti-fertility properties and is contraindicated in persons seeking to get pregnant. However, this effect has not been proven to be sufficient for the product to be used as a contraceptive, and it should not be relied on for such.

Cat's claw has chemicals that can reduce platelet aggregation and thin the blood. Check with your doctor first if you are taking coumadin or other blood-thinning drugs, and discontinue use one week to ten days prior to any major surgical procedure.

Cat's claw vine bark requires sufficient stomach acid to help break down the tannins and alkaloids during digestion and to aid in absorption. Avoid taking bark capsules or tablets at the same time as antacids. Avoid taking high tannin (dark-colored) liquid extracts and tinctures directly by mouth and dilute first in water or acidic juice (such as orange juice).

Large dosages of cat's claw (3–4 g doses at a time) have been reported to cause some abdominal pain or gastrointestinal problems, including diarrhea (due to the tannin content of the vine bark) in some people. The diarrhea or loose stools tend to be mild and go away with continued use. Discontinue use or reduce dosage if diarrhea persists longer than three or four days.

Drug Interactions

Due to its immune-stimulant effects, cat's claw should not be used with medications intended to suppress the immune system, such as cyclosporin or other medications prescribed following an organ transplant. (This theory has not been proven scientifically.)

Based upon *in vivo* rat studies, cat's claw may protect against gastrointestinal damage associated with non-steroidal anti-inflammatory drugs (NSAIDs) such as ibuprofen.

Cat's claw may potentiate coumadin and blood-thinning drugs.

Worldwide Ethnomedical Uses

Region	Uses
Colombia	for dysentery, gonorrhea
French Guiana	for dysentery
Peru	for abscesses, AIDS, arthritis, asthma, blood cleansing, bone pain, cancer, cirrhosis, diabetes, diarrhea, disease prevention, dysentery, fevers, gastric ulcers, gastritis, gonorrhea, hemorrhages, herpes, immune disorders, inflammations, intestinal disorders, menstrual irregularity, kidney cleansing, prostatitis, rheumatism, shingles, skin disorders, stomach disorders, ulcers problems, urinary tract disorders, tumors, wounds
Suriname	for dysentery, intestinal disorders, wounds
United States	for arthritis, cancer, colds, colitis, Crohn's disease, depression, diverticulitis, flu, gastritis, heart support, immune disorders, inflammation, irritable bowel syndrome, leaky gut, leukemia, rheumatism, skin disorders, shingles (herpes zoster), ulcers, viruses, wounds

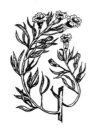

CATUABA		
HERBAL PROPERTIES AND ACTIONS		
Main Actions	**Other Actions**	**Standard Dosage**
• increases libido	• relieves pain	Bark
• calms nerves	• kills bacteria	**Infusion:** 1 cup one to three times daily
• reduces anxiety	• kills viruses	**Tincture:** 2–3 ml twice daily
	• dilates blood vessels	
	• relaxes blood vessels	

Family: Erythroxylaceae

Genus: *Erythroxylum*

Species: *catuaba*

Common Names: catuaba, cataguá, chuchuhuasha, tatuaba, pau de reposta, caramuru, piratançara, angelim-rosa, catiguá

Part Used: bark

Erythroxylum catuaba is a vigorous-growing, small tree that produces yellow and orange flowers and small, dark yellow, oval-shaped, inedible fruit. It grows in the northern part of Brazil in Amazonas, Para, Pernambuco, Bahia, Maranhao, and Alagoas. This catuaba tree belongs to the family Erythroxylaceae, whose principal genus, *Erythroxylum*, contains several species that are sources of cocaine. Catuaba, however, contains none of the active cocaine alkaloids.

A large amount of confusion exists today regarding the actual species of tree that is harvested in Brazilian forests and sold around the world as "catuaba." Experienced Brazilian harvesters will refer to two species: a "big catuaba" and a "small catuaba." The confusion thickens when relating these trees to approved botanical species names. "Small catuaba" is *Erythroxylum catuaba* (cataloged and accepted in 1936), which grows 2–4 m tall and sports yellow-to-orange flowers and—in Brazil—is referred to as *catuaba*. "Big catuaba," in the mahogany family, is *Trichilia catigua*, which grows 6–10 m tall, has cream-colored flowers and—in Brazil—is referred to as *catiguá* and *angelim-rosa*. Moreover, three other (unapproved) botanical names for catuaba are used incorrectly in herbal commerce today: *Juniperus brasiliensis* (which is thought to refer to "small catuaba"), and *Anemopaegma mirandum* and *Eriotheca candolleana*, which are completely different species altogether.

Anemopaegma is a huge tree in the Bignonia family, growing to 40 m tall and called *catuaba-verdadeira* in Brazil. This species of tree is now harvested and exported out of Brazil by inexperienced or unethical harvesters (resulting in the incorporation in herbal products sold in the U.S. today) as just "catuaba." *Erythroxylum catuaba* and *Trichilia catigua* are the preferred Brazilian herbal medicine species, with the longest documented history of use as "big and little catuaba." Both types are used interchangeably in Brazilian herbal medicine systems for the same conditions.

TRIBAL AND HERBAL MEDICINE USES

Catuaba has a long history of use in herbal medicine as an aphrodisiac. The Tupi Indians in Brazil first discovered the aphrodisiac qualities of the plant, and over the last few centuries have composed many songs praising its wonders and abilities. Indigenous and local peoples have used catuaba for generations. It is the most famous of all Brazilian aphrodisiac plants. In the Brazilian state of Minas there is a saying, "Until a father reaches 60, the son is his; after that, the son is catuaba's!"

In Brazilian herbal medicine today, catuaba is considered a central nervous system stimulant with aphrodisiac properties. A bark decoction is commonly used for sexual impotency, agitation, nervousness, nerve pain and weakness, poor memory or forgetfulness, and sexual weakness. According to Dr. Meira Penna, catuaba "functions as a stimulant of the nervous system, above all when one deals with functional impotence of the male genital organs . . . it is an innocent aphrodisiac, used without any ill effects at all."[1] In Brazil, it is regarded as an aphrodisiac with "proven efficacy" and, in addition to treating impotence, it is employed for many types of nervous conditions including insomnia, hypochondria, and pain related to the central nervous system (such as sciatica and neuralgia). In European herbal medicine, catuaba is considered an aphrodisiac and a brain and nerve stimulant. A bark tea is used for sexual weakness, impotence, nervous debility, and exhaustion. Herbalists and health practitioners in the United States use catuaba in much the same way: as a tonic for genital function, as a central nervous system stimulant, for sexual impotence,

Catuaba has a long history in herbal medicine as an aphrodisiac. The Indians in the Amazon have composed many songs praising its wonders and effects as a sexual stimulant.

general exhaustion and fatigue, insomnia related to hypertension, agitation, and poor memory. According to Michael van Straten, noted British author and researcher of medicinal plants, catuaba is beneficial to men and women as an aphrodisiac, but "it is in the area of male impotence that the most striking results have been reported" and "there is no evidence of side effects, even after long-term use."[2]

PLANT CHEMICALS

The chemical constituents found in catuaba include alkaloids, tannins, aromatic oils and fatty resins, phytosterols, cyclolignans, sequiterpenes, and flavonoids.[3–6] One Brazilian researcher documented (in 1958) that catuaba contained the alkaloid yohimbine (but it was unclear which species of tree he was studying).[3] A mixture of flavalignans, including cinchonain (also found in quinine bark), was isolated from the bark of *Trichilia catigua* and reported to have antibacterial and anticancerous properties.[6,7]

BIOLOGICAL ACTIVITIES AND CLINICAL RESEARCH

Research with animals show that catuaba can relieve pain and inhibit bacteria and viruses.

Clinical studies on catuaba also have shown results related to its antibacterial and antiviral properties. A 1992 study indicated that an extract of catuaba (*Erythoxlyum catuaba*) was effective in protecting mice from lethal infections of *Escherichia coli* and *Staphlococcus aureus,* in addition to inhibiting HIV significantly.[8] The study found that the pathway of catuaba's anti-HIV activity stemmed (at least partially) from the inhibition of HIV absorption into cells, and suggested that catuaba had potential against opportunistic infections in HIV patients.[8] A U.S. patent was granted (in 2002) to a group of Brazilian researchers for a catuaba bark extract (*Trichilia catigua*). This patent refers to animal studies that reported that it relieved pain and relaxed and dilated blood vessels in rats, rabbits, and guinea pigs.[9] A study published in 1997 reported that catuaba bark had significant pain-relieving activity *in vivo.*[10]

CURRENT PRACTICAL USES

To date, no toxicity studies have been published on catuaba—but its long history of use in Brazil has reported no toxicity or ill effects. In fact, according to Dr. Meira Penna, the only side effects are beneficial—erotic dreams and increased sexual desire! While no clinical research has validated the traditional use of catuaba as an aphrodisiac, it continues to be used widely for its ability to enhance sexual drive and increase libido in both men and women. In the last several years, its popularity has grown in the North American herbal market, with various products (especially libido formulas) now available in health food stores. Catuaba is also showing up in other formulas for depression, stress, and nervous disorders. (The jury's still out as to which species is being sold, however!) Interested consumers should seek a reputable manufacturer and product—with a verified plant source and botanical species for the herbal ingredient being sold.

Traditional Preparation	Generally, in Brazil, a standard infusion (bark tea) and an alcohol tincture are employed. Recommended usage is reported to be 1–3 cups of an infusion daily, or 2–3 ml of a standard alcohol tincture twice daily.
Contraindications	None known.
Drug Interactions	None known.

Worldwide Ethnobotanical Uses

Region	Uses
Brazil	as an aphrodisiac, central nervous system stimulant, and tonic; for exhaustion, fatigue, forgetfulness, frigidity, general pain, genitals, hypochondria, impotence, insomnia, nerve pain, nervousness, poor memory, sexual weakness, sleep, syphilis
Peru	for skin cancer
United States	as an aphrodisiac, stimulant, and tonic; for fatigue, impotency, insomnia, nervous exhaustion, nervous system weakness, pain, poor memory, sleep, weakness
Elsewhere	for brain, circulation, fatigue, genitals, impotence, low libido, nervous system

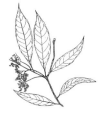

Family: Boraginaceae

Genus: *Cordia*

Species: *salicifolia, ecalyculata*

Common Names: chá de bugre, porangaba, cafezinho, café do mato, claraiba, café de bugre, cha de frade, louro-salgueiro, louro-mole, boid d'inde, bois d'ine, coquelicot, grao-do-porco, bugrinho, chá-de-negro-mina, laranjeira-do-mato, rabugem

Parts Used: leaves, fruit, bark

CHÁ DE BUGRE
HERBAL PROPERTIES AND ACTIONS

Main Actions
- decreases appetite
- reduces cellulite
- increases urination
- supports heart
- stimulates

Other Actions
- kills viruses
- reduces fever

Standard Dosage
Leaves

Infusion: 1 cup $\frac{1}{2}$ to 1 hour before meals

Tincture: 2–3 ml two to three times daily

Tablets/Capsules: 2–3 g twice daily

Chá de bugre is a small tree growing 8–12 m in height with a trunk 30–40 cm in diameter. It is indigenous to Brazil and can be found growing predominately in the Brazilian states of Minas Gerais, Bahia, Acre, and Goias. It is also found in tropical forest areas of Argentina and Paraguay. In Brazil, the tree is botanically classified as *Cordia salicifolia* and in Paraguay the same tree is classified as *Cordia ecalyculata*. In Brazil, it is commonly called *café do mato* (coffee of the woods) because it produces a red fruit resembling a coffee bean, which is roasted and brewed into tea as a coffee substitute.

TRIBAL AND HERBAL MEDICINE USES

Chá de bugre, which suppresses the appetite and reduces cellulite, is one of the most popular dieting aids in Brazil.

Chá de bugre products are highly commercialized as a weight-loss aid in Brazil, where tea bags, fluid extracts, and tinctures of chá de bugre are commonly seen in pharmacies, stores, and even in the beach-front eateries and refreshment stands along Rio de Janeiro's beaches (where bikinis rule!). It has long been a popular weight-loss product, which has been marketed as a diuretic and appetite suppressant, and believed to help prevent or reduce fatty deposits and cellulite. Several years ago, an enterprising Brazilian company re-launched a chá de bugre weight-loss product, calling it by its Indian name, *porangaba*, and market demand in Brazil has been fierce ever since. Dr. G.L. Cruz in his book, *Dictionary of the Plants Used in Brazil,* recommends chá de bugre as an excellent diuretic and weight-loss aid as well as a good general heart tonic, which can help stimulate circulation. It is also used in Brazil and Haiti as a tea to help relieve coughs, regulate renal function, and reduce uric acid, and externally to heal wounds.

PLANT CHEMICALS

Despite the popularity of chá de bugre in Brazil, very little has been done to analyze the phytochemicals in the plant. At present it is known to contain caffeine, potassium, allantoin, and allantoic acid. The red fruits or berries of chá de bugre (resembling a coffee bean) contain caffeine. The allantoin and allantoic acid may explain the traditional use of the plant for wound healing.[1] Main plant chemicals include allantoin, allantoic acid, caffeine, and potassium.

BIOLOGICAL ACTIVITIES AND CLINICAL RESEARCH

Research has validated chá de bugre's traditional use to support heart function.

Since chá de bugre is a commonly sold and popular natural product already, very little clinical research or interest has been shown to study the plant in Brazil. A Japanese university, however, has discovered some new uses for chá de bugre. In 1990, they demonstrated that a leaf extract reduced herpes virus penetration by 99 percent when they pretreated cells with the extract.[2] In 1994, they demonstrated that the herpes virus yield was reduced by 33 percent with as little as 0.25 mcg/ml, and also discovered that it had toxic activity against cancer cells (demonstrating a 40 percent inhibition), utilizing an extract of the branches and leaves.[3] Then, in 1997, research with rabbits and guinea pigs validated the traditional use of the plant as a heart tonic when cardiotonic and increased cardiovascular actions (using a leaf extract) was reported.[4]

CURRENT PRACTICAL USES

One certainly sees less cellulite on Rio's beaches than most American beaches, however, this phenomenon is probably *not* attributed to just chá de bugre! Whether it is called chá de bugre or porangaba, it will probably long be sold as a natural weight-loss aid in Rio and throughout Brazil. It is a great appetite suppressant—but rather than cutting off appetite all together (then causing intense hunger when it wears off at the wrong time) it gives one a sense of being full and satiated after eating only a few bites of food. This seems to promote much smaller meals, more often, which is what many practitioners believe is better for sustained weight loss and keeping the metabolism going throughout the day. It works best if taken thirty minutes to one hour prior to a meal. Chá de bugre is not widely available in the U.S. market today, but give it some time . . . these types of natural weight-loss aids are just as popular (and profitable) here as they are in South America—especially if they work.

Traditional Preparation One cup of a leaf infusion two to three times daily, thirty minutes before meals, or 2–3 ml of a 4:1 leaf tincture twice daily. If desired, 2–3 g of powdered leaf in tablets or capsules, one to three times daily, can be substituted.

Contraindications None reported.

Drug Interactions None reported.

Worldwide Ethnomedical Uses

Region	Uses
Brazil	as a circulatory stimulant, diuretic, and heart tonic; for arthritis, cellulite, circulatory insufficiency, cough, energy, fever, gout, kidney stones, obesity, renal insufficiency, rheumatism, wounds
Haiti	as a digestive stimulant, for obesity
Japan	as an antiviral, for herpes

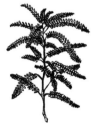

Family: Euphorbiaceae

Genus: *Phyllanthus*

Species: *niruri, amarus*

Common Names: chanca piedra, quebra pedra, stone-breaker, arranca-pedras, punarnava, amli, bhonya,

CHANCA PIEDRA
HERBAL PROPERTIES AND ACTIONS

Main Actions
- expels stones
- supports kidneys
- increases urination
- relieves pain
- protects liver
- detoxifies liver
- reduces spasms
- reduces inflammation
- kills viruses
- clears obstructions
- aids digestion
- reduces blood sugar
- lowers blood pressure
- lowers cholesterol

Other Actions
- kills bacteria
- treats malaria
- prevents mutation
- reduces fever
- mildly laxative
- expels worms

Standard Dosage
Whole herb

Infusion: 1 cup two to three times daily

Fluid Extracts: 2–4 ml two to three times daily

Capsules/Tablets: 1–2 g twice daily

bhoomi amalaki, bhui-amla, bhui amla, bhuianvalah, bhuimy-amali, bhuin-amla, bhumyamalaki, cane peas senna, carry-me-seed, creole senna, daun marisan, derriere-dos, deye do, erva-pombinha, elrageig, elrigeg, evatbimi, gale-wind grass, graine en bas fievre, hurricane weed, jar-amla, jar amla, kizha nelli, malva-pedra, mapatan, para-parai mi, paraparai mi, pei, phyllanto, pombinha, quinine weed, sacha foster, cane senna, creole senna, shka-nin-du, viernes santo, ya-taibai, yaa tai bai, yah-tai-bai, yerba de san pablo

Parts Used: entire plant

TRIBAL AND HERBAL MEDICINE USES

Chanca piedra has been called "stone breaker" because it has been used by indigenous peoples of the Amazon as an effective remedy to eliminate kidney stones for generations.

Chanca piedra is a small, erect, weed-like herb that grows 30–40 cm in height. It is indigenous to the rainforests of the Amazon and other tropical areas throughout the world, including the Bahamas, southern India, and China. *P. niruri* is quite prevalent in the Amazon and other wet rainforests, growing and spreading freely (much like a weed). *P. urninaria* and *P. sellowianus* are closely related to *P. niruri* in appearance, chemical structure, and history of use, but typically are found in the drier tropical climates of India, Brazil, and even Florida and Texas.

The *Phyllanthus* genus contains over 600 species of shrubs, trees, and herbs distributed throughout the tropical and subtropical regions of both hemispheres. Unfortunately, there remains a great deal of confusion among scientists regarding plant identification and, in many cases, plant misidentification makes evaluation of published information difficult. *P. amarus* and *P. sellowianus* are often considered a variety of *P. niruri,* or else no distinction is made among these three species, in published clinical research. Often, one name is indicated to be synonymous with another and, sometimes, both names are used interchangeably as if referring to one plant. It became so confusing that, in the 1990s, a major reorganization of the *Phyllanthus* genus was conducted which classified *P. amarus* as a type of *P. niruri.*

The Spanish name of the plant, *chanca piedra,* means "stone breaker" or "shatter stone." It was named for its effective use by generations of Amazonian indigenous peoples in eliminating kidney stones and gallstones. In Brazil, the plant is known as *quebra-pedra* or *arranca-pedras* (which also translates to "break-stone"). It is a leading and highly effective natural remedy for kidney stones throughout South America. In addition to kidney stones, the plant is employed in the Amazon for numerous other conditions by the indigenous peoples, including colic, diabetes, malaria, dysentery, fever, flu, tumors, jaundice, vaginitis, gonorrhea, and dyspepsia. Based on its long documented history of use in the region, the plant is generally used to reduce pain, expel intestinal gas, stimulate and promote digestion, expel worms, and as a mild laxative.

Chanca piedra has a long history in herbal medicine systems in every tropical country where it grows. For the most part, it is employed for similar conditions worldwide. Its main uses are for many types of biliary and urinary conditions including kidney and gallbladder stones; for hepatitis, colds, flu, tuberculosis, and other viral infections; liver diseases and disorders including anemia, jaundice, and liver cancer; and for bacterial infections such as cystitis, prostatitis, sexually transmitted diseases, and urinary tract infections. It is also widely used for diabetes and hypertension as well as for its diuretic, pain-relieving, digestive stimulant, antispasmodic, fever-reducing, and cellular-protective properties in many other conditions.

**PLANT
CHEMICALS**

Since the mid-1960s, chanca piedra has been the subject of much phytochemical research to determine the active constituents and their pharmacological activities. It is a rich source of plant chemicals, including many which have been found only in the *Phyllanthus* genus. Many of the "active" constituents are attributed to biologically active lignans, glycosides, flavonoids, alkaloids, ellagitannins, and phenylpropanoids found in the leaf, stem, and root of the plant. Common lipids, sterols, and flavonols also occur in the plant.

The main plant chemicals in chanca piedra include alkaloids, astragalin, brevifolin, carboxylic acids, corilagin, cymene, ellagic acid, ellagitannins, gallocatechins, geraniin, hypophyllanthin, lignans, lintetralins, lupeols, methyl salicylate, niranthin, nirtetralin, niruretin, nirurin, nirurine, niruriside, norsecurinines, phyllanthin, phyllanthine, phyllanthenol, phyllochrysine, phyltetralin, repandusinic acids, quercetin, quercetol, quercitrin, rutin, saponins, triacontanal, and tricontanol.

**BIOLOGICAL
ACTIVITIES
AND CLINICAL
RESEARCH**

It is little wonder that chanca piedra is used for so many purposes in herbal medicine systems: in clinical research over the years, the plant has demonstrated liver-protective, antilithic (expels stones), pain-relieving, hypotensive, antispasmodic, antiviral, antibacterial, diuretic, antimutagenic, and hypoglycemic activities. Due to the confusion among *P. niruri*, *P. amarus*, and *P. sellowianus* over the years (and the reclassification of the genus), the research reviewed herein will encompass that which has been reported on all three of these very similar species.

Clinical research validates chanca piedra's long-standing use for kidney stones: animal research suggests that it can eliminate as well as prevent the formation of kidney stones.

The first notable area of study has validated chanca piedra's long-standing traditional use for kidney stones. In 1990, the Paulista School of Medicine in São Paulo, Brazil, conducted studies with humans and rats with kidney stones. They were given a simple tea of chanca piedra for one to three months and it was reported that the tea promoted the elimination of stones.[1] They also reported a significant increase in urine output as well as sodium and creatine excretion. Subsequently, the medical school educated new doctors about the ability to treat kidney stones with this natural remedy and now it is found in many pharmacies throughout Brazil.

In a 1999 *in vitro* clinical study, a chanca piedra extract exhibited the ability to block the formation of calcium oxalate crystals (the building blocks of most kidney stones), which indicates that it might be a useful preventative aid for people with a history of kidney stones.[2] In a 2002 *in vivo* study, researchers seeded the bladders of rats with calcium oxalate crystals and treated them for forty-two days with a water extract of chanca piedra. Their results indicated that chanca piedra strongly inhibited the growth and number of stones formed over the control group.[3] Several of the animals even passed the stones which did form. In 2003, scientists again confirmed *in vitro* that chanca piedra could help prevent the formation of kidney stones, stating, "that it may interfere with the early stages of stone formation and may represent an alternative form of treatment and/or prevention of urolithiasis."[4]

Previously (in the mid-1980s), the antispasmodic activity of chanca piedra was reported. This led researchers to surmise that "smooth muscle relaxation within the urinary or biliary tract probably facilitates the expulsion of kidney or bladder calculi."[5] Researchers had already reported chanca piedra's antispasmodic properties[6] and smooth muscle relaxant properties (including a uterine relaxant effect) in earlier studies.[7] In 1990, Nicole Maxwell reported that Dr. Wolfram Wiemann (of Nuremburg, Germany) treated over 100 kidney stone patients with chanca piedra obtained in Peru and found it to be 94 percent successful in eliminating stones within a week or two.[8]

Chanca piedra is also used in herbal medicine for gallstones and, while no research has been performed that specifically validated this use, one study does indicate that chanca piedra has an effect on gallbladder processes. In a 2002 study, Indian researchers reported that chanca piedra increased bile acid secretion in the gallbladder and significantly lowered blood cholesterol levels in rats.[9] The beneficial effects of lowering cholesterol and triglyceride levels was also confirmed by another *in vivo* (rat) study in 1985.[10]

The plant's traditional use for hypertension has been explored by research, as well. The hypotensive effects were first reported in a dog study in 1952 (in which a diuretic effect was noted also).[7] The hypotensive effects were attributed to a specific phytochemical in chanca piedra called *geraniin* in a 1988 study.[11] In 1995, Indian researchers gave human subjects with high blood pressure chanca piedra leaf powder in capsules and reported a significant reduction in systolic blood pressure, and a significant increase in urine volume and sodium excretion.[12] Chanca piedra's diuretic effect in humans was recorded as far back as 1929[13] and, in India, a tablet of chanca piedra (called *Punarnava*) is sold as a diuretic.[14]

In the above 1995 study, researchers also reported that blood sugar levels were reduced significantly in human subjects studied.[12] Two other studies with rabbits[15] and rats[16] document the hypoglycemic effect of chanca piedra in diabetic animals. Yet another study documented chanca piedra with aldose reductase inhibition (ARI) properties.[17] Aldose reductases are substances that act on nerve endings exposed to high blood sugar concentration and can lead to diabetic neuropathy and macular degeneration. Inhibitors of these substances can prevent some of the chemical imbalances that occur, and thus protect the nerve. This ARI effect of chanca piedra was attributed, in part, to a plant chemical called *ellagic acid*. This well-studied plant chemical has been documented with many other beneficial effects in numerous clinical studies (over 300 to date).

Chanca piedra has demonstrated the ability to reduce cholesterol, blood pressure, and blood sugar, as well as to increase urination. This research in animals helps validate its uses in herbal medicine for hypertension, diabetes, and high cholesterol.

Chanca piedra has shown in the laboratory to be an effective pain-reliever: a single chemical in the plant was documented to be seven times more potent than aspirin or acetaminophen.

Another area of research has focused on the pain-relieving effects of chanca piedra. So far, researchers at this Brazilian university have published six studies on their findings. The first three studies reported strong and dose-dependent pain-relieving effects in mice given extracts of chanca piedra against six different laboratory-induced pain models.[18–20] In 1996, they isolated and tested chanca piedra's hypotensive plant chemical geraniin and reported that it was seven times more potent as a pain-reliever than aspirin or acetaminophen.[21] Their last two studies (published in 2000) continued to document chanca piedra's pain-relieving effects against normal pain models in mice, and, newly-tested nerve-related pain models.[22,23] Again, they related this effect to the geraniin plant chemical and reported its ability to inhibit several neurotransmitter processes that relay and receive pain signals in the brain.[23] Unlike aspirin (which can harm the mucousal lining of the stomach and cause ulcers), geraniin has been reported to have antiulcerous properties and to protect the gastric tract, instead.[24] This pain-relieving effect is probably why so many people taking chanca piedra for kidney stones (a *very* painful affair) report such quick relief, and long before chanca piedra could actually break down and expel a stone.

The liver-protecting activity of chanca piedra is another subject which has been established in clinical research with animals and humans. These effects have been attributed to (at least) two novel plant chemicals in chanca piedra named *phyllanthin* and *hypophyllanthin*. The researchers who reported the cholesterol-lowering effects also reported that chanca piedra protected rats from liver damage induced by alcohol and normalized a "fatty liver."[10] One *in vitro* study and four *in vivo* studies (with rats and mice) document that extracts of chanca piedra effectively protect against liver damage from various chemical liver toxins.[25–28] Two human studies reported chanca piedra's liver protective and detoxifing actions in children with hepatitis and jaundice. Indian researchers reported that chanca piedra was an effective single drug in the treatment of jaundice in children,[29] and British researchers reported that children treated with a chanca piedra extract for acute hepatitis had liver function return to normal within five days.[30] Researchers in China also reported liver protective actions when chanca piedra was given to adults with chronic hepatitis.[31]

Research suggests that chanca piedra can protect, detoxify, and even help regenerate the liver.

A 2000 study even documented that chanca piedra increased the life span of mice with liver cancer from thirty-three weeks (control group without treatment) to fifty-two weeks.[32] Another research group tried to induce liver cancer in mice that had been pre-treated with a water extract of chanca piedra. Their results indicated the chanca piedra extract dose-dependently lowered tumor incidence, levels of carcinogen-metabolizing enzymes, levels of liver cancer markers, and liver injury markers.[33] Both studies indicate that the plant has a better ability to prevent and slow down the growth of tumors, rather than a direct toxic effect or ability to kill cancer cells.

It may well be that chanca piedra's documented ability to stop cells from mutating plays an important factor in this reported anticancerous activity. In several animal studies (as well as within cell cultures), extracts of chanca piedra have stopped or inhibited cells (including liver cells) from mutating in the presence of chemical substances known to create cellular mutations and DNA strand breaks (which can lead to the creation of cancerous cells).[34–37] Again, one of these studies indicated that chanca piedra inhibited several enzyme processes peculiar to cancer cells' replication and growth—rather than a direct toxic effect of killing the cancer cell (sarcoma, carcinoma, and lymphoma cells were studied).[37] This cellular-protective quality was evidenced in other research, which indicated that chanca piedra protected against chemically-induced bone marrow damage in mice,[38] as well as against radiation-induced damage in mice.[39]

The last area of published research (which is the most extensive and the most confusing) concerns chanca piedra's antiviral properties. Both human and animal studies indicate that chanca piedra can protect the liver, even during hepatitis infection. Chanca piedra has also been reported to have direct antiviral activity in human, animal, and test tube studies against the hepatitis B virus. Over twenty clinical studies have been published to date about these effects, and the results have been inconsistent and confusing (unless thoroughly evaluated).

Hepatitis is enough of a worldwide concern to merit sifting through the disparate studies. Hepatitis B infection (HBV) is the leading cause of liver cancer worldwide—which is considered 100 percent fatal. Carriers of HBV are 200 times more likely to develop liver cancer decades after initial infection. Many people who contract HBV become chronic (and, often, asymptomatic) carriers of the disease while still being contagious to others. HBV is reported to be 100 times more infectious than HIV and, like HIV, is transmitted through blood transfusions, needles, sexual contact, and *in utero* (from mother to child in the womb). Statistics on HBV are staggering: one out of every 250 Americans are HBV carriers! The Center for Disease Control (CDC) estimates that 200,000 new U.S. cases of HBV infection per year are added to the current estimate of one million carriers in the U.S. (and an estimated 300 million worldwide). The CDC also reports that (in the U.S.) 3,000–4,000 annual deaths from cirrhosis and 1,000 deaths from liver cancer are HBV-related. So when Dr. Baruch Blumberg reported that chanca piedra could clear up the chronic carrier state of hepatitis B in 1988, it was a *big* deal. Dr. Blumberg was the winner of the 1963 Nobel Prize for discovering the HBV antigen in the first place. This led to the discovery that HBV was the primary cause of liver cancer and initiated the development of HBV vaccines.

Most of Blumberg's early research was carried out in India in collaboration with an Indian research group. Their first human study reported that a water extract of *Phyllanthus amarus* cleared the HBV surface antigen from twenty-two of thirty-seven chronic HBV patients in only thirty days (and they continued to test negative for nine months, at which time the report was published).[40] This same group had published several earlier *in vitro* studies as well as animal (woodchuck) studies. (Woodchucks respond to chronic HBV infection in much the same manner as do humans, which is why they are chosen for such research.) All reported similar and effective anti-HBV effects.[41,42] By that time, Blumberg was employed with the Fox Chase Cancer Center in Philadelphia; he, Fox Chase, and the Indian researchers filed two patents on the plant's ability to treat HBV and its antiviral properties in 1985 and 1988 (now calling the plant *P. niruri*).[43,44] The first patent was specific to HBV; the second stated that the plant's antiviral properties were achieved in part through a strong inhibition of reverse transcriptase (chemicals necessary for many types of viruses to grow) which made it possible to treat such retroviruses as HIV and sarcoma and leukemia viruses.

It was also during this time that the group developed a new and "better" extraction process. This process involved multiple, complicated extractions in which the plant was first soaked in cold water, then the resulting fluid was extracted first in hexane, then in benzene, then in methanol, and back into water. The group's documentation revealed, however, that they didn't know specifically what the active chemicals were in the final extract that provided the antiviral effects! While it was certainly a complicated and patentable process, much of the subsequent published research by this group throughout the 1990s using this new, patented "water extract" conflicted with their earlier studies, and was not as effective in the *in vivo* research for HBV. This caused much confusion as to whether chanca piedra (*P. niruri* or *P. amarus*) was an effective treatment or not. To add to the confusion, in 1994, a New Zealand research group prepared a chemically altered extract (of *P. amarus*) which was standardized to the geraniin chemical content (the chemical documented with analgesic and hypotensive properties). They started a double-blind HBV human trial, later discontinued it due to lack of response, and published another negative result study.

Meanwhile, a separate research group in China (where HBV is widespread) working with a straight water extract and/or herb powder published two positive studies showing good results with human HBV patients in 1994 and 1995.[45,46] Their second study suggested that different results were obtained through different *Phyllanthus* species of plants used (and that yet another species—*P. urinaria* provided the best anti-HBV results). The Chinese published a study in 2001 that compared thirty chronic HBV patients taking a chanca piedra extract to twenty-five patients taking interferon (the leading conventional drug used for HBV) for three months. Both treatments showed an equal effectiveness of 83 percent, but the chanca piedra group rated significantly higher in the normalization of liver enzymes and recovery of liver function than the interferon-treated group.[47] The researchers published yet another study in 2003 which attributed the anti-HVB effects mainly to four chemicals in chanca piedra: niranthin, nirtetralin, hinokinin, and geraniin.[48]

Finally, The Cochrane Hepato-Biliary Research Group in Copenhagen reviewed all the HBV published research (twenty-two randomized trials) and published an independent review of the results. It stated that treatment with "*Phyllanthus* herb" (they acknowledged the confusion among the various species used) had "a positive effect on clearance of serum HBsAg" (HBV surface antigen) comparable to interferon and was better than nonspecific treatment or other herbal medicines for HBV and liver enzyme normalization.[49] They also indicated that large trials were warranted due to these documented positive effects and the lack of standardization of research methods and plant species used in the various published studies to date.

In addition to hepatitis, chanca piedra also has been studied as an antiviral agent for HIV.

Focusing on HIV specifically, a Japanese research group reported that a simple water extract of *P. niruri* inhibited HIV-1 reverse transcriptase in 1992.[50] (Several conventional drugs used today against HIV are classified as "reverse transcriptase inhibitors.") They attributed this effect to a plant chemical in chanca piedra called *repandusinic acid A*. When they tested this chemical individually it demonstrated significant toxicity to HIV-1 at very small dosages (a 90 percent *in vitro* inhibition using only 2.5 mcg). Bristol-Myers Squibb Pharmaceutical Research Institute isolated yet another chemical in chanca piedra with anti-HIV actions—a novel compound that they named *niruriside* and described in a 1996 study.[51] A German research organization published their first study on chanca piedra and its application with HIV therapy (reporting a 70–75 percent inhibition of virus) in 2003.[52] In addition to these antiviral properties, the plant has also been documented as having other antimicrobial effects. Chanca piedra demonstrated *in vitro* antibacterial actions against *Staphylococcus, Micrococcus,* and *Pasteurella* bacteria[53,54] as well as *in vivo* and *in vitro* antimalarial properties,[55,56] which validates other traditional uses.

CURRENT PRACTICAL USES

Chanca piedra is a perfect example of a highly beneficial medicinal plant which is deserving of much more research—but one which is fraught with the typical problems of working with a complicated, chemically rich plant. Unless a major (and well-funded) pharmaceutical or research company can isolate a single, patentable chemical (or can come up with a patentable extraction process that actually works as well as a simple water extract) to justify the high cost of research, chanca piedra probably will remain in the "unproven herbal remedy" category. There just aren't enough non-profit dollars or government grant funds available to fund research on natural plant extracts that can't be patented. Since chanca piedra's many biological activities and benefits are attributed to many different chemicals (whose synergistic interactions are unclear), and most seem to be completely water soluble (no complicated and patentable manufacturing processes necessary), for-profit research dollars will probably be spent elsewhere. It is yet another perfect example that Mother Nature is infinitely a better chemist; the natural herb continues to work better than any man-made chemically altered (and patentable) extracts.

But what a natural remedy it is! With its applications for kidney stones and gallstones, cellular and liver protection, hypertension and high cholesterol, cancer prevention, and its pain-relieving and antiviral effects, it is gaining in popularity on many continents as an effective herbal remedy. It is also important to note that in all the research published over the last twenty years, no signs of toxicity or side effects have been reported in any of the human or animal studies, even in acute or chronic use.

Traditional Preparation

A standard herb infusion or weak decoction is prepared as the traditional remedy. Depending on what it's employed for, 1–3 cups are taken daily. Prevention and health maintenance dosages for kidney stones are reported by practitioners to be 1–3 cups weekly, while 3–4 cups daily are used to expel existing stones. Some pharmacies in Brazil and South America sell concentrated fluid extracts or water/glycerine extracts. Depending on the concentration of the extracts, 2–6 ml are taken two to three times daily. Since most of the active chemicals are water soluble (and broken down during digestion), 2–3 g in tablets or capsules twice daily can be substituted, if desired. Alcohol tinctures have not been traditionally used with chanca piedra (as the more fragile, water-soluble plant chemicals and sterols are thought to be damaged in alcohol).

Contraindications

Chanca piedra has demonstrated hypotensive effects in animals and humans. People with a heart condition and/or taking prescription heart medications should consult their doctor before taking this plant. It may be contraindicated for such individuals and their heart medications may need monitoring and adjusting.

Chanca piedra has been considered in herbal medicine to be abortive (at high dosages) as well as a menstrual promoter. While not studied specifically in humans or animals, animal studies do indicate it has uterine relaxant effects. It should therefore be considered contraindicated during pregnancy.

Chanca piedra has been documented with female anti-fertility effects in one mouse study (the effect was reversed forty-five days after cessation of dosing).[57]

While this effect has not been documented in humans, the use of the plant is probably contraindicated in women seeking pregnancy or taking fertility drugs. This effect has not been substantiated sufficiently to be used as a contraceptive, however, and should not be relied on for such.

Chanca piedra has demonstrated hypoglycemic effects in animals and humans. It is contraindicated for people with hypoglycemia. Diabetics should consult their doctor before taking this plant, as insulin medications may need monitoring and adjusting.

Chanca piedra has been documented, in human and animal studies, with diuretic effects. Chronic and acute use of this plant may be contraindicated in various other medical conditions where diuretics are not advised. Chronic long-term use of any diuretic can cause electrolyte and mineral imbalances; however, human studies with chanca piedra (for up to three months of chronic use) have not reported any side effects. Consult your doctor concerning possible side effects of long-term diuretic use if you choose to use this plant chronically for longer than three months.

Drug Interactions Chanca piedra may potentiate insulin and antidiabetic drugs. This plant contains a naturally-occurring phytochemical called geraniin. This chemical has been documented with negative chronotropic, negative inotropic, hypotensive, and angiotensin-converting enzyme inhibitor effects in animal studies with frogs, mice, and rats.[10] As such, this plant may potentiate antihypertensive drugs, Beta-blocker drugs, and other heart medications (including chronotropic and inotropic drugs).

Worldwide Ethnomedical Uses

Region	Uses
Amazonia	for bowel inflammation, colic, constipation, diabetes, digestion stimulation, dysentery, dyspepsia, edema, fever, flu, gallstones, gonorrhea, intestinal gas, itch, jaundice, kidney aliments, kidney stones, malaria, pain, proctitis, stomachache, tumor, urinary insufficiency, urinary tract disorders, vaginitis, worms, and to stimulate menstruation
Bahamas/ Caribbean	for bacterial infections, colds, constipation, fever, flu, hyperglycemia, spasms, stomachache, typhoid, urinary insufficiency, viral infections; as an appetite stimulant, laxative, liver detoxifier, liver protector, liver tonic
Brazil	for abortions, aches (joint), albuminuria, arthritis, bacterial infections, bile stimulant, biliary conditions, bladder problems, bladder stones, blood cleanser, cancer, catarrh (liver and kidney), cystitis, diabetes, digestion stimulation, edema, fever, gallbladder stimulation, gallstones, gastritis, gastrointestinal problems, gout, hepatitis, hypertension, hypoglycemic, inflammation, jaundice, kidney colic, kidney pain, kidney stones, liver disorders, liver support, malaria, obesity, pain, prostatitis, renal colic, renal problems, spasms, tonic, uric acid excess, urinary insufficiency, urinary problems, uterine relaxant, viral infections; and as a muscle relaxant and to promote perspiration

Haiti	for bowel inflammation, colic, digestion stimulation, digestive problems, fever, flu, indigestion, intestinal gas, malaria, spasms, stomachache, urinary insufficiency
India	for anemia, asthma, bronchitis, conjunctivitis, cough, diabetes, diarrhea, digestion stimulation, dysentery, fevers, edema, eye disorders, genitourinary disorders, gonorrhea, hepatitis, jaundice, lack of milk production, menstrual disorders, ringworm, scabies, thirst, tuberculosis, tumor (abdomen), urinary insufficiency, urogenital tract infections, vaginal discharge, warts
Malaysia	for caterpillar stings, constipation, dermatosis, diarrhea, itch, miscarriage, renal disorders, syphilis, urinary insufficiency, vertigo, and to stimulate menstruation
Peru	for gallstones, hepatitis, kidney pain, kidney problems, kidney stones, urinary infections, worms, and to stimulate menstruation
United States	for bile insufficiency, bronchitis, diabetes, fever, gallbladder problems, gallstones, gout, hepatitis, hypertension, kidney problems, kidney stones, liver disease, obstructions, pain, uric acid excess, urinary tract infections, viral infections
Elsewhere	for bile insufficiency, bruises, constipation, cough, cuts, diabetes, diarrhea, dysentery, dyspepsia, edema, eye diseases, fever, gallstones, gonorrhea, itch, jaundice, kidney disease, kidney stones, malaria, menstrual problems, pain, rectitis, sexually transmitted diseases, stomachache, tuberculosis, urinary insufficiency, urinary tract infections, vaginitis

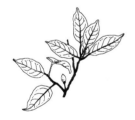

CHUCHUHUASI

HERBAL PROPERTIES AND ACTIONS

Main Actions
- reduces inflammation
- relieves pain
- relaxes muscles
- enhances immunity
- increases libido
- supports adrenals

Other Actions
- kills cancer cells
- prevents tumors
- stimulates digestion

Standard Dosage

Bark

Decoction: 1 cup two to three times daily

Tincture: 3–5 ml two to three times daily

Family: Celastraceae

Genus: *Maytenus*

Species: *krukovii*

Common Names: chuchuhuasi, chucchu huashu, chuchuasi, chuchasha, chuchuhuasha, chuchuaso, chuchumuasi, curi-caspi

Part Used: bark

Chuchuhuasi is an enormous canopy tree of the Amazon rainforest that grows to 30 m high. It has large leaves (10–30 cm), small white flowers, and extremely tough, heavy, reddish-brown bark. Several botanical names have been given to this species of tree. It is referenced as *Maytenus krukovii, M. ebenifolia, M. laevis,* and *M. macrocarpa;* however, all botanical names refer to the same tree. Chuchuhausi is indigenous to the tropical rainforests of Bolivia, Colombia, Ecuador, and Peru.

TRIBAL
AND HERBAL
MEDICINE USES

Indigenous people of the Amazon rainforest have been using the bark of chuchuhuasi medicinally for centuries. Its Peruvian name, chuchuhuasi, means "trembling back," which refers to its long-standing use for arthritis, rheumatism, and back pain. One local Indian remedy for arthritis and rheumatism calls for 1 cup of a bark decoction taken three times a day for more than a week. Local people and villagers along the Amazon believe that chuchuhuasi is an aphrodisiac and tonic, and the bark soaked in the local sugarcane rum (*aguardiente*) is a popular jungle drink that is even served in bars and to tourists (often called "go-juice" to relieve pain and muscle aches and to "keep going" during long treks in the rainforest). Local healers and *curanderos* in the Amazon use

Chuchuhuasi has long been used as a jungle remedy for arthritis, back pain and muscle spasms, as a healthy tonic to tone, balance and normalize the body, and as an aphrodisiac.

chuchuhuasi as a general tonic, to speed healing and, when combined with other medicinal plants, as a synergist for many types of illnesses. In Colombia, the Siona Indians boil a small piece of the bark (5 cm) in 2 liters of water until 1 liter remains, and drink it for arthritis and rheumatism. In the Ecuadorian rainforest, the Quijos Quichua Indians prepare a bark decoction for general aches and pains, rheumatism, sore muscles, menstrual pain, and stomachaches.

In the Peruvian Amazon, chuchuhuasi is still considered the best remedy for arthritis among both city and forest dwellers. It is also used as a muscle relaxant, aphrodisiac, and pain-reliever, for adrenal support, as an immune stimulant, and for menstrual balance and regulation. In Peruvian herbal medicine systems, chuchuhuasi alchohol extracts are used to treat osteoarthritis, rheumatoid arthritis, bronchitis, diarrhea, hemorrhoids, and menstrual irregularities and pain.

PLANT
CHEMICALS

Chuchuhausi is a powerhouse of plant chemicals—mostly triterpenes, favonols, and sesquiterpene alkaloids. Two of the more well-known chemicals in chuchuhuasi are *mayteine* and *maytansine*—alkaloids long documented (since the 1960s) with anti-tumor activity and which occur in other *Maytenus* plants as well. While these chemicals are found in chuchuhuasi, they don't occur in high enough amounts to really be therapeutic for cancer, however. Another rainforest *Maytenus* plant, espinheira santa (also featured in this book), is a much better source of these anticancerous chemicals. Other novel compounds found only in chuchuhuasi thus far include dammarane- and friedelane-type triterpenes, which are considered to be some of the plant's active constituents.[1-3]

The main plant chemicals found in chuchuhuasi include: agarofuran sesquiterpenes, canophyllol, catechin tannins, dammarane triterpenes, dulcitol, ebenifoline alkaloids, euojaponine alkaloids, friedelan triterpenes, krukovine triterpenes, laevisine alkaloids, macrocarpin triterpenes, maytansine, mayteine, maytenin, mebeverine, phenoldienones, pristimeran, proanthocyanidins, and tingenone (and its derivatives).

BIOLOGICAL ACTIVITIES AND CLINICAL RESEARCH

Chuchuhuasi's long history of use has fueled much clinical interest in the research community. In the 1960s, an American pharmaceutical company discovered potent immune-stimulating properties of a leaf extract and a bark extract, documenting that it increased phagocytosis (the ability of immune cells to attack bacteria and foreign cells) in mice.[4] Researchers in 1977 reported that alcohol extracts of the bark evidenced anti-inflammatory and analgesic activities in various studies with mice, which validated chuchuhuasi's traditional uses for arthritic pain.[5] Its anti-inflammatory action again was reported in the 1980s by an Italian research group. They reported that this activity (in addition to radiation protectant and anti-tumor properties) was at least partially linked to triterpenes and antioxidant chemicals isolated in the trunk bark.[6]

Scientists are just beginning to understand and to report why chuchuhuasi is effective for arthritis.

In 1993, a Japanese research group isolated another group of novel alkaloids in chuchuhuasi that may be responsible for its effectiveness in treating arthritis and rheumatism.[7] In the United States, a pharmaceutical company studying chuchuhuasi's anti-inflammatory and anti-arthritic properties determined that these alkaloids can effectively inhibit enzyme production of protein kinase C (PKC).[8] PKC inhibitors have attracted much interest worldwide, as there is evidence that too much PKC enzyme is involved in a wide variety of disease processes (including arthritis, asthma, brain tumors, cancer, and cardiovascular disease).[9] A Spanish research team found more new phytochemicals in 1998, one of which was cited as having activity against aldose reductase.[10] (This enzyme is implicated in nerve damage in diabetic patients.)

In the mid-1970s, Italian researchers tested a chuchuhuasi extract against skin cancers and identified its antitumorous properties.[11] They attributed these effects to two chemicals in chuchuhuasi called *tingenone* and *pristimerin*. Three groups found new and different sesquiterpene compounds in 1999, two of which showed marginal anti-tumor activity against four cell lines, and one of which was documented as effective against leishmaniasis (a tropical parasitic disease).[13–15] Other researchers found four more chemicals in the roots of chuchuhuasi (named *macrocarpins*) in 2000—three of which were documented as cytotoxic to four tumor cell lines.[12]

CURRENT PRACTICAL USES

If the constituents in chuchuhuasi responsible for inhibiting PKC can be synthesized, it is possible that a new arthritis drug will be developed. In the meantime, the natural bark of this important Amazon rainforest tree will continue to be an effective natural herbal remedy for arthritis, for adrenal support, and as an immune tonic—as it has been for centuries. It is best prepared as it has been traditionally: as an alcohol tincture or a decoction. It normally takes about three to four days of daily use to get a beneficial effect for arthritic pain, and up to a month or longer of daily use is necessary for adrenal support.

Traditional Preparation	Traditionally, 2–3 cups daily of a standard bark decoction or 2–4 ml of a standard tincture three times daily is used for this rainforest remedy.
Contraindications	None reported.
Drug Interactions	None reported.

Worldwide Ethnomedical Uses

Region	Uses
Brazil	for skin cancer
Colombia	as an aphrodisiac, pain-reliever, and for arthritis, rheumatism
Ecuador	for aches (menstrual, muscles), arthritis, fever, pain, rheumatism, stomachache, tumors (skin), and as an aphrodisiac
Peru	for aches (back, muscles), arthritis, bronchitis, cancer, diarrhea, dysentery, gastrointestinal disease, hemorrhoids, impotency, inflammation, influenza, menstrual disorders, nausea, osteoarthritis, pain, rheumatism, tumors, virility, and as an aphrodisiac

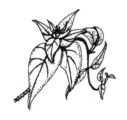

CIPÓ CABELUDO
HERBAL PROPERTIES AND ACTIONS

Main Actions	Other Actions	Standard Dosage
• relieves pain	• kills leukemia cells	Vines, Leaves
• reduces mucus	• kills cancer cells	**Infusion:** 1/2 cup twice daily
• increases urination	• calms nerves	**Tincture:** 5–10 ml twice daily
• thins blood		

Family: Asteraceae

Genus: *Mikania*

Species: *hirsutissima*

Common Names: cipó cabeludo, guaco-cabeludo, guaco peludo, cipó-almecega-cabeludo, erva dutra

Part Used: aerial parts

Cipó cabeludo is a very small, shrubby vine that grows only 13–18 cm tall and produces small, white flowers. A member of the *Mikania* genus (which comprises over 300 tropical species of climbing vines), it is indigenous to many parts of Brazil, including the Amazon region. It is also indigenous to Bolivia, Colombia, Costa Rica, Ecuador, French Guiana, Guyana, Honduras, Panama, Paraguay, Peru, Suriname, and Venezuela. In Brazil its common name is cipó cabeludo or guaco-cabeludo. It sometimes is confused with other *Mikania* vines that grow in the same regions—*Mikania guaco* or *M. cordifolia*—whose common name is "guaco" (which is also featured in this book).

TRIBAL AND HERBAL MEDICINE USES

Cipó cabeludo is widely used in Brazilian herbal medicine and highly regarded as a powerful diuretic. Its main documented uses are for cystitis, prostatitis, urethritis, gout, urinary tract infections, excessive mucus, gallstones, kidney stones, and to help lower uric acid levels in the urine and blood. It is a preferred natural remedy for nephritis and prostatitis and is considered helpful in removing excessive mucus from the urinary and bronchial tracts. It also is employed as a pain-reliever for neuralgia, chronic rheumatism and arthritis, and general muscle pain.

PLANT CHEMICALS

Chemical screening has revealed that cipó cabeludo contains coumarin, sesquiterpenes, flavonols, saponins, and kaurenoic acid derivatives.[1] These acid derivatives are chemicals that have been documented with various biological activities. Several of the known kaurenoic acids in cipó cabeludo (and other *Mikania* species) have demonstrated *in vitro* antibacterial properties against a broad range of bacteria in published research.[2,3] Cipó cabeludo (and other *Mikania* plants) contain the natural plant chemical *coumarin*. Coumadin (an anticoagulant prescription drug with blood-thinning effects) is derived and/or synthesized from this natural plant chemical. The main chemicals in this vine include coumarin, essential oils, flavonols, flavones, kaurenoic acid diterpenes, resins, saponins, and tannins.

BIOLOGICAL ACTIVITIES AND CLINICAL RESEARCH

This particular species of *Mikania* was described by a Brazilian researcher at the University of São Paulo in the early 1970s.[4,5] In the mid-eighties, other Brazilian researchers documented that an extract of cipó cabeludo had powerful molluscicidal effects (a lethal effect against adult snails) at only 10 ppm concentration.[6] This type of test generally is conducted on plants in the ongoing search for new products to treat the common and highly problematic tropical disease, schistosomiasis. More recently, cipó cabeludo has interested a research group in Japan. Their first study (in 1999) reported the discovery of two novel sesquiterpene chemicals, as well as nine other known compounds. They tested eleven of the isolated compounds against leukemia cells *in vitro* and reported that four of them "showed relatively strong cytotoxicity."[7] Their second (2000) study reported that cipó cabeludo contained five biologically active kaurenoic acids (which also occur in other *Mikania* species) as well as a novel one—which they named *mikanialactone*.[8]

Little research has been conducted thus far on cipó cabeludo; virtually none of its longstanding traditional uses have been confirmed by animal studies. Its use for various urinary infections may be related to the documented antimicrobial kaurenoic acid derivative chemicals found in the vine but, again, these

Preliminary research indicates cipó cabeludo has an anti-leukemic effect.

effects haven't been confirmed in animals or humans. One rat study in 2002 tested the anti-inflammatory effects of several *Mikania* species (some guaco species are known for their anti-inflammatory properties). While the researchers noted no anti-inflammatory effect for cipó cabeludo, they reported there were no signs of toxicity in rats at a dosage of 400 mg per kg of body weight with a standard leaf decoction.[9]

CURRENT PRACTICAL USES

Today, cipó cabeludo is mainly used in various products and formulas in Brazil for kidney problems and prostatitis. It is not widely known or used outside of Brazil and very few products are available in the U.S. market.

Traditional Preparation

In Brazilian herbal medicine, $\frac{1}{2}$ cup of a standard herb infusion once or twice daily, or 5–10 ml of a standard tincture daily is generally recommended.

Contraindications

Cipó cabeludo is used in herbal medicine as a diuretic. While these effects have not been confirmed scientifically, use of this plant may be contraindicated in various medical conditions where diuretics are not appropriate. Chronic long-term use of any diuretic can cause electrolyte and mineral imbalances as well as other medical problems and are generally not recommended; therefore, it is probably best to avoid chronic use of this plant.

While not substantiated scientifically, it is possible that cipó cabeludo may demonstrate a blood-thinning effect due to its coumarin content. Consult your doctor before using this plant if you are taking coumadin drugs (or if coumadin anticoagulant-type drugs are contraindicated for your condition).

Drug Interactions

Cipó cabeludo may potentiate coumadin and diuretic drugs.

Worldwide Ethnomedical Uses

Region	Uses
Brazil	for albuminuria, arthritis, cystitis, diarrhea, excessive mucus, gallstones, gastrointestinal disorders, gout, kidney stones, lumbago, menstrual colic, muscle pain, nephritis, neuralgia, pain, paralysis, prostatitis, renal disorders, rheumatism, urethritis, urinary insufficiency, urinary tract infections

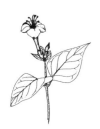

Family: Nyctaginaceae

Genus: *Mirabilis*

Species: *jalapa*

Common Names:
clavillia, four-o'clocks,
jalap, maravilla, bonina,
boa-noite, bonita, a'bbass,
beauty of the night, belle
de nuit, bella di notte,
buenas tardes, bunga
pukul empat, dondiego de
noche, false jalap, flower
of a'bbas, isabelitta,
morning rose, marvel of
Peru, nodja, noche buena,
numera, pathrachi, segera

Parts Used: roots, leaves,
flowers

CLAVILLIA		
HERBAL PROPERTIES AND ACTIONS		
Main Actions	Other Actions	Standard Dosage
• kills viruses	• kills parasites	Roots
• kills bacteria	• reduces spasms	**Infusion:** 1/2 cup twice daily
• kills fungi	• increases urination	**Tincture:** 1–2 ml twice daily
	• strongly laxative	**Capsules/Tablets:** 1 g twice daily
	• aids digestion	

Clavillia is a perennial herb that reaches a height of 50–100 cm from a tuberous root. Some cultivated hybrid species also can grow up to a meter in height. It produces beautiful flowers that usually open around four o'clock in the afternoon—hence its common name, *four o'clocks*. It is a popular ornamental plant grown worldwide for the beauty of its flowers (which can be white, red, pink, purple, or multicolored) and their sweet fragrance. It was officially botanically recorded in 1753, although it had already long been distributed as an ornamental plant throughout the tropics of the world. There is some disagreement about where it came from originally: Mexico, Chile, or India. Today, clavillia is naturalized throughout the tropics of South America, Latin America, France, and India. In Brazil the plant is known as *clavillia, maravilha,* or *bonina;* in Peru it is known as *jalapa* or *maravilla.* Hybrids of clavillia can be found in nurseries throughout the U.S. where they are sold as ornamental landscape plants.

TRIBAL AND HERBAL MEDICINE USES

The indigenous people of the Amazon enjoy the beauty of clavillia's flowers as much as city dwellers, and often plant it in their gardens. They employ the plant medicinally as well. Indigenous Peruvian people use a root decoction as a diuretic; the Shipibo-Conibo Indians put the flowers in baths to treat colds and flu. In Brazil, the Kayapo Indians inhale the powdered, dried flowers as a snuff for headaches, and use a root decoction to wash wounds and to treat such skin afflictions as leprosy. The Assuraní Indians in Brazil crush the seeds to use as a peppery condiment on foods, and grate the tuberous root into cold water and drink it for intestinal parasites. The tribal people of Orissa, India grind the roots of the plant into a paste with black pepper and take it orally for conjunctivitis. They also apply the juice of the leaves to fungal infections of the skin.

These indigenous practices impelled clavillia's presence in herbal medicine systems around the world. In Peru, the plant and/or tuber is used as a diuret-

Clavillia is used in many
tropical countries as an
herbal remedy for a
variety of viral, bacterial,
fungal, and parasitic
infections.

ic, laxative, and bowel cleanser. The juice of the flower is used to clear herpes lesions and for earaches. In Brazilian herbal medicine, a paste is made of the leaf and flower and applied to affections of the skin such as itchiness, eczema, herpes, skin spots, and skin infections. The juice of the root is dropped into the ear for earaches. Brazilians also use the root to combat worms, intestinal parasites, leucorrhea, edema, diarrhea, dysentery, abdominal colic, syphilis, and liver disorders. In Mexico, the entire plant is decocted and used for dysentery, vaginal discharge, infected wounds, and bee and scorpion stings. In the United States, the plant is used for mumps, bone fractures, and as a uterine stimulant to hasten childbirth.

PLANT CHEMICALS

Chemical analysis of clavillia shows that it is rich in many active compounds including triterpenes, proteins, flavonoids, alkaloids, and steroids. Of particular interest to researchers is a group of amino acid-based proteins, called *mirabilis antiviral proteins (MAPs)*. These chemicals have shown specific antiviral and antifungal actions. They are produced in the seeds, roots, and young shoots, and help the plant protect against various plant viruses and soil-borne fungi. In 1994, a Japanese tobacco company was awarded a U.S. patent on the MAPs in clavillia as being effective in protecting economically important crops (such as tobacco, corn, and potatoes) from a large variety of plant viruses (such as tobacco mosaic virus, spotted leaf virus, and root rot virus).[1] Researchers in Hong Kong isolated another MAP in the roots of clavillia with the same antiviral actions, and also noted, "The MAP demonstrated to possess abortifacient [abortion-causing] activity in pregnant mice, inhibitory effects on cell-free protein synthesis, and antiproliferative effects on tumor cells."[2] The MAPs found in clavillia have shown to inhibit cellular processes in viral cells.[3,4] The highest concentration of MAPs are found in the seeds of the plant, followed by the roots, then leaves.[5]

Chemicals in clavillia
have been patented
as antiviral agents.

The seeds, however, are a significant source of other peptide chemicals with actions similar to the neurotoxic peptides found in spider venom.[6] These peptides are in the same classification as (and act similarly to) another plant-derived toxic peptide, ricin (now being employed as a biological weapon). As compared with ricin, though, clavillia's peptides are only about one-thirtieth as toxic.[6] Because of this toxicity, though, the seeds are not generally used in herbal medicine systems (despite researchers' documentation of the significant antimicrobial actions attributed to them).[7–9]

Clavillia's main chemicals include alanine, alpha-amyrins, arabinose, beta amyrins, betalamic acid, betanin, brassicasterol, beta-sitosterols, 2-carbosyarabinitol, campesterol, daucosterol, d-glucan, dopamine, hexacosan-1-ol, indicaxanthin, isobetanin, 6-methoxyboeravinone C, methylabronisoflavone, mirabilis antiviral proteins, mirabilis peptides, miraxanthins, n-dotriacontane, n-hentri-acontane, n-heptacosane, n-hexacosane, n-nonacosane, n-octacosane, n-penta-cosane, n-pentatriacontane, n-tetracosane, n-tetratriacontane, n-triacontane, n-tricosane, n-tritriacontane, oleanolic acid, stigmasterol, tartaric acid, trigo-nelline, tryptophan, ursolic acid, and vulgaxanthin I.

BIOLOGICAL ACTIVITIES AND CLINICAL RESEARCH

Lab studies seem to suggest that the roots of clavillia provide the best action against fungi and *Candida*.

The plant and root have demonstrated other biological activities, in addition to the antiviral actions of the MAPs. In 2001, researchers found new phenolic com-pounds in clavillia which demonstrated *in vitro* action against the yeast *Candida albicans*.[10] A hot water extract of the flower, leaf, and root of clavillia has shown antifungal activity in another *in vitro* study.[11] Other research on the leaf and branches of clavillia did not confirm any antimicrobial actions, therefore, these properties are probably attributed only to the root of the plant.[12,13] In early research, the root of the plant (in water and ethanol extracts) also demonstrated mild uterine stimulant actions in rats, and antispasmodic actions in guinea pigs.[14]

CURRENT PRACTICAL USES

Clavillia, the lovely, sweet-smelling ornamental, has also earned its place in herbal medicine practices around the world; its array of biological activities continue to support its continued use worldwide for viruses, fungi, and yeast. As most research surrounding this plant's activity has occurred in the past ten years, additional findings regarding clavillia's power and versatility will like-ly explain more of its indigenous uses, and unearth new applications for it. Today, clavillia is generally employed as an antiviral herbal remedy for herpes, hepatitis, influenza, and other upper repiratory viruses, as well as for *Candida* and yeast infections.

Traditional Preparation

For viruses and *Candida*, generally $\frac{1}{2}$ cup of a standard root infusion or 1–2 ml of a 4:1 tincture is taken twice daily. If desired, 1 g of powdered root in capsules or tablets twice daily can be substituted.

Contraindications

The seeds of the plant contain neurotoxic chemicals and should not be ingested.
Chemicals found in clavillia have been documented to have abortive actions. Clavillia itself has been documented with a mild uterine stimulant effect; there-fore, its use during pregnancy is not advised.

Drug Interactions

None known.

Worldwide Ethnomedical Uses

Region	Uses
Brazil	for *Candida*, chagas disease, colic, constipation, contusions, diarrhea, dysentery, earache, eczema, edema, freckles, herpes, hives, itch, intestinal parasites, liver problems, pain, skin infections, skin problems, syphilis, vaginal discharge, urinary insufficiency, worms, wounds
Cuba	for herpes, intestinal parasites
Guatemala	for abscesses, aches, boils, bruises, conjunctivitis, dermatitis, fungal infections, gonorrhea, inflammation, mucosal lesions, ringworm, scrofula, skin problems, sores, ulcers (skin), vaginal discharge, vaginitis, wounds
India	for conjunctivitis, edema, fungal infections, inflammation, pain, swellings
Mexico	for bee stings, dysentery, scorpion stings, vaginal discharge, wounds
Peru	for constipation, dermatitis, earaches, herpes, urinary insufficiency
United States	for abortions, bone fractures, childbirth, mumps
Elsewhere	for abscesses, arthritis, boils, bowel cleansing, bruises, burns, colic, constipation, diabetes, digestion stimulation, dyspepsia, edema, fungal infections, gonorrhea, hepatitis, herpes, hypochondria, intestinal gas, intestinal parasites, libido stimulation, liver problems, menstrual irregularities, muscle pains, piles, pimples, sores, splenitis, strains, syphilis, thrush, tumors, urinary insufficiency, urogenital inflammation, urticaria, wounds, and as a tonic

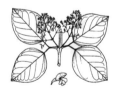

CLAVO HUASCA		
HERBAL PROPERTIES AND ACTIONS		
Main Actions	**Other Actions**	**Standard Dosage**
• increases libido	• relieves pain	Vine wood
• stimulates digestion	• expels gas	**Tincture:** 3–4 ml twice daily

Family: Bignoniaceae

Genus: *Tynanthus*

Species: *panurensis*

Common Names: clavo huasca, clove vine, white clove, cipó cravo, cipó trindade

Parts Used: vine wood, bark

Clavo huasca is a large, woody vine that grows up to 80 m in length and is indigenous to the Amazon rainforest and other parts of tropical South America. It produces very small, white flowers (which are pollinated by bees and butterflies) and elongated, flat, bean-like fruits. The vine bark and root have a distinctive, clove-like aroma (as do the leaves, somewhat), earning its common name *clove vine* or *white clove*. The vine, when cross-sectioned, has a distinctive "Maltese cross" design in the wood (with a darker, reddish color as the background and a golden color in the heartwood). Two species of plants are sold in herbal commerce as "clavo huasca"—the true *Tynanthus* vine, and another, completely different, *Mandevilla* genus vine.

TRIBAL AND HERBAL MEDICINE USES

The Shipibo-Conibo, Kayapó, and Assurini Indian tribes in the Amazon rainforest highly regard clavo huasca as an impotency remedy, for weak erections, and as an effective aphrodisiac for both men and women. It is also used as an adjunctive ingredient in various ayahuasca recipes (or taken shortly after taking the concoction) to settle the stomach. Ayahuasca is a phytochemically rich combination of plants brewed by Indian shamans to connect to the spirit world. Through a series of reactions among chemicals from several plants working together, a hallucinogenic plant extract is created. While clavo huasca is not itself a hallucinogen, the ayahuasca brew also can be quite purgative—causing vomiting and diarrhea. Clavo huasca is sometimes added to the brew or taken simultaneously to help reduce these effects.

Clavo huasca has a long history in the Amazon as an aphrodisiac for both men and women.

Clavo huasca is also widely regarded as an aphrodisiac for both men and women in Peruvian herbal medicine today. It is an ingredient in two famous herbal formulas for impotency and frigidity, which are sold widely in the herbal markets and stores in Peru as aphrodisiacs and for sexual potency. One is called *Siete Raices* ("seven roots") and the other is *Rompe Calzon* ("bust your britches"). In addition, this vine tincture is also employed for fever, aching muscles, and arthritis pain in Peruvian herbal medicine. The fresh sap or resin from the root of the plant is used as a toothache remedy—containing a chemical called *eugenol* that acts as a topical pain-reliever. As an aphrodisiac, clavo huasca is traditionally prepared by soaking the vine bark and wood in alcohol, or most commonly, the local sugarcane rum called *aguardiente*. In Brazilian herbal medicine, the plant is called *cipó cravo;* it is considered an excellent remedy for dyspepsia, difficult digestion, and intestinal gas (when brewed as a water decoction) and an aphrodisiac (when macerated in alcohol into a tincture).

PLANT CHEMICALS

Preliminary phytochemical analysis by Brazilian scientists have discovered an alkaloid they named *tinantina* as well as other alkaloids, tannins, tannic acids, eugenol, and other essential oils.

BIOLOGICAL ACTIVITIES AND CLINICAL RESEARCH

Despite its long and popular use in South America, there are no published clinical studies as yet on clavo huasca.

CURRENT PRACTICAL USES

Clavo huasca is still widely employed as a natural aphrodisiac for both men and women in South America today. It's reported to be highly effective, especially for pre-menopausal women (but not as effective for libido loss after menopause). This use has caught on in the U.S., and more clavo huasca products are now available in natural product stores. It is also showing up as an ingredient in various herbal libido formulas for men and women as well. For its aphrodisiac qualities, it is best prepared in its time-honored traditional method: as an alcohol tincture.

Traditional Preparation As a libido aid, 3–4 ml of a 4:1 tincture is taken twice daily. As a digestive aid and appetite stimulant, 1 cup of a vine wood or leaf infusion is prepared.

Contraindications None known.

Drug Interactions None reported.

Worldwide Ethnomedical Uses

Region	Uses
Brazil	as an aphrodisiac and appetite stimulant; for arthritis, digestive problems, dyspepsia, impotency, intestinal gas, pain, rheumatism, worms
Ecuador	as an aphrodisiac and for arthritis, fever, muscle aches, pain, rheumatism
Peru	as an aphrodisiac and pain-reliever; for arthritis, backaches, erectile dysfunction, fever, frigidity, impotency, muscle aches, rheumatism, toothache, virility
Elsewhere	as an aphrodisiac and for fever, toothache

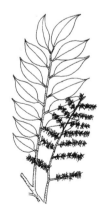

COPAIBA

HERBAL PROPERTIES AND ACTIONS

Main Actions
- relieves pain
- reduces inflammation
- kills germs
- kills bacteria
- kills fungi
- inhibits tumor growth
- dries secretions
- heals wounds
- protects gastric tract
- mildly laxative
- soothes and softens
- disinfects

Other Actions
- increases urination
- expels worms
- reduces acid
- suppresses coughs
- expels phlegm

Standard Dosage
Resin

Internal: 5–15 drops two or three times daily

External: apply diluted resin on affected areas

Family: Fabaceae

Genus: *Copaifera*

Species: *officinalis, langsdorffii, reticulata*

Common Names: copaiba, copaipera, cupayba, copauba, copal, balsam copaiba, copaiva, copaiba-verdadeira, Jesuit's balsam, copaibeura-de-Minas, cobeni, Matidisguate, matisihuati, mal-dos-sete-dias, aceite de palo, pau-de-oleo, básamo de copayba

Parts Used: resin, oil

Copaiba trees are considerably branched and grow from 15–30 m high. They produce many small, white flowers on long panicles and small fruit pods with two to four seeds inside. There are thirty-five species of *Copaifera*, found mainly in tropical South America (particularly in Brazil, Argentina, Bolivia, Guyana, Colombia, Peru, and Venezuela). Several different species are used as traditional medicines interchangeably: *C. langsdorffii* is found mostly in the *cerrados* of central Brazil, *C. reticulata* is indigenous to the Amazon region, and *C. officinalis* occurs widely throughout South America, including the Amazon.

The part of the tree that is often employed medicinally is the oleoresin that accumulates in cavities within the tree trunk. It is harvested by tapping or drilling holes into the wood of the trunk and collecting the resin that drips out, much in the same manner as harvesting maple syrup. A single copaiba tree can provide about 40 liters of oleoresin annually, making it a sustainable rainforest resource that can be harvested without destroying the tree or the forest in which it grows. When tapped, the initial oily resin is clear, thin, and colorless; it thickens and darkens upon contact with air. Commercially sold resins are a thick, clear liquid, with a color that varies from pale yellow to golden light brown. The variety gathered in Venezuela is said to be thicker and darker in color. Although it is often referred to as a balsam or oil, it is actually an oleoresin.

TRIBAL AND HERBAL MEDICINE USES

In Brazilian herbal medicine, copaiaba resin is used as a strong antiseptic and expectorant for the respiratory tract, as an anti-inflammatory and antiseptic for the urinary tract, as a topical anti-inflammatory agent for all types of skin disorders, and internally and externally for cancer and ulcers.

On the Rio Solimoes in northwest Amazonia, copaiba resin is used topically by indigenous tribes as a wound healer, to stop bleeding, for skin sores and psoriasis, and to treat gonorrhea. Healers and *curanderos* in the Amazon today use copaiba resin for all types of pain, for skin disorders and insect bites, and to cool inflammation.

In Brazilian herbal medicine systems, the resin is used as a strong antiseptic and expectorant for the respiratory tract (including bronchitis and sinusitis), as an anti-inflammatory and antiseptic for the urinary tract (for cystitis, bladder, and kidney infections), and as a topical anti-inflammatory agent for all types of skin problems. Copaiba resin is sold in gel capsules in stores and pharmacies in Brazil and recommended for all types of internal inflammation, stomach ulcers, and cancer. One of its more popular home-remedy uses in Brazil is as an antiseptic gargle for sore throats and tonsillitis (fifteen drops of resin in warm water). In Peruvian traditional medicine, three or four drops of the resin are mixed with a spoonful of honey and taken as a natural sore throat remedy. It is also employed in Peruvian herbal medicine systems to reduce inflammation and increase urination, and in the treatment of incontinence, urinary problems, stomach ulcers, syphilis, tetanus, bronchitis, catarrh, herpes, pleurisy, tuberculosis, hemorrhages, and leishmaniasis (applied as a plaster).

Copaiba resin was first recorded in European medicine in 1625 (brought back from the New World by the Jesuits and called *Jesuit's balsam*) and has been used there since in the treatment of chronic cystitis, bronchitis, chronic diarrhea, and as a topical preparation for hemorrhoids. In the United States, it was an official drug in the *U.S. Pharmacopeia* from 1820 to 1910. Noted ethnobotanist and author Mark Plotkin reports that copaiba oil has been used in the United States as a disinfectant, diuretic, laxative, and stimulant—in addition to being used in cosmetics and soaps. *The Encyclopedia of Common Natural Ingredients* cites that copaiba has diuretic, antibacterial, anti-inflammatory, expectorant, disinfectant, and stimulant activities.

PLANT CHEMICALS

The resin contains up to 15 percent volatile oil; the remaining materials are resins and acids. The active biological properties of copaiba resin are attributed to a group of phytochemicals called *sesquiterpenes* (over 50 percent of the resin may be sesquiterpenes), *diterpenes,* and *terpenic acids.* These chemicals include caryophyllene, calamenene, and copalic, coipaiferic, copaiferolic, hardwickic, and kaurenoic acids. Several of these chemicals are novel ones found only in copaiba.[1,2] Copaiba resin is the highest known natural source of caryophyllene, comprising up to 480,000 parts per million. Caryophyllene is a well-known plant chemical, which has been documented as having strong anti-inflammatory effects (among other actions).

Copaiba is the highest known source of the anti-inflammatory chemical, caryophyllene.

The main chemicals found in copaiba include: alloaromadendrene, alpha-bergamotene, alpha-cubebene, alpha-multijugenol, alpha-selinene, ar-curcumene, beta-bisabolene, beta-cubebene, beta-elemene, beta-farnesene, beta-humulene, beta-muurolene, beta-selinene, calamenene, calamesene, carioazulene, caryophyllenes, coipaiferic acid, copaene, copaiferolic acid, copalic acid, copaibic acids, cyperene, delta-cadinene, delta-elemene, enantio-agathic acid, gamma-cadinene, gamma-elemene, gamma-humulene, hardwickic acids, illurinic acid, kaurenoic acids, kaurenic acid, kolavenol 1, maracaibobalsam, methlyl copalate, paracopaibic acids, polyalthic acid, and trans-alpha-bergamotene.

BIOLOGICAL ACTIVITIES AND CLINICAL RESEARCH

Much of the clinical research performed to date has verified the traditional uses of copaiba. In 2002, researchers in Brazil confirmed that it was highly effective as a topical wound healer in animal studies.[2] Copaiba has long been used both internally and externally for inflammation of all sorts. Clinical research validates the resin's anti-inflammatory effects against various laboratory-induced inflammation in other animal studies.[4,5] The anti-inflammatory effects have been related to the sesquiterpene chemicals in copaiba oil, which scientists have noted can vary significantly—not only between different copaiba tree species, but also within a given species and, even among individual trees.[6] Sesquiterpene content can range anywhere from 30–90 percent. This may account for the results obtained by other Brazilian researchers who tested eight different commercial samples of copaiba oil, and only three of the eight demonstrated significant anti-inflammatory effects.[7] Of these sesquiterpenes, caryophyllene is the most well studied, demonstrating pain-relieving properties,[8] antifungal properties against nail fungus,[9] as well as anti-inflammatory and gastro-protective properties in other animal studies.[10]

The gastro-protective effects of caryophyllene documented in 1996 also help justify another traditional use of copaiba oil—as a natural remedy for stomach ulcers. In this animal study, not only did caryophyllene evidence significant anti-inflammatory effects without any damage to the stomach lining (most other non-steroidal anti-inflammatory agents cause stomach problems)—it actually significantly inhibited stomach injury induced by various chemicals.[10] Two years later, another Brazilian research group reported that giving natural copaiba resin to rats provided dose-dependent, significant protection against chemical- and stress-induced gastric damage and also evidenced an anti-ulcerous effect.[11]

Copaiba's traditional uses as an antiseptic for sore throat, upper respiratory, and urinary tract infections can be explained partly by the resin's antibacterial properties documented in the 1960s and 1970s.[12,13] Researchers again confirmed (in 2000 and 2002) that the resin as a whole (and, particularly, two of its diterpenes—copalic acid and kaurenic acid) demonstrated significant *in vitro* antibacterial activity.[14,15] One of copaiba's other chemicals, kaurenoic acid, has also demonstrated selective antibacterial activity in other recent studies.[16,17]

Another recent area of research on copaiba resin has focused on its anticancerous and anti-tumor properties. Researchers in Tokyo isolated six chemicals (clerodane diterpenes) in the oleoresin of copaiba in 1994 and tested them against carcinomas in mice to determine their anti-tumor activity. One particular compound, kolavenol, was twice as effective at increasing the lifespan in mice with carcinomas (by 98 percent) as the standard chemotherapy drug, 5-Fluorouacil (5-FU).[18] The natural resin also increased lifespan by 82 percent—which was still higher than 5-FU (which increased lifespan by 46 percent). Interestingly, the *in vivo* tests provided better anti-tumor effects than in previous test-tube studies. The Spanish team of researchers that documented copaiba's antimicrobial effects in 2002 also tested for *in vitro* anti-tumor effects. These scientists reported that another phytochemical in the resin, methlyl copalate, had *in vitro* activity against human lung carcinoma, human colon carcinoma, human melanoma, and mouse lymphoid neoplasm cell lines.[14] Brazilian researchers reported in 2002 that one of copaiba's active chemicals, kaurenoic acid, also inhibited the growth of human leukemic cells by 95 percent, and human breast and colon cancer cells by 45 percent *in vitro*.[19] Kaurenoic acid can comprise as much as 1.4 percent of the natural copaiba oleoresin.

Clinical research reveals that copaiba heals wounds, reduces pain and inflammation, and kills germs and bacteria on contact.

The newest research on copaiba suggests it contains chemicals which may have applications for cancerous tumors and leukemia.

CURRENT PRACTICAL USES

In all herbal medicine systems where it is employed, copaiba resin is taken internally only in very small dosages—usually only 5–15 drops (approximately ½–1 ml) one to three times daily. In large doses, it has been documented to cause nausea, vomiting, fever, and a measles-like skin rash. A French dermatologist reported that these side effects can also occur with the absorption of copaiba resin through the skin in sensitive individuals.[20] It has, however, been approved officially in the U.S. as a food additive and is used in small amounts as a flavoring agent in foods and beverages.[21] It has also been employed as a fixative in perfumes.

Today in the United States, copaiba resin is used mostly as a fragrance component in perfumes and in cosmetic preparations (including soaps, bubble baths, detergents, creams, and lotions) for its antibacterial, anti-inflammatory, and emollient (soothing and softening) properties. Natural health practitioners are just beginning to learn about the many ways that this important rainforest resource is employed in South American herbal medicine systems, and are beginning to incorporate them in their practices here. Used prudently and in small quantities, it is a wonderful natural remedy for stomach ulcers, inflammation of all kinds, nail fungus (applied topically), and for its documented wound-healing, antimicrobial, and anticancerous properties.

Traditional Preparation

In South America, 5–15 drops of the oleoresin in a cup of hot water is usually taken two to three times daily. It is applied directly to the skin for skin problems and wounds (normally prepared with one part copaiba resin to five parts glycerine or grapeseed oil). It is also employed topically as a massage oil for painful or inflamed muscles and joints—normally combined with another carrier oil (one part copaiba to ten parts carrier oil, such as almond or grapeseed oil). For nail fungus and skin cancer, the resin is applied full strength directly on the affected area(s) without diluting it in another oil or glycerine.

Contraindications

Avoid contact with eyes and mucous membranes, as the resin can act as an irritant. Those sensitive to the resin may experience a measles-like rash accompanied by irritation, itching, and/or tingling when using topically or taking internally. Discontinue use if these effects occur.

Do not take internally in large dosages (more than 5 ml). Large dosages have been reported to cause nausea, vomiting, fever, and rashes. Discontinue or reduce dosage if these effects occur. Do not take internally during pregnancy.

Drug Interactions

None reported.

Worldwide Ethnomedical Uses

Region	Uses
Amazonia	for coughs, excessive mucus, flu, gonorrhea, incontinence, inflammation, psoriasis, skin sores, syphilis, urinary tract disorders, wounds, and as a diuretic and disinfectant
Brazil	for bacterial infections, bladder infections, bronchitis, cancer, cough, cystitis, dandruff, dermatitis, dermatosis, diarrhea, dysentery, flu, gastric disorders, gonorrhea, hypertension, incontinence, inflammation, intestinal parasites, kidney inflammation, lung disorders, pain, pneumonia, psoriasis, respiratory problems, sinusitis, skin disorders, skin ulcers, sore throat, stomach ulcers, syphilis, tetanus, tumors, urinary infections, urinary inflammation, vaginal discharge, wounds, and as an antiseptic
Europe	for bladder irritation, bronchitis, chilblains, constipation, cystitis, diarrhea, edema, excessive mucus (bladder, vagina, respiratory tract), gonorrhea, hemorrhoids, intestinal gas, itch, sexually transmitted diseases, urinary inflammation, vaginal discharge; and as an antiseptic, diuretic, and stimulant
Peru	for bronchitis, diuretic, edema, excessive mucus, gonorrhea, hemorrhages, herpes, incontinence, inflammation, intestinal gas, insect bites, leishmaniasis, muscle pain, pleurisy, sexually transmitted diseases, syphilis, tetanus, tuberculosis, ulcers, urinary infections, vaginal discharge, wounds
United States	as an antibacterial, anti-inflammatory, disinfectant, diuretic, expectorant, laxative, stimulant
Elsewhere	for constipation, dermatitis, eczema, gonorrhea, sexually transmitted diseases, urinary insufficiency, wounds, and as a massage oil

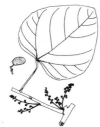

Family: Menispermaceae

Genus: *Chondrodendron*

Species: *tomentosum*

Common Names: curare, grieswurzel, pareira brava, pareira, vigne sauvage, uva-da-serra, uva-do-mato, ampihuasca blanca, antinupa, antinoopa, comida de venados, curari, ourari, woorari, worali, velvet leaf, ice vine, grieswurzel, urari

Parts Used: leaf, root

CURARE

HERBAL PROPERTIES AND ACTIONS

Main Actions	Other Actions	Standard Dosage
• increases urination • reduces fever • promotes menstruation	• blocks pain signals • relaxes muscles	Root **Decoction:** 1 cup twice daily

Curare is a South American vine native to the Amazon Basin. It is found growing in Brazil, Bolivia, Peru, French Guiana, Ecuador, Panama, and Colombia. This woody vine, sometimes 4 in. thick at its base, climbs a considerable height up into the canopy (up to 30 m high). Its large heart-shaped leaves have a soft silky underside made up of tiny white hairs, giving the plant the common name of *velvet leaf*. It has both male and female flowers, which are small, greenish-white, and grow in clusters. It produces an edible bittersweet fruit. The names *curare* and *woorari* are Indian names that refer to the poisons they prepare for their hunting darts and arrows. The actual name, *curare*, is a corruption of two Tupi Indian terms meaning "bird" and "to kill." *Chondrodendron tomentosum* or the curare vine is one of the main plants used by the Indians in the Amazon to prepare these arrow poisons.

TRIBAL AND HERBAL MEDICINE USES

Many different plants are used to prepare curare arrow poisons and many different recipes are used by different Indian tribes in the Amazon. Generally, the Indians in Venezuela and the Guianas use *Strychnos* plants as the main ingredient, and tribes in Peru, Ecuador, and Brazil use curare vine (*Chondrodendron tomentosum*) as the main ingredient in their poisons. In both cases, it usually is a combination of several different plants, and even snake and frog venom is sometimes added. The Sionas of Colombia, the Lamistas of Peru, and the Ketchwas of Ecuador use curare vine in the preparation of their poisons; they crush and cook the stems and roots of the vine, adding other plants and venomous animals. It is boiled down (sometimes for as long as two days) until it becomes a dark-colored syrup or paste. The resulting substance is then used to coat the darts of their blowguns and tips of hunting arrows. These poisons are not actually true toxins—rather they are potent muscle relaxants.

Curare is one of the main plants that Amazonian Indians use to prepare arrow poisons. These poisons are not actually true toxins—rather they are potent muscle relaxants.

Death from curare poison is caused by asphyxia (respiratory arrest) because the muscles become so relaxed that the muscles operating the diaphragm and lungs stop functioning. Interestingly, it only works if the poison gets into the bloodstream; ingesting curare poison (and even eating the meat of curare-poisoned animals) has no toxic effect since it is not absorbed in the stomach. It works well for the Indians because often their prey is high up in the canopy—the muscle-relaxant effect of the poison prevents the animal from fleeing and releases their grip on branches in the trees so they fall to the ground. The muscle-relaxing effect begins almost immediately upon hitting the bloodstream, but death from respiratory arrest can take a few minutes for birds and small prey, and up to twenty minutes or longer for larger mammals.

Curare vine also holds a place in herbal medicine systems. In Brazil and Peru the root of the vine is used to increase urination, reduce fever, and promote menstruation. It is also used to treat edema, kidney stones, and testicular inflammation. Externally, it is used for bruises and contusions. In Brazil the leaves are also crushed and applied externally for the treatment of poisonous snakebites. In homeopathy, the plant is used for inflammation of the urinary tract and enlarged prostate. Sir Walter Raleigh and several other early explorers reported on the Indian's use of curare vine in the 1500s and the plant became known in European herbal medicine systems. Maude Grieve, British author of the book *A Modern Herbal* (first published in 1931), reported that the plant acts as an antiseptic to the bladder for chronic inflammation of the urinary passages and recommended it for stones, vaginal discharges, rheumatism, jaundice, edema and water retention, and gonorrhea.

PLANT CHEMICALS

Curare vine is a rich source of alkaloids. The main alkaloid responsible for the muscle-relaxant actions (and why it works as an arrow poison) is called *d-*

tubocurarine. It was first isolated in 1897 and obtained in drug form in 1935. The alkaloid works by blocking the signals in the brain that tell the muscles to move—thereby rendering the whole body immobile to the point of becoming virtually paralyzed. It is not a toxin, and the effects generally wear off in about ninety minutes. In 1942, curare and d-tubocurarine were introduced into clinical anesthesia, starting the modern era of surgery. Today it is still sold as a prescription drug which is used as a general anesthetic and muscle relaxant in various types of surgeries (during which breathing can be controlled with machines).[1,2]

The main chemical responsible for curare's muscle-relaxant actions (and why it works as an arrow poison) is an alkaloid called *d-tubocurarine*. This chemical has been turned into a prescription drug, which is used as a general anesthetic and muscle relaxant during surgeries.

It is also used to treat paralysis caused by tetanus (which causes uncontrollable muscle contractions throughout the body). D-tubocurarine's chemical pathways and actions are also being evaluated for their role in blocking serotonin,[3] reducing vomiting,[4] alleviating drug withdrawal symptoms,[5,6] and for their anti-anxiety effects.[7] D-tubocurarine also stimulates the release of histamine. This release of histamine may cause lowered blood pressure due to relaxation of blood vessels.[8] Intravenous administration of d-tubocurarine causes rapid muscle relaxation, first affecting the toes, ears, and eyes, then the neck and limbs and finally respiration.

The main chemicals found in this rainforest vine include chondrocurarine, chondrocurine, chondodine, chondrofoline, curine, cycleanine, D-tubocurarine, isochondrodendrine, L-bebeerine, L-tubocurarine, N-benzyl-phthalimide, norcycleanine, pelonine, tomentocurine, and tubocurarine.

BIOLOGICAL ACTIVITIES AND CLINICAL RESEARCH

As is often the case in plant research—since scientists supposedly discovered the "main active chemical" in the plant so many years ago and turned it into a drug, further research on the natural plant was not forthcoming. Literally no clinical research has been conducted on the use of extracts of this natural vine as it is used in herbal medicine systems.

CURRENT PRACTICAL USES

Curare is yet another example of how the empirical knowledge of rainforest Indian tribes has been utilized by western science and the pharmaceutical industry. Since the strong muscle-relaxant chemicals in the plant are not absorbed in the stomach, oral extracts of the vine and root are considered "safe" in herbal medicine systems. Its uses today, however, are mainly limited to South America. A root decoction is generally prepared for persistent urinary tract infections, prostatitis, and testicular inflammation.

One U.S. manufacturer of herbal supplements does state that they use *Chondrodendron tomentosum* in a formula (for lowering blood sugar levels), however, they call it "abuta." Abuta and curare, are in fact, two different species of vines with very different uses in herbal medicine and different plant chemicals (and neither have been used for diabetes or blood sugar balancing). The real "abuta" vine is featured in this book as *Cissampelos pareira*. Even more confusing—the picture of the plant in their marketing materials is neither plant, but looks suspiciously like yet another rainforest vine: *Abuta grandifolia* (which has been used indigenously for diabetes). An experienced herbalist or botanist would wonder if this company even knew which plant they were actually using! As always, consumers should look for a reputable supplier of this plant and all medicinal plants coming from South America.

Traditional Preparation	Traditionally, 1 cup twice daily of a standard root decoction is taken, on an empty stomach.
Contraindications	Not to be used during pregnancy and breastfeeding. Curare may possibly reduce blood pressure; it should not be used in those with low blood pressure or those on medication to lower their blood pressure without careful attention to these possible effects.
Drug Interactions	None reported.

Worldwide Ethnomedical Uses

Region	Uses
Amazonia	for arrow poisons, fever, and as an antiseptic, diuretic, mild laxative
Brazil	for arrow poisons, bruises, contusions, earaches, edema, fever, kidney stones, mental disorders, snakebite, and to promote menstruation and increase urination
Germany	as a diuretic and tonic
Peru	for arrow poisons, earaches, edema, fever, kidney stones, urinary insufficiency, and to promote menstruation
Venezuela	for arrow poisons

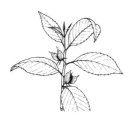

Family: Turneraceae

Genus: *Turnera*

Species: *aphrodisiaca, diffusa*

Common Names: damiana, damiane, oreganillo, the bourrique, Mexican damiana, Mexican holly, damiana de Guerrero

Parts Used: aerial parts, leaves

DAMIANA
HERBAL PROPERTIES AND ACTIONS

Main Actions	Other Actions	Standard Dosage
• increases libido	• reduces spasms	Leaves
• relieves depression	• dries secretions	**Infusion:** 1 cup two to three times daily
• reduces blood sugar	• stimulates digestion	**Fluid Extract:** 2–4 ml twice daily
• calms nerves	• increases urination	**Tablets/Capsules:** 3–4 g twice daily
	• mildly laxative	

Damiana is a small shrub that grows 1–2 m high and bears aromatic, serrate leaves that are 10–25 cm long. Small yellow flowers bloom in early to late summer, which are followed by small fruits with a sweet smell and fig-like flavor. The medicinal part of the plant is its leaves, which are harvested during the flowering season. Damiana is found throughout Mexico, Central America, and the West Indies, as well as in parts of South America. *Turnera diffusa* and *T. aphrodisiaca* are generally regarded as the same plant in herbal commerce. A closely related species, *T. ulmifolia*, is similar in appearance, but it has different traditional medicinal uses. The botanical Latin name of the plant, *Turnera aphrodisiaca*, describes its ancient use as an aphrodisiac.

TRIBAL AND HERBAL MEDICINE USES

Damiana was recorded to be used as an aphrodisiac in the ancient Mayan civilization, as well as for "giddiness and loss of balance." A Spanish missionary first reported that the Mexican Indians made a drink from the damiana leaves, added sugar, and drank it for its purported power to enhance lovemaking.

Damiana has a long history of use in traditional herbal medicine throughout the world. It is thought to act as an aphrodisiac, antidepressant, tonic, diuretic, cough suppressant, and mild laxative. It has been used for such conditions as depression, anxiety, sexual inadequacy, debilitation, bed-wetting, menstrual irregularities, gastric ulcers, and constipation. In Mexico, the plant also is used for asthma, bronchitis, neurosis, diabetes, dysentery, dyspepsia, headaches, paralysis, nephrosis, spermatorrhea, stomachache, and syphilis. Damiana first was recorded with aphrodisiac effects in scientific literature over 100 years ago.[1]

From 1888 to 1947, damiana leaf and damiana elixirs were listed in the National Formulary in the United States. For more than a century, damiana's use has been associated with improving sexual function in both males and females. The leaves are used in Germany to relieve excess mental activity and nervous debility, and as a tonic for the hormonal and central nervous systems.

Damiana first was recorded with aphrodisiac effects in scientific literature over 100 years ago, and for more than a century its use has been associated with improving sexual function in both males and females.

E. F. Steinmetz states that in Holland, damiana is renowned for its sexual-enhancing qualities and its positive effects on the reproductive organs.[2] The *British Herbal Pharmacopoeia* cites indications for the use of damiana for "anxiety neurosis with a predominant sexual factor, depression, nervous dyspepsia, atonic constipation, and coital inadequacy."

PLANT CHEMICALS

Damiana's chemical composition is complex and its components have not been identified completely. The leaves contain up to 1 percent volatile oil that is comprised of at least twenty constituents (including 1,8-cineole, p-cymene, alpha- and beta-pinene, thymol, alpha-copaene, and calamene). Damiana leaves also contain tannins, flavonoids, beta-sitosterol, damianin (a brown, bitter substance), and the glycosides gonzalitosin, arbutin, and tetraphyllin B.[2–4] Damiana has been reported to be non-toxic in humans and animals.[5]

The main constituents of damiana include: albuminoids, alpha-copaene, alpha-pinene, arbutin, barterin, beta-pinene, beta-sitosterol, calamenene, caoutchouc, chlorophyll, 1,8-cineole, cymene, cymol, damianin, essential oil, gamma-cadinene, gonzalitosin-i, hexacosanol-1, luteolin, quinovopyranosides, tannins, tetraphyllin b, thymol, triacontane, and trimethoxyflavones.

BIOLOGICAL ACTIVITIES AND CLINICAL RESEARCH

Several research studies and patents report that damiana may benefit women during menopause by relieving hot flashes, depression, and preventing weight gain.

Only one clinical study has been conducted to validate the traditional use of the plant for sexual dysfunction and impotence. In 1999, a group of researchers in Italy administered damiana to both sexually potent and sexually sluggish (or impotent) rats. The extract had no effect on sexually potent rats but, in the others, it increased the percentage of rats achieving ejaculation and made them more sexually active.[6] A U.S. patent was awarded in 2002 for a combination of herbs, including damiana, to "overcome natural inhibitors of human sexual response and allow for improved response and psychological effects."[7] Another U.S. patent was awarded for an herbal combination for females, with inventors reporting that damiana could "relieve anxiety, depression, headaches during menstruation, and exhaustion. Damiana also helps to balance female hormone levels and control hot flashes."[8] A 1998 *in vitro* clinical study reported that components in damiana bound to progesterone receptors in cultured human breast cancer cells, leading researchers to surmise that it had a neutral or anti-estrogenic activity.[9]

Central nervous system depressant activity has been attributed to damiana and verified by research.[10] Damiana also has been used in combination with other plants for its thermogenic activity.[11] Two U.S. patents have been filed on oral appetite suppressants containing damiana, citing its inclusion as an anti-anxiety and thermogenic substance.[12,13]

Damiana's traditional use for diabetes has been studied by scientists as well.

In 1984, Mexican researchers reported the hypoglycemic activity of the plant when a leaf infusion was given to diabetic mice.[14] This effect was re-verified in Mexico when the plant was prepared in the traditional manner (as an infusion) and given orally to hyperglycemic rats. This study reported that damiana reduced blood glucose levels as well.[15] A 2002 study, however, reported that an ethanol extract of damiana evidenced no hypoglycemic activity.[16] These conflicting studies suggest that the active "hypoglycemic" chemicals in damiana may be extracted in the traditional (hot water) process, and lost or not extracted in alcohol.

CURRENT PRACTICAL USES
With such an ancient history of traditional uses, it's not unusual that the plant appears in many books on herbal remedies published worldwide. Damiana is also widely available in most health food and natural product stores in a variety of forms—from tea blends, capsules, and tablets to liquid tinctures and extracts. Most herbalists prefer to use damiana in combination with other medicinal plants; therefore, it can be found in quite a few herbal combination formulas for sexual potency, weight loss, depression, hormonal balancing, and in overall tonics. Most of the damiana sold in herbal commerce today originates from Mexican and Latin American cultivation projects.

Traditional Preparation
The traditional remedy calls for 2–4 g of dried leaves infused in a cup of boiling water; 2–3 cups are taken daily. Alternatively, 2–4 ml of a liquid extract or 3–4 g of powdered leaf in tablets or capsules taken twice daily can be substituted, if desired.

Contraindications
Damiana has demonstrated mild hypoglycemic effects in animals. Persons with diabetes and hypoglycemia should use this plant with caution, as blood sugar levels should be monitored accordingly for this possible effect.

Damiana has a traditional use as an abortive and is contraindicated during pregnancy.

Drug Interactions
It may potentiate antidiabetic medications.

Worldwide Ethnomedical Uses

Region	Uses
Bahamas	for childbirth, headache, menstrual irregularities, urinary insufficiency
Brazil	for albuminuria, alcoholism, anorexia, asthenia, bronchitis, constipation, convalescence, debilitation, diabetes, diarrhea, digestive problems, dyspepsia, fertility problems, gallbladder disorders, impotence, indigestion, kidney problems, malaria, nervousness, nocturia, paralysis, respiratory ailments, rheumatism, syphilis, ulcers, urinary incontinence, vaginal discharge, weakness; and as an aphrodisiac, diuretic, and expectorant

Cuba	as an aphrodisiac, diuretic, and menstrual stimulant
England	for anxiety, constipation, depression, dyspepsia, hypochondria, neurosis, sexual debility, thymus problems, water retention
Germany	for depression, nervous debility, and as an aphrodisiac
Haiti	for colds, intestinal problems, sexually transmitted diseases, and as an aphrodisiac
Mexico	for asthma, bronchitis, colds, constipation, cough, diabetes, dysentery, dyspepsia, earaches, eye disorders, exhaustion, flu, headache, impotence, infections, infertility, inflammation, intestinal problems, malaria, menstrual disorders, nephritis, nervous disorders, neurosis, panacea, paralysis, stomachache, syphilis, urinary problems, vaginal dryness, weakness; and as an aphrodisiac, astringent, central nervous system depressant, diuretic, and expectorant
South America	for asthma, asthenia, bronchitis, cystitis, depression, impotence, urethritis; and as an antiseptic, aphrodisiac, expectorant, laxative, and stimulant
United States	for anxiety, constipation, cystitis, depression, frigidity, headaches, hypochondria, impotence, menstrual disorders, nervous disorders, sexual disorders; and as an adaptogen, aphrodisiac, diuretic, energizer, expectorant, stimulant, and tonic
Elsewhere	for anxiety, bladder problems, childbirth, colds, constipation, cough, cystitis, debilitation, depression, diabetes, diarrhea, dysentery, dyspepsia, fever, headache, hot flashes, impotence, infections, malaria, menopause, menstruation, nephritis, nervousness, neurasthenia, paralysis, renitis, sexual inadequacies, sexually transmitted diseases, stomachache, syphilis, ulcers; and as an aphrodisiac, diuretic, expectorant, stimulant, and tonic

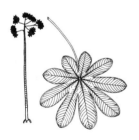

Family: Cecropiaceae

Genus: *Cecropia*

Species: *palmata, peltata, obtusifolia*

Common Names: embauba, trumpet tree, imbauba, umbauba, bois canon, bois trompette,

EMBAUBA
HERBAL PROPERTIES AND ACTIONS

Main Actions
- relieves asthma
- reduces spasms
- reduces inflammation
- kills bacteria
- kills fungi
- fights free radicals
- relieves pain
- strengthens heart
- lowers blood pressure
- reduces blood sugar

Other Actions
- dries secretions
- increases urination
- stimulates menstruation
- mildly laxative
- depresses central nervous system

Standard Dosage
Leaves

Infusion: 1 cup two to three times daily

Tablets/Capsules: 2–3 g twice daily

Embauba is native to Central and South America and the West Indies. It is a fast-growing, short-lived tree that springs up along riverbanks (where its seeds are deposited after annual flooding). It has large leaves (a foot wide) with a hol-

grayumbe, grayumbo, trompette, trompettier, yagruma, yagrumo, akowa, chancarpo, chancarro, guarumbo, guarumo, hormigo, hormiguillo, snakewood tree, pop-a-gun, tree-of-laziness, trompetenbaum, yaluma, certico, ambiabo, ambai, tree-of-sandpaper, palo lija

Part Used: leaves

TRIBAL AND HERBAL MEDICINE USES

Embauba is a popular and effective herbal remedy for asthma throughout South and Latin America.

low stem, and bears a cylindrical fruit with soft, sweet flesh around many small seeds. The tree, growing 5–10 m tall, often is inhabited by stinging ants that are attracted to the honey-like sap produced by the leaves. The symbiotic relationship with the ants is thought to protect the tree from leaf-eating insects. There are many closely related *Cecropia* species (including *C. peltata*, *C. palmata*, and *C. obtusifolia*) that may have different geographical locations yet are all very similar in appearance, chemical makeup, and traditional medicinal uses. *Cecropia* trees (nearly 100 tropical species in South and Latin America) are propagated by the many small fruit seeds they produce; bats, monkeys, and birds eat the succulent fruit and disperse the seeds in their droppings. Often, dense stands of trees can form that choke the growth of other plants anywhere that the canopy is disturbed.

Indian tribes in the Amazon use embauba for its anti-inflammatory properties—typically for rheumatic, kidney, and lung inflammations. The leaf is made into a tea and used widely for asthma and other upper respiratory complaints, as well as for diabetes. It also has been used for sores on the mouth and tongue. The Palikur indigenous people of Guyana wrap the large leaves around bone fractures, bruises and wounds, and use embauba to disinfect the genitalia and alleviate pain after childbirth.

In herbal medicine systems, embauba is used widely throughout Central and South America. In Brazil it is used for all types of respiratory complaints (such as asthma, bronchitis, coughs, whooping cough, and pneumonia). It is also used for diabetes, Parkinson's disease, kidney disorders, high blood pressure, and to increase the contraction strength of the heart muscle. It is considered effective against Parkinson's disease in Colombia, where it also is used as a substitute for digitalis-containing plants (digitalis is an active chemical found in plants and turned into a heart drug for various heart conditions), and to facilitate childbirth and menstruation. The leaf is used in Guatemalan herbal medicine systems for asthma, edema, rheumatism, diabetes, fever, atherosclerosis, and gonorrhea. The plant is popular in Mexico, where it is used for diabetes, coughs, inflammation, diarrhea, bladder irritation, asthma, obesity, liver disorders, high blood pressure, and warts.

In Cuba, virtually every part of the plant is employed in herbal medicine. The latex is considered corrosive and astringent, and is used topically against warts, calluses, herpes (and other sexually transmitted diseases), and skin ulcers. The bark is used to reduce mucus; the roots for bile complaints; and the fruit is considered emollient (soothing and softening the skin). The leaves are considered to reduce pain, and are used for asthma, liver disorders, edema, and to promote menstruation. In other parts of Latin America and the Amazon, it is often touted as a "cure" for asthma, after only a few weeks of taking a tea brewed from its leaves. (This has not been confirmed with any clinical research, however.)

PLANT CHEMICALS

Little research has been done to determine individual phytochemicals in embauba. In general, it is known to contain glycosides, lipids, alkaloids, flavonoids, tannins, cardenolids, triterpenes, polyphenols, steroids, and resins. A 2002 U.S. patent named ambain (a glycoside) and cecropin (an alkaloid) as the active plant chemicals in embauba that have cardiotonic and diuretic properties.[1] The flavonoids and proanthocyanidins in embauba recently were reported to inhibit angiotensin-converting enzyme (ACE) *in vitro*.[2] (ACE-inhibitors represent a class of pharmaceutical drugs used for hypertension which promote vasodilation and act as a diuretic.) The traditional use of embauba for high blood pressure might be explained if these chemicals can be demonstrated to inhibit ACE in humans and animals.

Chemicals in embauba have been reported to strengthen and tone the heart.

Main plant chemicals in embauba include ambain, arachidic acid, behenic acid, cecropin, cerotic acid, chlorogenic acid, isoorientin, leucocyanidin, lignoceric acid, polysaccharides, proanthocyanidins, stearic acid, and ursolinic acid.

BIOLOGICAL ACTIVITIES AND CLINICAL RESEARCH

Preliminary research is just beginning to explain and verify some of embauba's many uses in traditional medicine. Animal studies (with mice, rats, and guinea pigs) have shown that leaf extracts have pain-relieving, anti-inflammatory, and antispasmodic activities—which may explain, in part, its widespread traditional use in respiratory disorders.[3,4] Cuban researchers, however, reported that leaf infusions did not evidence any bronchodilator activity (in guinea pigs).[5] Other animal research has indicated that the plant can increase urination and lower blood pressure. One study reported that it increased urine flow in rats by 20 percent—without affecting the excretion of sodium and potassium.[6] Two different research groups (in Costa Rica and Mexico) reported that leaf extracts reduced blood pressure in rats.[7,8]

Animal studies confirm the anti-inflammatory, pain-relieving, and antispasmodic properties of embauba.

Another of embauba's traditional uses has been for diabetes. This use also has been studied in animals and verified by researchers. Water extracts of the leaf given to mice and rats were shown to lower blood sugar levels in two studies;[9,10] a hot water extract given to rabbits and dogs elicited the same blood-sugar-lowering effect.[11,12] One of these research groups attributed the hypoglycemic effect of the leaf, in part, to two flavone chemicals in embauba (isoorientin and chlorogenic acid) which, when tested individually, also demonstrated hypoglycemic activity in rats.[9]

Embauba has been reported to have *in vitro* antibacterial activity against various bacteria (such as *Staphylococcus, E. coli, Pseudomonas, Salmonella,* and

Shigella).[13,14] Water extracts seemed to have much more biological activity against bacteria than methanol or ethanol extracts *in vitro*. An ethanol extract of the leaf and stem was reported to have *in vitro* antifungal activity, but water extracts were inactive[15] (which suggests that antibacterial actions are derived from different chemicals than those providing antifungal actions). Embauba has also shown antioxidant activity with potent free-radical scavenging action.[16] In 2002 a U.S. patent was filed on various embauba extracts for use in cosmetics and dermatology. The patent reported the extracts had "pronounced action on lipolysis (fat-burning) which make them useful in slimming preparations, but also owing to their tightening effect, their smoothing properties and the improvement of the radiance of the skin."[1]

CURRENT PRACTICAL USES

It is hoped that researchers will continue to study embauba and validate more of its traditional uses—in particular, its use in respiratory disorders such as asthma and bronchitis. In the meantime, healthcare practitioners and herbalists around the world are utilizing this plant for not only respiratory disorders, but also for its cardiotonic and hypotensive properties, antidiabetic activity, and for its (yet-to-be-studied) use in Parkinson's disease. Generally, for upper respiratory problems and asthma, a standard leaf infusion is prepared and taken in 1 cup dosages two to three times daily. To help balance blood sugar levels, a cup of a leaf infusion is taken with each meal.

Traditional Preparation

Traditionally, $\frac{1}{2}$ to 1 cup of a standard leaf infusion is taken two to three times daily. If desired, 2–3 g of powdered leaf in tablets or capsules twice daily can be substituted.

Contraindications

Embauba has a traditional use of aiding childbirth and promoting menstruation. It should not be taken during pregnancy.

The plant has been reported in animal studies to have cardiotonic properties, increasing the strength of cardiac muscle contraction. It should not be used by anyone with a cardiac disorder unless monitored by a medical doctor. Embauba also has demonstrated hypotensive activity in animal studies. Those with low blood pressure or those on medication to lower their blood pressure should seek the advice of a qualified healthcare professional prior to using this plant.

Embauba has demonstrated a hypoglycemic effect in animals. It is contraindicated for persons with hypoglycemia. Diabetics should use this plant with caution as blood sugar levels should be monitored closely.

Drug Interactions

None reported in literature; however, embauba may potentiate cardiotonics (such as digitalis) as well as antihypertensive and ACE-inhibitor drugs. It may potentiate antidiabetic and insulin drugs.

Worldwide Ethnomedical Uses

Region	Uses
Amazonia	for asthma, bruises, childbirth, diabetes, fractures, inflammation, kidney problems, respiratory difficulties, rheumatic diseases, sores, wounds
Brazil	for asthma, bleeding, bronchitis, cancer, chagas disease, congestion, cough, diabetes, diarrhea, dysentery, edema, flu, gonorrhea, heart problems, hemorrhages, hemorrhoids, hypertension, liver support, malaria, Parkinson's disease, pneumonia, respiratory disorders, rheumatism, snakebite, ulcers, urinary insufficiency, urinary tract disorders, vaginal discharge, warts, wounds, and as an expectorant
Colombia	for childbirth, heart problems, menstrual difficulties, Parkinson's disease
Costa Rica	for arterial hypertension, urinary insufficiency
Cuba	for abscesses, aches, asthma, bile diseases, calluses, coughs, digestive, diuretic, dysentery, edema, fever, gonorrhea, heart conditions, herpes, liver disorders, pains, skin problems, sexually transmitted diseases, ulcers, warts
Guatemala	for asthma, atherosclerosis, diabetes, edema, fever, gonorrhea, heart support, hypertension, rheumatism, urinary insufficiency, and to promote perspiration
Mexico	for asthma, bladder problems, bites (scorpion, ants), burns, calluses, childbirth, chorea, corns, coughs, diabetes, diarrhea, dysentery, edema, fever, fractures, heart support, hepatitis, inflammation, liver support, nerve disorders, obesity, pulmonary problems, renal disorders, ulcers, urinary insufficiency, warts, wounds
Nicaragua	for abscesses, aches, coughs, diarrhea, digestive problems, fever, gastric, headache, intestinal disorders, liver support, pain, skin problems
Peru	for bleeding, diarrhea, energy, fever, heart support, Parkinson's disease, water retention, wounds
Trinidad	for bronchitis, cough, fever, flu, scorpion bite, snakebite
United States	for asthma, bronchitis, constipation, fungal infections, heart support, menstrual irregularities, pain, water retention
Venezuela	for constipation, heart support, inflammation, wounds
Elsewhere	for abscesses, aches, asthma, bronchitis, calluses, cancer, childbirth, corns, coughs, diabetes, diarrhea, digestive problems, dysentery, edema, fever, flu, fractures, gonorrhea, heart support, hematoma, hepatitis, herpes, hypertension, liver support, menstrual disorders, nerves, obesity, pain, scorpion bite, sexually transmitted diseases, skin problems, snakebite, warts, water retention, wounds, and as an antiseptic

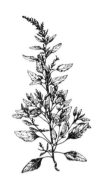

Family: Chenopodiaceae

Genus: *Chenopodium*

Species: *ambrosioides*

Common Names: epazote, wormseed, erva-de-santa maria, mastruço, apasote, paico, pazote, mexican tea, american wormseed, Jesuit's tea, payco, paiku, amush, camatai, cashua, amasamas, anserina, mastruz, sie-sie, jerusalem tea, Spanish tea, ambroisie du mexique, wurmsamen, hierba hormiguera

Parts Used: leaf, plant, seed

TRIBAL AND HERBAL MEDICINE USES

EPAZOTE		
HERBAL PROPERTIES AND ACTIONS		
Main Actions	**Other Actions**	**Standard Dosage**
• expels worms	• increases perspiration	Leaves
• kills parasites	• increases urination	**Decoction:** 1/2 cup once daily
• kills amebas	• increases breast milk	
• mildly laxative	• promotes menstruation	
• kills bacteria	• stimulates digestion	
• prevents ulcers	• calms nerves	
• repels insects	• mildly sedative	
	• heals wounds	
	• kills cancer cells	

Epazote is an annual herb that grows to about 1 m in height. It has multi-branched, reddish stems covered with small, sharply toothed leaves. Epazote bears numerous small yellow flowers in clusters along its stems. Following the flowers, it produces thousands of tiny black seeds in small fruit clusters. It is easily spread and re-grown from the numerous seeds it produces, which is why some consider it an invasive weed. The whole plant gives off a strong and distinctive odor.

Epazote is native to Mexico and the tropical regions of Central and South America, where it is commonly used as a culinary herb, as well as a medicinal plant. It has been widely naturalized throughout the world and can be found growing in parts of the southern United States. In Brazil, the plant's name is *erva-de-santa-maria* or *mastruço;* in Peru it is called *paico.* It is known throughout Mexico and Latin America as *epazote.* The Siona name of this plant means *worm remedy* and here in America it is referred to as *wormseed*—both referring to its long history of use against intestinal worms.

In the Yucatan, indigenous Indian groups have long used epazote for intestinal parasites, asthma, excessive mucus, chorea (a type of rheumatic fever that affects the brain), and other nervous afflictions. The Tikuna Indians in the Amazon use it to expel intestinal worms and as a mild laxative. The Siona-Secoya and Kofán Indian tribes in South America also use epazote for intestinal worms (usually by taking 1 cup of a leaf decoction each morning before eating for three consecutive days). The Kofán Indians also use the plant as a perfume—tying it to their arm for an aromatic bracelet. (However, most Americans consider the smell of the plant quite strong and objectionable—calling it *skunk-weed*!) Creoles use it as a worm remedy for children and a cold medicine for adults, while

the Wayãpi use the plant decoction for stomach upsets and internal hemorrhages caused by falls. In Piura, a leaf decoction is used to expel intestinal gas,
as a mild laxative, as an insecticide, and as a natural remedy for cramps, gout,
hemorrhoids, intestinal worms and parasites, and nervous disorders. Some
indigenous tribes bathe in a decoction of epazote to reduce fever and will also
throw a couple of freshly uprooted green plants onto their fires to drive mosquitoes and flies away.

*Epazote is a common
remedy for intestinal
worms and parasites
worldwide.*

In herbal medicine systems throughout Latin America, epazote is a popular
household remedy used to rid children and adults of intestinal parasites,
worms, and amebas. The plant is also used in cooking—it is said to prevent
intestinal gas if the leaves are cooked and/or eaten with beans and other common gas-forming foods. The leaves and seeds of epazote have long been used
in Central and South American medicine as a vermifuge (to expel intestinal
worms). In Brazilian herbal medicine, it is considered an important remedy for
worms (especially hookworms, round worms, and tape worms) and is also
used for coughs, asthma, bronchitis and other upper respiratory complaints, for
angina, to relieve intestinal gas, to promote sweating, and as a general digestive aid. It is used for similar conditions in Peruvian herbal medicine today.
Local people in the Amazon region in Peru also soak the plant in water for
several days and use it as a topical arthritis remedy. In other South American
herbal medicine systems, the plant is used for asthma, bronchitis, diarrhea,
dysentery, and menstrual disorders. Externally, it has been used as a wash for
hemorrhoids, bruises, wounds, contusions, and fractures.

The plant's ability to expel intestinal worms has been attributed to the essential oil of the seed and "Oil of Chenopodium" has been used for several centuries worldwide as a worm remedy. The oil was once in the *U.S. Pharmacopoeia*
as a drug used against amebas, roundworms, and hookworms. The therapeutic dose of the essential oil, however, does have other toxic effects; therefore it
fell from favor as an internal remedy many years ago. Intake of 10 mg of the oil
has been known to cause cardiac disturbances, convulsions, respiratory disturbances, sleepiness, vomiting and weakness, and even death.[1]

**PLANT
CHEMICALS**

Epazote is rich in chemicals called monoterpenes. The seed and fruit contain a
large amount of essential oil, which has a main active chemical in it called
ascaridole.[2,3] This chemical was first isolated in 1895 by a German pharmacist
living in Brazil and it has been attributed with most of the vermifuge (worm-
expelling) actions of the plant. Ascaridole has been also documented with sedative and pain-relieving properties,[4] as well as antifungal effects.[5] Application
of the oil topically was reported to effectively treat ringworm within seven to
twelve days in a clinical study with guinea pigs.[5] In other *in vitro* clinical stud-

ies, ascaridole was documented with activity against a tropical parasite called *Trypanosoma cruzi* [3] as well as strong antimalarial[6] and insecticidal actions.[7]

The main chemicals found in epazote include alpha-pinene, aritasone, ascaridole, butyric-acid, d-camphor, essential oils, ferulic-acid, geraniol, l-pinocarvone, limonene, malic-acid, menthadiene, menthadiene hydroperoxides, methyl-salicylate, myrcene, p-cymene, p-cymol, safrole, saponins, spinasterol, tartaric-acid, terpinene, terpinyl-acetate, terpinyl-salicylate, triacontyl-alcohol, trimethylamine, urease, and vanillic-acid.

BIOLOGICAL ACTIVITIES AND CLINICAL RESEARCH

A decoction and infusion of the plant was analyzed *in vitro* to determine if they had toxic effects. At various concentrations, the extracts caused cellular aberrations in the test tube, indicating possible toxic effects.[8] However, in the 1970s the World Health Organization reported that a decoction of 20 g of leaves rapidly expelled parasites without any apparent side effects in humans.[9] In 1996, extracts from the leaves of epazote were given to seventy-two children and adults with intestinal parasitic infections. A stool analysis was performed before, and eight days after, treatment. On average, an antiparasitic efficacy was seen in 56 percent of cases.[10] With respect to the tested parasites, epazote leaf extract was 100 percent effective against the common intestinal parasites, *Ancilostoma* and *Trichuris,* and 50 percent effective against *Ascaris.*[10]

Human studies confirm epazote is an effective natural parasite remedy.

In a study in 2001, thirty children (ages 3–14 years) with intestinal roundworms were treated with epazote. Doses given were 1 ml of extract per kg of body weight for younger children (weighing less than 25 pounds), and 2 ml of extract per kg of body weight in older children. One dose was given daily on an empty stomach for three days. Stool examinations were conducted before and fifteen days after treatment. Disappearance of the *Ascaris* eggs occurred in 86.7 percent, while the parasitic burden decreased in 59.5 percent.[11] In addition, this study also reported that epazote was 100 percent effective in eliminating the common human tapeworm (*Hymenolepsis nana*).

In other research, epazote has been documented with toxic effects against snails[12] and was shown to have an *in vitro* toxic action against drug-resistant strains of *Mycobacterium tuberculosis.*[13] In 2002, a U.S. patent was filed on a Chinese herbal combination containing epazote for the treatment of peptic ulcers. This combination (containing *Chenopodium* essential oil) was reported to inhibit stress-induced, as well as various chemical- and bacteria-induced ulcer formation.[14] The most recent research has documented the anticancerous and antitumorous properties of epazote. In one study, an extract of the entire plant of epazote showed the ability to kill human liver cancer cells in the test tube.[15] Another study reported that the essential oil of epazote (as well as its main chemical, ascaridole) showed strong antitumorous actions against numerous different cancerous tumor cells (including several multi-drug resistant tumor cell lines) in the test tube.[16]

CURRENT PRACTICAL USES Due to the toxicity of the essential oil (usually distilled from the seeds), the oil of this plant is no longer recommended for internal use. The leaves of the plant (containing smaller amounts of essential oil) is the preferred natural treatment for intestinal parasites in herbal medicine systems today throughout the world. It is best to find a source for only epazote leaves, as products sold as "whole herb" can contain a significant amount of seeds (and resulting essential oil) depending on when it was harvested. For intestinal worms and parasites, most herbalists and practitioners recommend $\frac{1}{2}$ cup of a standard leaf decoction taken in the morning on an empty stomach for three days in a row. On the fourth day, a mild laxative is given to evacuate the bowel (and the dead and dying parasites and worms). This is repeated two weeks later to address any worm eggs that may have survived and hatched.

Traditional Preparation For intestinal parasites, $\frac{1}{2}$ cup of a leaf decoction is taken once daily on an empty stomach for three days. A decoction of the leaves is employed (in $\frac{1}{2}$ cup dosages) for menstrual, respiratory, and digestive problems on an as-needed basis.

Contraindications The plant and essential oil should not be used during pregnancy and lactation. Not only does the plant have toxic activity, it has also been traditionally used to induce abortions.

While epazote has been used by indigenous tribes as a contraceptive, this use is not verified by clinical research (nor should it be relied on for such). However, the use of the plant is probably contraindicated for couples trying to get pregnant.

The oil of epazote is considered extremely toxic and should not be taken internally.

Drug Interactions None known.

Worldwide Ethnomedical Uses

Region	Uses
Belize	for digestive problems, hangovers, intestinal gas, intestinal parasites, and as a sedative
Brazil	for abortions, angina, bacterial infections, bronchitis, bruises, circulation problems, colds, coughs, contusions, digestive sluggishness, dyspepsia, falls, flu, fractures, gastric disorders, hemorrhages, hemorrhoids, increasing perspiration, insomnia, intestinal gas, intestinal parasites, laryngitis, menstrual difficulties, palpitations, sinusitis, skin parasites, skin inflammation, skin ulceration, spasms, throat inflammation, tuberculosis, worms, wounds, and as an insect repellent and sedative

Ecuador	for indigestion, intestinal gas, intestinal worms, slow digestion
Haiti	for parasites, skin sores, stomachache, worms, and as an antiseptic
Mexico	for colic, increasing perspiration, menstrual disorders, nerves, parasites, toothache, tumors, water retention, worms
Panama	for asthma, dysentery, worms
Peru	for abscesses, arthritis, birth control, blood cleansing, cholera, colic, contusions, cough, cramps, diabetes, diarrhea, digestive problems, dysentery, edema, excessive mucus, fractures, gastritis, gout, hemorrhoids, hysteria, increasing perspiration, indigestion, intestinal gas, liver support, lung problems, memory, menstrual disorders, nervousness, numbness, pain, paralysis, parasites, pleurisy, rheumatism, skin disorders, spasms, stomach pain, tumors, urinary tract inflammation, urinary infections, vaginal discharge, vomiting, water retention, worms, wounds; and as an antacid, antiseptic, insect repellent, and sedative
Trinidad	for amebic infections, asthma, childbirth, dysentery, dyspepsia, fatigue, fungal infections, lung problems, palpitations, sores, worms
Turkey	for asthma, digestive problems, menstrual difficulties, nervous disorders, worms
United States	for childbirth, increasing milk flow, menstrual disorders, nerves, pain, parasites, worms
Venezuela	for aiding digestion, worms
Elsewhere	for abortions, amebic infections, anemia, appendicitis, arthritis, asthma, breathing difficulty, bug bites, childbirth, cholera, colds, colic, conjunctivitis, coughs, cramps, dyspepsia, dysentery, fatigue, fever, fungal infections, hookworms, increasing perspiration, intestinal gas, intestinal parasites, intestinal ulceration, malaria, measles, menstrual irregularities, nervousness, neurosis, pains, palpitations, paralysis, rheumatism, roundworms, snakebite, stomach problems, spasms, tonic, tumor, water retention, worms; and as an antiseptic, insecticide, lactation aid, and sedative

River tributary in the Brazilian Amazon.

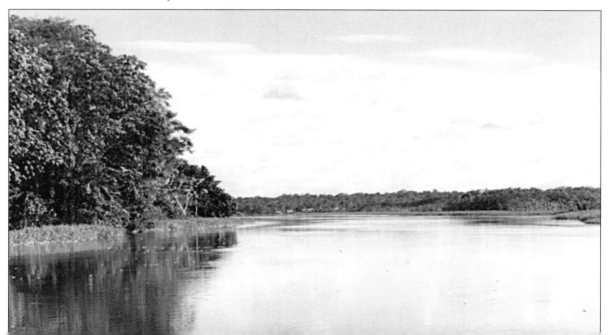

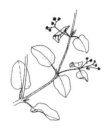

Family: Nyctaginaceae

Genus: *Boerhaavia*

Species: *diffusa, hirsuta*

Common Names:
erva tostão, erva toustao,
pega-pinto, hog weed, pig
weed, atikamaamidi,
biskhapra, djambo, etiponia,
fowl's lice, ganda'dar, ghetuli,
katkatud, mahenshi, mamauri,
ndandalida, oulouni niabo,
paanbalibis, patal-jarh,
pitasudu-pala, punar-nava,
punerva, punnarnava, purnoi,
samdelma, san, sant, santh,
santi, satadi thikedi, satodi,
spreading hog weed, tellaaku,
thazhuthama, thikri, touri-
touri, tshrana

Parts Used: whole herb,
roots

ERVA TOSTÃO
HERBAL PROPERTIES AND ACTIONS

Main Actions
- protects liver
- supports liver
- reduces inflammation
- relieves pain
- reduces spasms
- supports kidneys
- increases urination
- stops bleeding
- lowers blood pressure
- mildly laxative
- kills parasites

Other Actions
- detoxifies
- expels worms
- increases bile
- cleanses blood
- stops convulsions
- kills bacteria
- kills amebas
- kills viruses
- detoxifies
- stimulates milk flow

Standard Dosage
Leaves, Root

Decoction: 1 cup one to
three times daily

Tincture: 2 ml one to three
times daily

Capsules/Tablets: 500 mg–
2 g one to three times
daily

Erva tostão is a vigorous, low-growing, spreading vine with a long, tuberous taproot. It produces yellow and white flowers and is sometimes considered an invasive weed. It can be found in many tropical and warm-climate countries. Indigenous to Brazil, it is found in abundance along roadsides and in the forests in and near São Paulo, Rio de Janeiro, and Minas Gerais. Erva tostão is also indigenous to India, where it is found in abundance in the warmer parts of the country. Erva tostão is called *punarnava* in India, where it has a long history of use by indigenous and tribal people and in Ayurvedic herbal medicine systems.

TRIBAL AND HERBAL MEDICINE USES

The roots of erva tostão have held an important place in herbal medicine in both Brazil and India for many years. G. L. Cruz, one of Brazil's leading medical herbalists, reports erva tostão is "a plant medicine of great importance, extraordinarily beneficial in the treatment of liver disorders." It is employed in Brazilian herbal medicine to stimulate the emptying of the gallbladder, as a diuretic, for all types of liver disorders (including jaundice and hepatitis), gallbladder pain and stones, urinary tract disorders, renal disorders, kidney stones, cystitis, and nephritis. In Ayurvedic herbal medicine systems in India, the roots are employed as a diuretic, digestive aid, laxative, and menstrual promoter and to treat gonorrhea, internal inflammation of all kinds, edema, jaundice, menstrual problems, anemia, and liver, gallbladder, and kidney disorders. Throughout the tropics, erva tostão is considered an excellent natural remedy for guinea worms—a bothersome tropical parasite that lays its eggs underneath the skin of humans and livestock; the eggs later hatch into larvae or worms that eat the underlying tissue. The roots of the plant are normally softened in boiling water and then mashed up and applied as a paste or poultice to the affected areas to kill the worms and expel them from the skin.

PLANT CHEMICALS

Novel plant chemicals have been found in erva tostão, including flavonoids, steroids, and alkaloids, many of which drive its documented biological activities. The novel alkaloids found in erva tostão have been documented with immune modulating effects. In one study, the alkaloid fraction of the root evidenced a dramatic effect in reducing an elevation of cortisol levels under stressful conditions (cortisol is an inflammatory chemical produced in the body in an immune response).[1] Simultaneously, the alkaloids (and a whole root extract[2]) also prevented a drop in immune system performance indicating an adaptogenic immune modulation activity, which might suggest it could be helpful in preventing adrenal exhaustion.[1,2]

The main plant chemicals in erva tostão include alanine, arachidic acid, aspartic acid, behenic acid, boeravinone A through F, boerhaavic acid, borhavine, borhavone, campesterol, daucosterol, ecdysone, flavones, galactose, glutamic acid, glutamine, glycine, hentriacontane, heptadecyclic acid, histidine, hypoxanthine, liriodendrin, oleaic acid, oxalic acid, palmitic acid, proline, punarnavine, serine, sitosterols, stearic acid, stigmasterol, syringaresinol, threonine, triacontan, ursolic acid, and valine.

BIOLOGICAL ACTIVITIES AND CLINICAL RESEARCH

Many of erva tostão's traditional uses are being confirmed by clinical research.

Erva tostão has long been used in traditional medicine systems as a diuretic (to increase urination) for many types of kidney and urinary disorders. The diuretic action of erva tostão has been studied and validated by scientists in several studies. Researchers showed that low dosages (10–300 mg per kg of body weight) produced strong diuretic effects, while higher dosages (more than 300 mg/kg) produced the opposite effect—reducing urine output.[3] Later research verified these diuretic and antidiuretic properties, as well as the beneficial kidney and renal effects of erva tostão in animals and humans.[4–8] Research indicates that a root extract can increase urine output by as much as 100 percent in a twenty-four-hour period at dosages as low as 10 mg per kg of body weight.[4]

The worldwide use of erva tostão for various liver complaints and disorders was validated in three separate studies. These indicated that a root extract provided beneficial effects in animals by protecting the liver from numerous introduced toxins and even repairing chemical-induced liver and kidney damage.[8–10] In other clinical studies with animals, erva tostão extracts demonstrated smooth muscle and skeletal muscle stimulant activities in frogs and guinea pigs;[11] anti-inflammatory actions in rats;[4] hypotensive actions in dogs as well as *in vitro* hypotensive actions;[11] antispasmodic actions in frogs and guinea pigs;[11,12] analgesic activities in mice;[13] and antiamebic actions in rats.[14] In two studies with monkeys, a root extract was reported to reduce bleeding and uterine hemorrhaging commonly associated with wearing contraceptive IUDs.[15,16] The traditional use of erva tostão for convulsions was verified by scientists in two studies, demonstrating that a root extract provided anticonvulsant actions in mice.[17,18] *In vitro* testing of erva tostão confirmed its antibacterial properties against gonorrhea (another traditional use), as well as *Bacillus, Pseudomonas, Salmonella,* and *Staphylococcus*.[19–21] It was also shown to possess antiviral actions against several viral plant pathogens.[22]

CURRENT PRACTICAL USES

Many of these animal studies help to explain erva tostão's long history of different uses in natural medicine. Clearly, it has played an important role in the herbal practitioner's medicine chest of natural remedies for many maladies in both South America and India. It is an effective natural remedy, especially for the liver and kidneys, which is deserving of much more attention and use here in the United States. Several research groups studying various biological activities of erva tostão have shown the safety of the plant—indicating no toxicity of root and leaf extracts taken orally by mice at up to 5 g per kg of body weight.[9,13] Another group of scientists studied the effects of erva tostão on pregnant rats and reported that it had no abortive effects and no embryotoxic or teratogenic (fetal death or birth defect) activity.[23]

Traditional Preparation

For a general liver tonic, 1 cup of a whole herb or root decoction or 2 ml of a 4:1 tincture is taken once daily. This same dosage is taken two to three times daily for various liver and kidney disorders. For a natural diuretic, 500 mg of the root in capsules or tablets can be taken twice daily. As a menstrual aid (to reduce menstrual pain, cramping, and excessive bleeding) 1 cup of a whole herb or root decoction or 1–2 g in tablets or capsules can be taken two to three times daily as needed.

Contraindications

Both *in vivo* and *in vitro* studies have demonstrated the hypotensive properties of erva tostão. Those with heart problems such as low blood pressure, or those taking medications to lower their blood pressure, should not use this plant without the advice and supervision of a qualified health care practitioner as blood pressure levels should be monitored closely.

This herb has also demonstrated myocardial depressant activity[11] and should therefore not be taken by anyone with heart failure or those taking heart depressant medications unless under the direction and care of a qualified health care practitioner.

Drug Interactions Erva tostão may interfere with prescription diuretics and may potentiate cardiac depressant medications. Erva tostão has been documented in one *in vitro* study to have angiotensin-converting enzyme (ACE) inhibition action.[22] Therefore, this plant may potentiate ACE inhibitor drugs for high blood pressure. In one study, an oral dosage of 500 mg/kg (leaf extract) in mice inhibited barbiturates and decreased sleeping time.[13] Therefore, the use of this plant may decrease the effect of barbiturates.

Worldwide Ethnomedical Uses

Region	Uses
Brazil	for albuminuria, beri-beri, bile insufficiency, cystitis, edema, gallbladder problems, gallstones, gonorrhea, guinea worms, hepatitis, hypertension, jaundice, kidney disorders, kidney stones, liver disorders, liver support, nephritis, renal disorders, sclerosis (liver), snakebite, spleen (enlarged), urinary disorders, urinary retention
Guatemala	for erysipelas, guinea worms
India	for abdominal pain, anemia, ascites, asthma, blood purification, cancer, cataracts, childbirth, cholera, constipation, cough, debility, digestive sluggishness, dyspepsia, edema, eye problems, fever, gonorrhea, guinea worms, heart ailments, heart disease, hemorrhages (childbirth), hemorrhages (thoracic), hemorrhoids, inflammation (internal), internal parasites, jaundice, kidney disorders, kidney stones, liver disorders, liver support, menstrual disorders, renal insufficiency, rheumatism, snakebite, spleen (enlarged), urinary disorders, weakness; as a diuretic, expectorant, and lactation aid
Iran	for edema, gonorrhea, hives, intestinal gas, jaundice, joint pain, lumbago, nephritis; as an appetite stimulant, diuretic, and expectorant
Nigeria	for abscess, asthma, boils, convulsions, epilepsy, fever, guinea worms, and as an expectorant and laxative
West Africa	for abortion, guinea worms, menstrual irregularities, and as an aphrodisiac
Elsewhere	for childbirth, guinea worms, jaundice, sterility, yaws

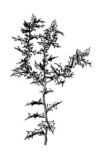

Family: Celastraceae

Genus: *Maytenus*

Species: *ilicifolia*

Common Names: espinheira santa, cancerosa, cangorosa, limaosinho, maiteno

Parts Used: leaves, bark, roots

ESPINHEIRA SANTA
HERBAL PROPERTIES AND ACTIONS

Main Actions	Other Actions	Standard Dosage
• reduces acid	• relieves pain	Leaves
• prevents ulcers	• kills germs	**Decoction:** 1 cup two to three times daily
• aids digestion	• cleanses blood	
• kills cancer cells	• increases urination	**Tablets/Capsules:** 2–3 g twice daily
• kills leukemia cells	• mildly laxative	
• inhibits tumors	• promotes menstruation	
• detoxifies	• reduces fertility	

Espinheira santa is a small, shrubby evergreen tree growing to 5 m in height with leaves and berries that resemble holly. It is native to many parts of South America and southern Brazil and it is even found in city landscapes for its attractive, holly-like appearance. With over 200 species of *Maytenus* distributed in temperate and tropical regions throughout South America and the West Indies, there are many *Maytenus* species that are indigenous to the Amazon region, which have been used medicinally by indigenous tribes.

TRIBAL AND HERBAL MEDICINE USES

This particular *Maytenus* species has not been used as extensively by the indigenous peoples in the Amazon region as other *Maytenus* trees in the area. It has been used by some native groups in Paraguay, where women use the plant as a contraceptive and fertility regulator, and to induce menstruation and abortions. Espinheira santa has a much longer and better documented history of use in urban areas and South American herbal medicine practices than in tribal areas, probably because of the types of illnesses that it treats. In Brazil, the leaves of the plant are brewed into a tea for the treatment of ulcers, indigestion, chronic gastritis, and dyspepsia (with a recorded history of use for these purposes dating back to the 1930s). The leaf tea is also applied topically to wounds, rashes, and skin cancer. In Brazilian pharmacies today, a topical ointment is made with espinheira santa and sold for skin cancer. In other herbal medicine systems in South America, espinheira santa for is used for anemia, stomach and gastric ulcers, cancer, constipation, gastritis, dyspepsia, liver disorders, and as a contraceptive. In Argentinean herbal medicine, the entire plant or leaves are infused or decocted for its antiseptic and wound healing properties and it is commonly used internally for asthma, respiratory and urinary tract infections, diarrhea, and to induce menstruation.

Espinheira santa is used for skin cancer, however its most popular use has been for the treatment of ulcers, indigestion, chronic gastritis, and dyspepsia.

PLANT CHEMICALS

Espinheira santa is a source for a group of well known chemicals (found in the leaf, bark, and roots of the tree) called *maytansinoids*. These chemicals represent a class of substances that have been studied since the early 1970s for their anti-tumorous and anticancerous activities and are today being developed into chemotherapy drugs. A different class of chemicals found in espinheira santa—triterpene chemicals called *cangorins*—have also evidenced significant antitumorous, antileukemic, and anticancerous properties.

> Espinheira santa contains many chemicals which have documented anticancerous actions.

The main plant chemicals include: atropcangorosin, cangoaronin, cangorins A through J, cangorinine, cangorosin A and B, celastrol, dispermol, dispermone, friedelan, friedelin, friedelinol, friedoolean, friedooleanan, ilicifolin, ilicifolinoside A through C, kaempferol trisaccharides, kaempferol disaccharides, maitenine, maytanbutine, maytanprine, maytansine, maytenin, maytenoic acid, maytenoquinone, pristimeriin, pristimerin, quercetin trisaccharides, quercitrin, salaspermic acid, tingenol, and tingenone.

BIOLOGICAL ACTIVITIES AND CLINICAL RESEARCH

Espinheira santa has been the subject of many clinical studies, fueled by its effectiveness in treating ulcers and even cancer, with research beginning as early as the mid-1960s. Toxicity studies in 1978 and 1991 showed no toxicity in rats and mice in dosages up to 1 g per kg of body weight.[1,2] Due to its reported traditional use as an abortive aid and contraceptive, researchers studied those aspects specifically but were unable to clinically validate these uses. In one study, a water extract fed to pregnant mice daily did not induce abortion and did not cause any fetus change.[2] Another research group injecting pregnant rats with leaf extracts (up to 100 mg/kg) reported that it did not cause abortive effects or toxic effects to the fetus, but did interfere in fertilization and implantation in non-pregnant rats.[3] A study in 2002 confirmed these results, again stating that a leaf extract had estrogenic actions, which suggested the anti-fertility effect may be the interference of uterine receptivity to the embryo, but did not induce abortions or have any embryotoxic effects.[4] It was also reported in 1998 by the same scientist that it had no effect in male mice on sperm production.[5]

> In a 1976 plant screening program by the National Cancer Institute, espinheira santa was reported to be toxic to cancer and leukemia cells at very low dosages.

Early research performed in Brazil in the 1970s revealed that espinheira santa, as well as a few other species in the *Maytenus* family, contains maytansinoid chemical compounds that showed potent anti-tumor and antileukemic activities *in vivo* and *in vitro* at very low dosages.[6–9] Then in a 1976 plant screening program by the National Cancer Institute (NCI), an alcohol and water extract of the leaves was documented with toxicity to cancer cells at very low dosages[10] and U.S. and European pharmaceutical companies began to show an interest in it. Two of the chemicals, named *maytansine* and *mayteine*, were extracted and tested in cancer patients in the United States and South America in the 1970s, following the NCI research.[11–15] Although there were some significant regressions in ovarian carcinoma and some lymphomas with maytansine,[15] further research was not continued due to the toxicity at the dosages used.[16] Research with the compound maytene revealed little-to-no toxicity[8,11,12] and validated its uses in traditional medicine for various types of skin cancers.[17,18] In the 1990s, Japanese researchers discovered a different set of compounds (triterpene chemicals) in espinheira santa which they named *cangorins* (cangorin A through J). These new chemicals showed cytotoxic and/or inhibitory activity against various leukemia and cancer tumor cells, and the researchers have published more than eight studies on their discovery and results.[19–26]

Animal studies suggest espinheira santa is as effective for ulcers as the two leading anti-ulcer drugs sold today.

Although espinheira santa is still used in South American traditional medicine for various types of cancer, its most popular use has been for the treatment of ulcers and digestive complaints. Its potent anti-ulcerous abilities were demonstrated in a 1991 study, which showed that a simple hot water extract of espinheira santa leaves was as effective as two of the leading anti-ulcer drugs, ranitidine (Zantac®) and cimetidine (Tagamet®). The same study showed that espinheira santa caused an increase in volume and pH of gastric juice.[27] In 1997, a Japanese research group filed a patent on the biologically active anti-ulcer compounds found in espinheira santa as a new anti-ulcer drug.[28]

CURRENT PRACTICAL USES

Espinheira santa is still widely sold in Brazilian stores and pharmacies today for stomach ulcers and cancer. With its popularity and beneficial results in South America, as well as its recent western research, espinheira santa is slowly becoming more popular and well known in the United States. Leaf infusions and/or leaf powder in capsules or tablets are currently being used for ulcers, as an antacid, as a laxative, as a colic remedy, to eliminate toxins through the kidneys and skin, to support kidneys, support adrenal glands, support digestive functions, and as an adjunctive therapy for cancer.

Traditional Preparation

One cup of a standard leaf decoction is taken two to three times daily (or with meals as a digestive aid). If desired, 2–3 g of leaf powder in tablets, capsules, or stirred into juice or water once or twice daily can be substituted. A standard leaf decoction can also be applied directly to the skin for topical use for wounds, rashes, and skin cancer.

Contraindications

Research suggests that water extracts of espinheira santa may have estrogenic effects and reduce fertility in females. Women seeking treatment for infertility, attempting to get pregnant, or those with estrogen-positive cancers should not use this plant.

Drug Interactions

One study involving mice injected with a water extract of leaves recorded barbiturate potentiation activity. However, the same study notes no potentiation activity when administered to mice orally.[1]

Worldwide Ethnomedical Uses

Region	Uses
Argentina	for abortions, asthma, cancer, diarrhea, increasing saliva, menstrual difficulties, respiratory tract infections, urinary tract infections, wounds, and as an antiseptic
Brazil	for asthma, bile disorders, cancer, digestive problems, gallbladder support, increasing saliva, inflammation, intestinal problems, pain, ulcers, wounds, and as an antiseptic and aphrodisiac
Paraguay	for abortions, birth control, libido, menstrual regulation
Elsewhere	for arthritis, asthma, cancer, contraceptive, digestive problems, rheumatism, spasms, tumors, water retention, wounds, and as an antiseptic

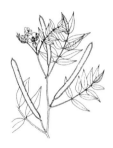

Family: Leguminosae

Genus: *Cassia*

Species: *occidentalis*

Common Names: fedegoso, fedegosa, yerba hedionda, brusca, guanina, martinica, platanillo, manjerioba, peieriaba, retama, achupa poroto, heduibda, folha-de-pajé, kasiah, khiyar shember, pois piante, shih chueh ming, sinamekki, tlalhoaxin, wang chiang nan, senting, kachang kota, menting

Parts Used: roots, leaves, seeds, bark, flowers

FEDEGOSO

HERBAL PROPERTIES AND ACTIONS

Main Actions
- protects liver
- detoxifies liver
- kills bacteria
- kills fungi
- kills parasites
- kills viruses
- expels worms
- enhances immunity
- cleanses blood
- kills germs
- detoxifies
- promotes perspiration
- mildly laxative

Other Actions
- relieves pain
- reduces inflammation
- kills cancer cells
- reduces spasms
- reduces fever
- reduces blood pressure
- kills insects

Standard Dosage

Leaves

Infusion: 1 cup twice daily

Tincture: 3–4 ml twice daily

Tablets/Capsules: 1–2 g twice daily

Fedegoso is a small tree that grows 5–8 m high and is found in many tropical areas of South America, including the Amazon. Indigenous to Brazil, it is also found in warmer climates and tropical areas of South, Central, and North America. It is in the same genus as senna (*C. senna*) and is sometimes called "coffee senna." It is botanically classified as both *Senna occidentalis* and *Cassia occidentalis*. Its seeds, found in long seed pods, are sometimes roasted and made into a coffee-like beverage. The *Cassia* genus comprises some 600 species of trees, shrubs, vines, and herbs, with numerous species growing in the South American rainforests and tropics. Many species have been used medicinally, and these tropical plants have a rich history in natural medicine. Various *Cas-*

sia plants have been known since the ninth or tenth centuries as purgatives and laxatives, including *Cassia angustifolia* and *Cassia senna.*

TRIBAL AND HERBAL MEDICINE USES

Fedegoso has been used as natural medicine in the rainforest and other tropical areas for centuries. Its roots, leaves, flowers, and seeds have been employed in herbal medicine around the world. In Peru, the roots are considered a diuretic, and a decoction is made for fevers. The seeds are brewed into a coffee-like beverage for asthma, and a flower infusion is used for bronchitis in the Peruvian Amazon. In Brazil, the roots of fedegoso are considered a tonic, fever reducer, and diuretic; they are used for fevers, menstrual problems, tuberculosis, anemia, liver complaints, and as a tonic for general weakness and illness. The leaves are also used in Brazil for gonorrhea, fevers, urinary tract disorders, edema, and menstrual problems. The Miskito Indians of Nicaragua use a fresh plant decoction for general pain, menstrual and uterine pain, and constipation in babies. In Panama, a leaf tea is used for stomach colic, the crushed leaves are used in a poultice as an anti-inflammatory, and the crushed fresh leaves are taken internally to expel intestinal worms and parasites. In many countries around the world, the fresh and/or dried leaves of fedegoso are crushed or brewed into a tea and applied externally for skin disorders, wounds, skin fungus, parasitic skin diseases, abscesses, and as a topical analgesic and anti-inflammatory natural medicine.

Virtually all parts of the fedegoso plant are used in herbal medicine systems around the world.

PLANT CHEMICALS

The *Cassia* plants are well known for a group of chemicals with strong laxative actions called *anthraquinones.* The most widely used species of *Cassia* in herbal medicine is known as *senna* (*Cassia senna* or *C. acutifolia*). The actions of the anthraquinones chemicals are the basis of senna's widespread use as a purgative and strong laxative. While fedegoso does contain a small amount of these anthraquinones, it was shown in a rat study not to have the same strong purgative and laxative effects as senna.[1]

The main plant chemicals in fedegoso include achrosine, aloe-emodin, anthraquinones, anthrones, apigenin, aurantiobtusin, campesterol, cassiollin, chryso-obtusin, chrysophanic acid, chrysarobin, chrysophanol, chrysoeriol, emodin, essential oils, funiculosin, galactopyranosyl, helminthosporin, islandicin, kaempferol, lignoceric acid, linoleic acid, linolenic acid, mannitol, mannopyranosyl, matteucinol, obtusifolin, obtusin, oleic acid, physcion, quercetin, rhamnosides, rhein, rubrofusarin, sitosterols, tannins, and xanthorin.

BIOLOGICAL ACTIVITIES AND CLINICAL RESEARCH

Fedegoso has been the subject of recent clinical research for its beneficial effects on the liver and immune system. In the late 1970s, two research groups published three studies citing the beneficial effects of fedegoso in human patients with liver toxicity, hepatitis, and even acute liver failure.[2-4] Other researchers followed up on those actions, publishing four different *in vivo* studies (mice and rats) from 1994 to 2001. These studies report that fedegoso leaf extracts have the ability to protect the liver from various introduced chemical toxins, normalize liver enzymes and processes, and repair liver damage.[5–8] Some of this research has also demonstrated significant immunostimulant activity by increasing humoral immunity and bone marrow immune cells in mice, and protecting them from chemically-induced immunosuppression.[8] These researchers and others also reported the antimutagenic actions of fedegoso.[5,8,9] In this research, fedegoso was able to prevent or reduce the mutation of healthy cells in the presence of laboratory chemicals which were known to mutate them.

Clinical studies in humans show fedegoso is benefical for liver and immune functions.

In other *in vivo* studies, fedegoso leaf extracts have demonstrated anti-inflammatory, hypotensive, smooth-muscle relaxant, antispasmodic, weak uterine stimulant, vasoconstrictor, and antioxidant activities in laboratory animals.[10,11] These documented actions certainly help to explain its uses in traditional medicine systems for menstrual cramps and other internal inflammatory conditions. Fedegoso has also been used for many types of bacterial, fungal, and parasitic infections for many years in the tropical countries where it grows. *In vitro* clinical research on fedegoso leaves over the years has reported active antibacterial, antifungal, antiparasitic, insecticidal, and antimalarial properties.[12–19]

CURRENT PRACTICAL USES

Although the seeds of fedegoso are used in herbal medicine in small amounts (and even roasted and brewed as a coffee substitute in some countries), several clinical studies have demonstrated the toxicity of the fresh and/or dried/roasted seeds. Ingestion of large amounts of the seeds by grazing animals has been reported to cause toxicity problems and even death in cows, horses, and goats. Due to the well-known and well-documented toxicity of these seeds, they are best avoided altogether. Toxicity studies on the aerial parts, leaves, and roots of fedegoso have been published by several research groups. These studies reported that various leaf and root extracts given to mice (administered orally and injected at up to 500 mg/kg) did not demonstrate any toxic effect or cause mortality.[5,6,19]

Health practitioners today are employing fedegoso in their practices much the same way it has been in traditional medicine for many years. It is an excellent natural remedy for bacterial and fungal infections and now is clinically shown to boost immune function simultaneously. As a liver tonic, science supports its beneficial action and use in various liver conditions including anemia, hepatitis, and liver damage (drug- or alcohol-induced). New research suggests, with its antimutagenic actions, fedegoso could possibly help keep damaged liver cells from turning into cancerous ones, as often happens with chronic hepatitis B and C infections.

Traditional Preparation The therapeutic dosage is reported to be 1 cup of a standard leaf infusion twice daily. If desired, 3–4 ml of a tincture twice daily or 1–2 g in tablets or capsules twice daily can be substituted.

Contraindications Fedegoso leaf extracts have demonstrated weak uterine stimulant activity and smooth-muscle relaxant actions in rats.[11] As such, the use of this plant is contraindicated during pregnancy.

Fedegoso has demonstrated hypotensive activity in dogs[11] and, as such, is probably contraindicated in people with low blood pressure. Individuals taking medications to lower their blood pressure should check with their doctor first before taking fedegoso (and monitor their blood pressure accordingly, as medications may need to be adjusted).

Long-term ingestion of small amounts and single high dosages of fedegoso seeds cause toxic reactions, including myodegeneration and death. Do not use fedegoso seeds without the supervision of a qualified professional who is familiar with the mechanisms, chemicals, actions, and toxicity of these seeds.

Drug Interactions It may potentiate the effects of antihypertensive drugs. Fedegoso has demonstrated significant antihepatotoxic (liver protective), hepatotonic (liver tonic), and hepatic detoxification (liver detoxifing) effects in animal and human studies. As such, the use of this plant might interfere with the metabolism of some drugs in the liver by increasing the clearance of them and/or reducing their half-life (which may reduce the effects of those drugs that require metabolization in the liver).

Worldwide Ethnomedical Uses

Region	Uses
Africa	for abscesses, bile complaints, birth control, bronchitis, bruises, cataracts, childbirth, constipation, dysentery, edema, erysipelas, eye infections, fainting, fever, gonorrhea, guinea worms, headache, hematuria, hemorrhages (pregnancy), hernia, increasing perspiration, inflammation, itch, jaundice, kidney infections, leprosy, malaria, menstrual disorders, pain (kidney), rheumatism, ringworms, scabies, skin diseases, skin parasites, sore throat, stomach ulcers, stomachache, swelling, syphilis, tetanus, worms, water retention, wounds
Amazonia	for abdominal pain, birth control, bile insufficiency, malaria
Brazil	for anemia, constipation, edema, fatigue, fever, gonorrhea, liver disorders, malaria, menstrual disorders, skin problems, tuberculosis, urinary disorders, water retention, weakness
Central America	for abortions, athlete's foot, birth control, constipation, diarrhea, fungal infections, headache, menstrual disorders, menstrual pain, pain, respiratory infections, ringworm, spasms, urinary insufficiency, urinary tract infections, uterine pain, worms
Haiti	for acne, asthma, burns, colic, constipation, edema, eye infections, gonorrhea, headache, malaria, rheumatism, skin rashes and infections, and to increase perspiration

India	for abscesses, bites (scorpion), constipation, diabetes, edema, fever, inflammation, itch, liver diseases, liver support, rheumatism, ringworm, scabies, skin diseases, snakebite, wounds
Mexico	for chills, digestive sluggishness, dyspepsia, earache, eczema, edema, fatigue, fever, headache, inflammation (skin), laxative, leprosy, nausea, pain, rash, rheumatism, ringworms, sexually transmitted diseases, skin problems, sores, stomachache, swelling, tumors, ulcers, water retention, worms, yellow fever
Panama	for colic, inflammation, spasms, stomach problems, worms, and as an antiseptic
Peru	for asthma, bronchitis, fever, liver problems, urinary insufficiency
Trinidad	for abortions, childbirth, colds, constipation, heart problems, inflammation, liver problems, palpitations
Venezuela	for asthma, colds, fever, intestinal gas, malaria, menstrual difficulties, skin problems, water retention
Elsewhere	for abdominal pain, abortions, bile insufficiency, birth control, bites (scorpion), childbirth, constipation, dermatosis, digestive problems, eczema, edema, eye infections, fevers, gonorrhea, headache, hemoglobin disorders, hemorrhage, hypertension, laxative, lice, liver disorders, malaria, menstrual disorders, pain, parasites, rheumatism, ringworms, scabies, skin disorders, snakebite, spasms, urinary insufficiency, worms, yellow fever

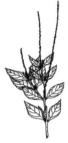

Family: Verbenaceae

Genus: *Stachytarpheta*

Species: *jamaicensis, cayennensis*

Common Names: gervâo, Brazilian tea, verbena cimarrona, bastard vervain, verbena azul, wild verbena, blue flower, rooster comb, jarbao, rat tail, porterweed, gewongan, rumput tahi babi, selaseh dandi (spotted basil)

Parts Used: plant, leaves

GERVÂO

HERBAL PROPERTIES AND ACTIONS

Main Actions
- reduces histamine
- suppresses coughs
- relieves spasms
- reduces acid
- prevents ulcers
- stimulates digestion
- protects gastric tract
- reduces inflammation
- expels worms
- protects liver
- dilates blood vessels
- kills larva

Other Actions
- relieves pain
- increases urination
- promotes menstruation
- reduces fever
- lowers blood pressure
- increases milk flow
- mildly laxative
- sedates
- promotes sweating
- heals wounds

Standard Dosage
Leaves
Infusion: 1/2 cup twice daily
Tincture: 2–3 ml twice daily
Tablets/Capsules: 1–2 g twice daily

Gervâo is a weedy annual (and sometimes perennial) herbaceous plant that grows 60–120 cm tall. It bears small reddish-purple to deep blue flowers that grow along tall stems that are favored by butterflies. It is indigenous to most parts of tropical America and, although some consider it a semi-invasive weed, it is sometimes cultivated as an ornamental plant for its true-blue flowers and striking deeply serrated, dark green leaves. Gervâo belongs to the large verbena family, which comprises about 100 genera and 2,600 species (including the common vervain and verbena plants). It is often referred to as "bastard vervain" or "wild verbena." While very similar to verbena and vervain in appearance and growth habits, gervâo is a different species of plant. Two very similar species of *Stachytarpheta* grow in the tropics and are used interchangeably (and share the same common names) in many countries' herbal medicine systems— *S. cayennensis* and *S. jamaicensis*.

TRIBAL AND HERBAL MEDICINE USES

Gervâo is widely used by indigenous peoples throughout the Amazon. The Créoles use the leaf tea for dysentery, while the Kofans in northwest Amazonia drink a decoction of the plant to relieve stomach pains. Indigenous peoples of Peru use the plant for diabetes and the Wayãpi and Palikur Indians in Guyana use the plant in baths to relieve colds and headaches. Other tribes in the Amazon prepare an infusion or decoction of the plant to take internally for fevers (including yellow fever), allergies, stomach problems, and intestinal parasites.

In Brazilian herbal medicine systems, the plant is considered to stimulate and aid digestion, suppress coughs, reduce fever, expel worms, increase perspiration, and promote menstruation. The natural remedy there is usually an infusion prepared with the leaves or entire aerial parts. It is employed today by Brazilian herbalists and practitioners as a stomach tonic; to stimulate the function of the gastrointestinal tract; for dyspepsia, allergies, asthma, and fevers; and for chronic liver problems. Gervâo is also used in Brazil as a diuretic for various urinary complaints and as a mild laxative for constipation. Externally it is used to clean ulcers, cuts, and wounds. In Cuban herbal medicine (where the plant is named *verbena cimarrona*) the plant is considered to be abortive, laxative, diuretic, and sedative and is used to reduce spasms, depress the central nervous system, promote menstruation, aid milk production, and reduce blood pressure.

Throughout the tropics where gervâo grows, it is a common herbal remedy for intestinal parasites, digestive complaints, and chronic liver disorders.

In the West Indies, gervâo commonly is employed to expel intestinal worms and other parasites; several commercial preparations sold in Jamaica for parasites contain gervâo. One popular preparation combines gervâo with graviola (*Annona muricata*) and epazote (*Chenopodium ambrosioides*) into a natural remedy for this purpose (both plants are featured in this book). Besides its long history of use as a parasite remedy (which was documented as early as 1898), gervâo also has been used by women in Jamaica and the West Indies for many types of menstrual disorders and female complaints. In many parts of the West Indies, a leaf tea is drunk after childbirth to restore health and to increase the supply of mother's milk. In Belize, a tea brewed from the aerial parts of the plant is taken for nervousness, heart conditions, stomachache, dyspepsia, neuralgia, cough, colds, fever, flu, and liver complaints. There the mashed leaves are also used in a poultice for boils and infected sores, and the leaf juice is taken internally for intestinal parasites.

PLANT CHEMICALS

The biological activity of the chemicals found in gervâo help explain the traditional uses of the plant for liver problems and respiratory complaints.

Gervâo contains flavonoids, terpenes, phenols, and steroids. Several of these plant chemicals have been documented with biological activities that may help explain the plant's indigenous uses (especially for liver ailments and respiratory problems). The first of these is an iridoid glycoside called *verbascoside* (also called *acetoside*), found in several plants in the *Verbenaceae* genus. In clinical research, this powerful antioxidant phytochemical has been documented with neuroprotective,[1] antiviral,[2] antibacterial,[3] liver protective,[4,5] cardioactive,[6] and antitumorous[7] effects. A flavonoid in gervâo called *scutellarein* has been documented with cardioprotective,[8] anti-inflammatory,[9] and antiviral[10] actions. Another flavonoid found in gervâo called *hispidulin* is also found in verbena and vervain and is considered one of the main "active" chemicals in all three plants. Hispidulin has been reported to have anti-asthmatic, bronchodilator, and antispasmodic properties;[11] liver detoxifing actions;[12] and to normalize sticky blood.[13]

The main plant chemicals in gervâo include: apigenol-7-glucuronide, alpha-spinasterol, gamma-amino butyric acid, chlorogenic acid, citral, dopamine, friedelin, geraniol, hentriacontane, hispidulin, ipolamiide, luteolol-7-glucuronide, n-dotriacontane, n-nonacosane, n-pentriacontane, n-tetratriancontane, n-triacontane, n-tritriacontane, salicylic-acid, scutellarein, stachytarphine, stigmasterol, tarphetalin, ursolic acid, and verbascoside.

BIOLOGICAL ACTIVITIES AND CLINICAL RESEARCH

Animal studies suggest gervâo relieves pain; reduces spasms and inflammation; reduces stomach acid and prevents ulcers; and acts as a laxative.

The first biological activity studies were published on gervâo in 1962 by researchers in India who reported that the plant demonstrated antispasmodic and vasodilator activities in several small animal studies.[14] In 1990, two clinical studies reported that leaf extracts evidenced larvicidal effects, which might help explain its long history of use for intestinal parasites.[15,16] In 1998, the anti-inflammatory and pain-relieving properties of gervâo were demonstrated in rats.[17] In this study, researchers pre-treated rats with gervâo and showed that it inhibited significantly their ability to induce inflammation with chemical agents. They isolated two chemicals in the plant (vebascoside and another iridoid chemical, ipolamiide) and tested them individually for these effects. These chemicals demonstrated a marked anti-inflammatory effect in rats (administered four hours after chemically inducing inflammation) of 94 percent and 70 percent, respectively. They attributed this effect, in part, to the extract (and its phytochemicals), which inhibited a histamine reaction.

Another area of research has verified gervâo's longstanding use for gastric and intestinal disorders. In a 1995 Brazilian study, a gervâo extract demonstrated anti-diarrhea effects in rats.[18] Another (1997) Brazilian study demonstrated antacid, anti-ulcer, and laxative effects in mice.[19] In this study, a water extract of the whole plant increased intestinal motility, protected against ulcers from various chemical agents, and inhibited gastric secretion. These researchers noted the same histamine-blocking properties in this ulcer model that was observed in the anti-inflammatory model, along with another possible pathways of action. They concluded that "whatever the mechanisms involved, the present data confirm the plant's effectiveness as antacid/antiulcer and laxative." In the mouse and rat studies performed thus far, no toxicity was noted when the plant was taken orally (at up to 2 g per kg of body weight).

CURRENT PRACTICAL USES

In herbal medicine today, gervâo is regarded as a safe, natural remedy when prepared in decoctions and infusions (taken orally or applied externally). A researcher in Panama, however (who injected mice with varying dosages of a leaf extract), reported toxic effects and even death at the highest dosages.[20] While gervâo is a well known and popular natural herbal remedy in South America for digestion and liver problems, colds, flu, asthma, and as a natural antihistamine and anti-inflammatory, practitioners in North America are just beginning to learn about its many uses. With its many applications, gervâo is sure to increase in popularity as more people learn of its many effective uses.

Traditional Preparation

One-half cup of a whole herb infusion is taken one to two times daily or 1–3 ml of a 4:1 tincture is taken twice daily. If desired, 1–2 g powdered herb in tablets, capsules, or stirred into juice or water daily may be substituted.

Contraindications

Gervâo has been used in herbal medicine as an abortive agent and, therefore, is probably contraindicated during pregnancy.

Gervâo has been documented with vasodilator properties in an animal study and, therefore, may lower blood pressure. Those with low blood pressure or those on antihypertensive medications should consult their doctor before using gervâo.

Stachytarpheta cayennensis (but not *S. jamaicensis*) has been reported to contain a small amount of naturally occurring salicylic acid. This phytochemical is the natural precursor to aspirin. Those allergic to aspirin should probably avoid using this plant product.

Drug Interactions

None reported, however the plant might potentiate heart and blood pressure medications.

Worldwide Ethnomedical Uses

Region	Uses
Amazonia	for asthma, fever, stomach pain
Bahamas	for abortions, asthma, bronchitis, chest colds, childbirth, itch, skin problems, sores, worms
Belize	for boils, colds, cough, fever, flu, heart problems, intestinal parasites, liver disorders, nervousness, neuralgia, sores, stomachache
Brazil	for acid reflux, allergies, amebic infections, arthritis, bile insufficiency, bronchitis, bronchial phlegm, chest pains, colds, constipation, contusions, cough, cuts, debilitation, diarrhea, digestive problems, dysentery, dyspepsia, eczema, edema, erysipelas, fever, flu, gastritis, gastrointestinal disorders, hemorrhoids, hepatitis, high blood pressure, hoarseness, intestinal parasites, liver disorders, liver support, lung problems, menstrual disorders, rheumatism, sexually transmitted diseases, skin problems, sores, stomachache, syphilis, tumors, ulcers, urinary complaints, water retention, worms, wounds, yellow fever, and to increase perspiration
Cuba	for abortions, constipation, depressing the central nervous system, diabetes, excessive mucus, fevers, hypertension, lactation aid, menstrual problems, spasms, urinary insufficiency
Haiti	for constipation, digestive complaints, edema, erysipelas, intestinal parasites, menstrual disorders, nerves, sores, tumors, worms, and as a sedative
India	for abortions, dysentery, fever, inflammation, rheumatism, skin ulcers
Mexico	for gonorrhea, menstrual difficulties, nerves, pain, syphilis, yellow fever, promoting perspiration
South America	for birth control, intestinal parasites, menstrual difficulties, worms
Trinidad	for blood cleansing, boils, chest colds, constipation, coughs, dysentery, eczema, eye disorders, eye wash, fever, flu, intestinal parasites, lactation stimulation, rashes, rectitis, stomach, vitiligo, worms
West Indies	for childbirth, intestinal parasites, lactation stimulation, menstrual disorders, skin parasites, worms
Elsewhere	for abortions, bile insufficiency, birth control, boils, bruises, cataracts, constipation, diabetes, diarrhea, dysentery, edema, erysipelas, fever, hair loss, headache, heart support, inflammation, intestinal parasites, liver disease, malaria, menstrual irregularities, nausea, rheumatism, rhinitis, sexually transmitted diseases, sores, sprains, stomach, tumors

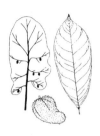

Family: Annonaceae

Genus: *Annona*

Species: *muricata*

Common Names: graviola, soursop, guanábana, guanábano, guanavana, guanaba, corossol épineux, huanaba, toge-banreisi, durian benggala, nangka blanda, cachiman épineux

Parts Used: leaves, fruit, seeds, bark, roots

GRAVIOLA
HERBAL PROPERTIES AND ACTIONS

Main Actions	Other Actions	Standard Dosage
• kills cancer cells	• relieves depression	Leaves
• slows tumor growth	• reduces spasms	**Infusion:** 1 cup three times daily
• kills bacteria	• kills viruses	
• kills parasites	• reduces fever	**Tincture:** 2–4 ml three times daily
• reduces blood pressure	• expels worms	
• lowers heart rate	• stimulates digestion	**Tablets/Capsules:** 2 g three times daily
• dilates blood vessels	• stops convulsions	
• sedates		

Graviola is a small, upright evergreen tree, 5–6 m high, with large, glossy, dark green leaves. It produces a large, heart-shaped, edible fruit that is 15–20 cm in diameter and green in color, with white flesh inside. Graviola is indigenous to most of the warmest tropical areas in South and North America, including the Amazon. The fruit is sold in local markets in the tropics, where it is called *graviola* in Brazil, *guanábana* in Spanish-speaking countries, and *soursop* in the United States. The fruit pulp is excellent for making drinks and sherbets and, though slightly sour-acidic, can be eaten out of hand.

TRIBAL AND HERBAL MEDICINE USES

All parts of the graviola tree are used in natural medicine in the tropics, including the bark, leaves, roots, fruit, and fruit seeds. Different properties and uses are attributed to the different parts of the tree. Generally, the fruit and fruit juice are taken for worms and parasites, to cool fevers, to increase mother's milk after childbirth, and as an astringent (drying agent) for diarrhea and dysentery. The crushed seeds are used against internal and external parasites, head lice, and worms. The bark, leaves, and roots are considered antispasmodic, hypotensive, and sedative, and a tea is made for various disorders toward those effects.

Graviola has a long, rich history of use in herbal medicine as well as a lengthy recorded indigenous use. In the Peruvian Andes, a leaf tea is used for catarrh (inflammation of mucous membranes) and the crushed seed is used to kill parasites. In the Peruvian Amazon the bark, roots, and leaves are used for diabetes and as a sedative and antispasmodic. Indigenous tribes in Guyana use a leaf and/or bark tea as a sedative and heart tonic. In the Brazilian Amazon a leaf tea is used for liver problems, and the oil of the leaves and unripe fruit is mixed with olive oil and used externally for neuralgia, rheumatism, and arthritis pain. In Jamaica, Haiti, and the West Indies, the fruit and/or fruit juice is used for fevers, parasites, and diarrhea; the bark or leaf is used as an antispas-

Over the last several years, graviola has become a popular complementary supplement for cancer.

modic, sedative, and nervine for heart conditions, coughs, flu, difficult child-birth, asthma, hypertension, and parasites.

Today, in the United States and Europe, graviola is sold as a popular adjunctive natural therapy for cancer. This use has stemmed from published research on graviola and its naturally occurring chemicals possessing anticancerous actions, rather than its established traditional uses in South America.

PLANT CHEMICALS

Many active compounds and chemicals have been found in graviola, as scientists have been studying its properties since the 1940s. Most of the research on graviola focuses on a novel set of chemicals called *Annonaceous acetogenins.* Graviola produces these natural compounds in its leaf and stem, bark, and fruit seeds. Three separate research groups have confirmed that these chemicals have significant antitumorous properties and selective toxicity against various types of cancer cells (without harming healthy cells). These groups have published eight clinical studies on their findings.[1-8] Many of the acetogenins have demonstrated selective toxicity to tumor cells at very low dosages—as little as 1 part per million. Four studies were published in 1998 which further specify the chemicals and acetogenins in graviola that are demonstrating the strongest anticancerous, antitumorous, and antiviral properties.[9-12]

Plant chemicals found in graviola have demonstrated the ability to kill cancer cells without harming healthy cells—including cancer cells which have developed a resistance to multiple chemotherapy drugs.

Annonaceous acetogenins are only found in the Annonaceae family (to which graviola belongs). These chemicals in general have been documented with antitumorous, antiparasitic, insecticidal, and antimicrobial activities.[13] Mode of action studies in three separate laboratories have recently determined that these acetogenins are superb inhibitors of enzyme processes that are only found in the membranes of cancerous tumor cells. This is why they are toxic to cancer cells but have no toxicity to healthy cells. Purdue University, in West Lafayette, Indiana, has conducted a great deal of the research on the acetogenins, much of which has been funded by The National Cancer Institute and/or the National Institutes of Health (NIH). Thus far, Purdue University and/or its staff have filed at least nine U.S. and/or international patents on their work around the antitumorous and insecticidal properties and uses of these acetogenins.

In 1997, Purdue University published information with promising news that several of the Annonaceous acetogenins "not only are effective in killing tumors that have proven resistant to anti-cancer agents, but also seem to have a special affinity for such resistant cells."[14] In several interviews after this information was publicized, the head pharmacologist in Purdue's research explained how this worked. As he explains it, cancer cells that survive chemotherapy can develop resistance to the agent originally used as well as to other, even unrelated, drugs. This phenomenon is called *multi-drug resistance* (MDR). One of the main ways that cancer cells develop resistance to chemotherapy drugs is by creating an intercellular pump, which is capable of pushing anticancer agents out of the cell before they can kill it. On average, only about two percent of the cancer cells in any given person might develop this pump—but they are the two percent that can eventually grow and expand to create multi-drug-resistant tumors. Some of the latest research on acetogenins reported that they were capable of shutting down these intercellular pumps, thereby killing multi-drug-resistant tumors. Purdue researchers reported that the acetogenins preferentially killed multi-drug-resistant cancer cells by blocking the transfer of ATP—the chief source of cellular energy—into them.[15]

A tumor cell needs energy to grow and reproduce, and a great deal more to run its pump and expel attacking agents. By inhibiting energy to the cell, it can no longer run its pump. When acetogenins block ATP energy to the tumor cell over time, the cell no longer has enough energy to operate sustaining processes—and it dies. Normal cells seldom develop such a pump; therefore, they don't require large amounts of energy to run a pump and, generally, are not adversely affected by ATP inhibitors. Purdue researchers reported that fourteen different acetogenins tested thus far demonstrate potent ATP-blocking properties (including several found only in graviola).[15] They also reported that thirteen of these fourteen acetogenins tested were more potent against MDR breast cancer cells than all three of the standard drugs (adriamycin, vincristine, and vinblastine) they used as controls.

The Annonaceous acetogenins discovered in graviola thus far include: annocatalin, annohexocin, annomonicin, annomontacin, annomuricatin A and B, annomuricin A through E, annomutacin, annonacin, annonacinone, annopentocin A through C, cis-annonacin, cis-corossolone, cohibin A through D, corepoxylone, coronin, corossolin, corossolone, donhexocin, epomuricenin A and B, gigantetrocin, gigantetrocin A and B, gigantetrocinone, gigantetronenin, goniothalamicin, iso-annonacin, javoricin, montanacin, montecristin, muracin A through G, muricapentocin, muricatalicin, muricatalin, muri-catenol, muricatetrocin A and B muricatin D, muricatocin A through C muricin H, muricin I, muricoreacin, murihexocin 3, murihexocin A through C, murihexol, murisolin, robustocin, rolliniastatin 1 & 2, saba-delin, solamin, uvariamicin I and IV, and xylomaticin.

BIOLOGICAL ACTIVITIES AND CLINICAL RESEARCH

In a 1976 plant screening program by the National Cancer Institute, graviola leaves and stem showed active toxicity against cancer cells, and researchers have been following up on these findings since.[16] Thus far, specific acetogenins in graviola and/or extracts of graviola have been reported to be selectively toxic *in vitro* to these types of tumor cells: lung carcinoma cell lines;[1,3–6] human breast solid tumor lines;[4] prostate adenocarcinoma;[9] pancreatic carcinoma cell lines;[1,9,12] colon adenocarcinoma cell lines;[1,2,12] liver cancer cell lines;[17–20] human lymphoma cell lines;[21] and multi-drug-resistant human breast adenocarcinoma.[22] Researchers in Taiwan reported in 2003 that the main graviola acetogenin, *annonacin,* was highly toxic to ovarian, cervical, breast, bladder and skin cancer cell lines at very low dosages, saying "annonacin is a promising anti-cancer agent and worthy of further animal studies and, we would hope, clinical trials."[23]

An interesting *in vivo* study was published in March of 2002 by researchers in Japan, who were studying various acetogenins found in several species of plants. First they inoculated mice with lung cancer cells. Then, one third received nothing (the control group), one third received the chemotherapy drug adriamycin, and one third received the main graviola acetogenin, annonacin (at a dosage of 10 mg/kg). At the end of two weeks, five of the six in the untreated control group were still alive and lung tumor sizes were then measured. The adriamycin group showed a 54.6 percent reduction of tumor mass over the control group—but 50 percent of the animals had died from toxicity (three of six). The mice receiving annonacin were all still alive, and the tumors were inhibited by 57.9 percent—slightly better than adriamycin—and without toxicity. This led the researchers to summarize: "This suggested that annonacin was less toxic in mice. On considering the antitumor activity and toxicity, annonacin might be used as a lead to develop a potential anticancer agent."[24]

Other studies over the years have validated some of graviola's other uses in herbal medicine. Several early studies demonstrated that the bark as well as the leaves had hypotensive, antispasmodic, anticonvulsant, vasodilator, smooth-muscle relaxant, and cardiodepressant activities in animals.[25,26] Researchers verified graviola leaf's hypotensive properties in rats again in 1991.[27] Several studies over the years have demonstrated that leaf, bark, root, stem, and seed extracts of graviola are antibacterial *in vitro* against numerous pathogens,[28–30] and that the bark has antifungal properties.[30,31] Graviola seeds demonstrated active antiparasitic properties in a 1991 study, which validated its long standing traditional use,[32] and a leaf extract showed to be active against malaria in two other studies (in 1990 and 1993).[33,34] The leaves, root, and seeds of graviola demonstrated insecticidal properties, with the seeds demonstrating strong insecticidal activity in an early 1940 study.[35] In a 1997 clinical study, novel alkaloids found in graviola fruit exhibited antidepressive effects in animals.[36]

CURRENT PRACTICAL USES

Cancer research is ongoing on these important *Annona* plants and plant chemicals, as several pharmaceutical companies and universities continue to

---

In test tube studies graviola has shown to be toxic to many types of cancer cells including lung, prostate, colon, breast, liver, pancreas, ovarian, skin, cervical, skin, and lymphoma cancer cells.

Other research indicates that graviola can lower blood pressure, reduce heart rate, dilate blood vessels, and reduce spasms and convulsions.

research, test, patent, and attempt to synthesize these chemicals into new chemotherapeutic drugs. In fact, graviola seems to be following the same path as another well-known cancer drug—Taxol. From the time researchers first discovered an antitumorous effect in the bark of the pacific yew tree and a novel chemical called taxol was discovered in its bark, it took thirty years of research by numerous pharmaceutical companies, universities, and government agencies before the first FDA-approved Taxol drug was sold to a cancer patient (which was based on the natural taxol chemical they found in the tree bark).

With graviola, it has taken researchers almost ten years to successfully synthesize (chemically reproduce) the main antitumorous chemical, annonacin. These acetogenin chemicals have a unique waxy center and other unique molecular energy properties, which thwarted earlier attempts, and at least one major pharmaceutical company gave up in the process. Now that scientists have the ability to recreate this chemical and several other active acetogenins in the laboratory, the next step is to change the chemical just enough (without losing any of the antitumorous actions in the process) to become a novel chemical, which can be patented and turned into a new (patented) cancer drug. (Naturally occurring plant chemicals cannot be patented.) Thus far, scientists seem to be thwarted again—every time they change the chemical enough to be patentable, they lose much of the antitumorous actions. Like the development of taxol, it may well take government agencies like the National Cancer Institute and the National Institutes of Health to step forward and launch full-scale human cancer research on the synthesized unpatentable natural plant chemical (which will allow any pharmaceutical company to develop a cancer drug utilizing the research, as happened with taxol) to be able to make this promising therapy available to cancer patients in a timely fashion.

In the meantime, many cancer patients and health practitioners are not waiting—they are adding the natural leaf and stem of graviola (with over forty documented naturally occurring acetogenins, including annonacin) as a complementary therapy to their cancer protocols. After all, graviola has had a long history of safe use as an herbal remedy for other conditions for many years, and research indicates that the antitumorous acetogenins are selectively toxic to just cancer cells and not healthy cells—and in miniscule amounts. While research confirms that these antitumorous acetogenins also occur in high amounts in the fruit seeds and roots of graviola, different alkaloid chemicals in the seeds and roots have shown some preliminary *in vitro* neurotoxic effects.[35] Researchers have suggested that these alkaloids might be linked to atypical Parkinson's disease in countries where the seeds are employed as a common herbal parasite remedy.[36] Therefore, using the seeds and root of graviola is not recommended at this time.

The therapeutic dosage of graviola leaf, (which offers just as high of an amount of acetogenins as the root and almost as much as the seed) is reported to be 2–3 g taken three or four times daily. Graviola products (capsules and tinctures) are becoming more widely available in the U.S. market, and are now offered under several different manufacturer's labels in health food stores. As one of graviola's mechanisms of action is to deplete ATP energy to cancer cells, combining it with other supplements and natural products that increase or enhance cellular ATP may reduce the effect of graviola. The main supplement that increases ATP is a common antioxidant called Coenzyme Q10 and for this reason, it should be avoided when taking graviola.

Graviola is certainly a promising natural remedy and one that again emphasizes the importance of preserving our remaining rainforest ecosystems. Perhaps—if enough people believe that the possible cure for cancer truly is locked away in a rainforest plant—we will take the steps needed to protect our remaining rainforests from destruction. One researcher studying graviola summarized this idea eloquently: "At the time of preparation of this current review, over 350 Annonaceous acetogenins have been isolated from 37 species. Our preliminary efforts show that about 50%, of over 80 Annonaceous species screened, are significantly bioactive and are worthy of fractionation; thus, this class of compounds can be expected to continue to grow at an exponential rate in the future, provided that financial support for such research efforts can be found. With the demise of the world's tropical rain forests, such work is compelling before the great chemical diversity, contained within these endangered species, is lost."[15]

Traditional Preparation

The therapeutic dosage is reported to be 2 g, three times daily, in capsules or tablets. A standard infusion (1 cup three times daily) or a 4:1 standard tincture (2–4 ml three times daily) can be substituted if desired.

Contraindications

Graviola has demonstrated uterine stimulant activity in an animal study (rats) and should therefore not be used during pregnancy.

Graviola has demonstrated hypotensive, vasodilator, and cardiodepressant activities in animal studies and is contraindicated for people with low blood pressure. People taking antihypertensive drugs should check with their doctors before taking graviola and monitor their blood pressure accordingly (as medications may need adjusting).

Graviola has demonstrated significant *in vitro* antimicrobial properties. Chronic, long-term use of this plant may lead to the death of friendly bacteria in the digestive tract due to its antimicrobial properties. Supplementing the diet with probiotics is advisable if this plant is used chronically.

One study with rats given a stem-bark extract intragastrically (at 100 mg/kg) reported an increase in dopamine, norepinephrine, and monomine oxidase activity, as well as an inhibition of serotonin release in stress-induced rats.[39]

Alcohol extracts of graviola leaf showed no toxicity or side effects in mice at 100 mg/kg; however, at a dosage of 300 mg/kg, a reduction in explorative behavior and mild abdominal constrictions were observed.[40] If sedation or sleepiness occurs, reduce the amount used.

Drug Interactions   None have been reported; however, graviola may potentiate antihypertensive and cardiac depressant drugs. See contraindications above.

Taking graviola in combination with Coenzyme Q_{10} and other agents that increase cellular ATP energy may reduce the effects of graviola.

Worldwide Ethnomedical Uses

Region	Uses
Brazil	for abscesses, bronchitis, chest problems, cough, diabetes, diarrhea, dysentery, edema, fever, intestinal colic, intestinal parasites, liver problems, nervousness, neuralgia, pain, parasites, rheumatism, spasms, worms
Caribbean	for chills, fever, flu, indigestion, nervousness, palpitations, rash, spasms, skin disease, and as a sedative
Curaçao	for childbirth, gallbladder problems, nervousness, and as a sedative and tranquilizer
Haiti	for coughs, diarrhea, digestive sluggishness, fever, flu, heart conditions, lice, nerves, parasites, pain, pellagra, sores, spasms, weakness, wounds, and as a lactation aid and sedative
Jamaica	for asthma, fevers, heart conditions, hypertension, nervousness, parasites, spasms, water retention, weakness, worms, and as a lactation aid and sedative
Malaysia	for boils, coughs, diarrhea, dermatosis, hypertension, rheumatism, and to reduce bleeding
Mexico	for chest colds, diarrhea, dysentery, fever, ringworm, scurvy, and to reduce bleeding
Panama	for diarrhea, dyspepsia, kidney, stomach ulcers, worms
Peru	for diabetes, diarrhea, dysentery, fever, hypertension, indigestion, inflammation, lice, liver disorders, parasites, spasms, tumors, ulcers (internal), and as a sedative
Trinidad	for blood cleansing, fainting, flu, high blood pressure, insomnia, palpitations, ringworms, and as a lactation aid
United States	for cancer, depression, fungal infections, hypertension, intestinal parasites, tumors
West Indies	for asthma, childbirth, diarrhea, hypertension, parasites, worms, and as a lactation aid
Elsewhere	for arthritis, asthma, bile insufficiency, childbirth, cancer, diarrhea, dysentery, fever, heart problems, kidney problems, lice, liver disorders, malaria, pain, ringworm, scurvy, stomach problems, and as a lactation aid and sedative

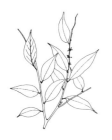

Family: Flacourtiaceae

Genus: *Casearia*

Species: *sylvestris*

Common Names: guacatonga, guassatonga, wild coffee, burro-kaa, café-bravo, cafeiillo, café silvestre, congonhas-de-bugre, corta-lengua, crack-open, dondequiera, erva-de-bugre, erva de pontada, guayabillo, mahajo, papelite, pau de lagarto, piraquina, raton, sarnilla, ucho caspi

Parts Used: bark, leaves, root

TRIBAL AND HERBAL MEDICINE USES

Indigenous peoples in the Amazon have long used guacatonga for snakebites and insect bites and stings. Scientists have reported that it is capable of neutralizing several types of bee and snake venoms.

GUACATONGA
HERBAL PROPERTIES AND ACTIONS

Main Actions	Other Actions	Standard Dosage
• protects stomach	• blocks pain signals	Leaves
• prevents ulcers	• neutralizes venom	**Infusion:** $1/2$ cup two to three times daily
• kills cancer cells	• kills viruses	
• slows tumor growth	• cleanses blood	**Tablets/Capsules:** 1–2 g twice daily
• relieves pain	• stops bleeding	
	• heals wounds	

Guacatonga grows as a shrub or small tree usually 2 or 3 m tall, but sometimes grows up to 10 m in undisturbed areas of the Amazon. In the clay soils of the Amazon, the plant has adapted for nutrient absorption and support by forming extensive lateral roots that are white, stiff, and covered with a corky bark. The tree produces small, white, cream, or greenish flowers (which smell like a mixture of honey and urine) crowded on short stalks on the leaf axils. After flowering it produces small fruits, 3–4 mm in diameter, which split open to reveal three brown seeds covered with a red-to-orange aril. Guacatonga grows wild throughout the tropics, adapting to both forests and plains. It is native to Cuba, Jamaica, Hispaniola, Puerto Rico, the Caribbean, Central America, and South America (including Brazil, Peru, Argentina, Uruguay, and Bolivia).

Guacatonga has a rich history in herbal medicine systems in nearly every tropical country where it grows. The Karajá Indians in Brazil prepare a bark maceration to treat diarrhea; the Shipibo-Conibo Indians of Peru use a decoction of the bark for diarrhea, chest colds, and flu. Other Indian tribes in Brazil mash the roots or seeds of guacatonga to treat wounds and leprosy topically. Indigenous peoples throughout the Amazon rainforest have long used guacatonga as a snakebite remedy. A leaf decoction is brewed that is applied topically and also taken internally. The same jungle remedy is used topically for bee stings and other insect bites. This native use found its way out of the rainforest and into current herbal medicine practices in cities and villages in South America. Its use has been validated by scientists in the last several years who documented the leaf extract as capable of neutralizing several types of bee and snake venoms.[1–3]

Guacatonga has a long history of use in Brazilian herbal medicine, documented in early folk medicine books as an antiseptic and wound healer for skin diseases (in 1939), as a topical pain-reliever (in 1941), and as an anti-ulcer drug (in 1958). It is currently used in Brazilian herbal medicine systems as a blood purifier, anti-inflammatory, and antiviral to treat rheumatism, syphilis, herpes, stomach and skin ulcers, edema, fevers of all kinds, diarrhea, and as a topical pain-reliever. It is also employed topically for burns, wounds, rashes, and such skin disorders as eczema. The natural herbal remedy calls for 20 g of dried leaves infused in 1 liter of water; quarter-cup amounts are taken orally two to three times daily.

The plant is also a popular herbal remedy employed in Bolivian herbal medicine, where it is considered to relieve pain, reduce inflammation, reduce stomach acid and prevent ulcers, stop bleeding, and heal wounds. There it is used to treat skin diseases, cancer, stomach ulcers, snakebite and bee stings, herpes, and in dental antiseptic mouthwash products.

PLANT CHEMICALS

The chemical makeup of guacatonga is quite complex. Scientists conducting the antivenin research discovered that the leaves and twigs of the plant contain a phytochemical called *lapachol*.[3] This is the well known and studied anticancerous/antifungal compound from which another rainforest plant, pau d'arco (*Tabebuia impetiginosa*), gained much renown. (Pau d'arco is also featured in this book.) While other researchers have been studying the anticancerous and antitumorous properties of guacatonga, a completely different set of phytochemicals has fueled their interest. These compounds, called *clerodane diterpenes*, are found abundantly in guacatonga and some have been patented as antisarcomic agents. Clerodane diterpenes have been documented with a wide range of biological activities ranging from insect antifeedants, to antitumorous, anticancerous, and antibiotic agents, to HIV replication inhibitors. Some of the clerodane diterpenes documented in guacatonga are novel chemicals which scientists have named *casearins* (A through S).

Novel chemicals in guacatonga have been patented as agents which kill sarcoma cancer cells.

Main plant chemicals in guacatonga include: caprionic acid, casearin A through S, casearia clerodane I through VI, casearvestrin A through C, hesperitin, lapachol, and vicenin.

BIOLOGICAL ACTIVITIES AND CLINICAL RESEARCH

The research on guacatonga's anticancerous properties began in 1988 by Japanese researchers from the Tokyo College of Pharmacy and Pharmacognosy. They published one preliminary trial in 1988 on their discovery of these novel clerodane diterpenes and their anticancerous and antitumorous activities. The study indicated that an ethanol extract of the leaf showed strong antitumorous activity in laboratory mice with sarcomas.[4] As soon as they made this discovery, they rushed to patent it, filing a Japanese patent for the casearin chemicals discovered as new antitumorous agents.[5] They published a follow-up study in 1990, again reporting their results from injecting mice with sarcomas with an ethanol extract of guacatonga leaves (100 mg per gram of body weight) and confirming their previous findings.[6] They then tested individual casearins against various human cancer cell lines and published two more studies in 1991 and 1992.[7,8] These studies reported newly isolated casearin chemicals and their antitumorous and anticancerous actions against various cancer tumor cells. Oddly, the Japanese researchers have not published any further studies and, since they had already filed patents, other research groups have not been forthcoming in funding research dollars on these patented antitumorous plant chemicals.

Animal studies on guacatonga reported a strong anti-tumor effect against sarcoma tumors.

In 2002, however, a well-known research group in North Carolina discovered three new casearins in the leaves and stems of guacatonga that the Japanese had not (and, obviously, hadn't patented). They named the new chemicals *casearvestrin A, B* and *C,* and published their first study in 2002, stating: "All three compounds displayed promising bioactivity, both in cytotoxicity assays against a panel of tumor cell lines and in antifungal assays."[9] Their research tested the new plant chemicals against human lung, colon, and ovarian tumor cells and indicated all three compounds had toxicity to cancer cells in very small amounts. This research was supported by a grant from the National Cancer Institute, National Institutes of Health (NCI) and performed by a non-profit biotech company, a large pharmaceutical company, and a major university. The NCI has also performed research in-house on clerodane diterpenoids found in another *Casearia* plant species documenting the anti-tumor properties of its novel diterpenoids[10] and another university research group has documented the anticancerous properties of this class of chemicals in a *Casearia* plant from the Madagascar rainforest as well.[11] It will be interesting to see if this diversified group will actually develop these chemicals into new effective chemotherapeutic agents; their research is ongoing.

Other research reveals that guacatonga provides equal effects as several anti-ulcer drugs and non-steroidal anti-inflammatory drugs.

All other research on the chemicals and activities of guacatonga has been performed by Brazilian research groups over the years. The first published toxicity study with rats indicated no toxicity with an ethanol extract of the leaves at 1,840 mg per kg.[12] This research group, at the University of São Paulo, studied the anti-ulcer properties of the plant (based on its long history of use as an effective herbal remedy for ulcers). They published two studies confirming these benefits. The first study with rats (in 1990) showed that a crude leaf extract reduced the volume of gastric secretion by 42 percent, but had little effect on pH. The extract also prevented lab-induced acute gastric mucosal injury which was equivalent to the anti-ulcer drug cimetidine (Tagamet®).[12] Ten years later they published a second rat study, documenting that a crude leaf extract protected the stomach lining without changing gastric pH and sped healing of acetic acid-induced chronic ulcers and *H. pylori* ulcers.[13]

Another Brazilian researcher documented that a bark-and-leaf infusion demonstrated pain relieving and mild anti-inflammatory properties in mice.[14] A university researcher followed up on the anti-inflammatory research, publishing in her dissertation that an extract of the leaves was as effective against inflammation in mice as the NSAID drugs Prioxicam® and Meloxicam®.[15] Leaf extracts have also been shown by two research groups to be active against common food poisoning bacteria strains, *Bacillus cerus* and *B. subtilis*, but inactive against such other common bacteria as *Staphylococcus*, *Streptoccoccus*, and *E. coli*.[16,17]

CURRENT PRACTICAL USES

It will be interesting to see what happens with guacatonga's ongoing cancer research—especially with sarcomas. These types of tumors typically grow very quickly, are resistant to many of the approved cancer drugs, and represent a bleak prognosis for most cancer patients. In the meantime, guacatonga is considered a safe plant and a great natural herbal remedy for ulcers, inflammation, and pain, and will continue to be used as a snakebite remedy throughout the Amazon jungles by the indigenous peoples. Although not widely available in the U.S. market yet, hopefully as more people learn of its beneficial uses, the market demand for it will increase.

Traditional Preparation

Twenty grams of dried leaves are infused in 1 liter of water and ¼-cup amounts are taken two to three times daily with meals as a digestive and anti-ulcer aid. Since most of the chemicals are water soluble, powdered leaves in tablets or capsules (1–2 g twice daily) can be substituted if desired. The above infusion can also be used topically for wounds, burns, skin rashes, and as a mouthwash after dental work or tooth extractions.

Contraindications   None known.

Drug Interactions   None reported.

Worldwide Ethnomedical Uses

Region	Uses
Bolivia	for blood cleansing, cancer, dental antiseptic mouthwash, inflammation, insect bites, pain, skin diseases, snakebite, tumors, ulcers, wounds, and to stop bleeding
Brazil	for blood cleansing, diarrhea, chest and body pains, eczema, fevers, flu, herpes, inflammation, leprosy, rheumatism, skin diseases, snakebite, syphilis, wounds, and as a male sexual stimulant
Colombia	for skin diseases, snakebite, ulcers, wounds
India	for snakebite
Peru	for diarrhea
Elsewhere	for leprosy, snakebite, wounds

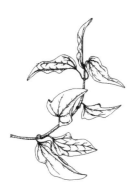

GUACO

HERBAL PROPERTIES AND ACTIONS

Main Actions	Other Actions	Standard Dosage
• suppresses coughs	• reduces fever	Leaves
• expels phlegm	• cleanses blood	**Infusion:** ½ cup three to
• dilates bronchial tubes	• heals wounds	four times daily
• arrests asthma	• promotes perspiration	**Tincture:** 3–4 ml three
• relieves pain	• increases urination	times daily
• kills bacteria	• kills protozoas	
• kills yeast		
• reduces inflammation		
• thins blood		

Family: Asteraceae

Genus: *Mikania*

Species: *cordifolia, glomerata, guaco*

Common Names: guaco, guace, bejuco de finca, cepu, liane Francois, matafinca, vedolin, cipó caatinga, huaco, erva das serpentes, coração de Jesus, erva-de-cobra, guaco-de-cheiro

Part Used: leaves

Mikania is the largest tropical genus of vines with over 300 species in the genus. The common name "guaco" is *quite* common; it is used for several species of *Mikania* vines that look very similar and are used for similar purposes. These include the South American species, *M. guaco,* found in Brazil, Peru, Venezuela, Bolivia, Colombia, and Ecuador; *M. cordifolia* which is found throughout South America as well as Guatemala, Honduras, Mexico, Costa Rica, and Panama; *M. glomerata* which is mostly found in Paraguay and Venezuela; and *Mikania laevigata* which has only been cataloged in Brazil thus far. All of these guaco plants are thornless shrubby vines reaching about 2 m in height and sprawling out 2 x 2.5 m wide. They produce wide bright green heart-shaped leaves and white to yellowish flowers. The leaves, when bruised or crushed, have a pleasant spicy scent reminiscent of pumpkin pie spice, and the flowers have a distinctive vanilla smell, especially after a rain.

TRIBAL AND HERBAL MEDICINE USES

Mikania cordifolia and *M. glomerata* are two plants in Brazil that are used interchangeably and oftentimes with no distinction between the two species; they are just referred to as *guaco.* Both have a long history of use by rainforest inhabitants. Brazilian Indians have an ancient tradition of using guaco for snakebites, preparing a tea with the leaves and taking it orally as well as applying the leaves or the stem juice (in a hurry) directly onto the snakebite. Other Amazonian rainforest Indian tribes have employed the crushed leaf stem topically on snakebites (as well as drinking the decoction of leaves and/or stem) and have used a leaf infusion for fevers, stomach discomfort, and for rheumatism. Indigenous people in the Amazon region in Guyana warm the leaves to put on skin eruptions and itchy skin. Several Indian tribes also believe if you crush the fresh aromatic leaves and leave them around your sleeping areas, the spicy scent will drive snakes away. For this reason and because of its long history as a snakebite remedy, it earned names in herbal medicine systems as "snake-vine" and "snake-herb."

In 1870, a Brazilian herbal drug called *Opodeldo de Guaco* was made from the leaf and stem of guaco that was considered a "saint's remedy" to treat bronchitis, coughs, and rheumatism. This "drug" is still a popular home remedy today throughout Brazil for the same purposes, but locals prepare it themselves by boiling guaco leaves into a tasty spicy cough syrup. The recipe calls for putting a handful of fresh leaves (or about 2 ounces dried leaves) in 6 cups of water and boiling until it is reduced to 2 cups. Then ¾ of a cup of sugar is added and it is boiled again for about twenty minutes into a syrup. The mixture is strained to remove the leaves, three soup-spoonfuls of honey are added, and the syrup is cooled, bottled, and stored in the refrigerator. As a cough syrup, one soup-spoonful is taken three times daily to help quiet coughs (and it is amazingly effective!).

In current herbal medicine systems in Brazil, guaco is well known and well regarded as an effective natural bronchodilator, expectorant, and cough suppressant employed for all types of upper respiratory problems including bronchitis, pleurisy, colds and flu, coughs, and asthma; as well as for sore throats, laryngitis, and fever. Guaco is also popular in Brazil as an anti-inflammatory, antispasmodic and pain-reliever for rheumatism, arthritis, intestinal inflammation, and ulcers. A decoction of the leaves is also employed externally for neuralgia, rheumatic pain, eczema, pruritus, and wounds.

> In current herbal medicine systems in Brazil, guaco is well known and well regarded as an effective natural bronchodilator, expectorant, and cough suppressant employed for all types of upper respiratory problems.

PLANT CHEMICALS

The main plant chemicals in guaco include caffeolylquinic acids, cinnamic acid, coumarin, glycosides, kaurenic acids, germacranolides, stigmasterol, tannins, and resins. Guaco is a significant source of the natural plant chemical, *coumarin* (as high as 11 percent in some guaco plants). Coumarin is used to produce the most commonly used anticoagulant and blood-thinning drug called coumadin. It is such a large source of coumarin, Brazilian research groups are studying the possibility of the commercial cultivation and extraction of coumarin from guaco leaves for pharmaceutical industry use.[1] Guaco also contain fourteen novel sesquiterpene chemicals that are called *germacranolides*.[2] This classification of plant chemicals has yielded some very biologically active antibacterial, insecticidal, anticancerous, and antitumorous agents obtained from plants; the actual activities of these novel guaco germacranolides are still being researched. At least three caffeoylquinic acids demonstrating *in vitro* anti-inflammatory activities[3] and two kaurenic acid chemicals with significant *in vitro* antibacterial activity[4] have been also been isolated in guaco leaves.

> Guaco contains a large amount of the blood-thinning chemical, coumarin.

BIOLOGICAL ACTIVITIES AND CLINICAL RESEARCH

Many of guaco's long-time traditional uses have been validated by scientists. Raul Coimbra wrote the first journal article validating the use of guaco as a bronchodilator and expectorant herbal drug in 1942.[5] In a 1984 Brazilian study, human volunteers were given a guaco leaf tea (*M. glomerata*), and researchers again reported the strong cough suppressant and bronchodilator effects.[6] Other researchers in Brazil published papers about the brochodilator and anti-inflammatory effects of guaco leaf extracts in 1992;[7–9] one scientist suggested that these actions could be attributed at least by half to the natural coumarin in the plant.[9] In 2002, a Brazilian research group reported that extracts of guaco leaves (*M. glomerata*) significantly inhibited histamine contractions and evidenced a relaxing effect of the trachea (throat) in guinea pigs (as well as isolated human bronchi *in vitro*). They summarized their findings by saying: "The results supported the indication of *M. glomerata* products for the treatment of respiratory diseases where bronchoconstriction is present."[10]

They also validated yet another indigenous use for snakebites; reporting that guaco significantly reduced swelling, edema, and related vasoconstriction in mice injected with snake venom.[10] Guaco's *in vitro* and *in vivo* anti-inflammatory activity had already been reported by three other studies,[11–13] the study in 2002 reporting an 81 percent inhibition of inflammation in rats.[13] In other recent research, a crude guaco leaf extract (*M. cordifolia*) demonstrated antiprotozoal activity in one study[14] and the same species evidenced one of the strongest antiprotozoal activity tested out of seventy-nine plant extracts tested in 2002 (against two protozoa: *Trichomonas vaginalis* and *Trypanosoma cruzi*).[15] In other research published in 2002, guaco was reported with *in vitro* antibacterial and anti-yeast actions against *Candida*.[16]

Clinical research validates guaco's long history of use for respiratory problems, snakebites, and inflammation.

CURRENT PRACTICAL USES

Guaco has long been regarded as a safe herbal remedy in Brazil. Toxicity studies with rats (in 2003) confirm that, even in high dosages (3.3 g per kg of body weight for fifty-two days), it does not have any toxic or anti-fertility effects.[17] While guaco is a widely popular and well-known Brazilian herbal remedy with Brazilian research validating much of its traditional uses, it is virtually unknown to North American consumers and health practitioners. It is deserving of much more attention here, especially for stubborn upper respiratory conditions, bronchitis, chronic coughs in general, and even the common cold or flu.

Traditional Preparation

In addition to the cough syrup detailed above, the traditional remedy is to take 2 cups of fresh leaves (or ½ cup dried leaves) and infuse them in a liter of water. A half-cup of this infusion is taken four times daily for rheumatism, respiratory problems, and coughs. A standard tincture is also sometimes employed for the same purposes at dosages of 3–4 ml three times daily. The leaf infusion may also be prepared as above and used as a topical wound healer and pain-reliever (although the fresh leaves are more effective for this purpose than using dried leaves).

Contraindications

In large dosages (two to three times the traditional remedy above) guaco has been reported to cause nausea, vomiting, and diarrhea.

Guaco contains a significant amount of coumarin, which is the plant chemical from which coumadin drugs are derived. Coumarin has an anticoagulant and blood thinning effect and the use of guaco may demonstrate anticoagulant effects due to the coumarin content. Consult with your physician before taking this plant if you are taking coumadin drugs or if coumadin anticoagulant type drugs are contraindicated for your condition.

Drug Interactions

May potentiate Warfarin® and other coumadin drugs.

Worldwide Ethnomedical Uses

Region	Use
Brazil	for albuminuria, appetite stimulation, arthritis, asthma, blood cleansing, bronchial constriction, bronchitis, cancer, cholera, colds, coughs, fever, gout, infections, influenza, intestinal problems, laryngitis, neuralgia, pain, pleurisy, pruritus, respiratory problems, rheumatism, snakebite, sore throat, syphilis, tonsillitis, wounds, and as an expectorant
Dominican Republic	for cholera, fever, flu
Guyana	for insect bite, itch, skin eruptions, snakebite
Haiti	for fever, malaria, syphilis
Mexico	for asthma, bites(dog), fever, malaria, menstrual irregularities, rheumatism, scorpion stings, sores, snakebite, spasm, stomach problems, tetanus, worms
Venezuela	for fever, snakebite, tumors
Elsewhere	for cholera, snakebite

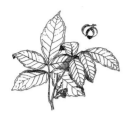

Family: Sapindaceae

Genus: *Paullinia*

Species: *cupana*

Common Names: guarana, guarana kletterstrauch, guaranastruik, quarana, quarane, cupana, Brazilian cocoa, uabano, uaranzeiro

Parts Used: fruit, seed

GUARANÁ
HERBAL PROPERTIES AND ACTIONS

Main Actions	Other Actions	Standard Dosage
• stimulates	• relieves pain	Seeds
• increases energy	• enhances memory	**Decoction:** 1 cup one to three times daily
• dilates blood vessels	• mildly laxative	
• increases urination	• increases libido	**Tincture:** 1–3 ml two to three times daily
• soothes nerves	• kills bacteria	**Tablets/Capsules:** 1–2 g one to three times daily
• fights free radicals	• thins blood	
• reduces weight		**Standardized Extracts:** Follow the label directions

Guaraná is a creeping shrub native to the Amazon (and particularly the regions of Manaus and Parintins). In the lushness of the Brazilian Amazon where it originates, it often grows to 12 m high. Its fruit is small, round, bright red in color, and grows in clusters. As it ripens, the fruit splits and a black seed emerges—giving it the appearance of an "eye," about which Indians tell legends.

TRIBAL AND HERBAL MEDICINE USES

The uses of this plant by the Amerindians predates the discovery of Brazil. South American Indian tribes (especially the Guaranis, from which the plant's name is derived) dry and roast the seeds and mix them into a paste with water. They then use it much the same way as chocolate—to prepare various foods, drinks, and medicines. The rainforest tribes have used guaraná mainly as a stimulant and as an astringent (drying agent) for treating chronic diarrhea. It is often taken during periods of fasting to tolerate dietary restrictions. Botanist James Duke cites past and present tribal uses in the rainforest: as a preventive for arteriosclerosis; as an effective cardiovascular drug; as a pain-reliever, astringent, stimulant, and tonic used to treat diarrhea, hypertension, fever, migraine, neuralgia, and dysentery.

Indians in the Amazon have long used guaraná as an energy tonic and for fevers, diarrhea, headaches, and cramps.

Over centuries, the many benefits of guaraná have been passed on to explorers and settlers. European researchers began studying guaraná (in France and Germany) in the 1940s, finding that Indians' uses to cure fevers, headaches, cramps, and as an energy tonic were well founded. Guaraná is used and well known for its stimulant and thermogenic action. In the United States today, guaraná is reputed to increase mental alertness, fight fatigue, and increase stamina and physical endurance. Presently, guaraná is taken daily as a health tonic by millions of Brazilians, who believe it helps overcome heat fatigue, combats premature aging, detoxifies the blood, and is useful for intestinal gas, obesity, dyspepsia, fatigue, and arteriosclerosis. The plant, considered an adaptogen, is also used for heart problems, fever, headaches, migraine, neuralgia, and diarrhea. Guaraná has been used in body care products for its toning and astringent properties, and to reduce cellulite. Guaraná also has been used as an ingredient in shampoos for oily hair and as an ingredient in hair-loss products. In Peru the seed is used widely for neuralgia, diarrhea, dysentery, fatigue, obesity, cellulite, heart problems, hypertension, migraine, and rheumatism.

Today the plant is known and used worldwide (and is the main ingredient in the "national beverage" of Brazil: Guaraná Soda!). Eighty percent of the world's commercial production of guaraná paste is in the middle of the Amazon rainforest in northern Brazil—still performed by the Guarani Indians, who wild-harvest the seeds and process them into paste by hand. The Brazilian government has become aware of the importance of the local production of guaraná through traditional methods employed by indigenous inhabitants of the rainforest. Since 1980, FUNAI (the National Indian Foundation) has set up a number of projects to improve the local production of guaraná. Now, under the direction of the FUNAI regional authority in Manaus, many cooperatives in the rainforest support indigenous tribal economies through the harvesting and production of guaraná.[1]

PLANT CHEMICALS

The first chemical examination of guaraná seeds was performed by the German botanist Theodore von Martius in the 1700s. He isolated a bitter, white crystalline substance with a remarkable physiological action. Von Martius named this substance *guaranine*, and it was later renamed *caffeine*. Many today still believe guaranine to be a unique phytochemical in guaraná. It is, however (according to chemists), caffeine.[2,3] As one group of researchers put it, guaranine is a product of crude laboratory processes and "should be considered nonexistent, being in reality impure caffeine."[4] Guaranine is probably just caffeine bound to a tannin or phenol. In living plants, xanthines (such as caffeine) are bound to sugars, phenols, and tannins, and are set free or unbound during the roasting process. See page 448 for a comparison of the caffeine content of guaraná seed to other popular plant beverage products. Guaraná seeds contain up to 4–8 percent caffeine (25,000 to 75,000 ppm), as well as trace amounts of theophylline (500 to 750 ppm) and theobromine (300 to 500 ppm).[5,6] They also contain large quantities of alkaloids, terpenes, tannins, flavonoids, starch, saponins, and resinous substances.[1,7]

Despite what marketers might tout, the chemical guaranine is really caffeine; guaraná is a significant source of natural caffeine.

The xanthine alkaloids (caffeine, theophylline, theobromine) are believed to contribute significantly to guaraná's therapeutic activity. In clinical studies, theophylline stimulates the heart[8] and central nervous system,[9] enhances alertness, and alleviates fatigue. It also has strong diuretic activity[9] and reduces constriction of the bronchials, making it useful in asthma.[8] Theobromine has similar effects. Certainly, many traditional uses of guaraná may be explained by its caffeine content. Among its many documented effects, caffeine has been shown to facilitate fat loss[10,11] and reduce fatigue.[9]

The main chemicals found in guaraná are adenine, allantoin, alpha-copaene, anethole, caffeine, carvacrol, caryophyllene, catechins, catechutannic acid, choline, dimethylbenzene, dimethylpropylphenol, estragole, glucose, guanine, hypoxanthine, limonene, mucilage, nicotinic acid, proanthocyanidins, protein, resin, salicylic acid, starch, sucrose, tannic acid, tannins, theobromine, theophylline, timbonine, and xanthine.

BIOLOGICAL ACTIVITIES AND CLINICAL RESEARCH

Toxicity studies with animals (in 1998) have shown that guaraná is non-toxic, even at high dosages (up to 2 g/kg of body weight).[12] Toxicity has been reported in only one human: a female who had an existing heart condition (mitrial valve prolapse).[13]

While the Indians have been using guaraná for centuries, western science has been slowly, but surely, validating that the indigenous uses are well-grounded. In 1989, a U.S. patent was filed on a guaraná seed extract, which was capable of inhibiting platelet aggregation (reducing sticky blood). The patent described guaraná's ability to prevent the formation of blood clots and to help in the breakdown of already-formed clots.[14] Clinical evidence was presented in conjunction with the 1989 patent and again in 1991 by a Brazilian research group that reported these anti-aggregation properties.[15,16] Once again, scientific validation is given to a plant used for centuries by the Indians as a heart tonic and to "thin the blood."

The use of guaraná as an effective energy tonic, for mental acuity, and to enhance long-term memory has been validated by scientists.

The use of guaraná as an effective energy tonic, for mental acuity, and to enhance long-term memory has been validated by scientists. In a 1997 *in vivo* study, guaraná increased physical activity of rats, increased physical endurance under stress, and increased memory with single doses as well as with chronic doses. Interestingly, the study revealed that a whole-seed extract performed more effectively than did a comparable dosage of caffeine or ginseng extract.[17] Another Brazilian research group has been studying guaraná's apparent effect of increasing memory,[18,19] thought to be linked to essential oils found in the seed.[20] The plant also was found to enhance memory retention and to have anti-amnesic activity in mice and rats.[17] A U.S. patent has been filed on a combination of plants (including guaraná) for promoting sustained energy and mental alertness "without nervousness or tension."[21] Guaraná (often in combination with other plants) also has been found to facilitate weight loss, by creating a feeling of fullness[22] and having a mild thermogenic effect.[23]

Guaraná has traditionally been used for headaches and migraines. A 1997 study found the plant to have pain-relieving activity,[24] which may explain its use for not only headaches but neuralgia, lumbago, and rheumatism. In 2001, a U.S. patent was filed on a combination of plants, including guaraná, to "relieve pain and other symptoms associated with migraines and headaches."[25]

Guaraná's antibacterial properties against *E. coli* and *Salmonella* have been documented as well.[26] Guaraná has also demonstrated antioxidant properties; researchers concluded, "Guaraná showed an antioxidant effect because, even at low concentrations (1.2 mcg/ml), it inhibited the process of lipid peroxidation."[12] In 1998, scientists demonstrated that a guaraná extract significantly increased the blood glucose levels and suppressed exercise-induced hypoglycemia in mice.[27]

CURRENT PRACTICAL USES

Guaraná's good health benefits and its standing as a natural stimulant has caused its popularity to grow steadily worldwide. It can be found under many labels and as an ingredient in many herbal formulas, energy drinks, and protein bars. Unfortunately, too many (unethical) manufacturers are simply adding the guaraná name to their labels to capitalize on its popularity—and adding chemical caffeine to their products instead. New standardized extracts of guaraná are available these days that "guarantee" and "standardize" the extract to the caffeine content. Unfortunately, many of these comprise a seed powder or extract to which caffeine has been added—rather than concentrating the caffeine through an extraction process of the natural seeds.

Recently, the Food and Drug Administration published results of their testing of twenty-four commercial guaraná products sold over the counter. They determined that "results and chromatographic profiles for 14 commercial products in solid dosage form indicate that a number of these products may not contain authentic guaraná as an active ingredient or contain less than the declared quantity of guaraná."[28] Consumers and manufacturers need to be aware of these inconsistencies to deal with reputable suppliers in purchasing guaraná products and supplements. Manufacturers buying guaraná extracts and standardized extracts should demand assays that show not only the caffeine content—but the theobromine and theophylline content as well. This will determine if the actual seed was concentrated into an extract. A good hint is to compare the prices of a supplement and a kilo of guaraná extract—if the extract is less than three to four times the cost of natural seed powder, it is likely a natural seed powder with some added caffeine.

Traditional Preparation

One-half to one cup seed decoction is taken one to three times daily or 1–3 ml of a 4:1 tincture twice daily; 1–2 g of powdered seed in tablets or capsules (or stirred into water or juice) one to three times daily can be substituted, if desired. Therapeutic dosages are reported to be 4–5 g daily. Relatively new to the U.S. market are guaraná extracts that are concentrated and standardized to the caffeine content (between 5 percent and 15 percent). Follow the labeled instructions and dosages for these products.

Contraindications   Not to be used during pregnancy or while breastfeeding. Guaraná contains caffeine and should not be used by those who are sensitive or allergic to caffeine or xanthines. Excessive consumption of caffeine is contraindicated for persons with high blood pressure, cardiac disorders, diabetes, ulcers, epilepsy, and other disorders.

Drug Interactions   May potentiate anticoagulant and blood-thinning medications such as Warfarin®. May have adverse effects if used with MAO-inhibitor medications.

Worldwide Ethnomedical Uses

Region	Uses
Amazonia	for arteriosclerosis, blood cleansing, cramps, diarrhea, dysentery, dyspepsia, fasting, fatigue, fever, headache, heart support, intestinal gas, malaria, obesity; and as an aphrodisiac, astringent, and stimulant
Brazil	for constipation, convalescence, central nervous system stimulation, depression, diarrhea, digestive problems, dysentery, exhaustion, fasting, fatigue, fever, gastrointestinal problems, headache, heart support, heat stress, intellect, intestinal gas, jet lag, lumbago, malaria, memory enhancement, menstrual problems, migraine, nervous asthenia, nervousness, neuralgia, rheumatism, skin disorders, stress, water retention. weakness; and as an adaptogen, antiseptic, aphrodisiac, appetite suppressant, and stimulant
Canada	for fever, libido enhancement, nervous disorders, and as a stimulant and tonic
Europe	for depression, diarrhea, exhaustion, fatigue, headache, heart support, migraine, nervous disorders, neuralgia, vaginal discharge, water retention, and as a stimulant and tonic
Latin America	for diarrhea, fatigue, hangovers, headaches, and as a stimulant
Mexico	for diarrhea and as a stimulant
Peru	for cellulite, convalescence, diarrhea, dysentery, fatigue, fever, heart support, hypertension, migraine, nerve support, neuralgia, obesity, paralysis, rheumatism; and as an aphrodisiac, astringent, stimulant, and tonic
South America	for arteriosclerosis, bowel problems, diarrhea, fever, heart support, nerve support, pain; and as an aphrodisiac, stimulant, and tonic
United States	for appetite suppression, athletic enhancement, concentration, diarrhea, endurance, exhaustion, fatigue, headaches, mental depression or irritation, migraine, nerve support, obesity, premenstrual syndrome, vaginal discharge, water retention; and as an aphrodisiac, stimulant, and tonic
Elsewhere	for convalescence, debility, diarrhea, dysentery, headache, lumbago, migraine, nerves, neuralgia, pain, rheumatism, water retention; and as an aphrodisiac, astringent, stimulant, and tonic

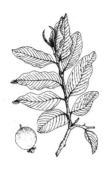

GUAVA
HERBAL PROPERTIES AND ACTIONS

Main Actions	Other Actions	Standard Dosage
• stops diarrhea	• depresses central nervous system	Leaves
• suppresses coughs	• lowers blood pressure	**Decoction:** 1 cup one to three times daily
• kills bacteria	• reduces blood sugar	
• kills fungi	• constricts blood vessels	
• kills yeast	• promotes menstruation	
• kills amebas		
• relieves pain		
• fights free radicals		
• reduces spasms		
• supports heart		

Family: Myrtaceae

Genus: *Psidium*

Species: *guajava*

Common Names: guava, goiaba, guayaba, djamboe, djambu, goavier, gouyave, goyave, goyavier, perala, bayawas, dipajaya jambu, petokal, tokal, guave, guavenbaum, guayave, banjiro, goiabeiro, guayabo, guyaba, goeajaaba, guave, goejaba, kuawa, abas, jambu batu, bayabas, pichi, posh, enandi

Parts Used: fruit, leaf, bark

Called *guayaba* in Spanish-speaking countries and *goiaba* in Brazil, guava is a common shade tree or shrub in home gardens in the tropics. It provides shade while the guava fruits are eaten fresh and made into drinks, ice cream, and preserves. In the richness of the Amazon, guava fruits often grow well beyond the size of tennis balls on well-branched trees or shrubs reaching up to 20 m high. Cultivated varieties average about 10 m in height and produce lemon-sized fruits. The tree is easily identified by its distinctive thin, smooth, copper-colored bark that flakes off, showing a greenish layer beneath.

Guava fruit today is considered minor in terms of commercial world trade but is widely grown in the tropics, enriching the diet of millions of people in such parts of the world. Guava has spread widely throughout the tropics because it thrives in a variety of soils, propagates easily, and bears fruit relatively quickly. The fruits contain numerous seeds that can produce a mature fruit-bearing plant within four years. In the Amazon rainforest, guava fruits are much enjoyed by birds and monkeys, which disperse guava seeds in their droppings and cause spontaneous clumps of guava trees to grow throughout the rainforest.

TRIBAL AND HERBAL MEDICINE USES

Guava may have been domesticated in Peru several thousand years ago; Peruvian archaeological sites have revealed guava seeds found stored with beans, corn, squash, and other cultivated plants. Guava fruit is still enjoyed as a sweet treat by indigenous peoples throughout the rainforest, and the leaves and bark of the guava tree have a long history of medicinal uses that are still used today.

The Tikuna Indians decoct the leaves or bark of guava as a cure for diarrhea. In fact, an infusion or decoction made from the leaves and/or bark has been used by many tribes for diarrhea and dysentery throughout the Amazon, and Indians also employ it for sore throats, vomiting, stomach upsets, vertigo, and to regulate menstrual periods. Tender leaves are chewed for bleeding gums and bad breath, and it is said to prevent hangovers (if chewed before drinking). Indians throughout the Amazon gargle a leaf decoction for mouth sores, bleeding gums, or use it as a douche for vaginal discharge and to tighten and tone vaginal walls after childbirth. A decoction of the bark and/or leaves or a flower infusion is used topically for wounds, ulcers, and skin sores. Flowers are also mashed and applied to painful eye conditions such as sun strain, conjunctivitis, or eye injuries.

In herbal medicine systems, guava is used for diarrhea, gastroenteritis, intestinal worms, gastric disorders, coughs, menstrual pain and hemorrhages, and edema.

Centuries ago, European adventurers, traders, and missionaries in the Amazon Basin took the much enjoyed and tasty fruits to Africa, Asia, India, and the Pacific tropical regions, so that it is now cultivated throughout the tropical regions of the world. Commercially the fruit is consumed fresh or used in the making of jams, jellies, paste or hardened jam, and juice. Guava leaves are in the *Dutch Pharmacopoeia* for the treatment of diarrhea, and the leaves are still used for diarrhea in Latin America, Central and West Africa, and Southeast Asia. In Peruvian herbal medicine systems today, the plant is employed for diarrhea, gastroenteritis, intestinal worms, gastric disorders, vomiting, coughs, vaginal discharges, menstrual pain and hemorrhages, and edema. In Brazil, guava is considered an astringent drying agent and diuretic and is used for the same conditions as in Peru. A decoction is also recommended as a gargle for sore throats, laryngitis, and swelling of the mouth, and used externally for skin ulcers and vaginal irritation and discharges.

PLANT CHEMICALS

Guava is rich in tannins, phenols, triterpenes, flavonoids, essential oils, saponins, carotenoids, lectins, vitamins, fiber, and fatty acids. Guava fruit is higher in vitamin C than citrus (80 mg of vitamin C in 100 g of fruit) and contains appreciable amounts of vitamin A as well.[1-3] Guava fruits are also a good source of pectin—a dietary fiber.[4-5] The leaves of guava are rich in flavonoids, in particular, quercetin. Much of guava's therapeutic activity is attributed to these flavonoids.[1,6] The flavonoids have demonstrated antibacterial activity.[6] Quercetin is thought to contribute to the anti-diarrhea effect of guava; it is able to relax intestinal smooth muscle and inhibit bowel contractions.[7] In addition, other flavonoids and triterpenes in guava leaves show antispasmodic activity.[8-9] Guava also has antioxidant properties which is attributed to the polyphenols found in the leaves.[4]

Guava leaves are a rich source of quercetin, a chemical which can relax intestinal smooth muscles, inhibit bowel constrictions, and be beneficial for diarrhea.

Guava's main plant chemicals include alanine, alpha-humulene, alpha-hydroxyursolic acid, alpha-linolenic acid, alpha-selinene, amritoside, araban, arabinose, arabopyranosides, arjunolic acid, aromadendrene, ascorbic acid, ascorbigen, asiatic acid, aspartic acid, avicularin, benzaldehyde, butanal, carotenoids, caryophyllene, catechol-tannins, crataegolic acid, D-galactose, D-galacturonic acid, ellagic acid, ethyl octanoate, essential oils, flavonoids, gallic acid, glutamic acid, goreishic acid, guafine, guavacoumaric acid, guaijavarin, guajiverine, guajivolic acid, guajavolide, guavenoic acid, guajavanoic acid, histi-dine, hyperin, ilelatifol D, isoneriucoumaric acid, isoquercetin, jacoumaric acid, lectins, leucocyanidins, limonene, linoleic acid, linolenic acid, lysine, mecocyanin, myricetin, myristic acid, nerolidiol, obtusinin, octanol, oleanolic acid, oleic acid, oxalic acid, palmitic acid, palmitoleic acid, pectin, polyphenols, psidiolic acid, quercetin, quercitrin, serine, sesquiguavene, tannins, terpenes, and ursolic acid.

BIOLOGICAL ACTIVITIES AND CLINICAL RESEARCH

The long history of guava's use has led modern-day researchers to study guava extracts. Its traditional use for diarrhea, gastroenteritis, and other digestive complaints has been validated in numerous clinical studies. A plant drug has even been developed from guava leaves (standardized to its quercetin content) for the treatment of acute diarrhea. Human clinical trials with the drug indicate its effectiveness in treating diarrhea in adults.[10] Guava leaf extracts and fruit juice have also been clinically studied for infantile diarrhea. In a clinical study with sixty-two infants with infantile rotaviral enteritis, the recovery rate was three days (87.1 percent) in those treated with guava, and diarrhea ceased in a shorter time period than controls. It was concluded in the study that guava has "good curative effect on infantile rotaviral enteritis."[4]

In a clinical study with sixty-two infants, researchers reported that guava has a good curative effect on infantile rotaviral enteritis. Human clinical trials also indicate it is effective in treating diarrhea in adults.

Guava has many different properties that contribute to its antidiarrheal effect: it has been documented with pronounced antibacterial, antiamebic, and antispasmodic activity.[12,13] It has also been shown to have a tranquilizing effect on intestinal smooth muscle, inhibit chemical processes found in diarrhea, and aid in the re-absorption of water in the intestines.[14-16] In other research, an alco-holic leaf extract was reported to have a morphine-like effect by inhibiting the gastrointestinal release of chemicals in acute diarrheal disease.[17] This morphine-like effect was thought to be related to the chemical quercetin. In addition, lectin chemicals in guava were shown to bind to *E. coli* (a common diarrhea-causing organism), preventing its adhesion to the intestinal wall and thus preventing infection (and resulting diarrhea).[18]

The effective use of guava in diarrhea, dysentery, and gastroenteritis can also be related to guava's documented antibacterial properties. Bark and leaf extracts have shown to have *in vitro* toxic action against numerous bacteria.[19] In several studies, guava showed significant antibacterial activity against such common diarrhea-causing bacteria as *Staphylococcus, Shigella, Salmonella, Bacil-lus, E. coli, Clostridium*, and *Pseudomonas*.[15,19-22] It has also demonstrated anti-fungal,[20] anti-yeast (*Candida*),[20] antiamebic,[23,24] and antimalarial[25] actions.

In a 2003 study with guinea pigs, Brazilian researchers reported that guava leaf extracts have numerous effects on the cardiovascular system which might be beneficial in treating irregular heat beat (arrhythmia).[1] Previous research indicated guava leaf provided antioxidant effects beneficial to the heart, heart protective properties, and improved myocardial function.[26] In two randomized human studies, the consumption of guava fruit for twelve weeks was shown to reduce blood pressure by an average eight points, decrease total cholesterol levels by 9 percent, decrease triglycerides by almost 8 percent, and increase "good" HDL cholesterol by 8 percent.[27,28] The effects were attributed to the high potassium and soluble fiber content of the fruit (however, 1–2 lbs. of fruit was consumed daily by the study subjects to obtain these results!). In other animal studies, guava leaf extracts have evidenced analgesic, sedative, and central nervous system (CNS) depressant activity,[29,30] as well as cough suppressant actions.[31] The fruit or fruit juice has been documented to lower blood sugar levels in normal and diabetic animals and humans.[32-34] Most of these studies confirm the plant's many uses in tropical herbal medicine systems.

CURRENT PRACTICAL USES

Guava, known as the poor man's apple of the tropics, has a long history of traditional use, much of which is being validated by scientific research. It is a wonderful natural remedy for diarrhea—safe enough even for young children. For infants and children under the age of 2, just a cup daily of guava fruit juice is helpful for diarrhea. For older children and adults, a cup once or twice daily of a leaf decoction is the tropical herbal medicine standard. Though not widely available in the U.S. market, tea-cut and powdered leaves can be obtained from larger health food stores or suppliers of bulk botanicals. Newer to the market are guava leaf extracts that are used in various herbal formulas for a myriad of purposes; from herbal antibiotic and diarrhea formulas to bowel health and weight loss formulas. Toxicity studies with rats and mice, as well as controlled human studies, show both the leaf and fruit to be safe and without side effects.

Traditional Preparation

The fruit and juice is freely consumed for its great taste, nutritional benefit and nutrient content, and as an effective children's diarrhea remedy. The leaves are prepared in a standard decoction and dosages are generally 1 cup one to three times daily.

Contraindications

Guava has recently demonstrated cardiac depressant activity and should be used with caution by those on heart medications. Guava fruit has shown to lower blood sugar levels and should be avoided by people with hypoglycemia.

Drug Interactions

None reported, however excessive or chronic consumption of guava may potentiate some heart medications.

Worldwide Ethnomedical Uses

Region	Uses
Amazonia	for diarrhea, dysentery, menstrual disorders, stomachache, vertigo
Brazil	for anorexia, cholera, diarrhea, digestive problems, dysentery, gastric insufficiency, inflamed mucous membranes, laryngitis, mouth (swelling), skin problems, sore throat, ulcers, vaginal discharge
Cuba	for colds, dysentery, dyspepsia
Ghana	for coughs, diarrhea, dysentery, toothache
Haiti	for diarrhea, dysentery, epilepsy, itch, piles, scabies, skin sores, sore throat, stomachache, wounds, and as an antiseptic and astringent
India	for anorexia, cerebral ailments, childbirth, chorea, convulsions, epilepsy, nephritis
Malaysia	for dermatosis, diarrhea, epilepsy, hysteria, menstrual disorders
Mexico	for deafness, diarrhea, itch, scabies, stomachache, swelling, ulcer, worms, wounds
Peru	for conjunctivitis, cough, diarrhea, digestive problems, dysentery, edema, gastritis, gastroenteritis, gout, hemorrhages, lung problems, premenstrual syndrome (PMS), shock, vaginal discharge, vertigo, vomiting, worms
Philippines	for sores, wounds, and as an astringent
Trinidad	for bacterial infections, blood cleansing, diarrhea, dysentery
Elsewhere	for aches, anorexia, bacterial infections, boils, bowel disorders, bronchitis, catarrh, cholera, chorea, colds, colic, convulsions, coughs, diarrhea, dysentery, dyspepsia, edema, epilepsy, fever, gingivitis, hemorrhoids, itch, jaundice, menstrual problems, nausea, nephritis, respiratory problems, rheumatism, scabies, sore throat, spasms, sprains, stomach problems, swelling, toothache, ulcers, worms, wounds; and as an antiseptic, astringent, and tonic

View from a villager's garden in the Peruvian high jungle.

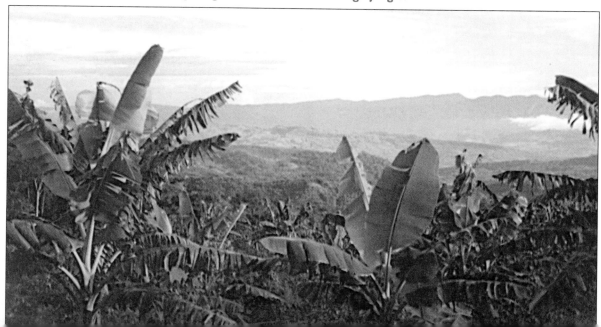

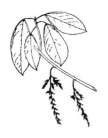

Family: Euphorbiaceae

Genus: *Alchornea*

Species: *castaneifolia*

Common Names:
iporuru, iporoni, iporuro,
ipururo, ipurosa,
macochihua, niando, pajaro

Parts Used: leaves, bark,
roots

IPORURU
HERBAL PROPERTIES AND ACTIONS

Main Actions
- relieves pain
- reduces inflammation
- increases libido

Other Actions
- kills fungi
- kills viruses
- prevents tumors

Standard Dosage
Leaves
Infusion: 1 cup two to three times daily
Maceration: 1/2 cup two to three times daily

Iporuru is a shrubby tree that reaches 8–10 m in height with light brown bark and violet flowers. It grows extensively in the lower elevations and flood plains of the Amazon River system in Peru, and is indigenous to the moist, tropical areas in Argentina, Bolivia, Brazil, Colombia, Paraguay, and Venezuela. Iporuru can be harvested only in the Amazon's dry season; it spends the rainy season underwater. The locals believe that the active medicinal properties found in the bark are present only during the dry season.

TRIBAL AND HERBAL MEDICINE USES

For centuries, the indigenous peoples of the Amazon have used the bark and leaves of iporuru for many different purposes and prepared it in various ways. The plant commonly is used with other plants during shamanistic training and, sometimes, is an ingredient in ayahuasca (a hallucinogenic, multi-herb decoction used by South American shamans). Throughout the Amazon, the bark or leaves are tinctured (generally with the local rum, called *aguardiente*) as a local remedy for rheumatism, arthritis, colds, and muscle pains. It is well known to the indigenous peoples of Peru for relieving the symptoms of osteoarthritis, and in aiding flexibility and range of motion. The Candochi-Shapra and the Shipibo Indian tribes use both the bark and roots for treating rheumatism. To prevent diarrhea, members of the Tikuna tribe take 1 tablespoon of bark decoction before meals. The pain-relieving properties of iporuru appear in topical treatments; crushed leaves are rubbed on painful joints and are beaten into a paste to apply to painful stingray wounds.

Iporuru is a well-known and highly regarded herbal remedy in the Amazon for arthritic pain and inflammation.

Today, iporuru remedies and products are sold in local markets and herbal pharmacies in Peru, where it is recommended highly for arthritis and rheumatism. In addition, locals prepare the leaves into a decoction for coughs. The leaves of iporuru are used in some parts of Peru to increase female fertility (mostly in cases where the male is relatively impotent). Richard Rutter, noted Peruvian ethnobotanist, insists that iporuru is widely used as an effective aphrodisiac and geriatric tonic for males. Throughout Peru it is regarded as a remedy for impotency as well as for balancing blood sugar levels in diabetics. Iporuru has been gaining popularity among North American athletes and health practitioners recently; reports state that iporuru provides nutritional support to muscle and joint structures. Here in the U.S., its reported analgesic and anti-inflammatory properties have begun to make it popular also to those suffering from arthritis and other joint problems.

PLANT CHEMICALS

Little research has been done to catalog completely the phytochemicals in iporuru. Initial screening has revealed it to contain steroids, saponins, phenols, flavonols, flavones, tannins, xanthones, and alkaloids. The anti-inflammatory properties of iporuru are attributed to a group of alkaloids, including one called *alchorneine*, which are found in the bark of iporuru as well as several other species of *Alchornea*.[1]

BIOLOGICAL ACTIVITIES AND CLINICAL RESEARCH

Likewise, there has been little clinical research on iporuru—despite its long history of use in South American herbal medicine. That which has been done, however, does help explain some of its traditional uses. Pharmacognosy students in Sweden documented that an ethanol extract of the stembark was capable of reducing lab-induced swelling and inflammation in rats when applied topically.[2] These researchers also reported that the extract was able to inhibit COX-1 prostaglandin synthesis.[2] Prostaglandins, produced by the activity of the enzyme cyclooxygenase (COX), are linked to inflammatory processes and diseases. (COX inhibitors are a class of anti-inflammatory and arthritis pharmaceutical drugs on the market.) This prostaglandin inhibition activity may, in part, explain the traditional use of iporuru for inflammatory joint and muscle disorders such as osteoarthritis, arthritis, and rheumatism. Other researchers in the U.S. confirmed these effects by injecting mice with an ethanol extract of iporuru and observing an anti-inflammatory effect against other chemical-induced inflammation.[3]

Scientists are just learning how iporuru reduces inflammation in research with animals: a mechanism similar to several leading arthritis drugs.

Other preliminary *in vitro* research (performed in Canada) has reported iporuru's antifungal, antiviral, and anti-tumor activities.[4] In their "crown gall tumor inhibition" assay (a preliminary laboratory test to predict anti-tumor activity), ethanol extracts and water extracts of the dried bark tested active in very small quantities. In another test to predict anti-tumor activity (an anticrustacean assay with *Artemia salina*), the ethanol extract tested active but the water extract was not active. Antimicrobial testing revealed that the ethanol extract demonstrated good antifungal activity against several fungal strains, but the water extract was inactive. Likewise, ethanol extracts evidenced better antiviral actions than those water-based. Neither the ethanol nor water extracts showed any antibacterial or anti-yeast actions against the strains they tested.

CURRENT PRACTICAL USES While iporuru will probably long remain in the South American herbalist's and shaman's medicine chest of natural remedies for impotency, arthritis, pain, and inflammation, its use by the rest of the world will be limited until more people and practitioners learn more about the plant and/or additional research is performed. Very few iporuru products are sold here in the U.S., and it is only available through a handful of companies (which mostly include it in multi-herb combination formulas).

Traditional Preparation The traditional impotency remedy in Peru calls for 1 cup of dried leaves to be macerated in 2 cups of water for one day, and two to three doses (of $\frac{1}{2}$ cup) are drunk daily. For diabetes, $\frac{1}{2}$ cup of dried leaves is infused in 4 cups of water, and 1 cup is drunk after each meal. As the leaves are prepared in standard infusions or cold macerations (indicating the beneficial chemicals providing the effects are water soluble), powdered leaves in capsules, tablets, or stirred into liquids can be substituted (1–2 g, two or three times daily).

Contraindications None known.

Drug Interactions None known.

Worldwide Ethnomedical Uses

Region	Uses
Amazonia	for aches (muscle), arthritis, colds, cough, diabetes, diarrhea, fertility, impotence, inflammation, pain, rheumatism
Canada	for arthritis, inflammation, muscle pains, rheumatism
Peru	for arthritis, bacterial infections, colds, cough, diabetes, diarrhea, flexibility, impotence, inflammation, muscle pains, osteoarthritis, pain, rheumatism, sterility
United States	for allergies, arthritis, athletic support, bacterial infections, constipation, inflammation, pain
Venezuela	for wounds

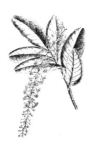

Family: Rutaceae

Genus: *Pilocarpus*

Species: *jaborandi,
microphyllus, pennatifolius*

Common Names:
jaborandi, Indian hemp,
jaborandi-do-norte, catai-
guacu, ibiratai, pimenta-
de-cachorro, arruda do
mato, arruda brava,
jamguarandi, juarandi

Part Used: leaf

TRIBAL AND HERBAL MEDICINE USES

JABORANDI		
HERBAL PROPERTIES AND ACTIONS		
Main Actions	**Other Actions**	**Standard Dosage**
• reduces glaucoma	• reduces inflammation	Leaves
• promotes perspiration	• increases milk flow	Not recommended.
• increases saliva		
• increases urination		
• increases heart rate		

Jaborandi refers to a 3–7 m high shrubby tree with smooth grey bark, large leathery leaves and thick, small, reddish-purple flowers. The leaves contain an essential oil, which gives off an aromatic balsam smell when crushed. Jaborandi is native to South and Central America and to the West Indies. Several *Pilocarpus* species are called jaborandi and used interchangeably in commerce and herbal medicine, including the main Brazilian species of commerce: *P. jaborandi,* and *P. microphyllus,* and the Paraguay species *P. pennatifolius.* All three tree species are very similar in appearance, chemical constituents, and traditional herbal medicine uses. The word *jaborandi* comes from the Tupi Indians and means "what causes slobbering" describing its ancient use in their rainforest herbal pharmacopeia.

In 1570, Gabriel Soares de Souza, a European observer, first recorded that the Guarani Indians of Brazil were using jaborandi to treat mouth ulcers. In the 1630s two Dutch West Indian Company scientists documented other Brazilian Indians using it as a tonic or panacea for colds and flu, a remedy against gonorrhea and kidney stones, and found that it was often used as an antidote to various poisons or toxins due to its ability to promote sweating, urination, and salivation. The indigenous tribes prized the pronounced sweat-inducing properties of the plant, particularly since they viewed sweating as a treatment in many diseases. The Indians also knew of the plant's ability to induce salivation; several tribes named the plant "slobber-mouth" in their own languages.

In folk medicine systems in the tropics where it grows, jaborandi has been used as a natural remedy for epilepsy, convulsions, gonorrhea, fever, influenza, pneumonia, gastrointestinal inflammations, kidney disease, psoriasis, neurosis, and as an agent to promote sweating. In Brazil, jaborandi has been used by herbalists for bronchitis, asthma, pneumonia, diphtheria, colds and flu, laryngitis, renal insufficiency, hepatitis, diabetes, kidney diseases, edema, and fever. An infusion or cold maceration of the leaves induces sweating within ten minutes—as much as 9 to 15 ounces of sweat can be excreted from a single dose! Externally it is used as a hair tonic, which is believed to open pores and clean hair follicles, prevent hair loss, and generally aid in the manageability of hair.

The Indians of the Amazon have used jaborandi for centuries for its ability to increase perspiration, salivation, and urination.

The introduction of jaborandi leaves to western medicine was in 1873, when Symphronio Coutinho, a Brazilian doctor, went to Paris for a European doctoral degree, taking with him samples of the leaves. The copious sweating and salivation brought about by the leaves attracted the attention of French physicians who began clinical research, publishing their first studies just one year later. The studies showed that jaborandi leaves "increases enormously the perspiration and saliva, and, in a much less degree, the secretion from the mucous membranes of the nose, the bronchial tubes, and the stomach and intestines."[1] By 1876, Jaborandi leaves were being employed in Europe in the treatment of many diseases including fever, stomatitis, colitis, laryngitis, bronchitis, influenza, pneumonia, and psoriasis.

PLANT CHEMICALS

Jaborandi is a perfect example of a plant that made the transition from Amazonian indigenous tribal use, to folklore use, and then into modern medicine based upon natural chemicals found in the plant. In 1875, two researchers independently discovered an alkaloid in jaborandi leaves, which was named *pilocarpine*. Tests revealed that pilocarpine was responsible for much of the biological activity of the plant—especially its ability to induce sweating and salivation, as well as to lower intraocular pressure in the eyes (making it an effective treatment in certain types of glaucoma).[2] In 1876, the isolated pilocarpine alkaloid was introduced to conventional ophthalmology for the treatment of glaucoma. The mixture of pilocarpine and another natural product, physostigmine, remains to this day one of the mainstay drugs in ophthalmology.

A chemical extracted from jaborandi in 1875 was turned into a drug for glaucoma and it is still used in mainstream medicine today.

Interestingly, scientists have never been able to fully synthesize the pilocarpine alkaloid in the laboratory; the majority of all pilocarpine drugs sold today are derived from the natural alkaloid extracted from jaborandi leaves produced in Brazil. Pilocarpine eye drops are still sold as a prescription drug worldwide for the treatment of glaucoma and as an agent to cause constriction of the pupil of the eye (useful in some eye surgeries and procedures).[3] In the treatment of glaucoma, pilocarpine causes the iris of the eye to contract, which leads to the opening of the space between the iris and the cornea and, in effect, relieves narrow-angle glaucoma.[4] It is even being used as a tool for the diagnosis of Alzheimer's disease in early stages; the eye constriction response to pilocarpine was found to be greater in Alzheimer's patients than in controls.[5]

Tablets of pilocarpine are also manufactured and prescribed to cancer patients to treat dryness of the mouth and throat caused by radiation therapy, as well as to patients with Sjögren's syndrome (an autoimmune disease in which immune cells attack the moisture-producing glands causing dry mouth and eyes).[3, 6–8] So as history shows, the Indians' "slobber-mouth" plant made it out of the jungles of the Amazon and into mainstream medicine and pharmaceutical use (for the identical uses the Indians employed it for). As usual, however, the Indians never realized any profits from the resulting manufacture and sales of several drugs over the last fifty years that have made use of their plant knowledge.

In addition to pilocarpine, jaborandi leaves contain terpenes, tannic acids, and other alkaloids. The natural leaf contains an average of 0.5 percent pilocarpine, plus similar amounts of other alkaloids such as isopilocarpine, jaborine, jaboridine, and pilocarpidine. The alkaloids in jaborandi (including pilocarpine) are a rather rare and unique type of alkaloid that are derived from histidine (an amino acid) and classified as imidazole alkaloids. The main chemicals found in jaborandi include 2-undecanone, alpha-pinene, isopilocarpidine, isopilocarpine, isopilosine, jaborine, jaborandine, jaboric, limonene, myrcene, pilocarbic acid, pilocarpidine, pilocarpine, pilosine, sandaracopimaradiene, and vinyl-dodecanoate.

BIOLOGICAL ACTIVITIES AND CLINICAL RESEARCH

There are well over a thousand clinical studies published on pilocarpine. As with most plant-based drugs, however, the use of the whole natural plant fell out of use as a natural remedy (and failed to attract further research efforts) in favor of the single isolated active ingredient that was turned into a prescription drug. The *PDR for Herbal Medicines* indicates that the effects of jaborandi leaves are as follows: increases the secretion of saliva, sweat, gastric juices and tears; and stimulates the smooth muscle of the gastrointestinal tract, bronchi, bile duct, and bladder.[9] Herbalists and natural health practitioners attribute the same biological activities for the plant as the main activities clinically validated for pilocarpine, but there is no actual clinical research on leaf extracts to support them or qualify them.

Another problem is trying to determine effective dosages of leaf extracts (in the absence of clinical research). The pilocarpine content of the leaf can vary—between different "jaborandi" tree species, as well as when using different harvesting methods, growth habitats, and even storage, handling, and drying methods of the harvested leaves. The pilocarpine chemical is fragile; dried jaborandi leaves have shown to lose as much as 50 percent of their pilocarpine content in as little as a year of storage.[10] Another alkaloid in the leaf, jaborine, has shown to counteract or decrease the effects of pilocarpine, which means that one cannot simply relate the effective dosage of a leaf extract based solely upon the pilocarpine content of the extract. Finally, one must consider that the long-standing documented use of pilocarpine is not with side effects, toxicity, or contraindications. Knowing at least an approximate amount of such an active chemical in a leaf extract is certainly necessary to help determine the extract's efficacy and safety.

The lethal dose of pilocarpine is reportedly 60 mg, which could correspond to as little as 5–10 g of the leaves.[9] Individuals with cardiac and circulatory problems may even have a lower lethal dosage. Reported side effects for non-lethal dosages of pilocarpine include vomiting, nausea, sweating, convulsions, increased heart rate, difficulty in breathing, and bronchial spasms.[3,9] Interestingly, a positive side effect of reported use of the pilocarpine eye solution drug was an improvement in sleep apnea and snoring in glaucoma patients.

CURRENT PRACTICAL USES

The use of jaborandi is best left in the hands of experienced herbalists and health practitioners, since pilocarpine has such pronounced biological activities and it occurs in significant amounts in the natural leaf. (The oral pilocarpine prescription drug, Salagen® is only 5 mg of pilocarpine, so very little is required for a pharmacological effect.) In recent years, demand by U.S. consumers for the natural leaf has been increasing, mainly fueled by the high cost of pilocarpine drugs and the rather new uses of it in cancer therapy (as a saliva enhancement agent). However, it still is not recommended to be used by the average layperson. The natural leaf is not widely available in the U.S. and importation of it as a natural product is a bit of a grey area since pilocarpine is sold as a regulated prescription drug. In fact, Brazil is the largest producer today of jaborandi leaves. However, 100 percent of Brazil's jaborandi leaf production goes into drug manufacture, including Merck Pharmaceuticals, who located a manufacturing plant in Brazil specifically for the processing and manufacture of their pilocarpine prescription drugs. Current laws in Brazil prohibit the export of jaborandi leaves as a natural product, as they regulate even the leaves as a drug.

Traditional Preparation

Not recommended.

Contraindications

Pilocarpine has shown to increase the rate of birth defects in animal studies. Jaborandi should not be taken during pregnancy or while breastfeeding.

Both jaborandi and pilocarpine may cause headaches and can irritate the stomach and cause vomiting and nausea. An overdose may cause such symptoms as flushing, profuse sweating and salivation, urinary frequency, nausea, rapid pulse, contracted pupils, diarrhea, or fatal pulmonary edema.

The plant may induce bradycardia. Those with cardiac or circulatory conditions should not take jaborandi.

Jaborandi may induce dehydration due to excessive perspiration and urination. If using jaborandi, electrolyte and fluid status must be monitored and maintained.

Drug Interactions Jaborandi may potentiate cardiac medications, diuretic medications, and cholinergic medications.

Worldwide Ethnomedical Uses

Region	Uses
Brazil	for asthma, bronchitis, colds, diabetes, diphtheria, dry mouth, edema, eye disorders, fever, flu, glaucoma, hair loss, hepatitis, laryngitis, nephritis, pleurisy, pneumonia, rheumatism, urinary insufficiency, and as an expectorant and to promote perspiration and salivation
England	for dry mouth, edema, hair loss, rheumatism, and to promote perspiration
Germany	for eye disorders, glaucoma, and to promote perspiration and salivation
Mexico	for edema, nephritis, pleurisy, rheumatism
Peru	to promote milk flow, perspiration, salivation, and urination
Elsewhere	for asthma, baldness, catarrh, deafness, diabetes, edema, glaucoma, intestinal problems, jaundice, lactation, nausea, nephritis, pleurisy, prurigo, psoriasis, renitis, rheumatism, syphilis, tonsillitis, and as an antidote (atropine and belladonna) and to promote perspiration and salivation

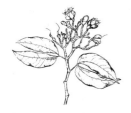

Family: Fabaceae

Genus: *Hymenaea*

Species: *courbaril*

Common Names: jatobá, stinking toe, algarrobo, azucar huayo, jataí, copal, Brazilian copal, courbaril, nazareno, Cayenne copal, demarara copal, gomme

JATOBÁ
HERBAL PROPERTIES AND ACTIONS

Main Actions
- kills fungi
- kills *Candida*
- kills mold
- increases energy
- kills bacteria
- stimulates digestion
- mildly laxative
- fights free radicals

Other Actions
- reduces spasms
- decongests bronchials
- dries secretions
- increases urination
- protects liver
- expels worms

Standard Dosage
Bark

Decoction: $1/2$–1 cup one to three times daily

Tincture: 1–3 ml twice daily

Jatobá is a huge canopy tree, growing to 30 m in height, and is indigenous to the Amazon rainforest and parts of tropical Central America. It produces bright green leaves in matched pairs, white, fragrant flowers that are pollinated by bats, and an oblong, brown, pod-like fruit with large seeds inside. The fruit is considered edible although hardly tasty; one of its common names, "stinking toe," is used to describe the smell and taste of the fruit! In the Peruvian Ama-

animee, pois confiture, guapinol, guapinole, loksi, South American locust

Parts Used: bark, leaves, fruit, resin

zon the tree is called *azucar huayo* and, in Brazil, *jatobá*. The *Hymenaea* genus comprises two dozen species of tall trees distributed in tropical parts of South America, Mexico, and Cuba.

Several species of *Hymenaea*, including jatobá, produce usable copal resins. At the base of the jatobá tree an orange, sticky, resinous gum collects, usually underground (however, the bark also produces smaller amounts of resin when wounded). The resin of *Hymenaea* trees converts to amber through a remarkable chemical process requiring millions of years. During this process, volatile plant chemicals leach out of the resin and other non-volatile chemicals bond together. This forms a hard polymer that is resistant to natural decay processes and the ravages of time. As portrayed in the *Jurassic Park* movies, amber of million-year-old *Hymenaea* trees have provided scientists with many clues to its prehistoric presence on earth as well as to the insects and other plants encased in it.

TRIBAL AND HERBAL MEDICINE USES

In the Amazon, jatobá's aromatic copal resin is dug up from the base of the tree and burned as incense, used in the manufacture of varnishes, used as a glaze for pottery, and is employed medicinally. Indians in the Amazon have long used the resin in magic rituals, love potions, and in wedding ceremonies. Although the name *Hymenaea* is derived from Hymen, the Greek god of marriage, it refers to the green leaflets that always occur in matching pairs, rather than the Indian's use of it in marriage ceremonies.

Jatobá's bark and leaves also have an ancient history of use with the indigenous tribes of the rainforest. The bark of the tree is macerated by the Karaja Indians in Peru and Créole people in Guyana to treat diarrhea. In Ka'apor ethnobotany, jatobá bark is taken orally to stop excessive menstrual discharge, applied to wounded or sore eyes, and used to expel intestinal worms and parasites. The bark is used in the Peruvian Amazon for cystitis, hepatitis, prostatitis, and coughs. In the Brazilian Amazon, the resin is used for coughs and bronchitis, and a bark tea is used for stomach problems as well as foot and nail fungus.

Jatobá bark tea is quite a popular drink among lumberjacks working in the forests in Brazil: it is a natural energy tonic that helps them to work long hours without fatigue.

With its long history of indigenous use, it would follow that jatobá has a long history of use in herbal medicine systems throughout South America. It was first recorded in Brazilian herbal medicine in 1930. The bark was described by Dr. J. Monteiro Silva who recommended it for diarrhea, dysentery, general fatigue, intestinal gas, dyspepsia, hematuria, bladder problems, and hemoptysis (coughing blood from the lungs). The resin was recommended for all types of upper respiratory and cardiopulmonary problems. In the mid-1960s an alcohol bark extract called *Vinho de Jatobá* was widely sold throughout Brazil as a tonic and fortificant, for energy, and for numerous other disorders.

In Brazilian herbal medicine today, jatobá bark and resin is still recommended for the same indications and problems as it has since 1930—and is documented to be a tonic, a digestive stimulant, astringent, antifungal, vermifuge (to expel intestinal worms), cough suppressant, and a wound healer. It is employed for diarrhea, prostatitis, cystitis, dysentery, intestinal colic, coughs, bronchitis, catarrh, asthma, and pulmonary weakness. Jatobá bark tea is still quite a popular drink among lumberjacks working in the forests in Brazil: it is a natural energy tonic that helps them to work long hours without fatigue. According to Dr. Silva, whomever drinks jatobá bark tea feels "strong and vigorous, with a good appetite, always ready to work."

In traditional medicine in Panama, the fruit is used to treat mouth ulcers, and the leaves and wood are used for diabetes. In the United States, jatobá is used as a natural energy tonic; for such respiratory ailments as asthma, laryngitis, and bronchitis; as a douche for yeast infections; and it is taken internally as a decongestant and for systemic *Candida* in the stomach and intestines. It is also used in the treatment of hemorrhages, bursitis, bladder infections, arthritis, prostatitis, yeast and fungal infections, cystitis, and is applied topically for skin and nail fungus. At present, none of the research has indicated that jatobá has any toxicity. One study highlighted the mild allergic effect that jatobá resin may have when used externally.[1]

PLANT CHEMICALS

Chemical analysis of jatobá shows that it is rich in biologically active compounds including diterpenes, sesquiterpenes, flavonoids, and oligosaccharides. The phytochemical makeup of jatobá is very similar to another resin-producing rainforest tree, copaiba, which is also featured in this book. Some of these same chemicals occurring in both plants (such as copalic acid, delta-cadinene, caryophyllene, and alpha-humulene) have shown to exhibit significant anti-inflammatory, antibacterial, antifungal, and anti-tumor activities in clinical studies.[2–6] In other research, another of jatobá's phytochemicals, astilbin, was shown in a 1997 clinical study to provide antioxidant and liver protective properties.[7,8]

Jatobá also contains terpene and phenolic chemicals which are responsible for protecting the tree from fungi in the rainforest.[9,10] In fact, the jatobá tree is one of the few trees in the rainforest that sports a completely clean trunk bark, without any of the usual mold and fungus found on many other trees in this wet and humid environment. These antifungal terpenes and phenolics have been documented in several studies over the years, and the antifungal activity of jatobá is attributed to these chemicals.[11–13]

The main chemicals found in jatobá include alpha-copaene, alpha-cubebene, alpha-himachalene, alpha-humulene, alpha-muurolene, alpha-selinene, astilibin, beta-bisabolene, beta-bourbonene, beta-copaene, betacubebene, beta-gurjunene, beta-humulene, beta-selinene, beta-sitosterol, calarene, carboxylic acids,

Jatobá contains chemicals that are responsible for protecting the tree from fungi in the rainforest. In fact, the jatobá tree is one of the few in the rainforest that sports a completely clean trunk bark, without any of the usual mold and fungus found on many other trees in this wet and humid environment.

caryophyllene, catechins, clerodane diterpenes, communic acids, copacamphene, copalic acid, cubebene, cyclosativene, cyperene, delta-cadinene, gamma-muurolene, gamma-cadinene, halimadienoic acids, heptasaccharides, kovalenic acid, labdadiene acids, octasaccharides, oligosaccharides, ozic acids, polysaccharides, selinenes, and taxifolin.

BIOLOGICAL ACTIVITIES AND CLINICAL RESEARCH

In addition to its antifungal properties, jatobá also has been documented to have anti-yeast activity against a wide range of organisms including *Candida*.[14,15] Other clinical studies have been performed on jatobá since the early 1970s which have shown that it has antimicrobial, molluscicidal (kills/controls snails and slugs), and antibacterial activities,[16–18] including *in vitro* actions against such organisms as *E. coli, Psuedomonas, Staphylococcus*, and *Bacillus*.[16] In addition, a water extract of jatobá leaves has demonstrated hypoglycemic activity, producing a significant reduction in blood sugar levels (which validates another traditional use).[19]

CURRENT PRACTICAL USES

Practitioners have long reported that jatobá bark has shown dramatic results with acute and chronic cystitis and prostatitis. Many practitioners today are discovering that these chronic conditions often can be fungal in nature rather than bacterial. The widespread use of antibiotics to treat these conditions can actually kill off friendly bacteria, which live off fungi—and increase the chances of a fungal problem or encourage fungal growth—even to the point of making the condition chronic. When these types of chronic prostatitis and cystitis cases react so quickly and dramatically to jatobá supplements, it is probably from jatobá's antifungal and anti-yeast properties at work, not its antibacterial properties.

Natural health practitioners in the United States are learning of jatobá's many uses and employing it as a natural remedy for prostatitis and cystitis, as a healthful tonic for added energy (without any caffeine or harmful stimulants), and for many fungal and yeast problems such as *Candida,* athlete's foot, yeast infections, and stubborn nail fungus. It is a wonderful, helpful natural remedy from an important and ancient rainforest resource.

Traditional Preparation

One-half to 1 cup bark decoction is taken one to three times daily or 1–3 ml of a 4:1 tincture twice daily. A strong bark decoction or standard tincture diluted with water and a small amount of cider vinegar is used topically for skin or nail fungi or employed as a douche for yeast infections.

Contraindications

Jatobá leaves have been documented to have a hypoglycemic effect and, as such, should be used under practitioner supervision by diabetics.

Drug Interactions

None reported.

Worldwide Ethnomedical Uses

Region	Uses
Amazonia	for eye problems, fatigue, fungal infections, menstrual discharge, worms
Brazil	for aches, anemia, arthritis, asthma, athlete's foot, bladder problems, bronchitis, bursitis, *Candida*, catarrh, colic, cough, cystitis, diarrhea, dysentery, dyspepsia, energy, fever, fungal infections, gastric sluggishness, hematuria, hemoptysis, hemorrhages, hepatitis, intestinal gas, laryngitis, lung problems, pains, prostatitis, skin disorders, stomachache, tuberculosis, urethritis, urinary insufficiency, urine retention, worms, wounds, yeast infections; and as an astringent, decongestant, digestive stimulant, and expectorant
Guatemala	for fever, mouth ulcers, rheumatism, and to promote sweating and urination
Haiti	for arthritis, asthma, bruises, catarrh, constipation, diarrhea, emphysema, headache, intestinal problems, kidney problems, respiratory problems, rheumatism, sores, spasms, stomachaches, and as an antiseptic
Mexico	for asthma, catarrh, rheumatism, sexually transmitted diseases, sores, and as a bowel stimulant
Panama	for asthma, diabetes, diarrhea, hypoglycemia, mouth ulcers, stomach problems
Peru	for coughs, cystitis, diarrhea, hepatitis, prostatitis
Venezuela	for fractures, lung problems, worms
Elsewhere	for asthma, beri-beri, bronchitis, cystitis, dyspepsia, indigestion, inflammation, laryngitis, malaria, pain (testicles/prostate), prostatitis, rheumatism, and as a digestion stimulant and expectorant

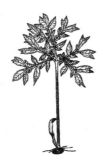

JERGÓN SACHA
HERBAL PROPERTIES AND ACTIONS

Main Actions	Other Actions	Standard Dosage
• kills viruses	• calms coughs	Rhizome
• neutralizes venom	• expels worms	**Tablets/Capsules:** 2–3 g two to three times daily
• reduces inflammation		**Tincture:** 3–5 ml twice daily

Family: Araceae

Genus: *Dracontium*

Species: *longipes, loretense, peruviuanum, asperum*

Common Names: jergón sacha, fer-de-lance, sacha jergón, hierba del jergón, erva-jararaca, jararaca, jararaca-taia,

Jergón sacha is a rainforest plant that consists of a single, giant, deeply-divided leaf borne from an underground tuber on a long, thick stem, which resembles the trunk of a sapling. When fertile, the flower stem emerges from the ground near the base of the plant and rises up to 2 m in height. At the end is a large, maroon spathe (a single, petal-like sheath) with bright red-orange, berry-like seeds crowded on a fleshy stalk inside. This bloom resembles that of a *caladium* or *dieffenbachia* plant—only much larger. While it is considered an herbaceous perennial, it's quite large for an herb—2–4 m tall! Thirteen species of *Dracontium* grow in the South and Latin American tropics. Four of these Amazonian species look almost identical and are used interchangeably in trop-

milho-de-cobra,
taja-de-cobra

Parts Used: tuber,
rhizome

ical herbal medicine systems: *Dracontium longipes, D. loretense, D. peruviuanum,* and *D. asperum.* While all four species are indigenous to the Amazon, *D. asperum* is more prevalent in the rainforests of Brazil, Suriname, and Guyana; *longipes, loretense,* and *peruviuanum* are more prevalent in Peruvian and Ecuadorian rainforests.

TRIBAL AND HERBAL MEDICINE USES

Ethnobotanically, jergón sacha is considered a signature plant: the plant's indigenous uses are directly related to its appearance. In this particular case, the trunk-like stem and its mottled coloring closely resembles a poisonous snake indigenous to the areas in which it grows. In Peru and Ecuador, the name of both snake and plant is *jergón sacha* and/or *fer-de-lance.* In Brazil, the snake is named *jararaca;* the plant, *erva-jararaca* (jararaca herb). These common names refer to the highly poisonous *Bothrops* genus of snakes, several species of which are indigenous to the Amazon (including the common *Bothrops jararaca,* for which the plant is named).

Throughout the rainforest,
jergón sacha is used to
treat snakebites, including
a particular species of
snake that resembles
the plant.

Local villagers as well as Indian tribes throughout the Amazon rainforest use the large tuber or rhizome of the jergón sacha plant as an antidote for the bite of these snakes. In such a case, the tuber is chopped up quickly, immersed in cold water, and drunk. More tuber is chopped finely and placed in a large banana leaf, which is then wrapped around the bite area. This poultice is changed every hour or two; more of the tuber is eaten every three to four hours. The efficacy of this remedy is reputed to be quite high if employed immediately (up to an hour) after being bitten. In remote areas of the Amazon where no means exist to preserve snake antivenin that requires refrigeration (its exorbitant cost notwithstanding), this generations-old remedy has been developed out of necessity. Indian tribes in Guyana also employ it as an antidote for stingray wounds, spider bites, and for poison dart and arrow wounds (where the poison, called *curare,* is prepared with poisonous plant and animal parts, including snake and/or frog venom). Other Indian cultures believe that beating the legs and feet with the leaves and/or stems of jergón sacha will prevent snakes from biting them.

Jergón sacha made its way out of the jungle and into herbal medicine systems of South America for other purposes. In addition to snakebite, the powdered tuberous rhizome is taken internally for asthma, menstrual disorders, chlorosis, and whooping cough in Brazilian herbal medicine. The root powder is used topically for scabies and the juice of the fresh rhizome is applied externally to treat sores caused by blowflies (and put directly on the site of a snakebite). The whole plant is also decocted and put in baths for gout. Jergón sacha is also well known in current Peruvian herbal medicine systems; tablets, capsules, and tinctures of the rhizome can be found in many natural pharmacies and stores. It is touted there as a natural remedy for HIV/AIDS, cancerous tumors, gastrointestinal problems, hernias (as a decoction applied topically), hand tremors, heart palpitations, and to enhance immune function.

The use of jergón sacha for AIDS and HIV in Peru was fueled by several newspaper articles published in Peruvian newspapers and magazines beginning in the early 1990s. The subject of the articles was a Peruvian physician, Dr. Roberto Inchuastegui Gonzales, who was president of the Committee of AIDS and Transmissible Diseases at the Peruvian Institute of Social Security in Iquitos, Peru. The media reported that, in experiments with AIDS patients conducted from 1989 to 1993, the doctor administered two plant extracts with remarkable results. One was a rhizome extract of jergón sacha (*D. peruviuanum*) as an antiviral, and the other was an extract of two cat's claw vines (*Uncaria tomentosa* and *U. guianensis*, which are also featured in this book) as immunostimulants. Dr. Inchuastegui reported that a majority of HIV patients treated had tested negative for the HIV virus and returned to normal lives after taking these two plant extracts for an average of six months. He has yet to publish any clinical trials. His work in Iquitos with AIDS patients has surfaced periodically in news and media reports over the last decade, which continues to purport the use of jergón sacha for HIV and other viruses. This has fueled the market in Peru for the sale of jergón sacha and, in the late 1990s, news of his work was disseminated in Eastern Europe.

Thousands of kilos of jergón sacha rhizome have since been exported annually to Poland, Russia, and other countries. This type of large-scale sales necessitated cultivation methods to be developed for the plant. Since the entire rhizome is harvested (which destroys the plant), it isn't sustainable for wild harvesting in the rainforest. In the last five years, two Peruvian universities have developed sound cultivation methods for replanting jergón sacha into the rainforest as it is harvested. New venues—old coca plantations and previously deforested lands—were developed for its new market as a cash crop for local farmers in organic cultivation programs.

PLANT CHEMICALS

Initial phytochemical screening indicates that the rhizome contains alkaloids, flavonoids, phenols, saponins, sterols, triterpenes, and starch; yet, none of these have been quantified or identified.

BIOLOGICAL ACTIVITIES AND CLINICAL RESEARCH

Despite the large and growing market for jergón sacha, not a single clinical study has been published on its actions. If jergón sacha's longstanding use as an effective snakebite remedy was clinically validated, it may explain its more recent use as an antiviral for HIV as well. The most recent class of drugs developed for HIV are called *protease inhibitors*. Protease inhibitors work by blocking an active component in HIV—its protease enzyme. With the protease enzyme blocked, HIV makes copies of its virus that are defective and can't infect new cells. In current (mainstream) HIV therapy, protease inhibitor drugs are usually combined with other antiviral drugs (which kill the virus directly) after the protease inhibitors have disabled its replication. Proteases are ubiquitously present in every cell of every living organism: they are enzymes that digest proteins.

It is well known that proteases are also main ingredients in snake venom. Typically the snakebite site is a necrotic area—the skin sloughs off due to action by proteases in the venom, which first turn the area bruised and swollen before digesting skin and tissue. The stronger the protease in the venom and its quantity relate directly to how much skin and tissue damage results at the site of the bite. For this reason, many herbal remedies that have been validated as snakebite remedies (especially those employed at the site of the bite) have been shown to be natural protease inhibitors also. In fact, many pharmaceutical company researchers bioprospecting for new chemicals and drugs in the Amazon are very interested in those plants the Indians employ as snakebite remedies for just this reason. It may be possible that Dr. Inchuastegui stumbled across one of these natural protease inhibitors in his work with HIV patients and jergón sacha. Clinical research is still required, however, to verify the mechanisms of action in jergón sacha against viruses and against snakebite and, particularly, if they are one and the same.

CURRENT PRACTICAL USES

Jergón sacha is one of the more unusual and interesting rainforest remedies coming from the Amazon today. Its signature plant status as a snakebite remedy is well known in South America and highly regarded. Without proper research to validate its traditional ethnomedical uses, however, it may take time for it to be a popular herbal remedy in North America. It is hoped that, with increasing sales in Peru and Eastern Europe for jergón sacha, someone will answer the call to perform this much-needed research—especially if it has applications for treating such deadly viruses as HIV.

Traditional Preparation

In Peruvian herbal medicine, 2–3 g of the dry powdered rhizome is taken two to three times daily, or 3–5 ml of a rhizome tincture twice daily is recommended.

Contraindications

None reported.

Drug Interactions

None reported.

Worldwide Ethnomedical Uses

Region	Uses
Brazil	for asthma, bites (snake, insect), chlorosis, gout, menstrual disorders, scabies, skin sores, whooping cough, worms, and as an antidote for poison arrow wounds
Ecuador	for snakebite
Guyana	as an antidote (poison arrow, stingray, spider, snake)
Mexico	for snakebite and urinary insufficiency
Panama	for snakebite
Peru	for AIDS, cancer, diarrhea, gastrointestinal problems, hernia, herpes zoster (shingles), HIV, immune enhancement, palpitations (heart), snakebite, tremors (hand), tumors, viral infections
Elsewhere	for snakebite

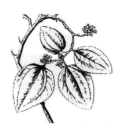

JUAZEIRO
HERBAL PROPERTIES AND ACTIONS

Main Actions	Other Actions	Standard Dosage
• reduces fever	• heals wounds	Bark
• kills bacteria	• dries secretions	**Decoction:** 1/2 cup two to three times daily
• prevents cavities	• increases urination	**Tincture:** Applied topically
• suppresses coughs	• supports heart	
• supports liver		

Family: Rhamnaceae

Genus: *Ziziphus*

Species: *joazeiro*

Common Names: juazeiro, joazeiro, raspa-de-jua, joá, juá, injuá, laranjinha-de-vaqueiro

Parts Used: bark, leaves

Juazeiro is a shrubby tree indigenous to the dry scrub-land areas called *caatingas* in the northeast of Brazil. It grows 5–10 m in height with a trunk that is 30–50 cm in diameter. It produces waxy leaves, small yellow flowers, and small, yellow, round, edible fruits (about 3–4 cm in size) that are favored by birds (especially parrots). Juazeiro is highly resistant to the seasonal droughts of the northeast, grows very slowly and is very long lived; 100-year-old specimens have been recorded. The tree is also native to the caatingas of Argentina, Bolivia, and Paraguay. In South America, the genus is referred to as *Zizyphus*; in North America it is classified as *Ziziphus*. It is a genus of about 100 species of deciduous or evergreen trees and shrubs distributed in the tropical and subtropical regions of the world. Interestingly, no matter where they are found, most all *Ziziphus* species on every continent are used in traditional medicine systems where they grow. The genus in general is recognized with potential pharmacological actions by scientists worldwide.

TRIBAL AND HERBAL MEDICINE USES

Juazeiro is one of the most respected trees in Brazil due to its numerous uses. The leaves and young branches are used as a high protein animal fodder (especially during severe droughts when not much else is available); the fruit is edible and sometimes turned into wine; the bark and leaves are used medicinally; and the wood is very durable and used for making furniture, farm implements, artistic wood carvings, and charcoal.

Juazeiro bark in used in South America to treat and prevent cavities and dental plaque. It is also used as a hair tonic and cleanser, which reportedly treats and prevents dandruff and seborrhea.

In Brazilian herbal medicine, the bark is decocted and used for liver complaints, headaches, dry coughs, bronchitis, upper respiratory infections, sore throats, urogenital disorders, and as a heart tonic. A bark decoction is also widely known and used by rural people in Brazil for fevers of all kinds. The inner bark is made into a paste (or prepared as a standard infusion) to treat and prevent cavities and dental plaque. The bark is infused or macerated and used as a hair tonic and cleanser, which reportedly treats and prevents dandruff and seborrhea. The bark is also prepared as a tincture and used externally for skin ulcers and other skin complaints. The leaves are prepared in an infusion and employed as a digestive aid for various complaints including dyspepsia, indigestion, and gastric ulcers. The fruit juice (which is rich in vitamin C) is used topically on the skin and face to treat acne and to soften the skin.

PLANT CHEMICALS

A large variety of triterpene, saponin, and alkaloid chemicals have been identified in juazeiro. The bark contains a large amount of saponins with natural foaming properties that are responsible for the formation of lather and its high cleansing power. For this reason, bark preparations have been used locally in shampoos and soaps. Juazeiro is a good source of a chemical called betulinic acid, as well as three novel ester derivatives of this acid which have only been found in juazeiro thus far.[1]

Betulinic acid has long been documented with moderate antibiotic activity, however, scientists discovered that the three ester derivatives demonstrated remarkable activity against gram-positive bacteria.[1,2] Betulinic acid has also demonstrated anticancerous activity in various clinical studies. Currently, betulinic acid is undergoing preclinical development for the treatment and prevention of malignant melanoma.[3] In one *in vivo* clinical study, mice grafted with human melanomas were administered betulinic acid, and tumor growth was completely inhibited without toxicity.[3] In other *in vitro* research, betulinic acid inhibited cultured carcinoma of the mouth and human melanoma cell lines.[4]

Main plant chemicals include: alkaloids, amfibine D, betulinic acid, betulinic acid derivatives, jujubogenine, saponins, and triterpenes.

BIOLOGICAL ACTIVITIES AND CLINICAL RESEARCH

Although its mechanism is still unknown, scientists have verified juazeiro's main traditional use for fevers. In an *in vivo* study with rabbits, the oral administration of a bark infusion reduced fevers that had been induced by bacterial toxins.[5] In Brazilian research, scientists have begun to validate its use for den-

Researchers have validated juazeiro's traditional use for fevers and cavities.

tal cavities; a bark decoction demonstrated strong activity against the common bacteria that forms dental plaque and cavities.[6] In addition, a juazeiro leaf extract was shown to reduce inflammation, provide pain relief, promote healing, and reduce secondary bacterial infections caused by guinea worms.[7] Guinea worms are the largest of the tissue parasites (which live under the skin) that afflict humans in tropical countries.

CURRENT PRACTICAL USES

In Brazil, juazeiro is a popular natural remedy to bring down fevers rapidly, especially where fevers are related to colds, flu, and upper respiratory infections. Natural health practitioners there administer it as a standard bark decoction. It is also a common ingredient in many natural body care products—in healing soaps for skin disorders, mouthwashes and toothpastes, skin care creams and lotions, hair tonics, and dandruff shampoos. In the U.S., juazeiro and its uses are virtually unknown. As more major U.S. body and hair care manufacturers are launching more natural formulas and herbal formulas in their product lines, it should only be a matter of time before juazeiro is discovered here and a market is created for it. Not only is it a great natural foaming agent, it provides natural antibiotic and healing properties for the skin and hair.

Traditional Preparation

In Brazil, juazeiro is prepared in different ways depending on what it is employed for. For fevers: 20 g of dried bark is decocted in 1 liter of water and ½ cup amounts are taken two to three times daily. This decoction is also used to prevent cavities by using it as a mouth gargle. In addition, 30 g of bark is left to soak in 1 liter of cold water for a day or two; this cold maceration is used as a hair tonic, a dandruff shampoo, and as a natural cleaning agent. The bark is prepared as a standard alcohol tincture to apply externally to wounds, ulcers, and skin rashes.

Contraindications

None known.

Drug Interactions

None known.

Worldwide Ethnomedical Uses

Region	Uses
Brazil	for bacterial infections, blood diseases, bronchitis, cavities, coughs, dandruff, debilitation, dental plaque, diabetes, digestive disorders, dysentery, dyspepsia, epilepsy, fevers, headache, heart support, intermittent fevers, jaundice, liver problems, seborrhea, skin disorders, soap, sore throat, stomach ulcers, urogenital infections, water retention, weakness, and as an expectorant and hair shampoo

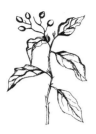

Family: Solanaceae

Genus: *Solanum*

Species: *paniculatum,*
insidiosum

Common Names:
jurubeba, jubeba,
juribeba, jupela, juripeba,
juuna, juvena,
jurubebinha, jurubeba-
branca, jurubeba-
verdadeira

Parts Used: leaves,
roots, fruit

TRIBAL AND HERBAL MEDICINE USES

Jurubeba leaf tea is a
very common household
remedy throughout Brazil
for hangovers. Brazilians
love to eat . . . a Brazilian
hangover usually means
relief is needed as much
from indigestion and
bloating from overeating as
from too much alcohol. It
is relied on there to speed
the digestive process and
promote gastric emptying
for just that reason.

JURUBEBA		
HERBAL PROPERTIES AND ACTIONS		
Main Actions	**Other Actions**	**Standard Dosage**
• reduces acid	• reduces inflammation	Leaves
• prevents ulcers	• decongests	**Infusion:** 1 cup two to three times daily
• stimulates bile	• increases urination	
• expels gas	• reduces fever	**Fluid Extract:** 3–4 ml two to three times daily
• supports heart	• clears obstructions	
• supports liver		**Tablets/Capsules:** 1–2 g two to three times daily
• lowers blood pressure		

Jurubeba is a small tree that grows up to 3 m high, with heart-shaped leaves that are smooth on top and fuzzy underneath. It produces a small, yellow fruit and lilac or white flowers. Both male and female jurubeba trees exist; the female grows slightly taller, has larger leaves, and bears fruit. The leaves and roots of both female and male specimens (as well as the fruit) are used interchangeably for medicinal purposes with equal effectiveness. Jurubeba is indigenous to Brazil as well as Paraguay and Argentina.

The indigenous uses of jurubeba are very poorly documented, but its uses in Brazilian herbal medicine have been described quite well. Jurubeba is listed as an official drug in the *Brazilian Pharmacopoeia* as a specific remedy for anemia and liver disorders. Jurubeba has long been used for liver and digestive disorders. In 1965, Dr. G. L. Cruz wrote that "the roots, leaves, and fruit are used as a tonic and decongestive. It stimulates the digestive functions and reduces the swelling of the liver and spleen. It is a good remedy against chronic hepatitis, intermittent fever, uterine tumors, and hydropsy." The leaves and roots are used in Brazilian medicine today as a tonic and for fevers, anemia, erysipelas, hepatitis, liver and spleen disorders, uterine tumors, irritable bowel syndrome, chronic gastritis, and other such digestive problems as sluggish digestion, bloating, and flatulence.

Jurubeba leaf tea is a very common household remedy throughout Brazil for hangovers. Brazilians love to eat . . . a Brazilian hangover usually means relief is needed as much from indigestion and bloating from overeating as from too much alcohol. It is relied on there to speed the digestive process and promote gastric emptying for just that reason. It is also sometimes employed externally in poultices to heal wounds and ulcers.

PLANT
CHEMICALS

Jurubeba's active constituents were first documented in the 1960s, when German researchers discovered novel plant steroids, saponins, glycosides, and alkaloids in the root, stem, and leaves.[1–3] The alkaloids were found more abundantly in the root, although also present in the stem and leaves.[3,4] Solanidine and solasodine were discovered in the leaves and fruit of jurubeba, which probably accounts for its liver-protective properties.[5–6] The compound solanin, also found in the plant, has been documented in clinical research to possess pain-relieving activity (possibly through its ability to block pain impulses in the nervous system).[7] The steroids and saponins were found in higher quantities in the root, while the leaves had the greatest amount of glycosides.[2,3,8] The plant also has been found to contain a large proportion of bitter properties, which were thought to contribute to its ability to stimulate digestion.[7,9]

The main plant chemicals in jurubeba include isojurubidin, isopaniculidin, jurubin, jurubidin, jurubilin, paniculin, paniculidin, paniculonin A, paniculonin B, painculogenin, solanin, solanidin, solasodine, and neochlorogenin.

BIOLOGICAL
ACTIVITIES
AND CLINICAL
RESEARCH

All of the clinical research on jurubeba has been done in Brazil—as the plant and its medicinal uses are not well known outside of Brazil. A 2002 study sought to validate the traditional use of the plant as a digestive aid. The root, stem, flower, leaf, and fruit of the plant were found to have anti-ulcer activity.[10] A water extract of the root, given orally to mice, inhibited gastric acid secretion induced by stress and various chemical agents, as well as prevented gastric lesions from developing.[10] Other extracts were found to inhibit gastric acid secretion in mice with the ulcer-causing bacteria *H. pylori*. In another study, rats with acetic acid-induced gastric ulcers were given a water extract of jurubeba.[7] The extract also enabled acceleration of chronic gastric lesion healing.[7] Researchers summarized, "Collectively, the results validate folk use of *Solanum paniculatum* plant to treat gastric disorders."[10]

Laboratory research reports that jurubeba can prevent ulcers, as well as help heal existing stomach ulcers.

Animal studies with cats have indicated that water extracts and alcohol extracts of jurubeba lowered blood pressure, while only the water extract increased respiration.[11,12] The plant also has been documented to have cardiotonic activity, as evidenced by a stimulant action to the heart in frogs.[11–12] This positive effect on the heart may be due to the alkaloid solanidine, which has been documented to have this activity.[13]

CURRENT
PRACTICAL USES

While jurubeba is a very popular natural remedy, its use has been mostly confined to South America. The plant has demonstrated little toxicity: a recent study showed that a water extract of the flower, fruit, leaf, stem, or root (given orally to mice at 2 g/kg) had no toxicity.[10] It is a great liver tonic and a wonderful remedy for many types of digestive disorders (especially for sluggish digestion), working quickly and efficiently, and is deserving of much more attention in the United States.

Traditional Preparation

One cup of a standard leaf infusion, or 3–4 ml of a fluid extract is taken one to three times daily (with or just after meals). If desired, 1–2 g of powdered leaves in tablets or capsules (or stirred into water or juice) with meals can be substituted.

Contraindications

The phytochemical solasodine has been documented to reduce sperm count and have an anti-fertility effect in male animals. While jurubeba itself has not been documented to have this action, males undergoing fertility treatment should probably avoid using this plant.

This plant has been documented to have mild hypotensive activity as well as a stimulating action on the heart. Those with cardiovascular disorders, low blood pressure, or those on blood-pressure-lowering medications should use this plant with caution and monitor these possible effects.

Herbalists in Brazil report that prolonged or chronic use of this plant may irritate the stomach lining in some individuals. Do not use chronically (daily) for longer than thirty days.

Drug Interactions

None known, but it may potentiate antihypertensive medications.

Worldwide Ethnomedical Uses

Region	Uses
Amazonia	for alcohol excess, digestive problems, inflammation, liver disorders, spleen inflammation, uterine tumors, water retention, and as a liver tonic
Brazil	for abscesses (internal), anemia, anorexia, bile insufficiency, bladder problems, bloating, blood cleansing, boils, catarrh, congestion, constipation, contusions, convalescence, cystitis, debility, diabetes, digestive sluggishness, dyspepsia, edema, erysipelas, fever, flatulence, gallbladder inflammation, gastric disorders, hangover, headache, heartburn, hepatitis, hives, irritable bowel syndrome, itch, jaundice, liver problems, malaria, menstrual disorders, nausea, skin disorders, spleen inflammation, tumors (uterine/abdominal), ulcers (stomach/skin), water retention, wounds, and as a liver tonic
United States	for alcohol excess, digestive sluggishness, gastric disorders, inflammation, spleen inflammation, stomach ulcers, water retention, and as a liver tonic

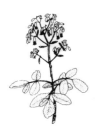

Family: Crassulaceae

Genus: *Kalanchoe*

Species: *brasiliensis, pinnata*

Common Names:
air plant, balangban, bruja, clapper bush, coirama, coirama-branca, coirama-brava, curtain plant, dipartenga, farine chaude, fel pavo, floppers, folha-da-costa, green love, hoja de aire, life leaf, live forever, mexican loveplant, miracle leaf, motta patti, paichecara, pashipadeh, paochecara, pirarucu, potagoja, sayao, saião, siempre viva

Parts Used: leaves, leaf juice

TRIBAL AND HERBAL MEDICINE USES

KALANCHOE		
HERBAL PROPERTIES AND ACTIONS		
Main Actions	**Other Actions**	**Standard Dosage**
• kills bacteria	• prevents ulcers	Leaves
• kills viruses	• increases urination	**Infusion:** 1 cup twice daily
• kills fungi	• lowers cholesterol	**Juice:** Applied topically two
• reduces fever	• constricts blood vessels	to three times daily
• heals wounds	• mildly sedative	
• suppresses coughs		
• blocks histamine		
• relieves pain		
• relaxes muscles		
• reduces inflammation		

Kalanchoe is a succulent perennial plant that grows 3–5 feet tall. Commonly known as "air plant," it has tall hollow stems, fleshy dark green leaves that are distinctively scalloped and trimmed in red, and bell-like pendulous flowers. Kalanchoe is botanically classified with two main Latin names which refer to the same plant: *Bryophyllum pinnatum* and *Kalanchoe pinnatum* (as well as various synonyms of both). This is the only *Kalanchoe* species found in South America, however, 200 other species of *Kalanchoe* are found in Africa, Madagascar, China, and Java. A number of species are cultivated as ornamentals in the U.S. and they are becoming popular tropical houseplants. In Brazil the plant goes by the common names of *saião* or *coirama* and in Peru it is called *hoja del aire* (air plant) or *kalanchoe*.

Kalanchoe is somewhat of a panacea to the indigenous peoples of the Amazon; they employ it for many different purposes. The Créoles use the lightly roasted leaves for cancer and inflammations, and a leaf infusion is a popular remedy for fevers. The Palikur mix the leaf juice with coconut oil or andiroba oil and then rub it on the forehead for migraines and headaches. To the Siona indigenous peoples, kalanchoe is known as "boil medicine" and they heat the leaves and apply them topically to boils and skin ulcers. Along the Rio Pastaza in Ecuador, natives use a leaf infusion for broken bones and internal bruises. In Peru, indigenous tribes mix the leaf with aguardiente (sugarcane rum) and apply the mixture to the temples for headaches; they soak the leaves and stems overnight in cold water and then drink it for heartburn, urethritis, and fevers. The root is also prepared as an infusion and used for epilepsy. Other tribes in the Amazon squeeze the juice from fresh leaves and mix it with mother's milk for earaches.

Throughout South America, kalanchoe has had a long history of use. It is commonly called the "miracle leaf" and "life leaf" for its remarkable healing properties. In Brazil, the plant is considered a sedative, wound healer, diuretic, anti-inflammatory, and cough suppressant. It is used for all sorts of respiratory conditions—from asthma and coughs to bronchitis. It is also employed for kidney stones, gastric ulcers, skin disorders, and edema of the legs. Externally, a leaf infusion or the leaf juice is used for headaches, toothaches, earaches, eye infections, wounds, ulcers, boils, burns, and insect bites. In Peru, the plant is employed for the same uses. In Mexico and Nicaragua, kalanchoe is used for similar purposes and also to promote menstruation and assist in childbirth.

Kalanchoe is called "miracle leaf" and "life leaf" throughout South America for its remarkable healing properties both internally and externally.

PLANT CHEMICALS

Kalanchoe is rich in alkaloids, triterpenes, glycosides, flavonoids, steroids, and lipids. The leaves contain a group of chemicals called *bufadienolides*, which are very active and have sparked the interest of scientists. They are very similar in structure and activity to two other cardiac glycosides, *digoxin* and *digitoxin* (drugs used for the clinical treatment of congestive heart failure and related conditions). Kalanchoe's bufadienolides have demonstrated in clinical research to possess antibacterial, antitumorous, cancer preventative, and insecticidal actions.[1–4]

The main plant chemicals found in kalanchoe include: arachidic acid, astragalin, behenic acid, beta amyrin, benzenoids, beta-sitosterol, bryophollenone, bryophollone, bryophyllin, bryophyllin A–C, bryophyllol, bryophynol, bryotoxin C, bufadienolides, caffeic acid, campesterol, cardenolides, cinnamic acid, clerosterol, clionasterol, codisterol, coumaric acid, epigallocatechin, ferulic acid, flavonoids, friedelin, glutinol, hentriacontane, isofucosterol, kaempferol, oxalic acid, oxaloacetate, palmitic acid, patuletin, peposterol, phosphoenolpyruvate, protocatechuic acid, pseudotaraxasterol, pyruvate, quercetin, steroids, stigmasterol, succinic acid, syringic acid, taraxerol, and triacontane.

BIOLOGICAL ACTIVITIES AND CLINICAL RESEARCH

Many of kalanchoe's traditional uses can be explained by the clinical research conducted thus far on the plant. The traditional use for infectious conditions (both internally and externally) is supported by research indicating kalanchoe leaves have antibacterial, antiviral, and antifungal activity.[5,6] The leaf and leaf juice have demonstrated significant *in vitro* antibacterial activity towards *Staphylococcus*, *E. coli*, *Shigella*, *Bacillus*, and *Pseudomonas*,[7–9] including several strains of multi-drug resistant bacteria.[9] A water extract of kalanchoe leaves (administered topically and internally) has been shown to prevent and treat leishmaniasis (a common parasitic disease in tropical countries which is transmitted by the bite of sand flies) in both humans and animals.[10,11] In addition to its antibacterial properties, kalanchoe's traditional uses for upper respiratory conditions and coughs might be explained by research demonstrating that the leaf juice has potent antihistamine and anti-allergic activity. In an *in vivo* study (with rats and guinea pigs) the leaf juice was able to protect against chemically induced anaphylactic reactions and death by selectively blocking histamine receptors in the lungs.[12]

Laboratory research is beginning to validate kalanchoe's long history of use for infections, fever, ulcers, and respiratory distress.

In another *in vivo* study, scientists validated kalanchoe's use for gastric ulcers; a leaf extract protected mice from such ulcer-inducers as stress, aspirin, ethanol, and histamine.[13] Other *in vivo* research confirms that kalanchoe can reduce fevers,[14,15] and provides anti-inflammatory, pain-relieving, and muscle relaxant effects.[14–18] Its anti-inflammatory effects have been partially attributed to the immunomodulatory and immune suppressant effect documented by scientists in several studies. In several *in vivo* and *in vitro* studies, researchers reported that extracts of the leaf and/or juice suppressed various immune reactions, including those which trigger an inflammatory response as well as a histamine response.[18–21] Kalanchoe has also shown sedative and central nervous system depressant actions in animal studies.[22] These effects were attributed partially to the leaf extract demonstrating the ability to increase the levels of a neurotransmitter in the brain called GABA (gamma aminobutyric acid).[22]

CURRENT PRACTICAL USES

With many of kalanchoe's traditional uses verified by animal research, it is not unusual that it continues to be a popular natural remedy throughout the tropics where the plant grows. From upper respiratory infections and coughs to stomach ulcers and infections of the skin, eyes, and ears it is widely known and used as "miracle leaf." The clinical research performed to date with animals indicate that the leaves are not toxic at dosages up to 5 g per kg of body weight (in rats).[17] However, there are a few reports of toxicity and even death when grazing animals (cows and goats) consumed excessive quantities of the leaves and flowers (estimated at 20 g per kg of body weight).[23,24]

Kalanchoe is not well known or widely available in the United States. While various hybrid species may be in plant stores and nurseries, these types of plants have been genetically modified for their qualities and appearance as ornamental plants and they shouldn't be used internally as a natural remedy.

Traditional Preparation

In the Amazon, 1 cup of a leaf infusion twice daily is generally used for upper respiratory infections, coughs, and fever. The leaf is rather juicy and succulent; the leaf is mashed up to obtain the juice, which is placed directly on cuts,

<table>
<tr><td>Contraindications</td><td>scrapes, boils, and other infected skin conditions and dropped into the ears or eyes for earaches and eye infections.</td></tr>
</table>

Contraindications	scrapes, boils, and other infected skin conditions and dropped into the ears or eyes for earaches and eye infections. The plant should not be used in pregnancy. Though not supported by clinical research, it has traditionally been used during childbirth and may stimulate the uterus.

Kalanchoe has documented immune modulating actions and should not be used chronically for long periods of time, or by those with a lowered immune system.

| **Drug Interactions** | Kalanchoe may potentiate barbiturates, cardiac glycosides such as digoxin and digitoxin, and central nervous system depressant medications. |

Worldwide Ethnomedical Uses

Region	Uses
Brazil	for abscesses, adenoids(infected), arthritis, athlete's foot, boils, bronchitis, bubos, burns, calluses, conjunctivitis, corns, coughs, dermatitis, dermatosis, earaches, eczema, edema, erysipelas, fever, glaucoma, headache, infections, inflammation, insect stings, intestinal problems, itch, kidney stones, lymphatic disorders, mouth sores, nervousness, respiratory infections, rheumatism, scurvy, skin problems, toothache, tuberculosis, tumor, ulcers, urinary insufficiency, warts, whooping cough, wounds, and as a sedative
Ecuador	for broken bones, bruises
Guatemala	for aches, diarrhea, pain, skin problems
India	for abdominal discomfort, boils, bruises, cholera, cuts, diabetes, diarrhea, dysentery, flatulence, headaches, kidney stones, indigestion, insect bites, scabies, sores, urinary insufficiency, wounds
Mexico	for eye infections, headaches, inflammation, menstrual disorders, pimples, wounds
Nicaragua	for aches, burns, childbirth, colds, coughs, fever, headache, pain, respiratory infections
Nigeria	for coughs, earaches, eczema, inflammation, pimples
Peru	for bacterial infections, boils, broken bones, bronchitis, cancer (lymphoma), conjunctivitis, coughs, earaches, eye infections, epilepsy, erysipelas, fever, gas, headache, heartburn, inflammation, intestinal problems, migraine, nausea, skin problems, sores, ulcers, urethritis
South America	for asthma, chest colds, earaches, headaches, sores, strains, tumors
United States	for chicken pox, fevers, stomachache
West Indies	for menstrual disorders, ulcers
Elsewhere	for arthritis, asthma, bruises, burns, constipation, diabetes, earaches, headaches, malnutrition, migraines, nephritis, paralysis, respiratory infections, rheumatism, sprains, swelling, ulcers, wounds

MACA
HERBAL PROPERTIES AND ACTIONS

Main Actions	Other Actions	Standard Dosage
• is nutritious	• increases fertility	Root
• increases energy		**Powder:** 1 tablespoon
• balances body systems		**Capsules/Tablets:** 5 g twice daily

Family: Brassicaceae

Genus: *Lepidium*

Species: *meyenii*

Common Names:
maca, Peruvian ginseng, maka, maca-maca, mace, peppergrass, maino, ayak chichira, ayuk willku

Part Used: root

Maca is a hardy perennial plant cultivated high in the Andes Mountains, at altitudes from 8,000 to 14,500 feet. It has one of the highest frost tolerances among native cultivated species. Maca has a low-growing, mat-like stem system, which can go unnoticed in a farmer's field. Its scalloped leaves lie close to the ground and it produces small, self-fertile, off-white flowers typical of the mustard family, to which it belongs. The part used is the tuberous root, which looks likes a large radish (up to 8 cm in diameter) and is usually off-white to yellow in color. Unlike many other tuberous plants, maca is propagated by seed. Although it is a perennial, it is grown as an annual; seven to nine months is required to produce the harvested roots.

The species *L. meyenii* was described by Gerhard Walpers in 1843. It has been suggested that the cultivated maca of today is not *L. meyenii* but a newer species *L. peruvianum* Chacón, based on various specimens collected since 1960 in the district of San Juan de la Jarpa, in Huancayo province of Peru. While most maca sold in commerce today still refers to the *L. meyenii* name, economic botanists believe most is *L. peruvianum*. In 1994, less than 50 hectares were devoted to the commercial cultivation of maca; by 1999, over 1,200 hectares were under production due to rising demand in the U.S. and abroad.

The area in which maca is found, high in the Andes, is an inhospitable region of intense sunlight, violent winds, and below-freezing weather. With its extreme temperatures and poor, rocky soil, the area rates among the world's worst farmland; yet, over the centuries, maca has evolved to flourish under these conditions. Maca was domesticated about 2,000 years ago by the Incas, and primitive cultivars of maca have been found in archaeological sites dating as far back as 1600 B.C.

TRIBAL AND HERBAL MEDICINE USES

To the Andean Indians and indigenous peoples, maca is a valuable commodity. Because so little else grows in the region, maca is often traded with communities at lower elevations for such other staples as rice, corn, green vegetables, and beans. The dried roots can be stored for up to seven years. Native Peruvians traditionally have utilized maca since pre-Incan times for both nutritional and medicinal purposes. It is an important staple in the diets of these people, as it has the highest nutritional value of any food crop grown there. It is rich in sugars, protein, starches, and essential nutrients (especially iodine and iron). The tuber or root is consumed fresh or dried. The fresh roots are considered a treat and are baked or roasted in ashes (in the same manner as sweet potatoes). The dried roots are stored and, later, boiled in water or milk to make a porridge. They also are made into a popular sweet, fragrant, fermented drink called *maca chicha*. In Peru even maca jam, pudding, and sodas are popular. The tuberous roots have a tangy, sweet taste and an aroma similar to that of butterscotch.

Maca is a high mountain root vegetable that is a staple crop; it is eaten daily by the Andean people, much like beans, rice, and potatoes.

This energizing plant is also referred to as Peruvian ginseng (although maca is not in the same family as ginseng). Maca has been used for centuries in the Andes to enhance fertility in humans and animals. Soon after the Spanish conquest in South America, the Spanish found that their livestock was reproducing poorly in the highlands. The local Indians recommended feeding the animals maca; so remarkable were the results that Spanish chroniclers gave in-depth reports. Even colonial records of some 200 years ago indicate that payment of (roughly) nine tons of maca was demanded from one Andean area alone for this purpose.

In Peruvian herbal medicine today, maca is reported to be used as an immunostimulant; for anemia, tuberculosis, menstrual disorders, menopause symptoms, stomach cancer, sterility (and other reproductive and sexual disorders); and to enhance memory. Maca has been growing in world popularity over the last several years due to several large U.S. marketing campaigns touting its energizing, fertility enhancement, hormonal balancing, aphrodisiac, and, especially, enhanced sexual performance properties. Other (anecdotal) herbal medicine uses in the U.S. and abroad include increasing energy, stamina, and endurance in athletes; promoting mental clarity; treating male impotence; and helping with menstrual irregularities, female hormonal imbalances, menopause, and chronic fatigue syndrome.

PLANT CHEMICALS

The nutritional value of dried maca root is high, resembling those of cereal grains such as maize, rice, and wheat. It contains 60–75 percent carbohydrates, 10–14 percent protein, 8.5 percent fiber, and 2.2 percent lipids.[1,2] The protein content of maca exists mainly in the form of polypeptides and amino acids (including significant amounts of arginine, serine, histidine, aspartic acid, glutamic acid, glycine, valine, phenylalanine, tyrosine, and threonine). It also has about 250 mg of calcium, 2 g of potassium, and 15 mg of iron in 100 g of dried root—and important amounts of fatty acids (including linolenic, palmitic, and oleic acids). Maca contains sterols (about 0.05 percent to 0.1 percent) and other vitamins and minerals.[1] In addition to its rich supply of essential nutrients, maca contains alkaloids, tannins, and saponins.[3] See the table on page 340 for a specific nutritional profile of dried maca root.

A chemical analysis conducted in 1981 showed the presence of biologically active aromatic isothiocyanates (a common chemical found in the mustard family of plants and shown to be a wood preservative and insecticide).[4] Chemical research shows maca root contains a chemical called *p-methoxybenzyl isothiocyanate,* which has reputed aphrodisiac properties.[4] At least four alkaloids are also present but have not yet been quantified. Fresh maca root contains about 1 percent glucosinolates—plant chemicals found in many plants in the family Brassicaceae (broccoli, cabbage, cauliflower, and other cruciferous vegetables).[5] While no novel glucosinolates have been reported in maca yet, several of the chemicals found in this group of known plant chemicals are documented to be cancer-preventive.[5]

Maca's main plant chemicals include alkaloids, amino acids, beta-ecdysone, calcium, carbohydrates, fatty acids, glucosinolates, iron, magnesium, p-methoxybenzyl isothiocyanate, phosphorus, potassium, protein, saponins, sitosterols, stigmasterol, tannins, vitamin B_1, vitamin B_2, vitamin B_{12}, vitamin C, vitamin E, and zinc.

Nutritional Profile of Dried Maca Root
(per 10 g serving: approximately 1 tablespoon)

Component	Amino Acids	Minerals	Vitamins	Fats/Lipids
Protein 1–1.4 g	Alanine 63.1 mg	Calcium 25 mg	B_2 39 mcg	Linoleic 72 mcg
Carbohydrates 6–7.5 g	Arginine 99.4 mg	Copper 0.6 mg	B_6 114 mcg	Palmitic 52 mcg
Fats (lipids) 220 mg	Aspartic acid 91.7 mg	Iron 1.5 mg	C 28.6 mg	Oleic 24.5 mcg
Fiber 850 mg	Glutamic acid 156.5 mg	Iodine 52 mcg	Niacin 565 mcg	
Ash 490 mg	Glycine 68.3 mg	Manganese 80 mcg		
Sterols 5–10 mg	Histidine 41.9 mg	Potassium 205 mg		
Calories 32.5	HO-Proline 26 mg	Sodium 1.9 mg		
	Isoleucine 47.4 mg	Zinc 380 mcg		
	Leucine 91 mg			
	Lysine 54.5 mg			
	Methionine 28 mg			
	Phenylalanine 55.3 mg			
	Proline 0.5 mg			
	Sarcosine 0.7 mg			
	Serine 50.4 mg			
	Threonine 33.1 mg			
	Tryptophan 4.9 mg			
	Tyrosine 30.6 mg			
	Valine 79.3 mg			

BIOLOGICAL ACTIVITIES AND CLINICAL RESEARCH

Maca's fertility-enhancing properties were reported as early as 1961, when researchers discovered that it increased fertility in rats.[6] Marketing and resulting sales of maca for sexual function has been fueled by clinical research since. The majority of this research, however, has been performed or funded by two main marketers of maca products in the U.S. and abroad! Also suspect to the independent scientific community are studies that "measure libido enhancement"—these are known to be highly subjective. Study protocols can also be easily orchestrated to provide desired outcomes and results; therefore, many trained industry and medical professionals note this brand of (product-sponsored) research with mild interest at best.

The first study reporting maca's effect on sexual function was published in 2000 (and performed by a marketer of maca) and described the beneficial effects of using maca in impotent mice and rats.[7] Another, published a year later, indicated similar effects in male rats.[8] Studies in 2001 reported a beneficial effect on male sperm production in rats[9] and improvement of sperm count and motility in nine healthy adult men.[10] In 2002, a study reported improved sexual performance in inexperienced male rats;[11] another "self-perception on sexual desire" test in healthy men reported aphrodisiac or libido enhancement effects.[12] In several of the rat and mice studies, the animals were administered up to 4 g per kg of body weight of a "concentrated maca extract" to achieve the reported results. This would (approximately) equate to a 300 g (10 oz.) dose for an average (170 lb.) man! None of these studies, however, indicated a possible mechanism of action—or related these observed effects to constituents or chemicals contained in maca root.

While maca is heavily marketed today as an alternative to estrogen replacement therapy, it simply will not perform as marketed. Independent research reports that maca has no hormonal effect in animal and human studies.

It may well be that maca's beneficial effects for sexual function and fertility can be explained simply by its high concentration of proteins and vital nutrients. Dried maca root contains about 10 percent protein—mostly derived from amino acids. Amino acids (the building blocks of proteins) are required in the diet to drive many cellular functions in the body—including sexual and fertility functions. Amino acids are required to manufacture neurotransmitters such as dopamine and noradrenaline. These substances transmit signals in the nervous system and play a major role in the process of sexual arousal and physical performance during sex. The main amino acids that these neurotransmitters require include phenylalanine, tyrosine, and histidine (all three of which are found in good supply in maca). The amino acid arginine, of which maca is a significant source, is thought to assist in the generation of nitric oxide—which is thought to counteract male impotence (although this is not clinically validated). Many libido- and sexual-enhancement health supplements on the market today contain arginine for this reason. Arginine has also clinically proven to play a role in male fertility through its action of increasing sperm production and motility.[13] It is highly likely that some of the sexual and fertility effects reported were due to maca's high arginine content.

The amino acid histidine also is found in maca root in high amounts. This amino acid plays an often-overlooked but important role in sexual function: during ejaculation and orgasm. The body utilizes histidine to produce histamine, and histamine in the corpus cavernosum (penile erectile tissue) ultimately is responsible for the way ejaculations happen.[14] Men suffering from premature ejaculation often show increased histamine activity; they may be helped by a simple antihistamine, or the amino acid methionine (which counteracts the formation of histamine from histidine). This is the same mechanism that explains a side effect of prescription antihistamines—aorgasmia (or the inability/difficulty to achieve an orgasm). Conversely, men and women having difficulties achieving orgasms may be helped by histidine supplementation—this may increase histamine levels in the sexual tract, which in turn makes orgasms and ejaculations easier.

An additional pro-sexual effect of histidine (as well as arginine) may lie in its vasodilating effect, increasing blood flow to the sex organs. Again, the significant, natural histidine content of maca may have played a role in the rat studies reporting a greater number of copulations. But it does make one wonder—is the benefit of additional copulations at the expense of shorter duration and/or premature ejaculation? Surely this subject is best suited for truly independent (and not product-sponsored) research.

Other benefits and anecdotal reports touting maca for hormonal balancing, endocrine and thyroid function enhancement, and even immune system enhancement, are likely related to maca's amino acid and nutrient content as well. The endocrine system drives many functions in the body, including the production of many types of hormones (which, in turn, regulate many other bodily processes). Although hormones are chemically diverse, they are constructed simply from amino acids and cholesterol. If given sufficient levels of starting materials (natural amino acids), the body may use them as needed to construct hormones, which keep the body in balance. Where diet and nutrition are poor (a common problem in the Andes, home to so few green, leafy vegetables), maca is a vital part of the diet—providing the necessary nutrients to keep the body healthy and functioning efficiently. The marketing claim made that maca actually increases testosterone or sex hormones has been clinically disproved. In a 2003 double-blind placebo human trial, men taking a maca root extract (1.5–3 g daily) evidenced no changes in any reproductive hormonal level tested, including testosterone (which actually showed a slight decrease!).[15]

CURRENT PRACTICAL USES Today, dried maca root is ground to powder and sold in capsules as a food supplement, and marketed to increase stamina (sexual and athletic) and fertility. Consumers bombarded with these marketing claims of hormonal balancing, thyroid stimulation (and resulting weight loss), sexual and athletic performance, and others need note: the indigenous uses to which marketers refer are in dosages by the ounce and pound daily—not just a few grams. No race of superhumans (with incredible sexual or athletic prowess) exists in the Andes, despite the fact that they eat, on average, five pounds of maca per week! When maca first made its debut in the press, in the late 1990s, it was touted to be the new "natural Viagra™" for men—sure to increase testosterone and sexual performance. After brisk sales, the market decreased because it simply didn't work as it claimed.

Several years later, and soon after the national media had a field day with the reported negative effects of conventional estrogen replacement therapy, marketers of maca shifted strategies and are today marketing maca as the "new HRT alternative" for women—sure to increase estrogen and treat menopause symptoms. Once again, maca sales are strong. Unfortunately, maca will not live up to this new marketing claim either.

There is no doubt—maca is a wonderful source of natural vital nutrients. The synergy of so many amino acids, vitamins, and minerals in their natural states may increase the assimilation, uptake, and utilization of them in the body. Consumers however, shouldn't expect "miracle cures" with maca—it's rather like taking a multi-vitamin supplement. Keep in mind that it is, in fact, a root vegetable and a main staple in the Andean indigenous diet (as beans, potatoes, and rice are elsewhere). Taking a few 500 mg capsules or tablets likely will not be of much benefit—or live up to wild marketing claims bandied about in the natural product market today.

The new standardized or concentrated extracts of maca available today are concentrating the extracts to the chemicals found only by the companies selling these products and funding the research. These chemicals and their biological effects have yet to be confirmed by independent studies. In the absence of true, independent science and research, consumers will be judging the efficacy and benefits of these extracts with the money spent for them.

The cultivation of maca is increasing in the highlands of the Andes to meet the growing demand worldwide; it is hoped that this demand will be sustained and not just another passing fad. In this severely economically depressed region, the market created for maca will offer new and important sources of income for the indigenous peoples of the Andes. About ten cultivars there produce maca with different-colored roots; most are the same, phytochemically. The cultivar *Lepidium peruvianum* Chacón has been identified in the major growing regions of the highlands and is the main variety of choice for expanded cultivation today. It will likely supply much of this new demand.

One of the main U.S. maca marketers (which funded much of the clinical research) has come under quite a bit of negative press recently in Peru (the world's exporter of maca), as well as in Europe and the U.S. The marketing company was granted plant-use patents in the U.S. (also pending in Europe and Australia) on the use of maca for fertility and aphrodisiac purposes. If these patents are enforced, it could prevent maca extracts of Peruvian origin from being imported into the United States and abroad. In 2002, a coalition of maca farmers and international activists was formed; its members purport that patenting indigenous knowledge is morally wrong and unacceptable. The coalition wants the Peruvian government and the World Intellectual Property Organization to condemn claims and patents such as these that steal traditional knowledge from farming communities and indigenous peoples.[16] After all—maca has been used by the indigenous people of the Peruvian Andes for centuries, and this marketing company learned of its uses through them.

Traditional Preparation	In the Andes, as much as a pound of fresh and/or dried maca root is eaten as a food in a single day. In herbal medicine in the United States, dried maca root tablets, capsules, and powders are generally recommended at dosages of 5–20 g daily. The dried root powder (a more economical choice than tablets or capsules) can be stirred into juice, water, or smoothies (2 tsp. of root powder are about 5.5 g). For standardized and concentrated extract products, follow the labeled instructions.
Contraindications	None reported.
Drug Interactions	None reported.

Worldwide Ethnomedical Uses

Region	Uses
Peru	for anemia, energy, fertility, food, impotence, memory, menopause, menstrual disorders, tuberculosis

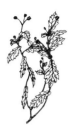

Family: Asteraceae

Genus: *Achyrocline*

Species: *satureoides*

Common Names:
macela, marcela, birabira, marcela-da-mata, hembra marcela, Juan blanco, macela-do-campo, marcela hembra, camomila-nacional, marcelita, mirabira, perpétua do mato suso, viravira, wira-wira, yatey-caa, yerba de chivo

Parts Used: aerial parts, leaves, flowers

TRIBAL AND HERBAL MEDICINE USES

In Brazilian herbal medicine, macela is prepared into a tea and used as a natural remedy for nervous colic, epilepsy, nausea, inflammation, liver and gastric problems, and as a mild sedative and pain-reliever.

MACELA		
HERBAL PROPERTIES AND ACTIONS		
Main Actions	**Other Actions**	**Standard Dosage**
• enhances immunity	• protects liver	Whole herb
• kills viruses	• prevents tumors	**Infusion:** 1 cup two to three times daily
• kills bacteria	• expels worms	
• relieves pain	• supports heart	**Capsules/Tablets:** 1–2 g two to three times daily
• reduces inflammation	• kills insects	
• fights free radicals	• promotes perspiration	**Tincture:** 2–3 ml twice daily
• reduces spasms	• regulates menstruation	
• stimulates bile		
• relaxes muscles		
• lowers blood sugar		
• stimulates digestion		
• mildly sedative		

Macela is a medium-sized aromatic annual herb that grows up to 1–1½ m high. It produces small white flowers with yellow centers and serrated green leaves. It is indigenous to much of tropical South America including Argentina, Bolivia, Brazil, Colombia, Ecuador, Guyana, Paraguay, Peru, Uruguay, and Venezuela. It often springs up on disturbed soils and some consider it a weed.

In Brazil, the plant is called *macela* or *marcela* and it has been used in herbal medicine for many years. Using the entire plant or just its flowers, a tea is prepared with 5 g of dried herb to 1 liter of boiling water. This infusion is used as a natural remedy for nervous colic, epilepsy, nausea, and gastric problems. It is also employed as an anti-inflammatory, antispasmodic, menstrual promoter, sedative, and pain-reliever for gastric disturbances, liver problems, diarrhea, and dysentery. This same infusion (or a slightly stronger one) is used externally for rheumatism, neuralgia, sore muscles, and even menstrual pain. The flowers are crushed and added to pillows as a natural sleeping aid (much in the same manner as the American hops flower). In Argentina, 20 g of fresh flowers are infused in 1 liter of hot water and taken to help regulate menstruation and for asthma; the aerial parts or entire plant is decocted as an aid for digestion and diabetes. In Uruguay, it is used in much the same way—for stomach, digestion, and gastrointestinal disorders; as a menstrual regulator; and as a sedative and antispasmodic. In Venezuela, the entire plant is infused or decocted and taken internally to treat diabetes, as a menstrual promoter, and to help overcome impotency. In Peru, the leaves are made into a tea for a cough suppressant to treat bronchitis; an infusion of the entire plant is used to treat diabetes (Type II).

PLANT CHEMICALS

Phytochemical analysis of macela, which began in the mid-1980s, shows that it is a rich source of flavonoids—including novel ones never seen before. Many of its active properties are attributed to these flavonoids as well as to other chemicals (called *terpenes*) isolated in the plant.[1,2]

The main plant chemicals found in macela include achyrocline polysaccharides, achyrofuran, auricepyrone, cadinene, caffeic acid, callerianin, calleryanin, caryatin, caryophyllene, chlorogenic acid, cineol, flavones, galangin, germacrene D, gnaphaliin, italidipyrone, lauricepyrone, luteolin, ocimene, pinene, pyrone, quercetagetin, quercetin, scoparol, scoparone, and tamarixetin.

BIOLOGICAL ACTIVITIES AND CLINICAL RESEARCH

Macela has been the subject of western research, and many of its long-time uses in herbal medicine have been validated by scientists. In animal studies with mice and rats, macela demonstrated pain relieving, anti-inflammatory, and smooth-muscle (gastrointestinal) relaxant properties internally without toxicity, in addition to anti-inflammatory and pain relief actions externally.[3,4] This may explain why macela has long been used effectively for many types of pain, gastrointestinal difficulties, menstrual cramps, and asthma.

In vitro studies have demonstrated that macela is molluscicidal (in a test used to ascertain its effectiveness against the tropical disease *schistosomiasis*), and active against *Salmonella, E. coli,* and *Staphylococcus.*[5–8] This could explain its long history of use for dysentery, diarrhea, and infections. It also has shown to be a strong antioxidant, to increases the flow of bile from the gallbladder, to help protect against liver damage, and to lower liver enzymes levels.[9–12] Again, this certainly supports its traditional uses for liver and gallbladder problems of various kinds.

In laboratory research with animals, macela has demonstrated the ability to reduce pain and inflammation as well as reduce spasms without toxicity.

Some of the *in vitro* antioxidant testing performed suggested that macela interfered in the degenerative processes of arteriosclerosis (it reduced blood stickiness, blood fats, and blood oxidation).[12] Macela has been used traditionally for diabetes throughout the tropics where it grows. Not until 2002 did researchers validate this use: a water extract of the entire plant exhibited blood-sugar-lowering activity in a mouse model of Type II diabetes. This hypoglycemic action was attributed to a novel plant chemical found in macela called *achyrofuran.*[13]

Other research on macela has concentrated on its antitumorous, antiviral, and immuno-stimulant properties. It passed the initial screening test used to predict anti-tumor activity in the mid-1990s by two separate research groups.[14,15]

In subsequent research, macela was reported to inhibit cancer cell growth *in vitro*,[16] and another research group showed that an extract of macela flowers inhibited the growth of cancer cells by 67 percent *in vitro*.[17] In 2002, researchers in Argentina studying macela reported a toxic effect against a human liver cancer cell line.[18] In the mid-1980s, German researchers extracted the whole dried plant and demonstrated that, in both humans and mice, it showed strong immunostimulant activity (by increasing phagocytosis and immune cell activity).[19,20] In 1996, researchers in Texas demonstrated its *in vitro* antiviral properties against HIV,[21] and Argentinean researchers found it to be active against *Pseudorabies* (a type of animal herpes virus).[22]

Toxicity studies indicate no toxicity in animals given macela orally, or even when water or ethanol extracts of the plant were injected into mice.[3,4] They did report, however, that a hot water extract potentiated the effects of barbiturates when injected (at a dose of 200 mg/kg).[3]

CURRENT PRACTICAL USES

With so many active biological properties documented thus far, macela should continue to be the subject of further research. Regardless, a simple macela tea (standard infusion) is still a highly effective natural remedy for many types of gastrointestinal complaints—especially where inflammation and spasms occur. Many practitioners in South and North America use macela for spastic colon, Crohn's disease, colitis, irritable bowel syndrome, and as a general digestive aid. In South America, it is still widely used to help regulate menstrual cycles. Although this has been done for many years with reported good results, this effect has not been studied by scientists.

Traditional Preparation

The therapeutic dosage is reported to be 1–2 g two or three times daily of dried whole herb and/or flowers. One cup of a whole herb infusion two to three times daily or 2–3 ml of a 4:1 tincture twice daily can be used.

Contraindications

This plant has been documented with hypoglycemic effects; people with hypoglycemia and/or diabetes should only use this plant under the care and direction of a qualified health care practitioner who can monitor blood glucose levels.

This plant has a long history of use as a menstrual promoter and regulator and its biological effects during pregnancy have not been studied or reported. While these traditional uses have not been clinically validated, pregnant women should still refrain from using this plant.

One study demonstrated barbiturate potentiation activity when a hot water extract of macela was injected in mice; it remains unclear if this effect is evident when taken orally. In herbal medicine systems, the plant is used as a sedative. Natural herb capsules, teas or tinctures might potentiate the effects of other sedatives and barbiturates. Use with caution when taking other prescription sedatives and pain killers.

Drug Interactions   Macela may potentiate insulin, diabetic medications, and also barbiturate drugs.

Worldwide Ethnomedical Uses

Region	Uses
Argentina	for asthma, diabetes, digestive disorders, menstrual regulation
Bolivia	for intestinal gas
Brazil	for appetite, bacterial infections, colds, colic, diabetes, diarrhea, digestive disorders, dysentery, epilepsy, flu, gallstones, gastritis, gastrointestinal disorders, headaches, inflammation, intestinal disorders, liver disorders, menstrual disorders, menstrual pain, nausea, neuralgia, pain, rheumatism, spasms; and as a sedative and to increase perspiration
Colombia	for gallbladder disorders, tumors
Paraguay	for bacterial infections, worms
Peru	for bronchitis, coughs, diabetes
Uruguay	for bacterial infections, digestive disorders, impotence, inflammation, menstrual disorders, spasms, and as a sedative
Venezuela	for diabetes, impotence, menstrual disorders

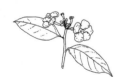

Family: Solanaceae

Genus: *Brunfelsia*

Species: *uniflora*

Common Names: manacá, manacán, chiric sanango, chuchuwasha,

MANACÁ

HERBAL PROPERTIES AND ACTIONS

Main Actions
- relieves pain
- reduces fever
- reduces inflammation
- detoxifies blood
- depresses central nervous system
- moderately sedative
- increases urination
- mildly laxative
- moves lymphatic fluid
- promotes menstruation

Other Actions
- prevents cellular mutations
- kills insects
- promotes perspiration
- lowers body temperature

Standard Dosage

Root

Decoction: 1/2 cup twice daily

Capsules/Tablets: 1 g twice daily

Tincture: 1–2 ml twice daily

manaka, vegetable mercury, managá caa, gambá, jeratacaca, bloom of the lent, camgaba, Christmas bloom, chuchuwasha, gerataca, geratacaca, good night, jerataca, moka pari, Paraguay jasmine, santa maria, umburapuama, white tree

Parts Used: root, bark, leaf

Manacá is a medium-sized, shrubby tree that grows to 8 m in height. It is often cultivated as an ornamental tree in the tropics, as it produces highly fragrant, pretty, white and purple flowers (which are sometimes employed in perfumes). It can be found in the Amazon regions of Brazil, Bolivia, Peru, Ecuador, Colombia, and Venezuela. In Brazil, manacá is known by several botanical names, including *Brunfelsia uniflora*, *B. hopeana*, and *Francisea uniflora*. In Europe, the plant is known and sold in herbal commerce as *Brunfelsia hopeana*. All refer to the same plant. Other plant relatives from Colombia and Ecuador include *Brunfelsia chiricaspi* (from its local name, chiricaspi, which means "tree of chills"), and *Brunfelsia grandiflora*, both of which are used by rainforest Indians as hallucinogens. However, due to the toxicity and unpleasant side effects, use of these plants appears to be on the wane. They are different plants than manacá—but sometimes are confused with manacá for their similar look, growth, and habit.

TRIBAL AND HERBAL MEDICINE USES

Manacá has a long history of indigenous use for both medicine and magic. Its Brazilian common name, *manacá*, originated with the Tupi Indians in Brazil; they named it after the most beautiful girl in their tribe, Manacán, for its lovely flowers. It is a sacred and spiritual plant used by shamans and *curanderos* in the potion *ayahuasca* (a sacred hallucinogen), in special initiation ceremonies, and for bad luck (the *chiricaspi* and *grandiflora* species are preferred for ayahuasca brews).

In the Amazon, manacá root is prepared into a tincture with *aguardiente* (rum) for rheumatism and sexually transmitted diseases. In Peru (where the local name of the plant is *chiricsanango*), indigenous peoples apply a decoction of leaves externally for arthritis and rheumatism; they also employ a root decoction for chills. One Amazonian *curandero* (near Pucallpa, Peru) uses a root tea for adult fevers, arthritis and rheumatism, back pain, common colds, bronchitis, lung disease and tuberculosis, snakebite, and as an enema for kidney disorders and ulcers. Indigenous tribes in the northwest Amazon utilize manacá to increase urination and perspiration in detoxification rituals. They also use it for fever, rheumatism, snakebite, syphilis, and yellow fever. *Curanderos* and herbal healers along the Amazon River in Ecuador use a root decoction to treat arthritis, rheumatism, colds and flu, uterine pain and cramps, sexually transmitted diseases, and to purify the blood—while using a poultice of the leaves as a topical pain-reliever.

In South American herbal medicine, the root of manacá is said to stimulate the lymphatic system. It has long been used for syphilis, earning the name *vegetable mercury* (mercury was once used to treat syphilis many years ago). In South American medicine systems today, manacá is considered to be an abortive, a lymph and blood cleanser, a topical anesthetic, diuretic, menstrual

Based on its long history of use in the Amazon, practitioners and herbalists in the United States now use manacá as a diuretic, laxative, and anti-inflammatory to treat arthritis and rheumatism, to treat sexually transmitted diseases, and to stimulate the lymphatic system and disperse uric acid.

promoter, laxative, sweat promoter, and narcotic. It is employed for arthritis, rheumatism, scrofula, and syphilis. In Brazil, herbalists use the root as a laxative and blood cleanser, for syphilis, rheumatism, scrofula, skin diseases, and to promote menstrual flow. Practitioners and herbalists in the United States use manacá as a diuretic, laxative, and anti-inflammatory to treat arthritis and rheumatism, sexually transmitted diseases, and to stimulate the lymphatic system and disperse uric acid. In Europe, the plant is used for arthritis, rheumatism, bronchitis, fevers, and snakebite.

PLANT CHEMICALS

A 1996 phytochemical study on the aerial parts of manacá revealed it contained such active compounds as benzenoids, terpenes, alkaloids, lactones, and lipids.[1] It is the root, though, that has been used primarily by indigenous peoples throughout the Amazon and by herbalists throughout the world. The root of manacá contains coumarins, alkaloids, lignans and sapogenins.[2–4] Active constituents include two alkaloids, manaceine and manacine, as well as scopoletin and aesculetin (types of coumarin chemicals). Manaceine and manacine are thought to be responsible for stimulating the lymphatic system, while aesculetin has demonstrated pain-relieving, liver detoxification, and anti-inflammatory activities in laboratory tests.[5] Scopoletin is a well-known phytochemical that has demonstrated analgesic, anti-inflammatory, antibacterial, anti-tumor, cancer preventive, antifungal, and antispasmodic activity in many different laboratory experiments.[6–10] It occurs in significant amounts in manacá.[8] A U.S. patent was awarded in 2002 for scopoletin's ability to inhibit nitric oxide production.[11] Nitric oxide is a reactive radical produced in the body and involved in inflammatory processes and in diseases such as asthma, heart disease, and erectile dysfunction.[12,13] These chemicals and their reported biological activities could help to explain many of manacá's uses in traditional herbal medicine systems.

Manacá contains a significant amount of *scopoletin*—a natural plant chemical documented with pain-relieving, anti-inflammatory, antibacterial, anti-tumor, cancer preventive, antifungal, and antispasmodic activity in many different laboratory experiments.

Manacá's main plant chemicals include aesculetin, alpha-ionone, alpha-terpineol, benzylbenzoate, benzylsalicylate, beta-bisabolene, beta-cyclocitral-brunfelsene, beta-damascenone, beta-eudesmol, beta-safranal, brunfelsene, brunfelsamidine, elemol, 2-ethylfuran, farnesol, farnesyl, geraniol, geranyl hopeanine, ionones, isobutylsalicylate, lavandulal, limonene, linalool, linoleic acid, linolenic acid, manaceine, manacine, mandragorine, methylfurans, methylanisoles, myrcene, myristic acid, n-decane, n-heneicosane, n-heptadecane, n-heptane, n-hexadecane, nerolidol, n-nonadecane, nonanes, n-octane, n-pentacosane, n-pentadecane, neophytadiene, n-tricosane, ocimene, pentadecanoic acid, palmitic acid, pinoresinols, salicylic acid esters, scopoletin, scopolin, and terpinolene.

BIOLOGICAL ACTIVITIES AND CLINICAL RESEARCH

Several animal studies confirm manacá's traditional uses for pain and inflammation.

Much more research is published on various chemicals found in manacá, rather than the plant itself. However, several animal studies do confirm some of its traditional uses—especially for pain and inflammation. In a 1991 clinical study with mice, manacá demonstrated pain-relieving and anti-inflammatory effects.[14] An earlier (1977) study reported that manacá root extracts evidenced marked anti-inflammatory actions in rats—as well as central nervous system depressant and fever-reducing actions.[15] Other root extracts administered to rats showed anti-inflammatory actions.[16] Leaf and root extracts of manacá also showed insecticidal actions (which may be attributed to naturally-occurring insecticidal chemicals nerolidol and farnesol).[17] Extracts of the twigs also have been documented to prevent cellular mutations.[18]

CURRENT PRACTICAL USES

In South America, manacá is respected as an important sacred and medicinal plant—mainly employed by shamans, healers, *curanderos*, herbal practitioners, and professionals. Due to its sedative effects and toxicity in large dosages, inexperienced non-professionals should refrain from self-treating or freely consuming this plant as a natural remedy; there are some contraindications and drug interactions that should be considered. This plant is best left in the hands of trained professionals (who can obtain the right species from reliable sources), and should be taken only in very small amounts and/or in proper combination with other plants.

Traditional Preparation

One-half cup root decoction one to two times daily, or 1–2 ml of a 4:1 tincture twice daily.

Contraindications

Manacá has a traditional use as an abortive. No clinical studies have been performed to indicate its safety during pregnancy; therefore, it is contraindicated for pregnant women.

Manacá root is reported to have toxicity in large doses—causing excessive salivation, vertigo, general anesthesia, partial paralysis of the face, swollen tongue, and disturbed vision.[5] Avoid dosages higher than the traditional remedy indicates.

Those allergic to aspirin (acetylsalicylic acid) should avoid using manacá. Manacá contains salicylate and several of its derivatives. Salicylate occurs naturally in plants; for some people, too much salicylate causes problems (known as "salicylate sensitivity" or "salicylate intolerance") without being allergic to aspirin. Do not use manacá if sensitive to salicylate.

Manacá root contains coumarins—plant chemicals known to thin the blood. Those taking blood-thinning medications such as coumadin should use manacá only under the direction and supervision of a qualified healthcare practitioner to monitor these effects.

The plant chemical scopoletin has been documented to inhibit monoamine oxidase.[19] Those taking monoamine oxidase (MAO) inhibitors should consult their healthcare practitioner before taking manacá.

Drug Interactions   None reported; however, manacá may potentiate blood-thinning medications such as Warfarin® and heparin. It may potentiate monoamine oxidase inhibitor drugs also.

Worldwide Ethnomedical Uses

Region	Uses
Amazonia	for arthritis, colds, detoxification, fever, flu, lymphatic disorders, rheumatism, sexually transmitted diseases, snakebite, syphilis, urinary insufficiency, uterine cramps, uterine disorders, yellow fever, and to increase perspiration
Brazil	for abortions, blood cleansing, constipation, fever, menstrual disorders, nausea, rheumatism, scrofula, sexually transmitted diseases, skin diseases, snakebite, syphilis, urinary disorders, urinary insufficiency, yellow fever, and to increase perspiration
Ecuador	for abortions, arthritis, cold, flu, lymph glands (swollen), malaria, pain, rheumatism, sexually transmitted diseases, snakebite, uterine problems, yellow fever
Europe	for arthritis, blood cleansing, bronchitis, fever, rheumatism, scrofula, snakebite, urinary insufficiency
Peru	for arthritis, back pain, bronchitis, chills, colds, fever, impotence, inflammation, kidney, lung disease, malaria, pain, rheumatism, sexually transmitted diseases, snakebite, syphilis, tuberculosis, ulcers, uterine cramps, yellow fever; as a diuretic, hallucinogen, and sedative and to increase perspiration
South America	for abortions, colds, fever, impotence, malaria, rheumatism, snakebite, yellow fever
United States	for menstrual disorders, pain, rheumatism, and to increase perspiration
Elsewhere	for abortions, arthritis, back pain, blood cleansing, bronchitis, cold, constipation, eczema, fever, gout, heat stroke, hypertension, inflammation, kidney problems, lung, lymphatic disorders, menstrual cramps, pain, rheumatism, scrofula, skin problems, snakebite, syphilis, tuberculosis, ulcers, urinary insufficiency, yellow fever and as a laxative

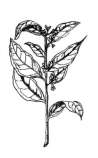

MUIRA PUAMA
HERBAL PROPERTIES AND ACTIONS

Main Actions	Other Actions	Standard Dosage
• increases libido	• is a male tonic	Root, bark
• promotes sexual function	• relieves pain	**Tincture:** 2–4 ml twice daily
• calms nerves	• reduces fatigue	**Decoction:** 1 cup daily
• relieves depression	• lowers blood pressure	
• enhances memory	• prevents ulcers	
• protects brain cells		

Family: Olacaceae

Genus: *Ptychopetalum*

Species: *olacoides, uncinatum*

Common Names: muira puama, potency wood, marapuama, marapama, muirat, muiratam, pau-homen, potenzholz

Parts Used: bark, roots

TRIBAL AND HERBAL MEDICINE USES

Muira puama is called "potency wood" because it is a highly regarded male sexual stimulant with a reputation as a powerful aphrodisiac in Brazil.

Muira puama, also called "potency wood," is a small tree that grows to 5 m high and is native to the Brazilian Amazon and other parts of the Amazon rainforest. The small, white flowers have a pungent fragrance similar to jasmine. The *Ptychopetalum* genus is a small one—only two species of small trees grow in tropical South America, and five in tropical Africa. The two South American varieties, *P. olacoides* (found in Brazil, French Guiana, Guyana, and Suriname) and *P. uncinatum* (found mainly in Brazil), are used interchangeably in South American herbal medicine systems. The *olacoides* variety is usually preferred, as it has a higher content of lupeol (one of the plant's active phytochemicals). A completely different species of Brazilian tree, *Liriosma ovata*, also goes by the common name of muira puama (and is often sold in commerce as such); however, it is a completely different tree with a different phytochemical makeup.[1]

Historically, all parts of muira puama have been used medicinally, but the bark and roots are the most utilized parts of the plant. It has long been used in the Amazon by indigenous peoples for a number of purposes. Native peoples along the Brazilian Amazon's Rio Negro river use the stems and roots from young plants as a tonic to treat neuromuscular problems; a root decoction is used in baths and massages for treating paralysis and beri-beri; and a root-and-bark tea is taken to treat sexual debility, rheumatism, grippe, and cardiac and gastrointestinal weakness. It's also valued there as a preventive for baldness. In Brazilian herbal medicine, muira puama still is a highly regarded sexual stimulant with a reputation as a powerful aphrodisiac. It has been in the *Brazilian Pharmacopoeia* since the 1950s.[2] It is used as a neuromuscular tonic for weakness and paralysis, dyspepsia, menstrual disturbances, chronic rheumatism (applied topically), sexual impotency, grippe, and central nervous system disorders.

Muira puama is employed around the world today in herbal medicine. Early European explorers noted the indigenous uses and the aphrodisiac qualities of muira puama and brought it back to Europe, where it has become part of herbal medicine in England. It is still listed in the *British Herbal Pharmacopoeia* (a noted herbal medicine source from the British Herbal Medicine Association); it is recommended there for the treatment of dysentery and impotence.[3] It is also used elsewhere in Europe to treat impotence, infertility, nerve pain, menstrual disturbances, and dysentery. In Germany, muira puama is employed as a central nervous system tonic, for hookworms, menstrual disturbances, and rheumatism. Muira puama has been gaining in popularity in the United States, where herbalists and health care practitioners are using it for impotence, depression, menstrual cramps and PMS, nerve pain, and central nervous system disorders.

PLANT CHEMICALS

Scientists began searching for the source of muira puama's efficacy in the 1920s.[4–6] Early researchers discovered that the root and bark were rich in fatty acids and fatty acid esters (the main one being behenic acid), essential oils (including beta-caryophyllene and alpha-humulene), plant sterols, triterpenes (including lupeol), and a new alkaloid—which they named *muirapuamine*.[7] Scientists resumed researching the plant's constituents and pharmacological properties in the late 1960s and continued into the late 1980s.[8–14] These studies indicated that the active constituents also included free long-chain fatty acids, sesquiterpenes, monoterpenes, and novel alkaloids.

The main plant chemicals found in muira puama include alpha-copaene, alpha-elemene, alpha-guaiene, alpha-humulene, alpha-muurolene, alpha-pinene, alpha-resinic acid, alpha-terpinene, arachidic acid, allo-aromadendren, behenic acid, beta-bisabolene, beta-caryophyllene, beta-pinene, beta-resinic acid, beta-sitosterol, beta-transfarnesene, borneol, campesterols, camphene, camphor, car-3-ene, caryophyllene, cerotic acid, chromium, coumarin, cubebene, delta-cadinene, dotriacontanoic acid, elixene, ergosterols, eugenol, essential oils, gamma-muurolene, hentriacontanoic acid, heptacosanoic acid, lignoceric acid, limonene, linalool, lupeol, melissic acid, montanic acid, muirapuamine, myrcene, nonacosanoic acid, para-cymene, pentacosanoic acid, phlobaphene, stigmasterols, trichosanic acid, and uncosanic acid.

BIOLOGICAL ACTIVITIES AND CLINICAL RESEARCH

In one of the early studies, researchers indicated that muira puama was effective in treating disorders of the nervous system and sexual impotence, and that "permanent effect is produced in locomotor ataxia, neuralgias of long standing, chronic rheumatism, and partial paralysis." [7] In 1930, Meira Penna wrote about muira puama in his book *Notas Sobre Plantas Brasileiras*. He cited physiological and therapeutic experiments conducted in France by Dr. Rebourgeon that confirmed the efficacy of the plant for "gastrointestinal and circulatory asthenia and impotency of the genital organs."[15]

The benefits of treating impotence with muira puama have been studied in two human trials in France, which reported that muira puama was effective in improving libido and treating erectile dysfunction. In one French study among 262 male patients who experienced lack of sexual desire and the inability to attain or maintain an erection, 62 percent of the patients with loss of libido reported that the extract of muira puama "had a dynamic effect," and 51 percent of patients with erectile dysfunction felt that muira puama was beneficial.[16] The second study evaluated positive psychological benefits of muira puama in 100 men with male sexual weakness.[17] The therapeutic dosage was 1.5 g of a muira puama extract daily. In their final report, researchers indicated muira puama could "enhance libido [in 85% of test group], increase the frequency of intercourse [in 100 %] and improve the ability to maintain an erection [in 90%]." [17]

The benefits of treating impotence with muira puama have been studied in two human trials in France, which reported that muira puama was effective in improving libido and treating erectile dysfunction.

In other recent clinical research, muira puama extracts have been reported to have adaptogenic, anti-fatigue, anti-stress, and beneficial effects on the central nervous system.[18,19] A specially prepared extract from the root of muira puama has been patented for its ability to "relieve physical and mental fatigue" and for "ameliorating a weakened constitution." [18] Researchers in Brazil documented a definite central nervous system effect of the bark in studies with mice.[19,20] The bark of muira puama also has demonstrated a mild, short-lived, hypotensive effect.[21] The root was found to inhibit stress-induced ulcers,[22] while the leaf demonstrated an analgesic effect.[23] Another U.S. patent has been filed on muira puama, citing that it can "reduce body fat percentage, increase lean muscle mass and lower cholesterol" in humans and animals with long-term use (and with no toxicity noted).[24] The newest research confirms muira puama's traditional use for memory and nervous disorders. Brazilian researchers reported in 2003 that an alcohol extract of muira puama facilitated memory retrieval in both young and aged mice and noted it may be beneficial for Alzheimer's patients.[25] Their next study, published in 2004, reported that an alcohol extract of muira puama protected and increased the viability of brain cells in mice (partly through an antioxidant effect), which may be beneficial for stroke victims.[26] Toxicity studies with mice, published in 1983, indicate no toxic effects.[27]

CURRENT PRACTICAL USES

While so-called aphrodisiacs have come and gone in history, muira puama has retained its stature and may well provide one of the more effective natural therapeutic approaches for erectile function and libido enhancement. Before trying to self-treat, however, men should always seek the advice of a health practitioner if suffering from erectile dysfunction or impotency; this often can be an early warning sign of vascular insufficiency and/or underlying heart problems.

To achieve the libido and potency effects of this particular plant, proper preparation methods must be employed. The active constituents thought to be responsible for muira puama's potency and libido effect are not soluble in water—taking bark or root powder in capsules or tablets will not be effective because these chemical cannot be digested or absorbed. High heat for at least twenty minutes with alcohol is necessary to free the volatile and essential oils, terpenes, gums, and resins found in the bark and root that have been linked to muira puama's beneficial effects.

Traditional Preparation   Since many of the most active principals are not water soluble it is best to prepared this plant as a tincture, using 2–4 ml of a 4:1 tincture twice daily. Boiling the tincture for twenty minutes will help facilitate extraction of the non-water-soluble chemicals. For its tonic effect, one of the traditional remedies is to gently simmer 1 teaspoon of root and/or bark in 1 cup of water for fifteen minutes and take $\frac{1}{2}$ to 1 cup daily.

Contraindications   None reported.

Drug Interactions   None reported.

Worldwide Ethnomedical Uses

Region	Uses
Amazonia	as an aphrodisiac and for baldness, beri-beri, cardiac weakness, central nervous system problems, diarrhea, flu, gastrointestinal problems, impotence, low libido, neuromuscular problems, paralysis, rheumatism, sexual debility, weakness
Brazil	as an aphrodisiac and appetite stimulant and for ataxia, baldness, beri-beri, central nervous system disorders, debility, depression, digestive problems, dysentery, dyspepsia, frigidity, gastrointestinal disorders, heart problems, hookworm, impotence, low libido, menopause, menstrual cramps, nerve problems, nervous exhaustion, neuralgia, neuromuscular problems, ovarian function, paralysis, poliomyelitis, premenstrual syndrome (PMS), rheumatism, stress, trauma, weakness (muscle)
Germany	as a central nervous system tonic and for hookworms, menstrual disturbances, rheumatism
Guyana	as an aphrodisiac, stimulant, and tonic, and for impotency
Europe	as an aphrodisiac and nerve tonic and for dysentery, impotence, infertility, menstrual disturbances, neurasthenia
United States	as an aphrodisiac and tonic and for central nervous system disorders, depression, impotence, menstrual problems, nerve pain, premenstrual syndrome (PMS)
Elsewhere	as an aphrodisiac and central nervous system stimulant and for baldness, dyspepsia, exhaustion, gastrointestinal weakness, impotency, infertility, low libido, menstrual irregularities, muscle paralysis, nerve pain, neuromuscular problems, paralysis, reproductive disorders, rheumatism, stress, trauma

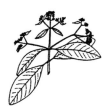

MULATEIRO		
HERBAL PROPERTIES AND ACTIONS		
Main Actions	**Other Actions**	**Standard Dosage**
• kills bacteria	• stops bleeding	Bark
• kills fungi		**Decoction:** $1/2$–1 cup two to
• heals wounds		three times daily
• fights free radicals		**Decoction:** Applied topically
• kills parasites		
• kills insects		
• repels insects		
• soothes skin		

Family: Rubiaceae

Genus: *Calycophyllum*

Species: *spruceanum*

Common Names: pau mulato, capirona, capirona negra, corusicao, palo mulato, uhuachaunin, ashi, capirona de bajo, haxo, asho, huiso asho nahua

Part Used: bark

Mulateiro is a fascinating multi-purpose canopy tree in the Amazon. It grows tall and straight up to a height of about 30 m, and has been long used as a source of good, high density lumber. It produces an abundance of small, white, aromatic flowers (from June to July), which are followed by elongated seedpods with three to five seeds inside. The tree propagates easily from the many seeds it produces. It can often be found near water, as it can survive common periodic flooding in the region.

Mulateiro is noted for its ability to completely shed and regenerate its bark on a yearly basis, making harvesting the bark a totally renewable and sustainable enterprise. The bark is smooth (as if polished) and changes colors throughout the year as it matures—going from a green tone to a brownish tone. *Calycophyllum* is a small genus with only about six species spread through tropical America; all are medium-sized to large trees. This particular species is indigenous to the Amazon basin in Brazil, Peru, Bolivia, and Ecuador. It is called *mulateiro* or *pau-mulato* in Brazil, and *capirona* in Peru.

TRIBAL AND HERBAL MEDICINE USES

Mulateiro bark is deeply ingrained in the native culture—from being used as an admixture in the *ayahuasca* rituals, to its many different uses in folkloric medicine. In the Amazon, a poultice made from the bark is used topically in treating cuts, wounds, and burns and believed to have antifungal and wound-healing qualities. The Indians also use a tea made from the bark on their bodies after bathing, and then sun-dry themselves. This forms a thin film covering their bodies believed to help fight the effects of aging, parasites, and fungal infections. Indigenous people of the Amazon also use a bark decoction to treat diabetes. They boil 1 kg of bark in 10 liters of water until 4 liters remain. It is believed that if this decoction is drunk every day (about 5 ounces daily) for three consecutive months that it is a "cure" for diabetes. Peruvian tribes also apply the powdered bark to fungal infections of the skin. They also prepare a bark decoction to treat skin parasites—especially "sarna negra"—a nasty little bug that lives under the skin, which is commonly found in the Amazon basin area.

Mulateiro is widely used in the Amazon for all types of skin conditions— from skin parasites and fungi to healing cuts, wounds, and burns.

In Peruvian herbal medicine today, mulateiro is used for many purposes. A bark decoction is used topically for eye infections and infected wounds as well as for skin spots, skin depigmentation, wrinkles, and scars. It stops bleeding quickly and is often applied to bleeding cuts. It's also thought to soothe insect bites and reduce bruising and swelling. The bark is decocted and used internally for diabetes and disorders of the ovaries. The resin is used for abscesses and skin tumors. Due to its beneficial effects to the skin, it is appearing as an ingredient in natural cosmetic products in Peru and Brazil.

PLANT CHEMICALS

Mulateiro bark contains a great deal of tannin chemicals, which give it an astringent or drying effect. Recently, the plant has been documented to contain a high content of phenols and organic acids, which have demonstrated antibacterial, antifungal, and insecticidal activity.[1] The isolated phenols have demonstrated strong antioxidant activity, which may explain its traditional use to stop the aging process of the skin.[1]

BIOLOGICAL ACTIVITIES AND CLINICAL RESEARCH

Only one clinical study has been published thus far on mulateiro; in 2001 researchers reported that it demonstrated strong antifungal activity *in vitro* against eleven common skin fungi and yeasts.[2] With this study, as well as the two groups of chemicals demonstrating antibacterial, antifungal, and insecticidal properties, scientists are just beginning to validate its traditional uses for various bacterial and fungal infections of the skin and as an insect repellent.

CURRENT PRACTICAL USES

Mulateiro is better known today as a rainforest hardwood tree which is logged in the Amazon and exported around the world for high density, durable lumber and building materials, than as a medicinal plant. It has recently sparked the interest of scientists and formulators of natural body care products in South America for its beneficial effect to the skin. Even a branch of the Brazilian government is currently working with researchers and manufacturers about these new possible uses and markets for mulateiro bark in the body care products industry. With the tree shedding its bark annually, this resource would be highly sustainable. If a sufficient market were established for this renewable resource, then landowners would not cut the trees down for the value of the lumber, and would protect them for the income realized by annual harvesting of the bark.

Traditional Preparation

For internal use, the standard remedy is $\frac{1}{2}$–1 cup of standard decoction two to three times daily. This decoction is also a common topical remedy for skin problems, wounds, skin fungus, and overall skin health. It is applied directly to the affected area several times daily and allowed to dry before covering.

Contraindications None known.

Drug Interactions None known.

Worldwide Ethnomedical Uses

Region	Uses
Amazonia	for burns, cuts, diabetes, fungal infections, skin parasites, wounds
Brazil	for skin problems and wounds, and as an antioxidant and cosmetic
Paraguay	for diabetes
Peru	for abscesses, anti-aging, bites (insect), bleeding, bruises, diabetes, eye infections, fungal infections, infections (skin), ovarian disorders, scabies, scars, skin parasites, skin problems, swelling, tumors, wounds, wrinkles, and as a contraceptive

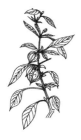

Family: Solanaceae

Genus: *Physalis*

Species: *angulata*

Common Names: mullaca, camapu, bolsa mullaca, cape gooseberry, wild tomato, winter cherry, juá-de-capote, capulí cimarrón, battre-autour, k'u chih, 'urmoa batoto bita, cecendet, dumadu harachan, hog weed, nvovo, polopa, saca-buche, thongtheng, tino-tino, topatop, wapotok

Parts Used: whole plant, leaves, roots

MULLACA

HERBAL PROPERTIES AND ACTIONS

Main Actions
- kills mycobacteria
- kills bacteria
- kills cancer cells
- kills leukemia cells
- kills viruses
- kills germs
- enhances immunity
- thins blood

Other Actions
- relieves pain
- reduces inflammation
- reduces spasms
- increases urination
- reduces fever
- expels phlegm

Standard Dosage

Whole plant

Infusion: ½–1 cup one to three times daily

Capsules/Tablets: 1–2 g twice daily

Tincture: 1–3 ml twice daily

Mullaca is an annual herb indigenous to many parts of the tropics, including the Amazon. It can be found on most continents in the tropics, including Africa, Asia, and the Americas. It grows up to 1 m high, bears small, cream-colored flowers, and produces small, light yellowish-orange, edible fruit sometimes referred to as cape gooseberry. The fruit is about the size of a cherry tomato, and like tomatoes, it contains many tiny edible seeds inside. Mullaca propagates easily from the seeds the fruit contains; spontaneous clumps of plants can be found along river banks and just about anywhere the soil is disturbed and the canopy is broken (allowing enough sunlight to promote its rapid growth).

**TRIBAL
AND HERBAL
MEDICINE USES**

Mullaca has long held a place in natural medicine in the tropical countries where it grows. Its use by rainforest Indians in the Amazon is well documented, and its edible sweet-tart fruits are enjoyed by many rainforest inhabitants, animal and human alike. Indigenous tribes in the Amazon use a leaf infusion as a diuretic. Some Colombian tribes believe the fruits and leaves have narcotic properties and also decoct them as an anti-inflammatory and disinfectant for skin diseases; others use a leaf tea for asthma. Indigenous peoples in the Peruvian Amazon use the leaf juice internally and externally for worms and the leaves and/or roots for earache, liver problems, malaria, hepatitis, and rheumatism. Indigenous tribes in the Brazilian Amazon use the sap of the plant for earaches and the roots for jaundice. Mullaca has also been used by indigenous peoples for female disorders. In the Solomon Islands, the fruit of mullaca is decocted and taken internally to promote fertility. A tea is made of the entire plant and/or the leaves in the West Indies and Jamaica to prevent miscarriages. In Peru, the leaf is infused and used to treat postpartum infections.

*In Brazilian herbal
medicine, mullaca is
employed for chronic
rheumatism; for skin
diseases and dermatitis;
as a sedative and diuretic;
for fever and vomiting;
and for many types of
kidney, liver, and
gallbladder problems.*

Mullaca is employed in herbal medicine systems today in both Peru and Brazil. In Peruvian herbal medicine, the plant is called *mullaca* or *bolsa mullaca*. To treat diabetes, the roots of three mullaca plants are sliced and macerated in $\frac{1}{4}$ liter of rum for seven days. Honey is added, and $\frac{1}{2}$ glass of this medicine is taken twice daily for sixty days. In addition, an infusion of the leaves is recommended as a good diuretic, and an infusion of the roots is used to treat hepatitis. For asthma and malaria, the dosage is 1 cup of tea made from the aerial parts of the plant. In Brazilian herbal medicine, the plant is employed for chronic rheumatism; for skin diseases and dermatitis; as a sedative and diuretic; for fever and vomiting; and for many types of kidney, liver, and gallbladder problems.

**PLANT
CHEMICALS**

Phytochemical studies on mullaca reveal that it contains many types of biologically active, naturally occurring chemicals including flavonoids, alkaloids, and many different types of plant steroids, some of which have never before been seen in science.[1-6] Mullaca has been the subject of recent clinical research (which is ongoing), based on the preliminary studies showing that it is an effective immune stimulant, is toxic to numerous types of cancer and leukemia cells, and that it has antimicrobial properties. The new steroids found in mullaca have received the most attention, and many of the documented anticancerous, antitumorous and antileukemic actions are attributed to these steroids.

Various extracts of mullaca, as well as these extracted plant steroids called *physalins*, have shown strong *in vitro* and *in vivo* (mice) activity against numerous types of human and animal cancer cells including lung, colon, nasophar-

Chemicals in mullaca have been the subject of ongoing clinical research, based on preliminary studies showing that they are effective immune stimulants, are toxic to numerous types of cancer and leukemia cells and that they have antimicrobial properties.

ynx, liver, cervix, melanoma and glioma (brain) cancer cells.[7–12] This cancer research began in the early 1980s with researchers in Thailand and the U.S.[7,8] and was verified with research performed at the University of Taiwan in 1992 (where they demonstrated a significant effect against five human cancer cell lines and three animal cancer cell lines).[9] Then in 2001, researchers at the University of Houston isolated yet another new chemical in mullaca which demonstrated remarkable toxicity against nasopharynx cancer cells, lung (adenocarcinoma) cancer cells, as well as leukemia in mice.[10] The same Taiwanese researchers had already published a separate study on mullaca's other antileukemic phytochemicals in 1992, reporting that two physalin chemicals inhibited the growth of five types of acute leukemia, including lymphoid (T & B), promyelocytic, myeloid, and monocytic.[11]

Other research in China and Russia independently demonstrated significant immunomodulatory effects against blastogenesis (a process triggered in leukemia), while boosting other immune functions, which might account for the antileukemic effects in mice seen by other researchers.[13–15] With tumor cells, research suggests that several of the steroidal chemicals in mullaca act on an enzyme level to arrest the normal cell cycle in cancer cells[16,17] as well as cause DNA damage inside of cancer cells (making them unable to replicate).[18,19]

The main plant chemicals isolated in mullaca thus far include ayanin, chlorogenic acid, choline, ixocarpanolide, myricetin, phygrine, physagulin A through G, physalin A through K, physangulide, sitosterol, vamonolide, withaminimin, withangulatin A, withanolide D, withanolide T, and withaphysanolide.

BIOLOGICAL ACTIVITIES AND CLINICAL RESEARCH

In addition to mullaca's anticancerous and antileukemic actions, several research groups have confirmed mullaca's antibacterial and antiviral activity. In 2002 and 2000, mullaca was shown to be active *in vitro* against several strains of mycobacteriums and mycoplasmas (both very stubborn types of bacteria which are not widely susceptible to standard antibiotics).[20,21] In addition to these actions, mullaca has demonstrated effective antibacterial properties *in vitro* against numerous types of gram positive and gram negative bacteria, including *Pseudomonas, Staphylococcus,* and *Streptococcus*.[22,23] Other research groups in Japan have been focusing on mullaca's antiviral actions and preliminary studies show that it is active *in vitro* against Polio virus I, Herpes simplex virus I, the measles virus, and HIV-I—demonstrating reverse transcriptase inhibitory effects.[24–27]

Mullaca has demonstrated in the laboratory to kill not only cancer cells—but also bacteria and viruses.

Mullaca has also been reported to reduce spasms in guinea pigs,[28] lower blood pressure in cats, and to contract isotonic muscles in toads.[29] In the test tube, mullaca was shown to have an anticoagulant effect.[30] Western scientists did somewhat validate the indigenous use for diabetes when they reported a mild hypoglycemic effect in mice fed a water extract of the root.[31] One must wonder what the results would have been if they had followed native customs and employed an alcohol extract instead.

CURRENT PRACTICAL USES

Interestingly enough, much of the clinical research has ignored the local and indigenous uses of the plant; thus, many of its effective uses in herbal medicine remain unexplained. Its tested antibacterial properties could validate its use as an antiseptic and disinfectant for skin diseases, and its use to treat gonorrhea. Its antiviral properties could well explain its long history of use for hepatitis, although scientists have not tested it specifically against hepatitis. Possibly the antispasmodic and muscle contractive properties documented for mullaca might explain its use for asthma and female disorders, as well. Yet, its widespread use throughout the rainforests for malaria and fevers remains unexplained by science.

Herbal practitioners in both South and North America today rely on mullaca for various bacterial and viral infections, and as a complementary therapy for cancer and leukemia. Although not widely available here in the U.S., it is found as an ingredient in various herbal formulas and in bulk supplies. The animal studies conducted to date indicate no toxicity at any of the dosages used, indicating that it is a safe natural remedy.

Traditional Preparation

Depending on what it is employed for, generally ½–1 cup of a whole herb infusion one to three times daily or 1–2 ml of a 4:1 tincture twice daily is used. If desired, 2–4 g of powdered whole herb (depending on body weight) in tablets or capsules or stirred into water or juice twice daily can be substituted (since the active sterol chemicals are completely water soluble).

Contraindications

One animal study indicates this plant may lower blood pressure[27] and one test tube study demonstrates a blood anticoagulant activity.[28] People with blood disorders such as hemophilia, those taking heart medications or blood thinners, or those with other heart problems such as low blood pressure should use this plant with the advice of a qualified health care practitioner.

Drug Interactions

None reported; however, see above contraindications.

Worldwide Ethnomedical Uses

Region	Uses
Brazil	for asthma, blood cleansing, dermatitis, earaches, fever, gallbladder problems, jaundice, kidney problems, liver disorders, malaria, nausea, rheumatism, skin diseases, urinary insufficiency
Central America	for fever, gonorrhea, malaria, skin diseases, and to prevent miscarriages

Colombia	for asthma, bacterial infections, inflammation, skin diseases
Japan	for colds, fever, strep throat, swelling, urinary insufficiency
Peru	for asthma, bacterial infections, diabetes, earaches, hepatitis, infection (postpartum), inflammation, itch, jaundice, liver problems, malaria, rheumatism, skin diseases, urinary insufficiency, worms
Taiwan	for cancer, fever, hepatitis, liver disease, tumors, urinary insufficiency
Trinidad	for bacterial infections, fever, indigestion, nephritis, rectitis
Suriname	for gonorrhea, jaundice, malaria, nephritis, urinary insufficiency
Elsewhere	for asthma, bacterial infections, boils, cancer, childbirth, diabetes, diarrhea, diuretic, edema, eye infections, fainting, fevers, hemorrhage (postpartum), infertility, inflammation, leukemia, malaria, nausea, pain, skin diseases, sleeping sickness, stomach problems, tumor (testicle); and as an antiseptic, expectorant, hemostatic

MULUNGU
HERBAL PROPERTIES AND ACTIONS

Main Actions
- relieves pain
- reduces anxiety
- calms nerves
- moderately sedative
- supports liver
- reduces blood pressure
- regulates heartbeat

Other Actions
- kills bacteria

Standard Dosage
Bark, root

Decoction: $1/2$ cup one to two times daily

Tincture: 1–2 ml one to two times daily

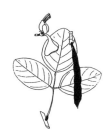

Family: Fabaceae

Genus: *Erythrina*

Species: *mulungu, crista-galli*

Common Names: mulungu, corticeira, murungu, muchocho, murungo, totocero, flor-de-coral, árvore-de-coral, amerikadeigo, ceibo, chilichi, chopo, hosoba deiko, pau-imortal, mulungu-coral, capa-homem, suiná-suiná

Part Used: bark

Mulungu is a medium-sized, well-branched tree that grows 10–14 m high. It produces a profusion of pretty, reddish-orange flowers (pollinated by hummingbirds) at the ends of the tree's many branches. The tree is sometimes called "coral flower," as the flowers resemble the color of orange coral. It produces black seedpods containing large, red-and-black seeds, which are sometimes used by indigenous peoples to make necklaces and jewelry. Mulungu is indigenous to Brazil, parts of Peru, and tropical areas in Latin America and, typically, is found in marshes and along riverbanks. The *Erythrina* genus comprises more than 100 species of trees and shrubs (mostly all heavily armed with spines or thorns) in the tropical and subtropical regions of both hemispheres. The mulungu tree (first recorded in 1829) is known by two botanical names, *Erythrina mulungu* and *Erythrina verna*. Another closely related species, *E. crista-galli*, is used interchangeably in South American herbal medicine systems and is found farther south on the South American continent. The flower of *E. crista-galli* is the national flower of Argentina.

TRIBAL
AND HERBAL
MEDICINE USES

In both North and South
American herbal
medicine systems,
mulungu is considered to
be an excellent sedative
to calm agitation and
nervous coughs and to
treat other nervous
system problems
including insomnia and
anxiety.

Several *Erythrina* tree species are used by indigenous peoples in the Amazon as medicines, insecticides, and fish poisons. Mulungu has long been used in Brazil by indigenous peoples as a natural sedative: it has been used to calm an overexcited nervous system and promote a restful sleep.

In both North and South American herbal medicine systems, mulungu is considered to be an excellent sedative to calm agitation and nervous coughs and to treat other nervous system problems including insomnia and anxiety. It also is widely used for asthma, bronchitis, gingivitis, hepatitis, inflammation of the liver and spleen, intermittent fevers, and to clear obstructions in the liver. In both Brazil and Peru, mulungu is used for epilepsy. Herbalists and practitioners in the United States use mulungu to quiet hysteria from trauma or shock, as a mild, hypnotic sedative to calm the nervous system, to treat insomnia and promote healthy sleeping patterns (by sedating overactive neurotransmitters), to regulate heart palpitations, and to treat hepatitis and liver disorders. Positive regulatory effects on heart palpitations and decreased blood pressure have been reported. Dr. Donna Schwontkowski, a chiropractor who has used Amazonian plants in her practice, recommends mulungu for hernias, stomachaches, and epilepsy—and to help augment milk flow as well.

PLANT
CHEMICALS

Research on the
chemicals found in
mulungu reveal they are
anti-inflammatory,
sedative, and regulate
the heart.

The chemicals in mulungu have been studied extensively; they have been found to comprise large amounts of novel flavonoids, triterpenes, and alkaloids. Much research has been performed on *Erythrina* alkaloids in the last decade, as they represent a group of very active chemicals with various properties and are almost always present in *Erythrina* species.[1] Thus far, alkaloids have been found in 78 of 107 species in the genus *Erythrina;* mulungu is documented with twenty isoquinoline alkaloids. Many of these have demonstrated anti-inflammatory, cardioactive, narcotic, and sedative activities.[1,2] One novel alkaloid discovered in mulungu is called *cristamidine.* Its positive effect on the liver was demonstrated in a 1995 clinical study with rats.[3] Mulungu's hypotensive and heart-regulatory activities were studied and attributed to its alkaloids.[4] Another alkaloid in mulungu (and other *Erythrina* plants), erysodine, has been documented with neuromuscular effects characteristic of curare arrow poisons. Two studies also indicate that it might be useful as an anti-nicotine drug, as it demonstrated actions as a competitive antagonist and to block nicotine receptors.[5,6] Interestingly, both of these studies were published by major (and competing) pharmaceutical companies!

The main plant chemicals in mulungu include alanine, arginine, aspartic acid, cristacarpin, cristadine, crystamidine, dimethylmedicarpin, erybidine, erycristagallin, erycristanol, erycristin, erydotrine, erysodienone, erysodine, erysonine, erysopine, erysotrine, erysovine, erystagallin A–C, erythrabyssin II, erythralines, erythramine, erythratine, eryvariestyrene, gamma-amino butyric acid, glutamic acid, hypaphorine lectins, n-nor-orientaline, oleanolic acid, oleanonic acid, phaseollidins, proteinases, sandwicensis, ursolic acid, and vitexin.

BIOLOGICAL ACTIVITIES AND CLINICAL RESEARCH

Research with animals suggests mulungu has a similar effect as a leading anti-anxiety drug.

The traditional use of mulungu for anxiety and stress has been validated by researchers in a 2002 study, where it was shown to alter anxiety-related responses.[7] An animal model (correlating to human generalized anxiety disorder, as well as panic disorder) was undertaken on a water-alcohol extract of mulungu. The researchers reported that the mulungu extract had an effect similar to the commonly-prescribed anti-anxiety drug diazepam.[7] It was suggested in this study that the alkaloids in *Erythrina* "may alter GABAergic neurotransmission." GABA (gamma-amino butyric acid) acts as a neurotransmitter in the brain; abnormalities with its function are implicated in diseases including epilepsy, anxiety, and depression.[8] Further research has validated the traditional use of mulungu as an antimicrobial agent for throat and urinary infections; mulungu has demonstrated antibacterial activity in two studies against *Staphylococcus aureus*, and antimycobacterial activity against *Mycobacterium fortuitum* and *Mycobacterium smegmatis*.[9,10]

CURRENT PRACTICAL USES

Mulungu is not very widely known or used in North America; it mostly appears as an ingredient in only a few herbal formulas for anxiety or depression. It is a wonderful rainforest medicinal plant that is deserving of much more attention in herbal medicine systems outside of South America. The main herbal remedy sold in America today for stress, anxiety, and as a general sedative is kava-kava. This plant, however, has had some negative press in recent years concerning possible negative effects to the liver. Since mulungu provides the same calming and stress-relieving effects (if not better), and actually has a positive effect on the liver, it is poised as the new replacement for this highly popular (and profitable) herbal supplement.

Traditional Preparation

One-half cup of a standard bark or root decoction or 1–2 ml of a 4:1 tincture once or twice daily.

Contraindications

This plant is a sedative and may cause drowsiness. In traditional medicine, the plant is used to lower blood pressure. Clinical research with animals has documented hypotensive actions. It is recommended that those on medications to lower blood pressure (and those with low blood pressure) use mulungu with caution and monitor their blood pressure accordingly.

Drug Interactions

None documented; however, mulungu may potentiate some anti-anxiety drugs (such as diazepam) and antihypertensive drugs.

Worldwide Ethnomedical Uses

Region	Uses
Argentina	for diarrhea, hemorrhoids, respiratory infections, urinary infections, and as an antiseptic and sedative
Brazil	for agitation, anxiety, asthma, bacterial infections, bronchitis, central nervous system disorders, convulsions, cough, cuts, epilepsy, fever, gingivitis, hepatitis, hysteria, inflammation, insomnia, liver problems, menopause, muscle pain, nervous tension, neuralgia, rheumatism, spleen disorders, stress, throat (sore), whooping cough, and as an antiseptic and sedative
Colombia	as a diuretic and sedative
Peru	for cystitis, epilepsy, eye irritations, hysteria, insomnia
United States	for central nervous system disorders, epilepsy, heart problems, hepatitis, hernia, high blood pressure, hysteria, insomnia, liver problems, stomachache, and as a lactation aid
Elsewhere	for edema, epilepsy, eye problems, headaches, heart problems, hepatitis, hernia, hypertension, hysteria, insomnia, liver problems, palpitations, rheumatism, spasms, stomach cancer, stomachache, urinary insufficiency, and as a sedative

When boats no longer float, they become houses. Nothing is discarded.

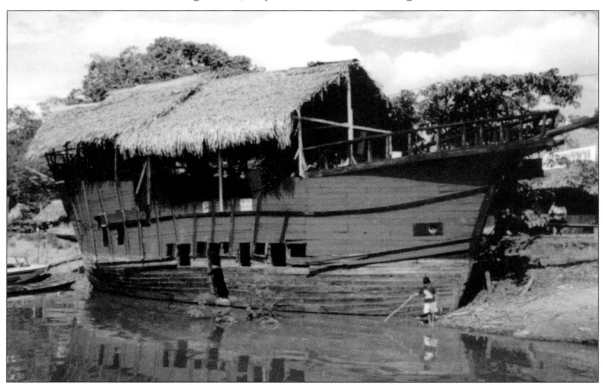

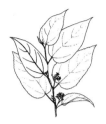

Family: Sterculiaceae

Genus: *Guazuma*

Species: *ulmifolia*

Common Names: mutamba, mutambo, embira, embiru, West Indian elm, guazima, guacima, guacimo, guasima de caballo, aquiche, ajya, guasima, cimarrona, guazuma, bolaina, atadijo, ibixuma, cambá-acã, bay cedar, bois d'homme, bois d'orme, bois de hetre, orme d'Amerique

Parts Used: bark, leaves, root

MUTAMBA		
HERBAL PROPERTIES AND ACTIONS		
Main Actions	**Other Actions**	**Standard Dosage**
• kills bacteria	• reduces inflammation	Bark
• kills fungi	• prevents ulcers	**Infusion:** 1 cup one to three times daily
• kills viruses	• supports heart	
• kills cancer cells	• stimulates digestion	**Capsules/Tablets:** 2 g twice daily
• cleanses blood	• protects liver	
• suppresses coughs	• reduces fever	**Tincture:** 2–3 ml twice daily
• fights free radicals	• promotes perspiration	
• lowers blood pressure		
• relaxes muscles		
• stops bleeding		
• heals wounds		

Mutamba is a medium-sized tree that grows up to 20 m high, with a trunk 30 to 60 cm in diameter. Its oblong leaves are 6 to 12 cm long, and the tree produces small white-to-light-yellow flowers. It produces an edible fruit that is covered with rough barbs and has a strong honey scent. Mutamba is indigenous to tropical America on both continents and found throughout the Amazon rainforest.

TRIBAL AND HERBAL MEDICINE USES

Mutamba is called *guasima* or *guacima* in Mexico, where it has a very long history of indigenous use. The Mixe Indians in the lowlands of Mexico use a decoction of dried bark and fruit to treat diarrhea, hemorrhages, and uterine pain. The Huastec Mayans of northeastern Mexico employ the fresh bark boiled in water to aid in childbirth, for gastrointestinal pain, asthma, diarrhea and dysentery, wounds, and fevers. Mayan healers in Guatemala boil the bark into a decoction to treat stomach inflammation and regular stomachaches. Mutamba was a magical plant to the ancient Mayans, who also used it against "magical illnesses" and evil spells. In the Amazon, indigenous people have long used mutamba for asthma, bronchitis, diarrhea, kidney problems, and syphilis. They use a bark decoction topically for baldness, leprosy, and various skin diseases.

Mutamba holds a place in herbal medicine systems in many tropical countries; chiefly the bark and leaves are used. In Belizean herbal medicine practices, a small handful of chopped bark is boiled for ten minutes in 3 cups of water and drunk for dysentery and diarrhea, for prostate problems, and as a uterine

In the Amazon, indigenous people have long used mutamba for asthma, bronchitis, diarrhea, kidney problems, and syphilis. They use a bark decoction topically for baldness, leprosy, dermatitis, and other skin conditions.

stimulant to aid in childbirth. A slightly stronger decoction is used externally for skin sores, infections, and rashes. In Brazilian herbal medicine practices, a bark decoction is used to promote perspiration, cleanse and detoxify the blood, and suppress coughs. There it is used for fevers, coughs, bronchitis, asthma, pneumonia, syphilis, and liver problems. A bark decoction is also prepared and is used topically to promote hair growth, to combat parasites of the scalp, and to treat various skin conditions. In Peru, the dried bark and/or dried leaves are made into tea (standard infusion) and used for kidney disease, liver disease, and dysentery. The bark is also used topically for hair loss. In Guatemala, the dried leaves of the tree are brewed into a tea and drunk for fevers, kidney disease, and skin diseases, as well as used externally for wounds, sores, bruises, dermatitis, skin eruptions and irritations, and erysipelas.

PLANT CHEMICALS

A chemical found in mutamba helps validate its long standing use in several countries for hair loss and baldness: researchers in Japan reported that this particular chemical was a safe topical hair-growing agent.

Mutamba bark is a rich source of tannins and antioxidant chemicals called *proanthocyanidins.* One in particular, *procyanidin B-2,* helps validate mutamba's long standing use in several countries for hair loss and baldness. In 1999, researchers in Japan reported that procyanidin B-2 was a safe topical hair-growing agent.[1] From 2000 to 2002, they published three *in vitro* and *in vivo* (in balding men) studies showing that procyanidin B-2 promoted hair cell growth and increased the total number of hairs on a designated scalp area.[2–4] Researchers have determined that mutamba bark is a rich source of this natural chemical compound.[5] Other independent research indicates that procyanidin B-2 also has antitumorous and anticancerous effects (even against melanoma) as well as lowers blood pressure and protects the kidneys.[6,7] The bark also contains a chemical called *kaurenoic acid,* which has been documented with antibacterial and antifungal properties in many studies over the years. The leaves of mutamba contain caffeine, however none has been found in the bark of the tree.

Mutamba's main plant chemicals include caryophyllene, catechins, farnesol, friedelin, kaurenoic acid, precocene I, procyanidin B-2, procyanidin B-5, procyanidin C-1, and sitosterol.

BIOLOGICAL ACTIVITIES AND CLINICAL RESEARCH

Mutamba's long history of effective uses in herbal medicine propelled researchers to begin studying its properties and activities in the laboratory (beginning in 1968). It has been the subject of numerous studies since. The first study published, which used various animals (rats, rabbits, guinea pigs, cats, and insects), reported that mutamba lowered heart rate and blood pressure, relaxed smooth muscles, and stimulated the uterus.[8] Two years later, another researcher reconfirmed the uterine stimulant effects in rats, validating its historical uses as a uterine stimulant and childbirth aid.[9] In eight different studies from 1987 to 2003, various leaf and bark extracts have clinically demonstrated remarkable antibacterial activity *in vitro* against several disease-causing pathogens, including *Bacillus, Staphylococcus, Streptococcus, E. coli,* and *Neisseria gonorrhea.*[10–17] One 2003 study also confirmed its antioxidant effects.[17] In a 1995 *in vitro* study, mutamba also demonstrated antiviral activity against Herpes simplex type 1.[18]

These studies could certainly explain why mutamba has been used so effectively in herbal medicine systems for many types of gastrointestinal problems, such sexually transmitted diseases as gonorrhea and syphilis, and upper respiratory conditions (pneumonia and bronchitis). Subsequent research focusing on particular chemicals found in mutamba documented their ability to interfere with an enzyme process by which bacteria and pathogens replicate.[5,19,20] Scientists showed that these chemicals interacted with a cholera toxin—preventing its toxicity and the resultant diarrhea.[5,20]

Traditionally, a decoction of mutamba leaves has been used in Mexico for diabetes. It has only been since 1998 that researchers in Mexico validated this indigenous use, publishing a study showing that a leaf extract significantly decreased hyperglycemia in rabbits.[21] Of particular note (in 1990), a Brazilian research group demonstrated that a crude extract of mutamba was toxic to cancer cells *in vitro,* exhibiting a 97.3 percent inhibition rate.[22] In another study in 2002, Belgium researchers reported the possible mechanism by which mutamba bark reduces hypertension—it inhibits an enzyme called *angiotensin II.*[23] Angiotensin inhibitors represent a classification of heart drugs (newer than the ACE inhibitors), which are now being prescribed to lower blood pressure.

Research over the years has indicated that mutamba possesses broad spectrum antibacterial and antiviral actions—validating its traditional uses for upper respiratory infections and sexually transmitted diseases.

CURRENT PRACTICAL USES

Research continues to document the unique properties and actions of this plant while validating its traditional uses. Mutamba is a favorite natural remedy among Central and South American health practitioners and the indigenous peoples of the Amazon. It is often turned to first for upper respiratory infections as it can quiet coughs, reduce fever, as well as provide antiviral and antibacterial actions. It will be interesting to see if anyone in North or South America follows up on the research concerning hair loss, and utilizes mutamba as a natural product for baldness and hair loss prevention. There certainly is a ready (and very profitable) market for products such as these—especially if they are effective!

Traditional Preparation

The traditional remedy for upper respiratory infections, asthma, and other respiratory problems is 1 cup of a standard bark decoction two to three times daily. For gastrointestinal problems and other conditions, the same bark decoction is used, or 2–3 ml of a 4:1 tincture twice daily, or 1–2 g of powdered bark daily in tablets or capsules (or stirred into water or juice) can be substituted, if desired. The same bark decoction is rinsed through the hair several times weekly as a natural remedy for hair loss.

Contraindications   Mutamba bark has been documented, in several animal studies, to have uterine stimulant activity, and it should not be taken during pregnancy.

Mutamba bark has been documented in animal studies to lower blood pressure. *In vitro* studies indicate that it can inhibit angiotensin II. People with a history of heart problems, those taking heart medications, or those with low blood pressure should not use this plant without the supervision and advice of a qualified health care practitioner.

Drug Interactions   None published; however, mutamba bark may potentiate the action of certain antihypertensive drugs.

Worldwide Ethnomedical Uses

Region	Uses
Belize	for childbirth, diarrhea, dysentery, infections, prostate problems, rashes, skin problems, sores, uterine problems
Brazil	for asthma, blood cleansing, bronchitis, coughs, dysentery, excessive mucus, fever, hair loss, hepatitis, liver problems, parasites (head), pneumonia, skin diseases, syphilis, ulcers, and to increase perspiration
Colombia	as a uterine stimulant
Cuba	for bruises, burns, colds, flu, hemorrhoids, urinary insufficiency, wounds
Dominican Republic	for dysentery, fertility (veterinary), lung problems, and to increase perspiration
Guatemala	for bruises, dermatitis, erysipelas, fevers, gonorrhea, kidney diseases, skin disorders (irritation, eruptions, inflammation, sores, ulcers), stomach inflammation, stomachache, wounds, and to increase perspiration
Haiti	for blood cleansing, cough, diabetes, diarrhea, digestive sluggishness, fever, flu, fractures, scurvy, skin problems, wounds
Jamaica	for diarrhea, elephantiasis, leprosy, malaria
Mexico	for asthma, chest problems, childbirth, constipation, diarrhea, dysentery, elephantiasis, fever, gastrointestinal problems, hemorrhages, infectious diseases, kidney problems, leprosy, malaria, rashes, skin problems, syphilis, uterine pain, wounds
Peru	for asthma, bronchitis, dermatitis, diarrhea, dysentery, elephantiasis, fever, hair loss, hepatitis, kidney disease, leprosy, liver disease, lung problems, malaria, syphilis
Venezuela	for syphilis, wounds, and to increase perspiration and lower body temperature
Elsewhere	for asthma, bleeding, bronchitis, chest problems, elephantiasis, hair loss, hypertension, kidney disorders, liver problems, obesity, skin problems, stomachaches, and to increase perspiration

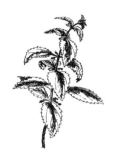

Family: Urticaceae

Genus: *Urtica*

Species: *dioica*

Common Names:
nettle, big string nettle, common nettle, stinging nettle, gerrais, isirgan, kazink, nabat al nar, ortiga, grande ortie, ortie, urtiga, chichicaste, brennessel, gross d'ortie, racine d'ortie

Parts Used: root, leaves

NETTLE

HERBAL PROPERTIES AND ACTIONS

Main Actions
- reduces allergies
- cleanses blood
- reduces inflammation
- relieves pain
- stops hair loss
- increases urination
- stops bleeding
- dilates blood vessels
- lowers blood pressure
- heals wounds

Other Actions
- stimulates digestion
- aids lactation
- promotes menstruation
- kills germs
- lowers body temperature
- expels worms

Standard Dosage
Leaves, Root

Infusion: 1 cup two to three times daily

Tablets/Capsules: 2–3 g two to three times daily

Tincture (root): 2–3 ml two to three times daily

Nettle, or stinging nettle, is a perennial plant growing in temperate and tropical wasteland areas around the world. The plant has been naturalized in Brazil and other parts of South America. It grows 2–4 m high and produces pointed leaves and white-to-yellowish flowers. Nettle has a well-known reputation for giving a savage sting when the skin touches the hairs and bristles on the leaves and stems. The genus name *Urtica* comes from the Latin verb *urere*, meaning "to burn," because of these stinging hairs. The species name *dioica* means "two houses" because the plant usually contains either male or female flowers.

TRIBAL AND HERBAL MEDICINE USES

In folk medicine nettle plants have been used as a diuretic, to build the blood, for arthritis, and for rheumatism. Externally, it has been used to improve the appearance of the hair, and is said to be a remedy against both oily hair and dandruff.

The plant has been widely used by herbalists around the world for centuries. In the first century, Greek physicians Dioscorides and Galen reported the leaf of nettle had diuretic and laxative properties and was useful for asthma, pleurisy, and spleen illnesses. Bandages soaked in a leaf and stem infusion were used in early American medicine to stop the bleeding of wounds; an account of this use was recorded by Dr. Francis P. Procher, a surgeon and physician in the Southern Confederacy during the Civil War. Nettle leaves were also recommended as a nutritious food and as a weight loss aid by the famous American plant forager and naturalist, Euell Gibbons.

In Brazilian herbal medicine, the entire plant is used for excessive menstrual bleeding, diarrhea, diabetes, urinary disorders, and respiratory problems including allergies. Externally, an infusion is used for skin problems. In Peru,

In Germany today, stinging nettle is sold as an herbal drug for prostate diseases and as a diuretic. It is a common ingredient in other herbal drugs produced in Germany for rheumatic complaints and inflammatory conditions (especially for the lower urinary tract and prostate).

nettle is used against a variety of complaints such as muscular and arthritis pain, eczema, ulcers, asthma, diabetes, intestinal inflammation, nosebleeds, and rheumatism. Externally, it is used for inflammations, sciatica, wounds, and head lice. In Germany today, stinging nettle is sold as an herbal drug for prostate diseases and as a diuretic. It is a common ingredient in other herbal drugs produced in Germany for rheumatic complaints and inflammatory conditions (especially for the lower urinary tract and prostate). In the United States, many remarkable healing properties are attributed to nettle and the leaf is utilized for different problems than the root. The leaf is used here as a diuretic, for arthritis, prostatitis, rheumatism, rheumatoid arthritis, high blood pressure, and allergic rhinitis. The root is recommended as a diuretic, for relief of benign prostatic hyperplasia (BPH) and other prostate problems, and as a natural remedy to treat or prevent baldness.

PLANT CHEMICALS

The stinging sensation of the leaf hairs is caused by several plant chemicals including formic acid, histamine, serotonin, and choline. In addition to these chemicals, nettle leaf is rich in minerals, chlorophyll, amino acids, lecithin, carotenoids, flavonoids, sterols, tannins, and vitamins. The root of the plant has other chemicals such as scopoletin, sterols, fatty acids, polysaccharides, and isolectins. Several of nettle's lectin chemicals have demonstrated marked antiviral actions (against HIV and several common upper respiratory viruses).[1,2] Other chemicals (flavonoids in the leaves and a lectin in the root) have been documented with interesting immune stimulant actions in preliminary research, which led researchers to suggest that the lectin might be useful in the treatment of systemic lupus.[3–7]

Nettle's main plant chemicals include acetophenone, acetylcholine, agglutinins, alkaloids, astragalin, butyric acid, caffeic acids, carbonic acid, chlorogenic acid, chlorophyll, choline, coumaric acid, folacin, formic acid, friedelins, histamine, kaempherols, koproporphyrin, lectins, lecithin, lignans, linoleic acid, linolenic acid, neoolivil, palmitic acid, pantothenic acid, quercetin, quinic acid, scopoletin, secoisolariciresinol, serotonin, sitosterols, stigmasterol, succinic acid, terpenes, violaxanthin, and xanthophylls.

BIOLOGICAL ACTIVITIES AND CLINICAL RESEARCH

Nettle's long-standing use as an anti-inflammatory aid for rheumatism and arthritis has been confirmed with clinical research. In several clinical studies (including a randomized double-blind placebo trial), nettle leaf extracts were documented with anti-inflammatory actions as well as being beneficial (and better than placebo) at relieving arthritis pain and inflammation in humans.[8–10] Research suggests that nettle's anti-inflammatory actions are attributed to its ability to interrupt the production and actions of inflammation-producing immune cells in the body (cytokines, prostaglandins, and leukotreines).[10–12]

Another randomized double-blind study was performed on nettle in 1990 which confirmed its traditional uses for allergies and rhinitis (a common inflammatory disorder causing sneezing, nasal congestion and discharge, and itchy skin and often triggered by allergies). In this study with sixty-nine patients, nettle extract again rated higher than placebo: 58 percent reported it relieved most all their symptoms and 48 percent stated it was more effective than other over-the-counter medications.[13] It was still being confirmed as a beneficial treatment for rhinitis ten years later when researchers then suggested the same sort of inflammatory immune cell suppression was responsible for the documented effects.[14]

Other animal studies with rats (in 2000 and 2002) reported that water extracts of nettle lowered blood pressure, reduced heart rate, and had notable diuretic actions.[15–17] One of the studies reported that a nettle root extract performed better than the control drug used (furosemide) at reducing blood pressure, increasing urine output, and increasing sodium excretion.[17] Earlier studies reported nettle had no effect on blood pressure in rats[18] but demonstrated a notable hypotensive effect in cats.[19] It was also shown to have a pain-relieving effect in mice,[19] a sedative effect in rats and mice,[19,20] as well as to inhibit drug-induced convulsions and lower the body temperature of rats.[20]

The last area of research on nettle focuses on its usefulness for prostate inflammation (prostatitis) and benign prostatic hyperplasia (BPH). In more than twenty clinical studies thus far, nettle root (and nettle combined with other herbs) has demonstrated an improvement of clinical symptoms in BPH and prostatitis. (Prostatitis is the inflammation of the prostate gland and surrounding tissues usually caused by bacteria. BPH is an age-related non-malignant enlargement of the prostate gland due to increased numbers of cells triggered to grow in the prostate.) While nettle's benefit for prostatitis is most probably related to its documented anti-inflammatory properties demonstrated in the arthritis and rhinitis research, its effect on BPH is quite different—it works on a hormonal level.

BPH, the most common disease of the prostate that generally affects men starting from the age of 40, actually occurs on a hormonal level. Androgens like testosterone as well as estrogens (such as estradiol and estrone) have been shown to cause BPH in animal studies.[21] While testosterone plays a role in BPH, it is rather the conversion of testosterone to the extremely potent dihydrotestosterone that is the problem (and this conversion naturally increases as men age for some unexplained reason). In excess, dihydrotestosterone causes pathological prostate growth.[22] Estrogens, which also increase as men age, influences prostate tissue by stimulating prostate cell growth.[23] These main hormones travel around the body in a free state, as well as bound to proteins.

One such protein is called *sex hormone binding globulin* (SHBG); its role is to maintain a dynamic hormonal balance in the body. SHBG binds or attaches to hormones and carries them to different receptor sites on cell membranes throughout the body, where they can be utilized in different ways. The effect it has depends on which hormone it binds to, and which receptor site it is carried to. For instance, in men, estrogen and dihydrotestosterone bound to SHBG are usually carried to the receptor sites on the prostate gland, and once there in excessive amounts, can stimulate prostate tissue cells to divide and grow rapidly—resulting in BPH.

Some of the more recent research on BPH and nettle indicates that nettle can interfere with or block a number of these hormone-related chemical processes in the body that are implicated in the development of BPH. In clinical research, nettle has demonstrated the ability to stop the conversion of testosterone to dihydrotestosterone (by inhibiting an enzyme required for the conversion), as well as to directly bind to SHBG itself—thereby preventing SHBG from binding to other hormones.[24,25] Other research also reveals that nettle can prevent SHBG that has already bound to a hormone from attaching to the receptor sites on the prostate,[26] as well as decrease the production of estrogens (estradiol and estrone) by inhibiting an enzyme required for their production.[27]

It all sounds a bit complicated, but basically, most of the complex intercellular processes required to trigger the prostate to grow new cells and enlarge seem to be inhibited by nettle. This is great news for men suffering from BPH (and there are millions)! Human and animal studies have confirmed these effects and benefits. In one study, a nettle root extract was shown to inhibit the growth of prostate cells by 30 percent in five days;[28] another reported it inhibited BPH in mice by 51.4 percent (which suggested it could be used as a preventative as well as a treatment).[29] In a study with 134 men with BPH, 300 mg of nettle root (with 25 mg of another plant called *Pygeum*) reduced retained urine (blocked by enlarged prostates) and reduced frequent urination at night (a bothersome symptom of BPH) in twenty-eight days.[30] A randomized double-blind clinical trial was conducted with 543 BPH patients who were given a combination of saw palmetto and nettle root or a drug called *finasteride*.[31] The average urine flow increased in both groups, while urinary urgency and frequency decreased in both groups. Other BPH symptoms also decreased in both groups, and, as usual, fewer side effects were reported by those taking the herbal combination than those taking the drug.

It also should be noted that these same androgen hormones have profound effects on scalp and body hair in both males and females. Hair loss in both men and women has been linked to excessive dihydrotestosterone (DHT) levels.[32] While no clinical studies have been conducted yet on the use of nettle in treating DHT-related hair loss and male pattern balding, research does indicate that nettle root can prevent the conversion of testosterone to DHT. Interestingly, a U.S. patent has recently been filed on an herbal combination containing nettle root for the treatment of male pattern baldness.[33] More research is sure to follow, as this is a highly popular and profitable area of research.

CURRENT PRACTICAL USES

Over the last several years, more consumers and practitioners have been learning of nettle's many uses for prostate problems, arthritis and inflammation in general, allergies, and hair loss, and it follows that more nettle products are showing up on the shelves in stores. Nettle root, nettle leaf, and whole herb (leaf, stem, and root) products in tablets, capsules, and tinctures are now widely available at most health food stores at very reasonable prices. Consumers just need to remember that the root is much better for BPH and hair loss, while the leaf is better for inflammation (including prostatitis), allergies, and as a natural diuretic for people with hypertension.

Unfortunately, consumers (and even natural product manufacturers) overlook these important distinctions between the root and leaf when searching for natural remedies and products. Nettle is now an ingredient in many herbal formulas for prostate health, which are sold in the U.S. market. Pay close attention to the ingredients stated on the labels however; the root is needed for BPH, and the leaves will provide much better results for prostatitis. As a general preventative to prostate problems, and for maintaining healthy prostate functions as well as male hormonal levels, clinical research suggests the root will work better than the leaf as well.

Traditional Preparation

Both the root and the leaves are traditionally prepared as infusions. Dosages depend on what one is taking it for. In herbal medicine systems, as a healthy prevention to prostate difficulties or to maintain prostate health, $\frac{1}{2}$ cup of a root infusion two to three times weekly is recommended (2–3 ml of a root tincture or 2–3 g of powdered root in capsules or tablets can be substituted if desired). The natural remedy for BPH is $\frac{1}{2}$ cup of a root infusion two to three times daily for thirty to ninety days (2–3 ml of a root tincture or 2–3 g in capsules or tablets two to three times daily can be substituted if desired). For allergies, inflammation, and hypertension: 1 cup of a leaf infusion is taken twice daily in traditional medicine systems. This also can be substituted by taking 3–4 g of leaf tablets/capsules twice daily.

Contraindications

Nettle has been documented in animal studies to lower blood pressure and heart rate. Those with heart conditions should seek the advice and supervision of a health practitioner to determine if nettle is suitable for their condition and to monitor its effects.

Nettle has been documented to have diuretic effects. Chronic use of this plant may be contraindicated in various medical conditions where diuretics are not advised. Chronic long-term use of any diuretic can cause electrolyte and mineral imbalances. Consult your doctor if you choose to use this plant chronically for longer than thirty days concerning possible side effects of long-term diuretic use.

Drug Interactions   Nettle may potentiate heart medications as well as diuretic drugs.

Worldwide Ethnomedical Uses

Region	Uses
Belize	for childbirth, diarrhea, dysentery, prostate problems, rashes, skin problems, sores
Brazil	for asthma, bleeding, bronchitis, cough, diabetes, diarrhea, dysentery, fever, liver support, lung problems, menstrual disorders, pneumonia, skin disorders, ulcers, urinary problems, and to increase perspiration
Cuba	for bruises, burns, flu, hemorrhoids, urinary insufficiency, wounds
Dominican Republic	for dysentery, fertility (veterinary), lung problems, and to increase perspiration
Germany	for arthritis, inflammation, prostate diseases, rheumatism, urinary insufficiency, urinary tract disorders
Greece	for asthma, inflammation, pleurisy, spleen disorders, urinary insufficiency, and as a laxative
Guatemala	for bruises, dermatitis, erysipelas, fever, gonorrhea, kidney disease, skin disease, skin irritation/eruptions, sores, ulcers, wounds, and to increase perspiration
Haiti	for blood purification, coughs, diarrhea, digestive problems, fever, flu, fractures, scurvy, skin problems, wounds
India	for eczema, nosebleeds, skin eruptions, uterine hemorrhages
Mexico	for asthma, chest problems, childbirth, constipation, diarrhea, dysentery, elephantiasis, fever, gastrointestinal disorders, hemorrhages, kidney problems, leprosy, malaria, rashes, skin problems, syphilis, uterine disorders, wounds
Peru	for arthritis, asthma, bleeding, diabetes, dysentery, hair, head lice, hemorrhoids, inflammation, intestinal inflammation, kidney stones, liver disease, muscle pain, nasal ulcers, pain, respiratory problems, rheumatism, sciatica, swelling, urinary insufficiency, wounds, as a diuretic and expectorant, and to increase perspiration
United States	for allergies, arthritis, BPH, bleeding, hair loss, hypertension, inflammation, prostatitis, rhinitis, sinusitis, urinary insufficiency, wounds
Venezuela	for syphilis and wounds, to lower body temperature, and increase perspiration
Elsewhere	for aches, allergic rhinitis, asthma, bacterial infections, baldness, bleeding, bronchitis, bruises, burns, cancer, catarrh, chest problems, childbirth, cholecystitis, constipation, cough, dandruff, diarrhea, dyspnea, edema, elephantiasis, epilepsy, fever, gout, hair loss, hemorrhages, hypertension, insanity, iron-deficiency anemia, kidney stones, leprosy, liver diseases, lung problems, menstrual disorders, neuralgia, obesity, osteoarthritis, pain, paralysis, prostate disorders, rheumatism, skin diseases, sprains, stomach problems, swelling, tumors, urinary insufficiency, urinary problems, uterine disorders, worms, wounds, and to promote perspiration

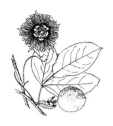

Family: Passifloraceae

Genus: *Passiflora*

Species: *incarnata, edulis*

Common Names: maracujá, passionflower, carkifelek, charkhi felek, maypop, maypop passionflower, saa't gulu, ward assa'ah, zahril aalaam, granadilla, passionvine, maracoc, apricot-vine, saa't gulu, ward assa'ah, zahril aalaam

Parts Used: vine, leaves, stem, fruit

TRIBAL AND HERBAL MEDICINE USES

In many countries around the world, the use of passionflower leaves to tranquilize and settle edgy nerves has been documented for over 200 years.

PASSIONFLOWER
HERBAL PROPERTIES AND ACTIONS

Main Actions
- relieves pain
- reduces anxiety
- relieves depression
- reduces inflammation
- stops convulsions
- reduces spasms
- calms nerves
- mildly sedative
- tranquilizes

Other Actions
- kills germs
- enhances libido
- increases urination
- lowers blood pressure
- expels worms

Standard Dosage
Leaves
Infusion: 1 cup two to three times daily
Tablets/Capsules: 1–3 g two to three times daily

Passionflower is a hardy woody vine that grows up to 10 m long and puts off tendrils, enabling it to climb up and over other plants in the rainforest canopy. It bears striking, large white flowers with pink or purple centers. The flowers gave it the name passionflower (or *flower of passion*) because Spanish missionaries thought they represented some of the objects associated with the Crucifixion of Christ. The vine produces a delicious fruit which is about the size of a large lemon, wrinkling slightly when ripe. Passionflower, called *maracujá* in the Amazon, is indigenous to many tropical and semi-tropical areas—from South America to North America. There are over 200 species of passionflower vines; the most prevalent species in the Amazon are *Passiflora edulis* and *P. incarnata*.

Passion fruit is enjoyed by all rainforest inhabitants—humans and animals alike. Several species of *Passiflora* have been domesticated for the production of their edible fruit. The yellow, gelatinous pulp inside the fruit is eaten out of hand, as well as mixed with water and sugar to make drinks, sherbet, jams and jellies, and even salad dressings. Indigenous tribes throughout the Amazon have long used passionflower leaves for its sedative and pain-relieving properties; the fruit is used as a heart tonic and to calm coughs.

Passionflower was first "discovered" in Peru by a Spanish doctor named Monardes in 1569 who documented the indigenous uses and took it back to the Old World where it quickly became a favorite calming and sedative herb tea. Spanish conquerors of Mexico and South America also learned its use from the Aztec Indians, and it eventually became widely cultivated in Europe. Since its introduction into European herbal medicine systems, passionflower has been extensively used as a sedative, antispasmodic, and nerve tonic. The leaf infusion was introduced in North American medicine in the mid 1800s as a sedative through native and slave use in the South. It was also used for headaches, bruises, and general pain by applying the bruised leaves topically to the affected area. In many countries in Europe, the U.S., and Canada, the use of passionflower leaves to tranquilize and settle edgy nerves has been documented for over 200 years. It also has been employed for colic, diarrhea, dysentery, menstrual difficulties, insomnia, neuralgia, eye disorders, epilepsy and convulsions, and muscle spasms and pain.

PLANT CHEMICALS

Chemical analysis of passionflower indicates it contains three main groups of active chemicals: alkaloids, glycosides, and flavonoids. Interestingly, when the glycosides and flavonoids are isolated and tested individually, they have demonstrated the opposite effects for which the plant is commonly used. Only when the two groups of chemicals are combined as a whole herb, do researchers observe the plant's sedative effect.[1–3] Passionflower also contains naturally occurring serotonin, as well as a chemical called *maltol,* which has documented sedative effects (and which might explain the natural calming properties of passionflower).[4] A group of harmane alkaloids in passionflower have demonstrated antispasmodic activity and the ability to lower blood pressure.[4] In addition, a flavonoid named *chrysin* has demonstrated significant anti-anxiety activity.[5,6]

Main plant chemicals include alkaloids, alpha-alanine, apigenin, aribine, chrysin, citric acid, coumarin, cyclopassifloic acids A-D, cyclopassiflosides I-VI, diethyl malonate, edulan I, edulan II, flavonoids, glutamine, gynocardin, harmane, harmaline, harmalol, harmine, harmol, homoorientin, isoorientin, isoschaftoside, isovitexin, kaempferol, loturine, lucenin-2, lutenin-2, luteolin, n-nonacosane, orientin, passicol, passiflorine, passifloric acid, pectin, phenolic acids, phenylalanine, proline, prunasin, quercetin, raffinose, sambunigrin, saponarin, saponaretin, saponarine, schaftoside, scopoletin, serotonin, sitosterol, and stigmasterol.

BIOLOGICAL ACTIVITIES AND CLINICAL RESEARCH

After almost 100 years of study, the sedative, antispasmodic, and analgesic effects of this tropical vine have been firmly established in science.

Passionflower (as well as its harmane alkaloids) have been the subject of much scientific research. After almost 100 years of study the sedative, antispasmodic, and analgesic effects of this tropical vine have been firmly established in science. The analgesic effects of passionflower were first clinically documented in 1897, while the sedative effects were first recorded in 1904.[7,8] Antispasmodic, anti-anxiety, and hypotensive actions of passionflower leaves were clinically validated in the early 1980s.[9] An extract of the fruit demonstrated anti-inflammatory[10] and tranquilizing effects[11] in animal studies. Also, a leaf extract has shown to have diuretic activity in rats.[12]

Passionflower has traditionally been used as an aphrodisiac, and recent clinical studies with mice have verified this use as well. In a 2003 study, a leaf extract was reported to improve overall sexual function, and increase sperm count, fertilization potential, and litter size.[13] Its traditional use for coughs has been confirmed as well. In a 2002 study with mice, a passionflower leaf extract was shown to be comparable to the cough suppressant action of codeine.[14]

CURRENT PRACTICAL USES

Passionflower is widely employed by herbalists and natural health practitioners around the world today for its sedative, nervine, anti-spasmodic, and analgesic effects. In the United States, *P. incarnata* is the species most used to treat insomnia, muscle cramps, hysteria, neuralgia, menstrual cramps, and PMS, and as a pain-reliever in various conditions. In Europe, it is employed for nervous disorders, insomnia, spasms, neuralgia, alcoholism, hyperactivity in children, rapid heartbeat, headaches, and as a pain-reliever and antispasmodic. In South America, *P. edulis* is the species most used as a sedative, diuretic, and antispasmodic, and for convulsions, alcoholism, headaches, insomnia, colic in infants, diarrhea, hysteria, neuralgia, menopausal symptoms, and hypertension. In South America, the fruit juice is also used as a natural remedy to calm hyperactive children, as well as for asthma, whopping cough, bronchitis, and other tough coughs. In Peruvian traditional medicine today, passionfruit juice is used for urinary infections and as a mild diuretic.

Passionflower leaves are classified as "Generally Regarded as Safe" by the FDA. They are the subject of various European monographs for medicinal plants and are generally regarded as safe even for children and infants.[15]

Traditional Preparation

The leaves are typically prepared in standard infusions. Dosages are 1 cup taken two to three times daily, or 2–3 g in tablets or capsules two to three times daily can be substituted, if desired.

Contraindications

None reported.

Drug Interactions

None reported.

Worldwide Ethnomedical Uses

Region	Uses
Brazil	for alcoholism, anxiety, arthritis, asthma, bronchitis, constipation, convulsions, cough, delirium, depression, diarrhea, flu, gout, headache, hemorrhoids, hyperactivity, hypertension, hysteria, infantile convulsions, insomnia, irritability, menopause, menstrual disorders, nerve pain, nervous disorders, rheumatism, stress, ulcers, urinary insufficiency, whopping cough, worms (intestinal); and as an anti-inflammatory, antispasmodic, heart tonic, pain-reliever, and sedative
England	for anxiety, eye problems, headaches, hypertension, hysteria, insomnia, muscle problems, nerve pain, nerve weakness, pain, restlessness, spasms, and as a relaxant and tranquilizer

Europe	for agitation, anxiety, asthma, insomnia, irritability, menopause, menstrual disorders, nervousness, pain, palpitations, restlessness, stress
Peru	for epilepsy, heart problems, hypertension, insomnia, muscular spasms, nervousness, tetanus, and as an aphrodisiac and sedative
South America	for burns, colic, depression, diarrhea, dysentery, epilepsy, eruptions, eye disorders, headache, hemorrhoids, hyperactivity, hypertension, hysteria, inflammation, insomnia, menopause, menstrual disorders, nerve pain, nervousness, neurosis, pain, seizures, skin problems, spasms, worms; and as an aphrodisiac, diuretic, and sedative
Turkey	for epilepsy, insomnia, menstrual disorders, neuralgia, neurosis, spasms, and as a sedative
United States	for agitation, anxiety, asthma, burns, depression, diarrhea, epilepsy, headache, hypertension, hysteria, inflammation, insomnia, menstrual disorders, mood disorders, nervous complaints, neuralgia, seizures, shingles, spasms; and as an aphrodisiac, pain-reliever, sedative, and tranquilizer
Elsewhere	for anxiety, asthma, epilepsy, heart problems (palpitation, tachycardia), hypertension, hysteria, insomnia, menstrual disorders, mood disorders, neuralgia, nicotine addiction, pain, sexual dysfunction, shingles, spasms

PATA DE VACA
HERBAL PROPERTIES AND ACTIONS

Main Actions	Other Actions	Standard Dosage
• lowers blood sugar	• expels worms	Leaves
• improves diabetes	• kills snails	**Infusion:** 1 cup two to three times daily
• cleanses blood	• tones body systems	
• increases urination		**Capsules/Tablets:** 2 g two to three times daily
• lowers cholesterol		
• lowers triglycerides		
• fights free radicals		

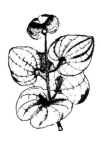

Family: Leguminosae

Genus: *Bauhinia*

Species: *forficata*

Common Names: pata de vaca, casco de vaca, mororó, pata de boi, unha de boi, unha de vaca, unha-de-anta

Parts Used: Leaves

TRIBAL AND HERBAL MEDICINE USES

Pata de vaca is a small tree that grows 5–9 m tall. Its leaves are 7–10 cm long and shaped like a cow's hoof, which is distinctive to the *Bauhinia* genus. Its Brazilian name, *pata de vaca*, translates to *cow's foot*. It produces large, drooping white flowers and a brown seedpod resembling that of mimosa. It can be found in the rainforests and tropical parts of Peru and Brazil, as well as in tropical zones of Asia, eastern Paraguay, and northeastern Argentina. It is quite prevalent in Rio de Janeiro and Brazil's Atlantic rainforest to the south. The *Bauhinia* genus comprises about 500 species of shrubs, small trees, and lianas in the tropics—most of which bears the distinctive cow's hoof shaped leaves.

The indigenous uses of pata de vaca are not well documented, but it has long held a place in Brazilian herbal medicine. It has been described as hypoglycemic, a blood purifier, and a diuretic, and has been used for over sixty years

Pata de vaca is a popular remedy in Brazil for diabetes and has been named "vegetable insulin."

to balance blood sugar levels in diabetics. It is considered a good blood cleanser, and a leaf decoction is used internally and externally for elephantiasis and snakebite, as well as other skin problems (including those of a syphilitic nature). It is a highly regarded treatment for diabetes, even being called "vegetable insulin." As such, it is used in South America to help balance blood sugar levels and to alleviate other symptoms of diabetes (such as polyuria, kidney disorders, and other urinary problems). Pata de vaca leaves and tea bags are common items on pharmacy shelves in South America; traditionally, a leaf tea (standard infusion) is drunk after each meal to help balance sugar levels.

PLANT CHEMICALS

Scientists have studied the constituents of pata de vaca and quantified them, however; little research has been done to determine which novel chemicals have biological activity. The leaves do contain a well-known antibacterial chemical called *astragalin* as well as flavonoids, alkaloids, and glycosides. The leaves are also a good source of a flavonoid called *kaempferitrin*. This chemical has been reported to help repair kidney cell damage,[1] and to have a diuretic effect.[2] The main plant chemicals in pata de vaca include astragalin, bauhinoside, beta-sitosterol, flavonols, flavonoids, glycosides, guanidine, heteroglycosides, kaempferitrin, organic acids, quercitrosides, rhamnose, and saponins.

BIOLOGICAL ACTIVITIES AND CLINICAL RESEARCH

Pata de vaca's ability to lower blood sugar was first reported by a Brazilian researcher in an *in vivo* 1929 clinical study, which was followed by another *in vivo* (dog) study in 1931.[3,4] The same Brazilian researcher published another study in 1941, reporting the blood sugar-lowering effects of pata de vaca in humans, dogs, and rabbits.[5] A study was funded in 1945 to determine the active constituents responsible for its activity.[6] Since a simple leaf tea was shown to help balance sugar levels, it became a popular natural remedy, however, no subsequent studies were done for many years due to a lack of funding for non-proprietary remedies and drugs.

In the mid-1980s, however (when herbal remedies again were popular), pata de vaca's continued use as a natural insulin substitute was reiterated in two Brazilian studies. Both studies reported *in vivo* hypoglycemic actions in various animal and human models.[7,8] Chilean research in 1999 reported the actions of pata de vaca in diabetic rats. Their study determined that pata de vaca was found to "elicit remarkable hypoglycemic effects," and brought about a "decrease of glycemia in alloxan diabetic rats by 39%."[9] In 2002, two *in vivo* studies on the blood sugar-lowering effects of pata de vaca were conducted by two separate research groups in Brazil. The first study reported "a significant blood glucose-lowering effect in normal and diabetic rats."[10] In the second study, 150 g of the leaf (per liter of water) was given to diabetic rats as their drinking water. Researchers reported that, after one month, those receiving pata de vaca had a "significant reduction in serum and urinary glucose and urinary urea" as compared to the control group.[11]

Clinical studies from 1929 up to the present verify and validate pata de vaca's benefits for diabetes. The most recent studies suggest it lowers not only blood sugar, but cholesterol as well.

In 2004, a research group reported that pata de vaca again lowered blood sugar in rats and also reduced triglycerides, total cholesterol, and HDL-cholesterol levels in diabetic rats, stating, "These results suggest the validity of the clinical use of B. forficata in the treatment of diabetes mellitus type II."[12] Other Brazilian researchers reported in 2004 that pata de vata, as well as a single chemical extracted from the leaves called *kaempferitrin*, significantly lowered blood sugar in diabetic rats at all dosages but lowered blood sugar in normal rats only at the highest dosages.[13] They also documented an antioxidant effect. Toxicity studies published in 2004 indicate there were no toxic effects in either normal or diabetic rats,[14] including pregnant diabetic rats.[15]

CURRENT PRACTICAL USES

Pata de vaca continues to be a popular natural medicine in South America for diabetes, and clinical research there supports its use. A standard infusion is brewed and drunk after each meal, and pata de vaca is often combined with pedra hume caá (another South American plant featured in this book) for this after-meal tea. North American practitioners and herbalists are now using it in their practices for diabetes, hyperglycemia, and polyuria.

Traditional Preparation

In South America, 1 cup of a standard leaf infusion is taken three times daily with or after meals for diabetes. If desired, 2 g in tablets or capsules three times daily can be substituted.

Contraindications

Pata de vaca lowers blood sugar levels. It is contraindicated in those with hypoglycemia. Diabetics who wish to use this plant should seek the advice and supervision of a qualified health care practitioner as blood sugar levels will need to be monitored carefully, and medications may need adjustments.

Drug Interactions

Pata de vaca will potentiate antidiabetic and insulin medications.

Worldwide Ethnomedical Uses

Region	Uses
Amazonia	for diabetes, diarrhea, and as a tonic
Brazil	for blood cleansing, central nervous system disorders, cystitis, diabetes, diarrhea, elephantiasis, hyperglycemia, intestinal worms, kidney problems, kidney stones, leprosy, obesity, polyuria, skin disorders, snakebite, syphilis, urinary diseases, and as an astringent and diuretic
Chile	for diabetes
Peru	for diabetes and as a tonic
Elsewhere	for diabetes and as a uterine relaxant

PAU D'ARCO
HERBAL PROPERTIES AND ACTIONS

Main Actions
- kills bacteria
- kills fungi
- kills cancer cells
- kills leukemia cells
- kills viruses
- relieves pain
- reduces inflammation
- kills parasites
- fights free radicals
- reduces tumors

Other Actions
- thins blood
- enhances immunity
- mildly laxative
- relieves rheumatism
- dries secretions

Standard Dosage
Bark, Heartwood

Decoction: ¹/₂–1 cup two to four times daily

Tincture: 2–3 ml two to three times daily

Capsules/Tablets: not recommended

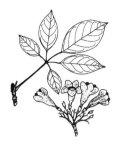

Family: Bignoniaceae

Genus: *Tabebuia*

Species: *impetiginosa*

Common Names: pau d'arco, ipê, ipê roxo, lapacho, tahuari, taheebo, trumpet tree, ipê-contra-sarna, tabebuia ipê, tajy

Parts Used: bark, heartwood

Pau d'arco is a huge canopy tree native to the Amazon rainforest and other tropical parts of South and Latin America. It grows to 30 m high and the base of the tree can be 6–10 feet in diameter. The *Tabebuia* genus includes about 100 species of large, flowering trees that are common to South American cities' landscapes and are known for their beauty. The tree also is popular with timber loggers—its high-quality wood is some of the heaviest, most durable wood in the tropics. Pau d'arco wood is widely used in the construction of everything from houses and boats to farm tools. The common name *pau d'arco* (as well as its other main names of commerce, *ipê roxo* and *lapacho*) is used for several different species of *Tabebuia* trees that are used interchangeably in herbal medicine systems. *T. impetiginosa* is known for its attractive purple flowers and often is called "purple lapacho." It has been the preferred species employed in herbal medicine. It is often referred to by its other botanical name, *Tabebuia avellanedae*; both refer to the same tree. Other pau d'arco species produce pink (*T. heptaphylla*), yellow (*T. serratifolia* and *T. chrysantha*) or white (*T. bahamensis*) flowers. Though many of these species may have a similar phytochemical makeup, they are different species of trees.

TRIBAL AND HERBAL MEDICINE USES

Pau d'arco has a long and well-documented history of use by the indigenous peoples of the rainforest. Indications imply that its use may actually predate the Incas. Throughout South America, tribes living thousands of miles apart have employed it for the same medicinal purposes for hundreds of years. Several Indian tribes of the rainforest have used pau d'arco wood for centuries to make their hunting bows; their common names for the tree mean "bow stick" and "bow stem." The Guarani and Tupi Indians call the tree *tajy*, which means "to have strength and vigor." They use the bark to treat many different conditions and as a tonic for the same strength and vigor it puts into their bows. Pau d'arco is recorded to be used by forest inhabitants throughout the Amazon for malaria, anemia, colitis, respiratory problems, colds, cough, flu, fungal infections, fever, arthritis and rheumatism, snakebite, poor circulation, boils, syphilis, and cancer.

In North American herbal medicine, pau d'arco is considered to be antioxidant, antiparasitic, antimicrobial, antifungal, antiviral, antibacterial, anti-inflammatory, and laxative, as well as to have anticancerous and pain-relieving properties.

Pau d'arco also has a long history in herbal medicine around the world. In South American herbal medicine, it is considered to be astringent, anti-inflammatory, antibacterial, antifungal, and laxative; it is used to treat ulcers, syphilis, urinary tract infections, gastrointestinal problems, *Candida* and yeast infections, cancer, diabetes, prostatitis, constipation, and allergies. It is used in Brazilian herbal medicine for many conditions including cancer, leukemia, ulcers, diabetes, candidiasis, rheumatism, arthritis, prostatitis, dysentery, stomatitis, and boils. In North American herbal medicine, pau d'arco is considered to be analgesic, antioxidant, antiparasitic, antimicrobial, antifungal, antiviral, antibacterial, anti-inflammatory, and laxative, as well as to have anticancerous properties. It is used for fevers, infections, colds, flu, syphilis, urinary tract infections, cancer, respiratory problems, skin ulcerations, boils, dysentery, gastrointestinal problems of all kinds, arthritis, prostatitis, and circulation disturbances. Pau d'arco also is employed in herbal medicine systems in the United States for lupus, diabetes, ulcers, leukemia, allergies, liver disease, Hodgkin's disease, osteomyelitis, Parkinson's disease, and psoriasis, and is a popular natural remedy for *Candida* and yeast infections. The recorded uses in European herbal medicine systems reveal that it is used in much the same way as in the United States, and for the same conditions.

PLANT CHEMICALS

The chemical constituents and active ingredients of pau d'arco have been well documented. Its use with (and reported cures for) various types of cancers fueled much of the early research in the early 1960s. The plant contains a large amount of chemicals known as *quinoids*, and a small quantity of benzenoids and flavonoids. These quinoids (and, chiefly, anthraquinones, furanonaphthoquinones, lapachones, and naphthoquinones) have shown the most documented biological activity and are seen to be the center of the plant's efficacy as an herbal remedy. In the 1960s, plant extracts of the heartwood and bark demonstrated marked antitumorous effects in animals, which drew the interest of the National Cancer Institute (NCI). Researchers decided that the most potent single chemical for this activity was a naphthoquinone chemical named *lapachol* and they concentrated solely on this single chemical in their subsequent cancer research. In a 1968 study, lapachol demonstrated highly significant activity against cancerous tumors in rats.[1]

Cancer research
on several powerful
chemicals in pau d'arco
has been ongoing since
the 1960s.

By 1970, NCI-backed research already was testing lapachol in human cancer patients. The institute reported, however, that their first Phase I study failed to produce a therapeutic effect without side effects—and they discontinued further cancer research shortly thereafter.[2] These side effects were nausea and vomiting (very common with chemotherapy drugs) and anti-vitamin K activity (the main concerns being this causes anemia and an anticoagulation effect). Interestingly, other chemicals in the whole plant extract (which, initially, showed positive anti-tumor effects and very low toxicity) demonstrated positive effects on vitamin K and, conceivably, compensated for lapachol's negative effect. Once again, instead of pursuing research on a complex combination of at least twenty active chemicals in a whole plant extract (several of which had anti-tumor effects and other positive biological activities), research focused on a single, patentable chemical—and it didn't work as well.

Despite NCI's abandonment of the research, another group developed a lapachol analog (which was patentable) in 1975. One study reported that this lapachol analog increased the life span of mice inoculated with leukemic cells by over 80 percent.[3] In a small, uncontrolled, 1980 study of nine human patients with various cancers (liver, kidney, breast, prostate, and cervix), pure lapachol was reported to shrink tumors and reduce pain caused by them—and three of the patients realized complete remissions.[4]

The phytochemical database housed at the U.S. Department of Agriculture has documented lapachol as being anti-abscess, anticarcinomic, antiedemic, anti-inflammatory, antimalarial, antiseptic, antitumorous, antiviral, bactericidal, fungicidal, insectifugal, pesticidal, protisticidal, respiratory depressant, schistosomicidal, termiticidal, and viricidal.[5] It's not surprising that pau d'arco's beneficial effects were seen to stem from its lapachol content. But another chemical in pau d'arco, beta-lapachone, has been studied closely of late—and a number of recent patents have been filed on it. It has demonstrated in laboratory studies to have activities similar to lapachol (antimicrobial,[6] antifungal,[7] antiviral,[8] antitumorous,[4] antileukemic,[9] and anti-inflammatory[10]), with few side effects. In one of these studies on beta-lapachone and other quinones in pau d'arco, researchers reported: "Because of their potent activity against the growth of human keratinocytes, some lapachol-derived compounds appear to be promising as effective antipsoriatic agents."[10] In a 2002 U.S. patent, beta-lapachone was cited to have significant anticancerous activity against human cancer cell lines including: promyelocytic leukemia, prostate, malignant glioma, colon, hepatoma, breast, ovarian, pancreatic, multiple myeloma cell lines and drug-resistant cell lines.[11] In yet another U.S. patent, beta-lapachone was cited with the *in vivo* ability to inhibit the growth of prostate tumors.[9]

The main plant chemicals in pau d'arco include: acetaldehydes, alpha-lapachone, ajugols, anisic acid, anthraquinones, benzoic acids, benzenes, beta-lapachone, carboxaldehydes, chromium, chrysanthemin, dehydro-alpha-lapachone, dehydroisolapachone, deoxylapachol, flavonoids,furanonaphthoquinones, hydrochlorolapachol, 2-hydroxy-3-methyl-quinone, 6-hydroxy-mellein, iso-8-hydroxy-lariciresinol, kigelinone, lapachenol, lapachenole, lapachol, lapachones, menaquinones, 4-methoxyphenol, naphthoquinones, paeonidin-3-cinnamyl-sophoroside, phthiolol, quercetin, tabebuin, tectoquinone, vanillic acid, vanillin, veratric acid, veratric aldehyde, and xyloidone.

BIOLOGICAL ACTIVITIES AND CLINICAL RESEARCH

In addition to its reported anti-tumor and antileukemic activities, pau d'arco clearly has demonstrated broad spectrum actions against a number of disease-causing microorganisms, which supports its wide array of uses in herbal medicine. Antimicrobial properties of many of pau d'arco's active phytochemicals were demonstrated in several clinical studies, in which they exhibited strong *in vitro* activity against bacteria, fungi, and yeast (including *Candida, Aspergillus, Staphylococcus, Streptococcus, Helicobacter pylori, Brucella,* tuberculosis, pneumonia, and dysentery).[12–17]

Laboratory studies over the years reveal that pau d'arco has a broad-spectrum action against various bacteria, viruses, yeast, and fungi, which supports its traditional uses against so many types of diseases.

In addition to its isolated chemicals, a hot water extract of pau d'arco demonstrated antibacterial actions against *Staphylococcus aureus,*[18] *Helicobacter pylori*[19] (the bacteria that commonly causes stomach ulcers), and *Brucella.*[20] A water extract of pau d'arco was reported (in other *in vitro* clinical research) to have strong activity against eleven fungus and yeast strains.[21] Pau d'arco and its chemicals also have demonstrated *in vitro* antiviral properties against various viruses, including herpes I and II, influenza, polio virus, and vesicular stomatitis virus.[22–24] Its antiparasitic actions against various parasites (including malaria, schistosoma, and trypanosoma) have been confirmed as well.[22,25,26] Finally, bark extracts of pau d'arco have demonstrated anti-inflammatory activity and have shown success against a wide range of induced inflammation in mice and rats.[27]

CURRENT PRACTICAL USES

Pau d'arco is an important resource from the rainforest with many applications in herbal medicine. Unfortunately, its popularity and use have been controversial due to varying results obtained from its use. For the most part, these seem to have been caused by a lack of quality control—and confusion as to which part of the plant to use and how to prepare it. Many species of *Tabebuia,* as well as other completely unrelated tree species exported today from South America as "pau d'arco," have few to none of the active constituents of the true medicinal species.

Pau d'arco lumber is in high demand in South America. The inner bark shavings commonly exported to the U.S. and Europe are actually by-products of the South American timber and lumber industries. At least ten species of *Tabebuia* are logged commercially in South America for lumber purposes alone. When these logs arrive at lumber mills, the identifying leaves and flowers (which distinguish the tree species) are long gone—it's all just "pau d'arco." This may explain varying species of pau d'arco bark being sold as herbal products—and their resulting (diminished) quality. Even mahogany shavings from the same sawmill floors in Brazil are swept up and sold around the world as "pau d'arco" (due to the similarity in color and odor of the two woods).[28] In 1987, a chemical analysis of twelve commercially available pau d'arco products revealed only one product containing lapachol—and only in trace amounts.[29] As lapachol concentration typically is 2–7 percent in true pau d'arco, the study surmised that the products were not truly pau d'arco, or that processing and transportation had damaged them. Additionally, most pau d'arco research has centered on the heartwood of the tree.

Most of the commercially available products, though, contain just the inner bark of the tree—which is stripped off at sawmills when the heartwood is milled into lumber for construction materials. Laboratory analysis has always confirmed that the lapachol content is in higher concentration in the heartwood than the bark. Finally, many consumers and practitioners are unaware that, for the best results when extracting these particular active chemicals (even after obtaining the correct species), the bark and/or wood must be boiled at least ten to fifteen minutes—rather than brewed as a simple tea or infusion (lapachol and the other quinoids are not very water soluble).

It is therefore not surprising that consumers and practitioners are experiencing spotty results with commercially available pau d'arco products. With its many effective applications, however, it would behoove consumers to take the time to learn about the available products and suppliers, and find a reliable source for this important medicinal plant from the rainforest. Relatively new in the marketplace are standardized extracts of pau d'arco (that guarantee the amount of lapachol and/or naphthoquinones). In such a product, it would be unclear if other active quinones and phytochemicals have been extracted (and to what extent) in these chemically altered products. Although the natural wood and bark are quite effective when the correct species is used and prepared properly, the new standardized extracts may be the safer (yet more expensive) purchase for most laypersons and general consumers concerned about quality but who don't have the time to research each product.

There have been no reports of human toxicity when a whole-bark decoction or tincture of pau d'arco is used. The oral 50 percent lethal dosage (LD^{50}) for lapachol is reported to be 1.2–2.4 g/kg (body weight) in rats and 487–621 mg/kg in mice. Signs of toxicity in humans (vomiting/diarrhea) were reported at oral dosages of 1,500 mg daily (and higher) of pure lapachol. However, even at these dosages, no bone marrow, liver, or kidney toxicity was noted. Good quality pau d'arco (*Tabebuia impetiginosa*) contains an average of 4 percent lapachol (or 40 mg of lapachol per gram of pau d'arco bark/wood).

Traditional Preparation	From ½–1 cup bark and/or heartwood decoction is taken orally two to four times daily. (Do not prepare an infusion/tea for this plant—it will not be as effective.) This decoction also is employed traditionally as a douche for yeast infections (use once daily for three consecutive days) and is used topically on the skin for skin fungi (such as nail fungus and athlete's foot).
Contraindications	There have been no reports in the literature of contraindications when a whole-bark decoction or tincture is used. However, at least one isolated phytochemical in pau d'arco, lapachol, has demonstrated abortive properties and retarded fetal growth in animal studies. As there are no studies confirming the safety of traditional bark decoctions used by pregnant women (nor is there documentation in traditional medicine systems of women using this plant during pregnancy), the use of pau d'arco during pregnancy is not recommended.
	Large single dosages of pau d'arco decoctions (more than 1 cup) may cause gastrointestinal upset and/or nausea. Do not use in high doses unless under the advice of a qualified health practitioner; reduce dosage if nausea occurs.
Drug Interactions	None reported.

Worldwide Ethnomedical Uses

Region	Uses
Amazonia	for colds, cough, fever, flu, leishmaniasis, sores, urinary tract infections
Argentina	for diarrhea, respiratory infections, urinary tract infections
Bahamas	for backaches, gonorrhea, incontinence, toothache, urinary disorders
Brazil	for allergies, arthritis, asthma, athlete's foot, bacterial infections, bed-wetting, boils, bursitis, cancer, cancer pain, *Candida*, circulation (poor), colds, colitis, constipation, cystitis, diabetes, dysentery, eczema, fever, flu, fungal infections, gastritis, gingivitis, gonorrhea, hemorrhages, hemorrhoids, hernia, herpes, Hodgkin's disease, immune disorders, impetigo, inflammation, itch, leishmaniasis, leukemia, liver disorders, malaria, parasites, prostatitis, psoriasis, respiratory problems, rheumatism, ringworm, scabies, skin problems, snakebite, sore throat, stomach problems, stomatitis, syphilis, tendonitis, ulcers, urinary tract infections, uterine disorders, vaginal discharge, varicose veins, warts, wounds; and as an astringent, blood builder, diuretic, pain-reliever, and tonic
Costa Rica	for cancer, colds, fever, headaches, snakebites
Mexico	for anemia, fever

South America	for allergies, anemia, arthritis, bacterial infections, boils, cancer, *Candida*, circulation problems, colds, colitis, constipation, cough, cystitis, diabetes, diarrhea, dysentery, fever, flu, fungal infections, gastritis, gastrointestinal problems, inflammation, malaria, pharyngitis, prostatitis, respiratory diseases, snakebites, syphilis, ulcers, urinary disorders
United States	for allergies, arthritis, bacterial infections, boils, cancer, *Candida*, circulation disturbances, colds, constipation, diabetes, dysentery, fevers, flu, fungal infections, gastrointestinal problems, Hodgkin's disease, inflammation, leukemia, liver disease, lupus, osteomyelitis, parasites, Parkinson's disease, prostatitis, psoriasis, respiratory problems, skin ulcerations, syphilis, ulcers, urinary tract infections, viral infections, warts; and as an anti-inflammatory, antioxidant, and pain-reliever

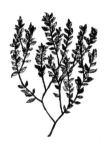

PEDRA HUME CAÁ
HERBAL PROPERTIES AND ACTIONS

Main Actions
- lowers blood sugar
- improves diabetes
- increases urination
- protects nerves

Other Actions
- fights free radicals
- dries secretions

Standard Dosage
Leaves
Infusion: 1 cup two to three times daily with meals
Tablets/Capsules: 1–2 g two to three times daily with meals

Family: Myrtaceae

Genus: *Myrcia*

Species: *salicifolia, uniflorus, sphaerocarpa*

Common Names: pedra hume caá, pedra-ume-caá, vegetable insulin

Parts Used: aerial parts, leaves

TRIBAL AND HERBAL MEDICINE USES

Pedra hume caá is another important rainforest remedy for diabetes.

Pedra hume caá is a medium-sized shrub that grows in drier regions of the Amazon and other parts of Brazil. It has small, green leaves and large, orange-red flowers. A member of the myrtle family, it is one of more than 150 species of *Myrcia* indigenous to tropical South America and the West Indies. In Brazil, the common name *pedra hume caá* refers to three species of *Myrcia* plants that are used interchangeably—*Myrcia salicifolia, M. uniflorus,* and *M. sphaerocarpa.*

Pedra hume caá has been used by indigenous tribes in the rainforest for diabetes, diarrhea, and dysentery. The Taiwanos tribe (in northwest Amazonia) considers the leaves to be astringent (dries secretions) and uses it for persistent diarrhea. It has had a place in Brazilian traditional medicine for many years. Dr. G. L. Cruz, a leading Brazilian practitioner and herbalist, nicknamed it "vegetable insulin" in 1965. Dr. Cruz noted in his book *Livro Verde das Plantas Medicinais e Industriais do Brasil* that "one uses all parts of the plant in infusions, decoctions or extracts to combat diabetes. Specialists that have made careful study of medicinal plants affirm that the regular use of this plant produces surprising results in the treatment of this ailment, as in a short space of time the sugar disappears from the urine. Hence the name 'vegetable insulin.'"

Pedra hume has long been used by people in remote areas where insulin and diabetes medications simply aren't available.

Even decades later, Dr. Cruz and other Brazilian researchers and practitioners are recording the actions and uses of pedra hume caá for diabetes in much the same manner. It remains a very popular natural remedy for diabetes throughout South America; traditional use is a simple leaf tea with a pleasant, slightly sweet taste taken with meals. It is also used for diarrhea, hypertension, enteritis, hemorrhages, and mouth ulcers.

PLANT CHEMICALS

Phytochemical analysis of pedra hume caá reveals a high content of flavonoids, flavonols, and flavanones. In 1998, Japanese researchers reported the discovery of several novel and biologically active phytochemicals. These new flavanone glucosides were named *myrciacitrins I and II*; the new acetophenone glucosides were named *myrciaphenones A and B.*[1] Their published study reported that a methanol extract of pedra hume caá (as well as these novel chemicals) demonstrated potent inhibitory activities on aldose reductase and alpha-glucosidase.

Research reveals that pedra hume caá is indeed beneficial for diabetes. It not only balances blood sugar levels—chemicals in the plant also interfere with various processes that can cause diabetic complications like neuropathy and macular degeneration.

Aldose reductase inhibitors (ARIs) are substances that act on nerve endings exposed to high blood sugar concentration to prevent some of the chemical imbalances that occur, and thus protect the nerves. Alpha-glucosidase inhibitors delay the digestion and subsequent absorption of sugar in the gastrointestinal tract. For this reason, the novel compounds in pedra hume caá that act upon aldose and glucosidase were seen to be (at least partially) responsible for pedra hume caá's blood sugar-balancing properties.[1] Various ARIs (both synthetic and natural) are being studied by researchers; it is believed that these compounds may be helpful in reducing or preventing some side effects of diabetes—including diabetic neuropathy and macular degeneration.

Other flavonoids found in pedra hume caá (notably quercitrin, myricitrin, guaijaverin, and desmanthin) also have shown in numerous studies to inhibit aldose reductase and xanthine oxidase (xanthine oxidase inhibitors block the production of uric acid).[2–5] The main plant chemicals documented in pedra hume caá include: beta-amyrin, catechin, desmanthin, gallic acid, ginkgoic acid, guaijaverin, mearnsitrin, myrciacitrin I–V, myrciaphenone A, myrciaphenone B, myricitrin, and quercitrin.

BIOLOGICAL ACTIVITIES AND CLINICAL RESEARCH

Brazilian scientists have documented leaf extracts of pedra hume caá with hypoglycemic activity since 1929.[6–10] Two clinical studies published in the 1990s again demonstrated its hypoglycemic activity and confirmed its traditional use for diabetes. In a 1990 double-blind placebo clinical study with normal and Type II diabetic patients, pedra hume caá (3 g powdered leaf daily) demonstrated the ability to lower plasma insulin levels in the diabetic group.[11] In a 1993 study, 250 mg/kg of a leaf extract demonstrated the ability to reduce appetite and thirst and to reduce urine volume, urinary excretion of glucose, and urea in diabetic rats. The extract also inhibited the intestinal absorption of glucose. This study concluded that "aqueous extracts of *Myrcia* have a beneficial effect on the diabetic state, mainly by improving metabolic parameters of glucose homeostasis."[12]

CURRENT PRACTICAL USES Pedra hume caá continues to be one of the more popular natural remedies for diabetes throughout South America, where it is widely known. The studies with animals and humans have confirmed its safety, and no toxic effects or side effects were noted. It is hoped that, with the growing diabetes epidemic in North America, health practitioners here will look for natural alternatives and incorporate this wonderful rainforest remedy into their natural health practices. These tropical shrubs grow very quickly and growth is encouraged by pruning. A single shrub can be harvested of its leaves by hard pruning four times a year or more, producing approximately 50–60 kg of leaves annually. It is truly a wonderful and sustainable resource the rainforest offers!

Traditional Preparation One cup of leaf infusion two to three times daily is taken with meals. If desired, 1–2 g of leaf powder in tablets or capsules with meals can be substituted.

Contraindications Pedra hume caá has been documented to lower blood sugar levels in animal and human studies. It is contraindicated in those with hypoglycemia. Diabetics who wish to use this plant should seek the advice and supervision of a qualified health care practitioner, as blood sugar levels will need to be monitored carefully and medications may need adjustments.

Pedra hume caá has been used in South American herbal medicine for hypertension. This use has not been substantiated or confirmed by clinical research. Those with low blood pressure and/or those on medications to lower their blood pressure should use this plant with caution and closely monitor these possible effects.

Drug Interactions Pedra hume caá will potentiate antidiabetic medications and insulin drugs, and may potentiate high blood pressure medications.

Worldwide Ethnomedical Uses

Region	Uses
Amazonia	for diabetes, diarrhea, and as an astringent
Brazil	for diabetes, diarrhea, dysentery, enteritis, heart problems, hemorrhages, hypertension, mouth ulcers, and as an astringent and diuretic

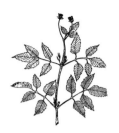

Family: Asteraceae

Genus: *Bidens*

Species: *pilosa*

Common Names:
picão preto, carrapicho, amor seco, pirca, aceitilla, cadillo, chilca, pacunga, cuambu, erva-picão, alfiler, clavelito de monte, romerillo, saltillo, yema de huevo, z'aiguille, jarongan, ketul, pau-pau pasir, Spanish needles, bident herisse, herbe d'aiguille, zweizahn, mozote, beggar's tick

Parts Used: whole herb

PICÃO PRETO
HERBAL PROPERTIES AND ACTIONS

Main Actions
- kills bacteria
- kills viruses
- kills germs
- kills leukemia cells
- kills yeast
- reduces inflammation
- protects liver
- prevents ulcers
- inhibits stomach acid
- helps diabetes
- reduces spasms
- fights free radicals

Other Actions
- dries secretions
- increases urination
- inhibits tumors
- lowers blood sugar
- promotes menstruation
- expels worms
- stimulates digestion

Standard Dosage
Whole herb
Decoction: ½–1 cup twice daily
Tablets/Capsules: 2 g twice daily
Tincture: 2–3 ml twice daily

Picão preto is a small, erect annual herb that grows to 1 m high. It has bright green leaves with serrated, prickly edges and produces small, yellow flowers and black fruit. Its root has a distinctive aroma similar to that of a carrot. It is indigenous to the Amazon rainforest and other tropical areas of South America, Africa, the Caribbean, and the Philippines. It is often considered a weed in many places. It is a southern cousin to *Bidens tripartita*, the European bur marigold, which has an ancient history in European herbal medicine. In Brazil, the plant is most commonly known as *picão preto* or *carrapicho;* in Peru it is known as *amor seco* or *pirca.*

TRIBAL AND HERBAL MEDICINE USES

Picão preto has a long history of use among the indigenous people of the Amazon, and virtually all parts of the plant are used. Generally, the whole plant is uprooted and prepared in decoctions or infusions for internal use, and/or crushed into a paste or poultice for external use. In the Peruvian Amazon, picão preto is used for aftosa (foot-and-mouth disease), angina, diabetes, menstrual disorders, hepatitis, laryngitis, intestinal worms, and for internal and external inflammations. In Piura region of Peru, a decoction of the roots is used for alcoholic hepatitis and worms. The Cuna tribe mixes the crushed leaves with water to treat headaches. Near Pucallpa, Peru, the leaf is balled up and applied to a toothache; the leaves also are used for headaches. In other parts of the Amazon, a decoction of the plant is mixed with lemon juice and used to treat angina, hepatitis, sore throat, and water retention. The Exuma tribe grinds the sun-dried leaves with olive oil to make poultices for sores and lacerations and, in Tonga, an infusion of the flowers is used to treat upset stomach in food poisoning.

In Peruvian herbal medicine picão preto is employed to reduce inflammation, increase urination, and to support and protect the liver.

In Peruvian herbal medicine picão preto is employed to reduce inflammation, increase urination, and to support and protect the liver. It is commonly used there for hepatitis, conjunctivitis, abscesses, fungal infections, urinary infections, as a weight loss aid, and to stimulate childbirth. In Brazilian herbal medicine it is used for fevers, malaria, hepatitis, diabetes, sore throat, tonsillitis, obstructions in the liver and other liver disorders, urinary infections, and vaginal discharge and infections. An infusion or decoction of the entire plant is often gargled for tonsilitis and pharyngitis. Externally it is used for wounds, fungal infections, ulcers, diaper rash, insect bites, and hemorrhoids. Brazilian herbalists also report using picão preto to normalize insulin and bilirubin levels in the pancreas, liver, and blood. In Mexico, the entire plant or leaf is used to treat diabetes, stomach disorders, hemorrhoids, hepatitis, nervous problems, and fever. It is used as a gargle for mouth blisters, and the juice of the plant is used in an external poultice for kidney and liver inflammation.

PLANT CHEMICALS

Picão preto is rich in flavonoids, terpenes, phenylpropanoids, lipids, and benzenoids. Even as early as 1979 and 1980, scientists demonstrated that specific chemicals found in the herb were toxic to bacteria and fungi.[1,2] Many of the flavonoids in picão preto have been documented with antimalarial activity.[3] In 1991, Swiss scientists isolated several known phytochemicals with antimicrobial and anti-inflammatory properties, which led them to infer that the presence of these compounds "may rationalize the use of this plant in traditional medicine in the treatment of wounds, against inflammation and against bacterial infection of the gastrointestinal tract."[4] New bioactive phytochemicals, discovered in 1996, showed activity against transformed human cell lines.[5]

The plant chemicals in picão preto include aesculetin, behenic acid, beta-sitosterol, borneol, butanedioic acid, butoxylinoleates, cadinols, caffeine, caffeoylic acids, capric acid, daucosterol, elaidic acid, erythronic acids, friedelans, friedelins, germacrene D, glucopyranoses, glucopyranosides, inositol, isoquercitrin, lauric acid, limonene, linoleic acids, lupeol, luteolin, muurolol, myristic acid, okanin-glucosides, palmitic acid, palmitoleic acid, paracoumaric acids, phenylheptatriynes, phytenoic acid, phytol, pilosola A, polyacetylenes, precocene I, pyranoses, quercetin, sandaracopimaradiols, squalene, stigmasterols, tannic acid, tetrahydroxyaurones, tocopherolquinones, tridecapentaynenes, tridecatetrayndienes, and vanillic acid.

BIOLOGICAL ACTIVITIES AND CLINICAL RESEARCH

Picão preto has been the subject of recent clinical research that has supported many of its uses in herbal medicine. A research group in Taiwan reported that a picão preto extract was capable of protecting the liver of rats from various introduced toxins known to cause liver injury.[6] This research group had previously demonstrated picão preto's anti-inflammatory actions in animals a year earlier (in 1995).[7] In 1999, a Brazilian research group confirmed the anti-inflammatory activities in mice and attributed them to an immune modulation effect (noting the extract reduced the amount of pro-inflammatory immune cells in human blood in a previous study).[8] In addition, other research demonstrated that a picão preto extract inhibited prostaglandin-synthesis and cyclooxygenase (COX) activities.[9] Both are chemical processes in the body that are linked to inflammatory diseases (and provide the focus for COX inhibitor classes of anti-inflammatory and arthritis pharmaceutical drugs).

Picão preto was shown to be better than two prescription anti-ulcer drugs in animal studies.

Other areas of research have validated picão preto's traditional use for ulcers and diabetes. Extracts of the leaf (as well as the entire plant) have clinically shown to protect rats against chemical- and bacteria-induced gastric lesions and ulcers and, also, to reduce gastric acid secretion.[10–12] The activity noted in these studies was higher than that shown by two prescription anti-ulcer drugs. Other *in vivo* studies with rats and mice have demonstrated that picão preto has hypoglycemic activity and is able to improve insulin sensitivity, which validates its long history in herbal medicine for diabetes.[13–15] Researchers (in 2000) attributed the plant's hypoglycemic properties to a group of glucoside chemicals found in the aerial parts of the plant.[16] Picão preto was also documented to prevent hypertension in rats fed a high-fructose diet, and to lower the resulting (elevated) blood pressure and triglyceride levels.[17,18] In hypertensive rats (including high dietary salt-induced hypertension), extracts of the plant significantly lowered blood pressure—without having an effect on heart rate and urine volume.[19] A leaf extract was also shown to have smooth-muscle relaxant activity on the heart.[20]

Picão preto has long been used in traditional medicine systems for infections of all kinds: from such upper respiratory tract infections as colds and flu to urinary tract infections and sexually transmitted diseases—and even infected wounds on the skin. Research has begun to confirm these uses in several *in vitro* microbial studies. In 1991, scientists in Egypt first documented picão preto's antimicrobial activity against various pathogens.[4] Other *in vitro* studies have demonstrated its antibacterial activity against a wide range of bacteria including *Klebsiella pneumonia*, *Bacillus*, *Neisseria gonorrhea*, *Pseudomonas*, *Staphylococcus*, and *Salmonella*.[5,21–25]

Extracts of the leaf also have been documented to have antimycobacterial activity towards *Mycobacterium tuberculosis* and *M. smegmatis*.[26,27] A water extract of the leaf has shown significant anti-yeast activity towards *Candida albicans*.[23] Much of picão preto's antimicrobial actions have been attributed to a group of chemicals called *polyacetylenes*, which includes a chemical called *phenylheptatriyne*. Phenylheptatriyne has shown strong *in vitro* activity against numerous human and animal viruses, bacteria, fungi, and molds in very small amounts.[1,5,28–30]

In the tropics, picão preto is also used for snakebite and malaria; research has confirmed these uses as well. Several studies have confirmed the plant's antimalarial activity; it reduced malaria in animals by 43–66 percent,[3,31] and *in vitro* by 90 percent.[3,32] With regard to its status as a traditional snakebite remedy, one research group confirmed that a picão preto extract could protect mice from lethal injections of neurotoxic snake venom.[33]

The last area of research has focused on picão preto's anticancerous possibilities. Early research, in various *in vitro* assay systems designed to predict anti-tumor activity, indicated positive results in the early 1990s.[34,35] Picão preto first was reported to have antileukemic actions in 1995.[36] Then researchers from Taiwan reported (in 2001) that a simple hot water extract of picão preto could inhibit the growth of five strains of human and mouse leukemia at less than 200 mcg per ml *in vitro*.[37] They summarized their research by saying that picão preto "may prove to be a useful medicinal plant for treating leukemia."

CURRENT PRACTICAL USES

Picão preto, one of South America's well-known medicinal plants, is widely used for numerous conditions. Many of its indigenous uses for inflammation, hypertension, ulcers, diabetes, and infections of all kinds are being validated and verified by modern research. Unfortunately, little is known of it in herbal medicine practices in the U.S.—and it is not widely available here. In South America, it is considered a safe plant to use; in the various animals studies performed to date, no toxic effects have been reported. Specific toxicology studies have shown no toxicity when dosages of (up to) 1 g per kg of body weight were injected into mice.[38]

Traditional Preparation

In the tropics, generally 1 cup of a standard decoction is taken one to three times daily, depending on the condition that is being treated. If desired, 2–3 ml of a 4:1 tincture twice daily, or 2–3 g of powdered herb in tablets, capsules, or stirred into water (or juice) twice daily can be substituted.

Contraindications

Picão preto has evidenced weak uterine stimulant activity in guinea pigs.[38] As such, it should probably be avoided during pregnancy.

This plant contains several coumarin derivatives. Coumarins are a group of chemicals that thin the blood. Those on blood thinning medications such as Warfarin® should use picão preto with caution and monitor these possible effects.

The plant has been documented to lower blood sugar levels in several animal studies. Those with hypoglycemia or diabetes should monitor their blood sugar levels closely if they use picão preto.

Picão preto has been documented with hypotensive activity in several animal studies. People with heart conditions and those taking antihypertensive drugs should consult their doctors prior to using this plant to monitor these possible effects (as medications may need adjustment).

Drug Interactions   None clinically documented in humans; however, the use of this plant may potentiate antidiabetic, anticoagulant, and antihypertensive drugs (based on animal studies).

Worldwide Ethnomedical Uses

Region	Uses
Africa	for bleeding, blood clots, burns, cataracts, colitis, conjunctivitis, constipation, diarrhea, earache, eye disorders, food poisoning, hemorrhages, inflammation, malaria, pneumonia, postpartum hemorrhage, respiratory infections, rheumatism, sores, stomach pains, tuberculosis, worms, wounds, yaws, and as an antiseptic
Amazonia	for angina, chills, diabetes, dysentery, edema, eye disorders, headache, hepatitis, jaundice, laryngitis, malaria, menstrual disorders, parasites, sore mouth, sore throat, stomachache, toothache, urinary insufficiency, worms, wounds
Bahamas	for cancer, fever, heat rash, intestinal gas, itch, lacerations, skin sores, water retention, wounds
Brazil	for breast engorgement, cough, diabetes, diaper rash, dysentery, fever, fungal infections, gonorrhea, hemorrhoids, hepatitis, inflammation, insect bites, jaundice, lactation aid, liver obstructions, lung disorders, malaria, parasites, pharyngitis, rheumatism, sclerosis (glands), scurvy, sore throat, tonsillitis, toothache, ulcers, urinary infections, urinary insufficiency, vaginal discharge, vaginal infections, wounds; and as an antiseptic, astringent, and liver tonic
Dominican Republic	for chest problems and toothaches, and to promote menstruation, milk production, salivation, urination
Ghana	for allergies, bleeding, earaches, eye infections, hives
Haiti	for angina, catarrh, diabetes, foot-and-mouth disease, mental disorders, milk production, nervous shock, stomatitis, tonsillitis, vomiting
Mexico	for blood clots, chest problems, diabetes, fever, gastroenteritis, hemorrhoids, inflammation, jaundice, kidney, liver disorders, mouth blisters, nervous problems, snakebite, stomach problems, and as an antiseptic and diuretic
Panama	for colds, headache, intestinal disorders, prostate tumors, rheumatism
Peru	for abscesses, angina, anuria, baldness, bile stimulation, childbirth, chills, conjunctivitis, cystitis, diabetes, dysentery, edema, fever, foot-and-mouth disease, fungal infections, headache, hemorrhage, hepatitis, inflammation, jaundice, lacerations, laryngitis, liver problems, liver support, menstrual disorders, mouth sores, nephritis, nervous system disorders, obesity, pain, parasites, rheumatism, sexually transmitted diseases, sores, sore throat, tonsillitis, toothache, urinary infections, urinary insufficiency, worms, wounds
Elsewhere	for abortions, bleeding, blood cleansing, boils, bronchitis, burns, cancer, *Candida,* colds, colic, colitis, conjunctivitis, coughs, cuts, diabetes, diarrhea, dysentery, eye problems, fever, flatulence, flu, food poisoning, gout, hair loss, hepatitis, hyperglycemia, hypertension, inflammation, intestinal infections, liver diseases, menstrual promotion, parasites, respiratory infections, rheumatism, skin problems, snakebite, stomach disorders, styptic, sweat promotion, thrush, toothache, ulcerative colitis, ulcers, urinary infections, urinary problems, worms, wounds; and as an antiseptic, astringent, diuretic

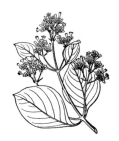

Family: Rubiaceae

Genus: *Cinchona*

Species: *officinalis, ledger-iana, succirubra, calisaya*

Common Names: quinine bark, quina, quinine, kinakina, China bark, cinchona bark, yellow cinchona, red cinchona, Peruvian bark, Jesuit's bark, quina-quina, calisaya bark, fever tree

Parts Used: bark, wood

TRIBAL AND HERBAL MEDICINE USES

QUININE
HERBAL PROPERTIES AND ACTIONS

Main Actions	Other Actions	Standard Dosage
• treats malaria	• relieves pain	Bark
• kills parasites	• kills bacteria	**Decoction:** $1/2$ cup one to three times daily
• reduces fever	• kills fungi	
• regulates heartbeat	• dries secretions	**Tablets/Capsules:** 2 g twice daily
• stimulates digestion	• calms nerves	
• kills germs		**Tincture:** 1–2 ml two to three times daily
• reduces spasms		
• kills insects		

The *Cinchona* genus contains about forty species of trees. They grow 15–20 m in height and produce white, pink, or yellow flowers. All cinchonas are indigenous to the eastern slopes of the Amazonian area of the Andes, where they grow from 1,500–3,000 m in elevation on either side of the equator (from Colombia to Bolivia). They can also be found in the northern part of the Andes (on the eastern slopes of the central and western ranges). They are now widely cultivated in many tropical countries for their commercial value, although they are not indigenous to those areas.

Cinchona, or quinine bark, is one of the rainforest's most famous plants and most important discoveries. Legend has it that the name *cinchona* came from the countess of Chinchon, the wife of a Peruvian viceroy, who was cured of a malarial type of fever by using the bark of the cinchona tree in 1638. It was supposedly introduced to European medicine in 1640 by the countess of Chinchon, even before botanists had identified and named the species of tree. Quinine bark was first advertised for sale in England in 1658, and was made official in the *British Pharmacopoeia* in 1677. Physicians gave credit to the drug and, because of its effectiveness with malaria, it was recognized officially even while the identity of the tree species remained unknown. Several years after the "Countess's powder" arrived in England, it arrived in Spain. There, quinine bark was used by the Jesuits very early in the group's history and due to the influence of the Company of Jesus, the newly named "Jesuit's powder" became known all over Europe. When the plant was finally botanically classified almost one hundred years later in 1737, botanists still named it after the countess for her contribution.

Throughout the mid-1600s to mid-1800s, quinine bark was the primary treatment for malaria and it evidenced remarkable results. It was also used for fever, indigestion, mouth and throat diseases, and cancer.

Throughout the mid-1600s to mid-1800s, quinine bark was the primary treatment for malaria and it evidenced remarkable results. It was also used for fever, indigestion, mouth and throat diseases, and cancer.

Natural quinine bark is still employed in herbal medicine systems around the world today. In Brazilian herbal medicine, quinine bark is considered a tonic, a digestive stimulant, and fever reducer. It is used for anemia, indigestion, gastrointestinal disorders, general fatigue, fevers, malaria, and as an appetite stimulant. Other folk remedies in South America cite quinine bark as a natural remedy for cancer (breast, glands, liver, mesentery, spleen), amebic infections, heart problems, colds, diarrhea, dysentery, dyspepsia, fevers, flu, hangover, lumbago, malaria, neuralgia, pneumonia, sciatica, typhoid, and varicose veins. In European herbal medicine, the bark is considered antiprotozoal, antispasmodic, antimalarial, a bitter tonic, and a fever reducer. There it is used as an appetite stimulant; for hair loss; alcoholism; liver, spleen, and gallbladder disorders; and to treat irregular heartbeat, anemia, leg cramps, and fevers of all kinds. In the U.S., quinine bark is used as a tonic and digestive aid; to reduce heart palpitations and normalize heart functions; to stimulate digestion and appetite; for hemorrhoids, varicose veins, headaches, leg cramps, colds, flu, and indigestion; and for its astringent, bactericidal, and anesthetic actions in various other conditions.

PLANT CHEMICALS

In 1820 two scientists, Pelletier and Caventou, isolated an alkaloid chemical in the bark that provided the highest antimalarial effect, and named it *quinine*. Once discovered, methods were developed to extract only the quinine alkaloid from the natural bark to sell as an antimalarial drug.

In addition to the quinine alkaloid, another alkaloid chemical called *quinidine* was discovered to have beneficial effects for the heart. Quinidine, a compound produced from quinine, is still used in cardiology today, sold as a prescription drug for arrhythmia.

The South American rainforests benefited from the income generated by harvesting cinchona bark for the extraction of this alkaloid from the bark for the manufacture of quinine drugs. In the middle of the nineteenth century, though, seeds of *Cinchona calisaya* and *Cinchona pubescens* were smuggled out of South America by the British and the Dutch. The *calisaya* species was planted and cultivated in Java by the Dutch and the *pubescens* species was cultivated in India and Ceylon by the British. However, the quinine content of these species was too low for high-grade, cost effective, commercial production of quinine. The Dutch then smuggled seeds of *Cinchona ledgeriana* out of Bolivia, paying $20 for a pound of seeds, and soon established extensive plantations of quinine-rich cinchona trees in Java. They quickly dominated the world production of quinine and, by 1918, the majority of the world's supply of quinine was under the total control of the Dutch "kina burea" in Amsterdam. Huge profits were reaped—but Bolivia and Peru, from which the resource originated, saw none of it.

The upheavals of the Second World War led to changes in the market, which still remain in effect today. When Java was occupied by the Japanese in 1942, the Allies' supply of quinine was cut off. South American sources of cinchona trees and quinine bark were once again in demand, but new plantations were planted by the Allies in Africa as well. This dire shortage of quinine fueled research for developing and producing a synthetic version of the quinine alkaloid, rather than relying on the natural bark. In 1944, scientists were able to synthesize the quinine alkaloid in the laboratory. This led to various synthesized and patented quinine drugs which were manufactured by several pharmaceutical companies and were of course, highly profitable.

Today, Indonesia and India still cultivate cinchona trees; however Africa, with the expansions of the old WWII plantations, has emerged as the leading supplier of quinine bark. Much lower on the list of producers are the South American countries of Peru, Bolivia, and Ecuador, still struggling to compete. Although all cinchona species are good sources of quinine, *C. succirubra* and *C. ledgeriana* are the species containing the highest amount of quinine alkaloids—which is why they are the species of choice for cultivation today.

The cardiac effects of cinchona bark were noted in academic medicine at the end of the seventeenth century. Quinine was used sporadically through the first half of the eighteenth century for cardiac problems and arrhythmia and it became a standard of cardiac therapy in the second half of the nineteenth century. Another alkaloid chemical called *quinidine* was discovered to be responsible for this beneficial cardiac effect. Quinidine, a compound produced from quinine, is still used in cardiology today, sold as a prescription drug for arrhythmia. The sales demand for this drug still generates the need for harvesting natural quinine bark today, because scientists have been unsuccessful in synthesizing this chemical without utilizing the natural quinine found in cinchona bark.

The main plant chemicals found in quinine include aricine, caffeic acid, cinchofulvic acid, cincholic acid, cinchonain, cinchonidine, cinchonine, cinchophyllamine, cinchotannic acid, cinchotine, conquinamine, cuscamidine, cuscamine, cusconidine, cusconine, epicatechin, javanine, paricine, proanthocyanidins, quinacimine, quinamine, quinic acid, quinicine, quinine, quininidine, quinovic acid, quinovin, and sucirubine.

BIOLOGICAL ACTIVITIES AND CLINICAL RESEARCH

Interestingly enough, natural quinine extracted from quinine bark and the use of natural bark tea and/or bark extracts are making a comeback in the management and treatment of malaria. Malaria strains have evolved that have developed a resistance to the synthesized quinine drugs. It was shown in early studies that an effective dose of natural quinine bark extract elicited the same antimalarial activity as an effective dose of the synthesized quinine drug.[1] Scientists are now finding that these new strains of drug-resistant malaria can be treated effectively with natural quinine and/or quinine bark extracts. As evolving pathogens develop widespread resistance to our standard antibiotics, antivirals, and antimalarial drugs, it is of little wonder that the use of the natural medicine in quinine bark is being revisited, even by such giants as the World Health Organization.

A recent use for quinine drugs has been for the treatment of muscle spasms and leg cramps. A 1998 study documented the beneficial effects of quinine for leg cramps, with tinnitus being the only documented side effect.[2] In 2002, a double-blind placebo study was undertaken in which ninety-eight people with nocturnal leg cramps were given 400 mg of quinine daily for two weeks.[3] The results stated that quinine administered at this dose effectively reduced the frequency, intensity, and pain of leg cramps without relevant side effects. This use has fueled the natural product market and more people are looking for natural quinine bark as an alternative to the synthesized prescription drugs.

CURRENT PRACTICAL USES

Quinine bark is harvested today much as it has been for hundreds of years. The tree trunks are beaten and the peeling bark is removed. The bark partially regenerates on the tree and, after a few years and several cycles of bark removal, the trees are uprooted and new ones are planted. The commercial quinine market today is difficult to calculate. It is thought that 300–500 metric tons of quinine alkaloids are extracted annually from 5,000–10,000 metric tons of harvested bark. Nearly half of the harvest is directed to the food industry for the production of quinine water, tonic water, and as an FDA-approved bitter food additive. The remainder is utilized in the manufacture of the quinidine prescription drug. Quinine is very bitter tasting and commercially sold tonic waters often use quinine as their bitter ingredient/component. Commercially produced tonic water usually contains around 100–300 parts per million quinine and up to a maximum allowable concentration of 70 mg of quinine per liter.

The history of the cinchona tree provides a perfect example of how a natural product can go from folklore and indigenous use into world trade—and then into the drug market. It is also indicative of how indigenous peoples and countries with important natural resources are pirated.

The long-standing natural remedy for quinine bark usually calls for 1 cup of boiling water to be poured over approximately 1–2 g of ground or chopped natural bark and allowed to steep for ten minutes. A cupful of this infusion is drunk half an hour before meals to stimulate the appetite, or after meals to treat digestive disorders. The use of pure quinine at large dosages can be toxic. The reported therapeutic oral dose for quinine alkaloids in adults is between 167–333 mg three times per day.[2] Reportedly, a single dose of 2–8 g of pure quinine alkaloids taken orally may be fatal to an adult.[2] Natural bark teas prepared in the traditional manner, however, have a long history of use without toxic effects. A cup of traditional quinine bark tea would provide approximately 100 mg of total alkaloids, including quinine (based upon an average of 5 percent total alkaloid content in the raw bark).

The history of the cinchona tree provides a perfect example of how a natural product can go from folklore and indigenous use into world trade—and then into the drug market. It's also indicative of how indigenous peoples and countries with important natural resources are too often pirated and left out of the profit loop by industrialized nations and rich, multinational, profit-driven organizations. Despite the fact that quinine and quinidine drugs were patented and sold, Peru and Bolivia—from which the discovery was made and the resources extracted—did not share in the patents or resulting profits. Their natural resources were smuggled out, and profitable world markets were created from them. These were poor, developing nations without multinational backing or investment capital—and ended up at the bottom of the heap while competing in a global market for resources indigenous to their countries.

While governments are making inroads and there are new laws concerning biodiversity and intellectual property rights to correct this situation, business still has a long way to go to "do the right thing." Ideally, if natural quinine bark makes a comeback in the growing natural products industry or new drugs are developed for these drug-resistant strains of malaria, these new laws will protect the natural resources of these developing nations.

Traditional Preparation One-half cup bark decoction is taken one to three times daily, or 1–2 ml of a 4:1 tincture twice daily. If desired, 1–2 g daily of powdered bark in tablets or capsules can be substituted.

Contraindications Quinine bark contains naturally occurring quinine alkaloids. These quinine alkaloids are sold as prescription drugs with numerous side effects and warnings documented in the literature. Do not exceed the quinine bark natural remedy amounts shown above unless you are under the care and advice of a qualified health care practitioner who is familiar with the warnings, side effects, and contraindications of higher therapeutic levels of quinine alkaloids.

Drug Interactions May potentiate blood-thinning medications such as Warfarin.[®]

Worldwide Ethnomedical Uses

Region	Uses
Brazil	for anemia, anorexia, debility, digestive sluggishness, dyspepsia, fatigue, fevers, gastrointestinal disorders, indigestion, malaria
Europe	for alcoholism, anemia, cramps, debility, diarrhea, enlarged spleen, fevers, flatulence, gallbladder disorders, hair loss, irregular heartbeat, leg cramps, liver disorders, malaria, muscle pain, protozoal infections, and as an antiseptic and appetite stimulant

Mexico	for malaria and as an antiseptic, astringent, and tonic
United States	for bacterial infections, colds, digestive disorders, dyspepsia, fevers, flu, headaches, heart palpitations, hemorrhoids, leg cramps, malaria, pain, varicose veins, viral infections; and as an appetite stimulant, astringent, and cardiotonic
Venezuela	for cancer and malaria
Elsewhere	for amebic infections, bacterial infections, carditis, colds, cough, dandruff, diarrhea, digestive sluggishness, dysentery, dyspepsia, fever, flu, glandular disorders, hangovers, hemorrhoids, lumbago, malaria, neuralgia, pain, pinworms, pneumonia, sciatica, septic infections, sore throat, stomatitis, tumor (glands), typhoid, varicose veins; and as a contraceptive, insecticide, insect repellent, stimulant, and uterine tonic

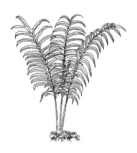

SAMAMBAIA
HERBAL PROPERTIES AND ACTIONS

Main Actions
- protects brain cells
- protects skin cells
- reduces inflammation
- relieves psoriasis
- modulates immune function
- suppresses coughs
- reduces phlegm
- fights free radicals
- is natural sunscreen

Other Actions
- cleanses blood
- increases urination
- lowers blood pressure
- promotes perspiration

Standard Dosage
Leaves, Rhizome

Infusion: ½–1 cup one to three times daily

Tablets/Capsules: 1–2 g twice daily

Tincture: 2–3 ml twice daily

Family: Polypodiaceae

Genus: *Polypodium*

Species: *decumanum, leucotomos, aureum*

Common Names: samambaia, calaguala, anapsos, huayhuashi-shupa, cotochupa, mirane, temakaje

Parts Used: rhizome, aerial parts

Samambaia is a fern that grows in the rainforests of South America, as well as in drier tropical forests in Latin America. The Polypody family contains three-quarters of all ferns—over 6,000 species of plants, mostly native to the tropics of both hemispheres. There are seventy-five species of plants in the *Polypodium* genus, many of which have been used medicinally for centuries. The name is derived from *poly,* meaning "many," and *podus,* meaning "foot," for the many foot-like divisions of the root or rhizomes of polypody ferns. *Polypodium leucotomos* (also classified as *Polypodium aureum*) and *Polypodium decumanum* are indigenous to the Honduran rainforests but also can be found throughout the South American tropics and in parts of Latin America and the Caribbean. In Brazil, the common name is *samambaia;* in Mexico and other Spanish-speaking tropical countries, the plant is known as *calaguala.*

TRIBAL AND HERBAL MEDICINE USES

Samambaia, like most ferns, has an intricate, creeping root system; it is this rhizome, as well as the fronds or leaves, that is used most medicinally. The plant historically has been used by the indigenous peoples of Honduras for malignant tumors, rheumatoid arthritis, and psoriasis. In the Amazon rainforest, a maceration of the rhizome is used for fever; grated fresh, it is made into a tea for whooping cough and kidney problems. The Boras Indians (in the Peruvian Amazon) prepare the leaves in a drink for coughs. The Witotos Indians (in the northwest Amazon) use the rhizome for treating coughs. Other Peruvian indigenous tribes use the rhizome for problems of the pancreas. Indigenous groups in Latin America use the rhizome and leaves for many different maladies including cancer, psoriasis, peptic ulcers, kidney problems, diarrhea, arthritis, and pains in joints and tendons. It is generally considered throughout the Amazon to be a general tonic, to detoxify the body, and to support the immune system.

> Indigenous groups in Latin America use the rhizome and leaves of samambaia for many different maladies including cancer, psoriasis, peptic ulcers, kidney problems, diarrhea, arthritis, and pains.

Many types of ferns are used in traditional medicine around the world. Most, including samambaia, are considered a tonic, blood cleanser, expectorant, and are used for numerous upper respiratory conditions. In Honduran traditional medicine systems today, samambaia commonly is used for tumors, psoriasis, atopic dermatitis, vitiligo, rheumatoid arthritis, and arthritis. In Brazilian traditional medicine, samambaia is considered a blood cleanser, sweat promoter, tonic, and expectorant; it is widely used for coughs, bronchitis, colds and flu, and other upper respiratory problems—as well as for rheumatism and skin problems (including psoriasis and dermatitis). In Peruvian herbal medicine, the rhizome is used for coughs, fevers, and urinary infections, as well as skin problems such as psoriasis, boils, ulcers, and abscesses.

PLANT CHEMICALS

Samambaia contains flavonoids, alkaloids, and lipids. It is a rich source of lipids and fatty acids, and its therapeutic activity is attributed to these groups of chemicals. Within its lipids are a group of chemicals called *sulphoquinovosyldiacylglycerols,* which have been documented and patented as part of the plant's "active" chemicals.[1]

The main plant chemicals identified in samambaia thus far include adenosine, alkaloids, arachidonic acid, arabinopyranosides, calagualine, ecdysone, ecdysterone, eicosapentaenoic acid, elaidic acid, juglanin, kaempferols, linoleic acid, linoleic acids, linolenic acids, melilotoside, oleic acid, polypodaureine, ricinoleic acid, rutin, selligueain, and sulphoquinovosyldiacylglycerols.

BIOLOGICAL ACTIVITIES AND CLINICAL RESEARCH

Toxicity studies on samambaia with mice and rats have demonstrated no toxicity in acute or chronic dosages;[2] in humans, oral doses greater than 1,000 mg have not shown toxicity.[3]

There has been a great deal of scientific interest in *Polypodium* plants, mostly focusing on their ability to treat psoriasis. In the mid-1970s, rhizome extracts of samambaia were first reported to decrease the over-growth of skin cells and skin thickening, and reduce the severity and extent of skin lesions in psoriasis patients.[4] In the early 1980s, a company in Spain produced an herbal drug from a water extract of samambaia (*P. leucotomos*) rhizome and named it *Anapsos*. Since that time it has been a prescription drug registered by the Health Ministry of Spain for the treatment of psoriasis. Clinical research also has been published on Anapsos since then (including various double-blind placebo human trials) indicating it to be an effective treatment for psoriasis—as well as dermatitis and vitiligo (with a three to six month course of treatment required).[5–12]

The mechanism of action in treating psoriasis is thought to be related to the modulation of certain cellular processes found in inflammation and psoriatic skin. Scientists have shown that psoriatic skin has abnormally high quantities of chemicals produced in the body called *leukotriene* and *PAF* (platelet-activating factor). Both are implicated in the cause and progression of psoriasis. In clinical research, samambaia (and/or some of its novel chemicals) have shown to be effective in blocking excess leukotriene production[13] as well as excess PAF.[14–16] Psoriasis is also considered an autoimmune disease (as many of the immune cells are overstimulated, while others are suppressed). Extracts of samambaia have clearly demonstrated in clinical studies to possess some of the specific immune modulating effects needed to treat the imbalances in the immune system that are peculiar to psoriasis.[9,10,16–22] Additionally, extracts of samambaia have been documented to have a direct anti-inflammatory activity in mice, rats, and humans with psoriasis.[1,23]

Some of the more recent research on samambaia has focused on other chronic and degenerative diseases. A U.S. patent was filed (in 2001) on a samambaia rhizome extract that indicated its suitability in the treatment of AIDS- and cancer-related wasting syndrome, reporting marked benefits in several non-randomized human studies with cancer and AIDS patients.[24] In 1997, a U.S. patent was filed on a samambaia leaf and rhizome extract capable of treating brain disorders such as Alzheimer's disease and dementia.[25] The patent and several *in vivo* clinical studies indicate samambaia protects against brain cell degeneration, promotes repair of damaged brain cells, and has a protective effect to brain cells.[25–29] This was discovered when psoriasis patients in Europe taking Anapsos (who also had Alzeimer's) reported an improvement in their Alzheimer's symptoms. This led the drug manufacturer to fund clinical trials on its use for brain disorders. In a double-blind placebo human trial (in 2000), researchers reported that a dosage of 360 mg per day of Anapsos given to patients with senile dementia improved cognitive per-

> Samambaia has clearly demonstrated in clinical studies to possess some immune modulating effects needed to treat the imbalances in the immune system that are peculiar to psoriasis.

> The newest research on samambaia reports that it can protect and repair brain cells. Samambaia extracts are now sold in Europe as herbal drugs for the treatment of Alzheimer's disease and dementia.

formance, increased the blood supply to the brain, and also increased the electrical impulses in the brain.[30] The results were better with Alzheimer's patients and those with mild dementia than those with severe dementia and extensive brain cell degeneration. Anapsos now is used in Spain and Europe for the treatment of Alzheimer's and dementia.[31]

The same protective effects to brain cells seem to extend to skin cells as well. A 1997 U.S. patent was filed on an extract of samambaia, which indicated it is effective in preventing sunburn and skin damage (taken internally, as well as applied topically prior to exposure).[3] Its protective effect against ultraviolet radiation was reported to be due, in part, to an antioxidant effect.[32] One of the *in vivo* human studies confirming this activity was performed at Massachusetts General Hospital's dermatology department.[33] Another study (with hairless mice), conducted at Harvard medical school in 1999, reported that a samambaia extract applied topically helped to avoid skin damage and sun-associated skin aging, as well as reduced the number of UV-induced skin tumors in mice.[34]

The Harvard researchers published a human study in 2004 reporting that samambaia evidenced "substantial benefits of skin protection" to prevent sunburn and prevent skin aging when it was taken internally (at 7.5 mg/kg).[35] Based on some *in vitro* studies, other university student researchers suggested that samambaia may help prevent sun damage and skin aging at low dosages while higher dosages may actually reverse the loss of normal elastic fibers associated with intrinsic aging of the skin.[36] A pharmaceutical company in Spain has also published a study indicating that samambaia is suitable to use as a preventative treatment for sunburn and skin damage.[37]

The last area of research concerns samambaia's possible uses for cancer. Researchers at M. D. Anderson Cancer Center in Houston, Texas published their first study on samambaia and one of its main chemicals (calagualine) in 2003. They reported that some of the intercellular processes blocked during psoriasis (NF-kappaB and tumor necrosis factor chemicals) also evidenced the ability to block and suppress inflammation, tumor formation, and tumor growth.[38]

CURRENT PRACTICAL USES It is likely that scientists will continue studying samambaia and why it works; meanwhile, natural health practitioners around the world will continue to employ it for many purposes, without knowing which specific chemicals are creating the beneficial effects. In addition to psoriasis, vitiligo, and Alzheimer's, health practitioners in the United States are using samambaia for coughs, bronchitis, chest colds, flu, and disorders of the respiratory tract, skin, and immune systems—much as it has been used in indigenous herbal medicine systems for years. With the newer research indicating uses for cellular repair—for both skin cells and brain cells, as well as cancer prevention—it is only a matter of time before samambaia shows up as an ingredient in the widely popular anti-aging products being marketed to the aging "baby-boomers" market.

Traditional Preparation

One-half to 1 cup leaf or root infusion is taken one to three times daily, or 2–3 ml of a 4:1 tincture or fluid extract twice daily. Traditionally, a simple, cold maceration of the rhizome and leaves is used; therefore, 1–2 g daily of powdered root or leaf in tablets or capsules can be substituted, if desired.

Contraindications

Reports indicate that samambaia may enhance the effects of the heart drug digitalis (a medication commonly used to increase the force of heart contractions in those diagnosed with certain conditions).[31] It is therefore contraindicated in combination with digitalis, and persons with any heart condition should seek the advice of a qualified health practitioner prior to using samambaia.

Drug Interactions

Samambaia may potentiate the effects of digitalis and/or other digitalis-type prescription heart drugs. The absorption of samambaia is reported to be reduced in the presence of antacids.

Worldwide Ethnomedical Uses

Region	Uses
Amazonia	for cancer, coughs, detoxification, fever, immune disorders, kidney problems, pancreatic disorders, psoriasis, rheumatism, whooping cough
Brazil	for blood cleansing, bronchitis, colds, coughs, flu, gout, psoriasis, respiratory disorders, rheumatism, skin disorders; and as an expectorant, tonic, and to increase perspiration
Colombia	for coughs
Honduras	for arthritis, cancer, dermatitis, joint pains, kidney disorders, psoriasis, rheumatoid arthritis, stomach ulcers, tendon pain, tumors
Mexico	for coughs, fever, respiratory problems, and to increase perspiration
Peru	for abscesses, boils, cough, fever, psoriasis, skin disorders, ulcers (skin), urinary infections, whooping cough
United States	for Alzheimer's, bronchitis, colds, cough, dermatitis, detoxification, eczema, flu, gout, hypertension, immune disorders, psoriasis, respiratory disorders, rheumatism, skin disorders, and to increase perspiration and urination
Venezuela	for sexually transmitted diseases and as a laxative
Elsewhere	for bronchitis, cancer, colds, coughs, fever, flu, gout, hypertension, immune disorders, kidney problems, psoriasis, respiratory disorders, rheumatism, skin disorders, tonic, tumors, urinary insufficiency

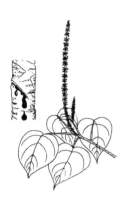

SANGRE DE GRADO *"DRAGON'S BLOOD"*
HERBAL PROPERTIES AND ACTIONS

Main Actions	Other Actions	Standard Dosage
• heals wounds	• kills cancer cells	Resin
• stops bleeding	• prevents tumor growth	**Internal:** 10–15 drops one
• kills bacteria	• stops cellular mutations	to two times daily
• kills germs		**External:** Apply to affected
• kills fungi		area twice daily
• kills viruses		
• relieves diarrhea		
• reduces inflammation		
• relieves itching		

Family: Euphorbiaceae

Genus: *Croton*

Species: *lechleri, salutaris, draco*

Common Names: sangre de grado, sangre de drago, dragon's blood, drago, sangue de drago, sangue de agua

Parts Used: bark, resin/sap

Sangre de grado is a medium- to large-sized tree that grows from 10–20 m high in the upper Amazon region of Peru, Ecuador, and Colombia. Although tall, the trunk is usually less than 30 cm in diameter and is covered by smooth, mottled bark. It has large, heart-shaped, bright green leaves and unique, greenish-white flowers on long stalks. Its Peruvian name, *sangre de grado,* means "blood of the dragon" (in Spanish). In Ecuador, it's named *sangre de drago* (which means "dragon's blood" as well). When the trunk of the tree is cut or wounded, a dark red, sappy resin oozes out as if the tree is bleeding—earning this local name. The genus *Croton* is a large one, with 750 species of trees and shrubs distributed across the tropical and subtropical regions of both hemispheres. *Crotons* are rich in active alkaloids, and several species are well-known medicinal plants used as laxatives and tonics.

TRIBAL AND HERBAL MEDICINE USES

For centuries, the sangre de grado resin has been painted on wounds to stop bleeding, to accelerate healing, and to seal and protect injuries from infection. The sap dries quickly and forms a barrier, much like a "second skin."

Sangre de grado's red sap or latex (and also its bark) has a long history of indigenous use in the rainforest and in South America. The earliest written reference dates its use to the 1600s, when Spanish naturalist and explorer P. Bernabé Cobo found that the curative power of the sap was widely known throughout the indigenous tribes of Mexico, Peru, and Ecuador. For centuries, the sap has been painted on wounds to staunch bleeding, to accelerate healing, and to seal and protect injuries from infection. The sap dries quickly and forms a barrier, much like a "second skin." It is used externally by indigenous tribes and local people in Peru for wounds, fractures, and hemorrhoids, internally for intestinal and stomach ulcers, and as a douche for vaginal discharge. Other indigenous uses include treating intestinal fevers and inflamed or infected gums, in vaginal baths before and after childbirth, for hemorrhaging after childbirth, and for skin disorders.

Sangre de grado resin and bark are used in traditional medicine in South America today in much the same manner as indigenous ones. In Peruvian herbal medicine, it is recommended for hemorrhaging, as an antiseptic vaginal douche and, topically, for healing wounds. It is also used internally for ulcers in the mouth, throat, intestines, and stomach; as an antiviral for upper respiratory viruses, stomach viruses, and HIV; internally and externally for cancer and, topically, for skin disorders, insect bites, and stings. In Brazilian traditional medicine, the sap currently is used for wounds, hemorrhaging, diarrhea, mouth ulcers, and as a general tonic.

PLANT CHEMICALS

Sangre de grado resin or sap is a storehouse of phytochemicals, including proanthocyanidins (antioxidants), simple phenols, diterpenes, phytosterols, and biologically active alkaloids and lignans. Scientists have attributed many of the biologically active properties of the sap (especially its wound-healing capacity) to two main "active" constituents: an alkaloid named *taspine*, and a lignan named *dimethylcedrusine*.

Of course, botanists, herbalists, and naturopaths would disagree with such reductionist conclusions (and often do); in this particular case, the matter is actually proven by science. Noted author and ex-USDA economic botanist Dr. James Duke summed this up eloquently, saying,

> *I like the comments on dragon's blood, and would add one further note: in addition to the proanthocyanadins (including Pycnogenol) and taspine, there's another active ingredient—dimethylcedrusine. While each of these alone— dimethylcedrusine, Pycnogenol and taspine—was shown to effectively heal wounded rats (with squares of skin exfoliated, i.e., peeled off) by European scientists, the whole dragon's blood was shown to speed healing four times faster. The whole was better than the sum of its parts. Synergy makes the whole herb stronger; diversity makes the rainforest stronger.[1]*

While several chemicals in the resin have been scientifically documented with would-healing actions, the natural crude resin was shown to be four times more effective at healing wounds than any isolated chemical.

The taspine alkaloid from sangre de grado was first documented with anti-inflammatory actions in 1979.[2] In 1985, taspine was documented with anti-inflammatory, antitumorous (against sarcomas), and antiviral actions.[3]

The main plant chemicals in sangre de grado include alpha-calacorene, alpha-copaene, alpha-pinene, alpha-thujene, beta-caryophyllene, beta-elemene, beta-pinene, betaine, bincatriol, borneol, calamenene, camphene, catechins, cedrucine, crolechinic acid, cuparophenol, D-limonene, daucosterol, dihydrobenzofuran, dimethylcedrusine, dipentene, eugenol, euparophenol, gallocatechin, gamma-terpinene, gamma-terpineol, hardwickiic acid, isoboldine, korberin A and B, lignin, linalool, magnoflorine, methylthymol, myrcene, norisoboldine, p-cymene, proanthocyanidins, procyanidins, resin, tannin, taspine, terpinen-4-ol, and vanillin.

The wound-healing action of sangre de grado resin was first related to the taspine alkaloid in 1989.[4] Several later studies also concentrated on the wound-healing[5] and antitumorous properties of taspine.[6] The lignan dimethyl-cedrusine was isolated by scientists in 1993 and was shown to play a central role in sangre de grado's effective wound-healing action.[7] This Belgian study revealed that the crude resin stimulated contraction of wounds, helped in the formation of a crust/scab at the wound site, regenerated skin more rapidly, and assisted in the formation of new collagen. This was the study to which Dr. Duke referred in documenting that the crude resin was found to be four times more effective at wound healing and collagen formation than its isolated chemicals (and healed wounds ten to twenty times faster than using nothing at all).[7]

Sangre de grado's traditional use for wounds has been confirmed by scientists. In laboratory studies with animals the crude resin reportedly stimulated contraction of wounds, helped in the formation of a crust/scab at the wound site, regenerated skin more rapidly, and assisted in the formation of new collagen.

The Belgian scientists also determined that taspine was active against herpes virus in this study. In 1994 other phytochemicals were found, including phenolic compounds, proanthocyanadins, and diterpenes, which showed potent antibacterial activity (against *E. coli* and *Bacillus subtilis*) as well as wound-healing properties.[8] Another study documented sangre de grado's antioxidant effects[9] and researchers in Canada documented its antifungal properties.[10]

Another important traditional use of the sap was verified by clinical research in a 2000 study designed to evaluate its gastrointestinal effects. Researchers concluded that "Sangre de grado is a potent, cost-effective treatment for gastrointestinal ulcers and distress via antimicrobial, anti-inflammatory, and sensory afferent-dependent actions."[11] In 2002, these same researchers reported that sangre de grado evidenced an *in vitro* effect against stomach cancer and colon cancer cells as well.[12] In 2003, Italian researchers reported that the resin inhibited the growth of a human myelogenous leukemia cell line and also prevented cells from mutating in test tube studies.[13]

Extracts of sangre de grado have demonstrated antiviral activity against influenza, parainfluenza, herpes simplex viruses I and II, and hepatitis A and B.[7,8,14,15] The antiviral and anti-diarrhea properties of sangre de grado have come to the attention of the pharmaceutical industry over the last ten years. A U.S.-based pharmaceutical company has filed patents on three pharmaceutical preparations that contain antiviral constituents and novel chemicals (a group of plant flavonoids they've named SP-303), extracted from the bark and resin of sangre de grado. Their patented drugs include an oral product for the treatment of respiratory viral infections, a topical antiviral product for the treatment of herpes, and an oral product for the treatment of persistent diarrhea. These products have been the subject of various human clinical trials. Although the immunomodulating effects of sangre de grado have not been the subject of targeted research yet, some researchers believe that the anti-inflammatory, anti-microbial, and antioxidant activities may provide nonspecific immune enhancement effects as well.[16]

Sangre de grado resin and bark (as well as some of its chemicals) have been patented and made into prescription drugs for viruses, including herpes, upper respiratory viruses, and stomach viruses.

More recently, several scientific tests have been conducted on a proprietary sangre de grado product (made into a skin balm), which was also based on traditional uses. They reported that in pest control workers, a sangre de grado balm was preferred over placebo, for the relief of itching, pain, discomfort, swelling, and redness in response to wasps, fire ants, mosquitoes, bees, cuts, abrasions, and allergic plant reactions (poison ivy and others).[17] Subjects reported relief within minutes, and that it provided pain relief and alleviated symptoms (itching and swelling) for up to six hours. These reported effects in humans, as well as several other tests they conducted in animals and in vitro models of inflammation, led them to conclude that sangre de grado prevents pain sensation by blocking the activation of nerve fibers that relay pain signals to the brain (therefore functioning as a broad-acting pain killer), as well as blocking the tissue response to a chemical released by nerves that promotes inflammation.

CURRENT PRACTICAL USES

Research has confirmed many of the indigenous uses of this powerful rainforest plant. It is a wonderful, sustainable rainforest resource that warrants consumer attention as it becomes more widely available in the marketplace. Applied directly to the affected area, it is helpful for all types of cuts, scrapes, external wounds, bites, stings, rashes, and skin problems, including skin and nail fungi. James E. Williams, OMD, sums up sangre de grado's many uses by natural health practitioners, stating

> There is a wide range of potential applications for sangre de grado, including as a broad-spectrum anti-diarrheal agent from causes such as side effects of drugs, chemotherapy or radiation treatment, microbial infections of the intestine, traveler's diarrhea, and viral-induced diarrhea as in AIDS. It may also have other uses in gastrointestinal disorders such as irritable bowel syndrome and ulcerative diseases. Its cytotoxic effects make it a possible antitumor agent and its cicatrizant properties provide wound-healing potential. In addition, the antimicrobial and anti-inflammatory effects of sangre de grado make it a useful compound in the clinical treatment of chronic viral diseases and as a natural antibacterial agent.[15]

In addition, several health practitioners in the U.S. indicate benefits in using sangre de grado resin internally for diabetic neuropathy because of its previously documented effects on nerve endings, nerve pain, and nerve inflammation. Benefits have also been reported with diabetes-related skin ulcers and sores (applied topically), which have refused to heal using other methods.

Traditional Preparation For external use, the resin/sap is rubbed directly on the affected area several times daily and allowed to dry. Please note: the resin is red! It will temporarily stain the skin a reddish-brown (which will wash off), but it will permanently stain clothing. Rubbing the resin in the palm of the hand first or directly where applied will thicken the resin into a thin, lighter colored paste, which helps form a second skin on top of a wound or rash and reduces staining. For internal use, the traditional remedy is 10–15 drops in a small amount of liquid, taken one to three times daily (be prepared, however; it tastes quite dreadful).

Contraindications None reported.

Drug Interactions None reported.

Worldwide Ethnomedical Uses

Region	Uses
Brazil	for bacterial infections, blood cleansing, cancer, digestive disorders, fever, fungal infections, hemorrhages, stomach ulcers, tumors, ulcer (mouth), wounds, and for its astringent (drying) effects
Dominican Republic	for wounds, and to stop bleeding
Ecuador	for cancer, inflammation, wounds
Mexico	for fever, infected gums, wounds
Peru	for cancer, diabetes, diarrhea, eczema, fractures, fungal infections, gastrointestinal problems, hemorrhages, hemorrhoids, infected gums, infections, insect bites, laryngitis, rheumatism, skin cancer, skin rashes, throat problems, toothache, tumors, ulcers (intestinal, mouth, stomach), vaginal discharge, vaginal infections, vaginitis, wounds, and as an antiseptic
United States	for cancer, diabetic neuropathy, eczema, fungal infections (skin, nail, foot), hemorrhages, inflammation, insect bites, itching, pain, rashes, ulcers (intestinal, mouth, skin, stomach), wounds, and as an antiseptic

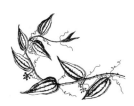

SARSAPARILLA
HERBAL PROPERTIES AND ACTIONS

Main Actions	Other Actions	Standard Dosage
• detoxifies organs	• relieves pain	Root
• cleanses blood	• kills fungus	**Decoction:** 1/2–1 cup two to three times daily
• aids absorption	• reduces inflammation	
• kills bacteria	• kills germs	**Tablets/Capsules:** 1–2 g twice daily
• stimulates digestion	• reduces fever	
• increases urination	• modulates immune system	**Tincture:** 2–3 ml twice daily
• protects liver	• kills free radicals	
• promotes perspiration	• relieves rheumatism	

Family: Smilacaceae

Genus: *Smilax*

Species: *officinalis, aristolochiaefolia, glabra, febrifuga, ornata, regelii, japicanga*

Common Names: sarsaparilla, salsaparrilha, khao yen, saparna, smilace, smilax, zarzaparilla, jupicanga

Part Used: root

Sarsaparilla is a brambly, woody vine that grows up to 50 m long, with paired tendrils for climbing (often high into the rainforest canopy). It produces small flowers and black, blue, or red berry-like fruits which are eaten greedily by birds. *Smilax,* a member of the lily family, is native to tropical and temperate parts of the world and comprises about 350 species worldwide. It is native to South America, Jamaica, the Caribbean, Mexico, Honduras, and the West Indies. The name *sarsaparilla* or *zarzaparilla* comes from the Spanish word *zarza* (bramble or bush), *parra* (vine), and *illa* (small)—a small, brambled vine.

The stems of many *Smilax* species are covered with stickers and, sometimes, these vines are cultivated to form impenetrable thickets (which are called *cat-briers* or *greenbriers*). The root, used for medicinal purposes, is long and tuberous—spreading 6–8 feet—and is odorless and fairly tasteless. Many species of *Smilax* around the world share the name *sarsaparilla;* these are very similar in appearance, uses, and even chemical structure. These include *S. officinalis, S. japicanga,* and *S. febrifuga* from South America (Brazil, Ecuador and Colombia); *S. regelii, S. aristolochiaefolia,* and *S. ornata* from Mexico and Latin America; and *S. glabra* from China. Sarsaparilla vine should not be confused with the large sasparilla and sassafras trees (the root and bark of which were once used to flavor root beer). While sarsaparilla has been used as an ingredient in root beer and other beverages, it is used for its foaming properties—not for its flavoring properties.

TRIBAL AND HERBAL MEDICINE USES

Sarsaparilla root has been used for centuries by the indigenous peoples of Central and South America for sexual impotence, rheumatism, skin ailments, and as a general tonic for physical weakness. It has long been used by tribes in Peru and Honduras for headaches and joint pain, and against the common cold. Many shamans and medicine men in the Amazon use sarsaparilla root internally and externally for leprosy and other skin problems (such as psoriasis and dermatitis). Leprosy can be common in areas where the disease is carried by armadillos (and in the Amazon, armadillos are "on the menu" in indigenous diets). Sarsaparilla root also was used as a general tonic by indigenous tribes in South America, where New World traders found it and introduced it into European medicine in the 1400s.

> Many shamans and medicine men in the Amazon use sarsaparilla root internally and externally for leprosy and other skin problems (such as psoriasis and dermatitis).

European physicians considered sarsaparilla root a tonic, blood purifier, diuretic, and sweat promoter. A *Smilax* root from Mexico was introduced into European medicine in 1536, where it developed a strong following as a cure for syphilis and rheumatism.[1] Since this time, *Smilax* roots have had a long history of use for syphilis and other sexually transmitted diseases throughout the world. With its reputation as a blood purifier, it was registered as an official herb in the *U.S. Pharmacopoeia* as a syphilis treatment from 1820 to 1910. From the 1500s to the present, sarsaparilla has been used as a blood purifier and general tonic and also has been used worldwide for gout, syphilis, gonorrhea, rheumatism, wounds, arthritis, fever, cough, scrofula, hypertension, digestive disorders, psoriasis, skin diseases, and cancer.

PLANT CHEMICALS

Sarsaparilla contains the plant steroids sarsasapogenin, smilagenin, sitosterol, stigmasterol, and pollinastanol; and the saponins sarsasaponin, smilasaponin, sarsaparilloside, and sitosterol glucoside, among others.[2] The majority of sarsaparilla's pharmacological properties and actions have been attributed to these steroids and saponins. The saponins have been reported to facilitate the body's absorption of other drugs and phytochemicals,[2,3] which accounts for its history of use in herbal formulas as an agent for bioavailability and to enhance the power and effect of other herbs.

> Sarsaparilla has been marketed (fraudulently) to contain testosterone and/or other anabolic steroids. While it is a rich source of natural plant steroids and saponins, it never has been proven to have any anabolic effects, nor has testosterone been found in sarsaparilla.

Saponins and plant steroids found in many species of plants (including sarsaparilla) can be synthesized into human steroids such as estrogen and testosterone. This synthesis has never been documented to occur in the human body—only in the laboratory. Yet, plant steroids and their actions in the human body have been a subject of much interest, sketchy research and, unfortunately, disinformation—mainly for marketing purposes. Sarsaparilla has been marketed (fraudulently) to contain testosterone and/or other anabolic steroids. While it is a rich source of natural plant steroids and saponins, it never has been proven to have any anabolic effects, nor has testosterone been found in sarsaparilla or any other plant source thus far.[2,4]

Flavonoids in sarsaparilla have been documented to have immune modulation and liver protective activities.[7] A U.S. patent was awarded in 2003 describing these flavonoids to be effective in treating autoimmune diseases and inflammatory reactions through their immunomodulating effects.[8] Sarsasapogenin and smilagenin were subjects of a 2001 U.S. patent which reported that these *Smilax* steroids had the ability to treat senile dementia, cognitive dysfunction, and Alzheimer's disease.[9] In the patent's animal studies references, smilagenin reversed the decline of brain receptors in aged mice and restored the receptor levels to those observed in young animals, reversed the decline in cognitive function, and enhanced memory and learning.[9] These studies, however, have not been published in any peer-reviewed journals—only in the context of the patent, thus far.

Sarsaparilla's main plant chemicals include acetyl-parigenin, astilbin, beta-sitosterol, caffeoyl-shikimic acids, dihydroquercetin, diosgenin, engeletin, essential oils, epsilon-sitosterol, eucryphin, eurryphin, ferulic acid, glucopyranosides, isoastilbin, isoengetitin, kaempferol, parigenin, parillin, pollinastanol, resveratrol, rhamnose, saponin, sarasaponin, sarsaparilloside, sarsaponin, sarsasapogenin, shikimic acid, sitosterol-d-glucoside, smilagenin, smilasaponin, smilax saponins A–C, smiglaside A–E, smitilbin, stigmasterol, taxifolin, and titogenin.

BIOLOGICAL ACTIVITIES AND CLINICAL RESEARCH

Clinical research has validated the traditional use of sarsaparilla for skin conditions such as psoriasis, eczema, acne, and leprosy. In 1942, it was reported in the *New England Journal of Medicine* to improve the condition of psoriasis dramatically. The results of a clinical study with ninety-two patients was detailed, which reported that it improved psoriasis lesions in 62 percent of cases and completely cleared lesions in 18 percent of cases.[10] One of the possible mechanisms of action in psoriasis is sarsaparilla's blood cleansing properties. Individuals with psoriasis have been found to have high levels of endotoxins circulating in the bloodstream (endotoxins are cell wall fragments of normal gut bacteria).[11] Sarsaponin, one of sarsaparilla's main steroids, was found to bind to these endotoxins and remove them, thus improving psoriasis.[10]

Laboratory studies suggest that sarsaparilla can bind to toxins and remove them from the blood—confirming its long standing traditional use as a blood purifier.

This endotoxin-binding action is probably why the root has been used for centuries as a "blood purifier." Other health conditions associated with high endotoxin levels include eczema, arthritis, and ulcerative colitis. Sarsaparilla's effective use in the treatment of leprosy has been documented in a 1959 human trial.[12] The effectiveness of sarsaparilla in the treatment of adolescent acne caused by excessive androgens has received some experimental support as well.[10]

A 2001 U.S. patent was filed on sarsaparilla (*Smilax china*) for psoriasis and respiratory diseases.[13] This patent cited clinical observations and studies with children and human adults with *Psoriasis vulgaris*, pustular psoriasis, erythroderma psoriaticum lesions, and associated itching—reporting marked clinical improvements with dosages of 3–6 g daily. It also reported that, upon discontinuation of sarsaparilla after only two months of treatment, there was further gradual remission of lesions and no side effects. In addition, this patent indicated sarsaparilla was shown to be a preventative and therapeutic agent for respiratory and allergic diseases such as acute bronchitis, bronchial asthma, asthmatic bronchitis, and chronic bronchitis. Again, these studies and observations reported in the patent have yet to be published in any peer-reviewed journals.

Sarsaparilla has long been used in the treatment of syphilis. Clinical observations in China demonstrated that sarsaparilla was effective (according to blood tests) in about 90 percent of acute and 50 percent of chronic cases.[2] In the 1950s the antibiotic properties of sarsaparilla were documented;[14,15] other studies documented its antifungal and antimycobacterial activities.[16,17] Its anti-inflammatory activity has been demonstrated in several *in vitro* and *in vivo* studies, using different laboratory-induced models of arthritis and inflammation.[18,19] One of these studies attributes the beneficial effect for arthritis to sarsaparilla's immune modulatory action.[19] Sarsaparilla also has demonstrated liver protective effects in rats, with researchers concluding that it is able to prevent immune-mediated liver injury.[7,8,20] Improvement of appetite and digestion has been noted with sarsaparilla, as well as its diuretic actions in humans.[21] The root has been reported to have stimulatory activity on the kidneys in humans and, in chronic nephritis, it was shown to increase the urinary excretion of uric acid.[22,23]

CURRENT PRACTICAL USES

Sarsaparilla is becoming more widely available in health food stores, with a variety of tablets, capsules, and tincture products sold today. Most of the sarsaparilla root in herbal commerce today comes from cultivation projects in Mexico and Latin America, as well as China. In naturopathic and herbal medicine, it is used mostly in combination with other herbs for its tonic, detoxifying, blood purifying, and lymph-cleansing properties. In retail stores and products, it can be found as an ingredient in various herbal remedies made for skin disorders, libido enhancement, hormone balancing, and sports nutrition formulas. It's also commonly used in herbal preparations as a synergist or bioavailability aid—as it is thought that the saponins in sarsaparilla root increase the absorption of other chemicals in the gut. No known toxicity or side effects have been documented for sarsaparilla; however, ingestion of large dosages of saponins may cause gastrointestinal irritation.[4,5,6]

Traditional Preparation

One-half to 1 cup of a standard root decoction is taken two to three times daily. Alternatively, 1–2 g of root powder in tablets or capsules twice daily, or 2–3 ml of a standard tincture or fluid extract may be taken twice daily.

Contraindications

Large doses may cause gastrointestinal upset.

Drug Interactions   Sarsaparilla may increase the absorption of some drugs and compounds. Some report that it can increase the absorption of digitalis drugs while accelerating the elimination of hypnotic drugs.[2]

Worldwide Ethnomedical Uses

Region	Uses
Argentina	for rheumatism, and to increase libido and perspiration
Brazil	for acne, anorexia, arthritis, blood purification, digestive disorders, eczema, fever, gallstones, gout, hives, kidney problems, kidney stones, impotence, leprosy, muscle weakness, psoriasis, rheumatism, sexually transmitted diseases, skin disorders, sterility, syphilis, ulcers, urinary insufficiency; and as an aphrodisiac, laxative, and to increase perspiration
China	for abscesses, arthritis, boils, cystitis, diarrhea, digestive disorders, dysentery, enteritis, fever, malaria, mercury poisoning, rheumatism, rheumatoid arthritis, skin problems, sores, syphilis, urinary insufficiency, and as an aphrodisiac and tonic
England	for abscesses, anorexia, antiseptic, blood cleansing, cancer, dysentery, eczema, fatigue, gout, immune enhancement, impotence, infections, inflammation, itching, leprosy, mercury poisoning, muscle weakness, premenstrual syndrome (PMS), psoriasis, rheumatism, rheumatoid arthritis, sexually transmitted diseases, skin problems, syphilis; and as an aphrodisiac, antiseptic, diuretic, tonic, and to increase perspiration
Europe	for arthritis, inflammation, kidney problems, psoriasis, rheumatism, sexually transmitted diseases, skin problems, sweat promotion, urinary disorders, urinary insufficiency
Latin America	for aches, acne, arthritis, colds, digestive disorders, fever, gout, impotence, pain, psoriasis, rheumatism, sexually transmitted diseases, skin problems, sweat promotion, syphilis, weakness, and as an aphrodisiac and tonic
Mexico	for arthritis, blood purification, burns, cancer, digestive disorders, dyspepsia, eczema, fever, gonorrhea, inflammation, leprosy, nephritis, rash, rheumatism, scrofula, sexually transmitted diseases, skin problems, syphilis, and to increase perspiration and urination
United States	for acne, arthritis, bladder problems, blood purification, burns, cancer, convalescence, coughs, diabetes, digestive disorders, eczema, eye infections, fatigue, fever, gonorrhea, gout, herpes, hives, hypertension, impotence, infertility, inflammation, itching, kidney problems, laxative, liver protection, pleurisy, premenstrual syndrome (PMS), psoriasis, rheumatism, scrofula, sexually transmitted diseases, shingles, skin problems, stomach disorders, stress, sweat promotion, syphilis, tuberculosis, ulcerative colitis, ulcers, urinary disorders, urinary insufficiency, vaginal discharge, warts, wounds, and as an expectorant
Elsewhere	for abscesses, arthritis, asthma, boils, burns, cancer, colds, conjunctivitis, cystitis, dysentery, dyspepsia, eczema, edema, epilepsy, gonorrhea, gout, herpes, impotence, inflammation, intestinal gas, kidney problems, leprosy, lymph inflammation, malaria, menstrual disorders, psoriasis, rashes, sexually transmitted diseases, stimulant, tonic, toothache, tumor, urogenital diseases, wounds; and as an aphrodisiac, stimulant, and tonic

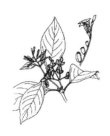

SCARLET BUSH
HERBAL PROPERTIES AND ACTIONS

Main Actions	Other Actions	Standard Dosage
• relieves pain	• reduces spasms	Leaves
• reduces inflammation	• kills parasites	**Infusion:** 1 cup two to three times daily
• heals wounds	• enhances immunity	
• kills bacteria	• increases urination	**Decoction:** Apply topically to affected area
• reduces fever		
• kills fungi		**Tincture:** 1–2 ml two to three times daily
• lowers body temperature		

Family: Rubiaceae

Genus: *Hamelia*

Species: *patens, erecta*

Common Names: scarlet bush, corail, ix-canan, koray, ponasi, polly red head, red head, sanalo-todo, uvero, hummingbird bush, firebush, Texas firecracker

Part Used: entire plant

Scarlet bush is a small, fast growing, semi-woody bush that can be found throughout South America including the Amazon basin. It grows up to 3 m in height and has red tinged, deeply veined leaves about 10–20 cm long. It produces a showy mass of tubular, bright reddish-orange flowers—earning its name of *scarlet bush* or *fire bush*. It also produces a showy fruit; the edible juicy berry turns from green to yellow, to red, and finally, black when ripe. In Mexico, the ripe berry is turned into wine. The plant is indigenous to most all of South America, the West Indies, Mexico, and even southern Florida.

Due to its beauty and adaptability from hot and dry climates to hot and humid climates, it has been gaining in popularity over the last few years as a landscape plant in parts of the lower United States, including Texas, Florida, and California. In Texas (the southern half), it makes a great 4–5 foot mound of bright red flowers from early summer until late fall; the leaves turn bright red in the fall before shedding, then it freezes to the ground in the winter and re-sprouts each spring. It can be found in southern plant nurseries these days being sold under such names as Texas firecracker bush, fire bush, polly red-head, and of course, scarlet bush. It makes a beautiful addition to any Southern garden and attracts butterflies and hummingbirds.

Scarlet bush belongs to the Madder family (Rubiaceae), to which another important rainforest plant belongs: cat's claw. Several of the same active chemicals can be found in both plants, and some of their traditional medicinal uses are similar as well.

TRIBAL AND HERBAL MEDICINE USES

Its Mayan name, *Ix-canan*, means "guardian of the forest." Indigenous people in Belize use the plant to prepare a natural remedy to treat all types of skin problems including sores, rashes, wounds, burns, itching, cuts, skin fungus, and insect stings and bites. The remedy is prepared by boiling a double handful of leaves, stems, and flowers in two gallons of water for ten minutes.

After it cools, it's applied liberally to the affected area. This same remedy is also drunk as a tea to relieve menstrual cramps. The Choc Indians in Panama drink a leaf infusion for fever and bloody diarrhea; the Ingano Indians of northwest Amazonia prepare a leaf infusion for intestinal parasites. Indigenous tribes in Venezuela chew on the leaves to lower body temperature to prevent a sun or heat stroke. In the Peruvian Amazon, the leaves are used by the indigenous people for dysentery, fevers, rheumatism, and scurvy. Leaves are also warmed or prepared into a poultice and applied externally as a pain-reliever for bruises, strains, sprains, and other painful or inflamed conditions.

In some parts of Latin America, scarlet bush is a common topical remedy for sores, rashes, wounds, burns, itching, cuts, skin fungus, and insect stings and bites. Farther South, the leaves are used to lower body temperature to prevent a sun or heat stroke.

In Peruvian herbal medicine systems today, the scarlet bush is used to reduce inflammation, relieve pain, and to expel intestinal worms. It is also used there for dysentery, fevers, itchy conditions, skin diseases, rheumatism, parasites, and scurvy. In Brazil, the root is used as a diuretic, while the leaves are used for scabies and headaches. In Latin American herbal medicine systems, scarlet bush is widely used for many affections including skin problems, diarrhea, fever, postpartum pain, and menstrual disorders. In Cuba, the leaves are used externally for headaches and sores while a decoction is taken internally for rheumatism. In Mexico, it is widely used externally to staunch the flow of blood and heal wounds.

PLANT CHEMICALS

Scarlet bush is rich in active phytochemicals including alkaloids and flavonoids. It contains several of the same oxindole alkaloids as cat's claw (*Uncaria tomentosa*) including *pteropodine* and *isopteropodine;* both have been highly studied and even patented as effective immune stimulants.[1,2] These two chemicals have also recently shown to have a positive modulating effect on brain neurotransmitters (called 5-HT(2) receptors)[3] that are targets for drugs used in treating a variety of conditions including depression, anxiety, eating disorders, chronic pain conditions, and obesity.[4] Three new oxindole alkaloids have also been discovered in scarlet bush which have never been classified before; they've been named *Hamelia patens* alkaloid A, B, and C.[5] Scientists in India discovered that scarlet bush leaves contain small amounts (0.05 percent) of ephedrine—a stimulant alkaloid that has received some negative press.[6] In addition, the aerial parts of the plant have been found to contain rosmarinic acid, a phytochemical that has demonstrated immune modulating and antidepressant activity.[7–9]

Scarlet bush contains two of the alkaloid chemicals for which cat's claw (another famous rainforest plant) is well known. These two chemicals have been patented as effective immune stimulants.

The main plant chemicals documented in scarlet bush thus far include apigenin, ephedrine, flavanones, isomaruquine, isopteropodine, maruquine, narirutins, oxindole alkaloids, palmirine, pteropodine, rosmarinic acid, rumberine, rutin, seneciophylline, speciophylline, and tannin.

BIOLOGICAL ACTIVITIES AND CLINICAL RESEARCH

Much of the clinical research on scarlet bush has validated the traditional uses of the plant. In animal studies (with rats), scarlet bush leaf extracts demonstrated analgesic, diuretic, and hypothermic actions.[10] External use of the leaf in mice showed significant anti-inflammatory activity comparable to that of a prescription anti-inflammatory drug used as a control.[11] Scientists in two different countries have documented scarlet bush's antibacterial and antifungal properties against a wide range of fungi and bacteria in several *in vitro* studies.[12–14] The plant has also been documented with diuretic effects and was shown to inhibit the growth of tumor and bacteria cells.[10,15]

CURRENT PRACTICAL USES

A decoction or infusion of the leaves of scarlet bush is generally used internally or externally for bacterial and fungal infections, as well as for its anti-inflammatory and pain-reducing properties. Typically, if the remedy is taken internally, an infusion is employed; a leaf decoction is prepared for external use. Try planting a beautiful scarlet bush in the garden—while working in the garden on hot days, chew on one of the leaves like the rainforest Indians do; it has remarkable hypothermic/cooling actions, which will help keep the body from overheating.

The use of this plant in herbal medicine systems has been reported to be safe and non-toxic when taken orally at the traditional remedy dosages. Only one of the animal studies published thus far indicated toxicity: when they injected a methanol extract of scarlet bush leaves into mice at high dosages (1.5 g per kg of body weight).[10]

Traditional Preparation

One cup of a standard decoction or leaf infusion is taken two to three times daily. If desired, 1–2 ml of a 4:1 alcohol tincture can be substituted. A decoction of the leaves is also applied topically to wounds, rashes, burns, and skin fungus, and is widely used in the tropics to stop wounds from bleeding.

Contraindications

None known.

Drug Interactions

None known.

Worldwide Ethnomedical Uses

Region	Uses
Amazonia	for cancer, cholera, constipation, diarrhea, dysentery, erysipelas, fever, headaches, jaundice, malaria, scurvy, skin disorders, sores, wounds
Belize	for burns, cuts, fungal infections, insect bites and stings, itch, menstrual cramps, rashes, skin problems, sores, wounds

Brazil	for headaches, scabies
Costa Rica	for migraines
Cuba	for headaches, rheumatism, sores
Guatemala	for dysentery, menstrual disorders
Haiti	for abortions, anemia, headaches, menstrual disorders, nervous shock, rage
Mexico	for skin problems, sores, wounds (bleeding)
Panama	for bites (snake and insect), diarrhea, fever, postpartum pain
Peru	for blood cleansing, constipation, dysentery, fever, inflammation, itching, pain, pharyngitis, rheumatism, scurvy, skin problems, worms, wounds
Venezuela	for headaches, jaundice, sunstroke, syphilis
Elsewhere	for cancer, constipation, diarrhea, dysentery, erysipelas, fever, fungal infections, headaches, insect bites, jaundice, malaria, menstrual disorders, migraine, ovarian disorders, pain, rheumatism, skin problems, uterine disorders

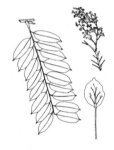

Family: Simaroubaceae

Genus: *Simarouba*

Species: *amara, glauca*

Common Names: simarouba, gavilan, negrito, marubá, marupá, dysentery bark, bitterwood, paradise tree, palo blanco, robleceillo, caixeta, daguilla, cedro blanco, cajú-rana, malacacheta, palo amargo, pitomba, bois amer, bois blanc, bois frene, bois negresse, simaba

Parts Used: bark, wood, leaves

SIMAROUBA

HERBAL PROPERTIES AND ACTIONS

Main Actions
- kills parasites
- kills amebas
- kills bacteria
- kills viruses
- relieves dysentery
- kills leukemia cells
- treats malaria
- reduces tumor growth
- expels worms

Other Actions
- relieves pain
- reduces fever
- promotes menstruation
- hydrates skin
- promotes perspiration

Standard Dosage
Bark

Decoction: 1 cup two to three times daily

Tincture: 5–10 ml twice daily

Simarouba is a medium-sized tree that grows up to 20 m high, with a trunk 50–80 cm in diameter. It produces bright green leaves 20–50 cm in length, small white flowers, and small red fruits. It is indigenous to the Amazon rainforest and other tropical areas in Mexico, Cuba, Haiti, Jamaica, and Central America.

TRIBAL AND HERBAL MEDICINE USES

The leaves and bark of simarouba have long been used as a natural medicine in the tropics. Simarouba was first imported into France from Guyana in 1713 as a remedy for dysentery. When France suffered a dysentery epidemic from 1718 to 1725, simarouba bark was one of the few effective treatments.[1] French explorers "discovered" this effective remedy when they found that the indigenous Indian tribes in the Guyana rainforest used simarouba bark as an effective treatment for malaria and dysentery—much as they still do today. Other indigenous tribes throughout the South American rainforest use simarouba bark for fevers, malaria, and dysentery, as a hemostatic agent to stop bleeding, and as a tonic.

Simarouba goes by the common name of "dysentery bark" in several countries. It has been used for several centuries as an effective natural remedy for amebic dysentery and diarrhea.

Simarouba also has a long history in herbal medicine in many other countries. In Cuba, where it is called *gavilan,* an infusion of the leaves or bark is considered to be astringent, a digestion and menstrual stimulant, and an antiparasitic remedy. It is taken internally for diarrhea, dysentery, malaria, and colitis; it is used externally for wounds and sores. In Belize, the tree is called *negrito* or *dysentery bark.* There the bark (and occasionally the root) is boiled in water to yield a powerful astringent and tonic used to wash skin sores and to treat dysentery, diarrhea, stomach and bowel disorders, hemorrhages, and internal bleeding. In Brazil, it is employed much the same way against fever, malaria, diarrhea, dysentery, intestinal parasites, indigestion, and anemia. In Brazilian herbal medicine, simarouba bark tea has long been the most highly recommended (and most effective) natural remedy against chronic and acute dysentery.

PLANT CHEMICALS

The main active group of chemicals in simarouba are called *quassinoids,* which belong to the triterpene chemical family. Quassinoids are found in many plants and are well known to scientists. The antiprotozoal and antimalarial properties of these chemicals have been documented for many years. Several of the quassinoids found in simarouba, such as ailanthinone, glaucarubinone, and holacanthone, are considered the plant's main therapeutic constituents and are the ones documented to be antiprotozal, antiamebic, antimalarial, and even toxic to cancer and leukemia cells.

The main plant chemicals in simarouba include ailanthinone, benzoquinone, canthin, dehydroglaucarubinone, glaucarubine, glaucarubolone, glaucarubinone, holacanthone, melianone, simaroubidin, simarolide, simarubin, simarubolide, sitosterol, and tirucalla.

BIOLOGICAL ACTIVITIES AND CLINICAL RESEARCH

After a two hundred-year documented history of use for dysentery, its use for amebic dysentery was finally validated by conventional doctors in 1918. A military hospital in England demonstrated that the bark tea was an effective treatment for amebic dysentery in humans.[2] The Merck Institute reported that simarouba was 91.8 percent effective against intestinal amebas in humans in a 1944 study[3] and, in 1962, other researchers found that the seeds of simarouba showed active anti-amebic activities in humans.[4] In the 1990s, scientists again documented simarouba's ability to kill the most common dysentery-causing organism, *Entamoeba histolytica*,[5] as well as two diarrhea-causing bacteria, *Salmonella* and *Shigella*.[6]

Scientists first looked at simarouba's antimalarial properties in 1947, when they determined a water extract of the bark (as well as the root) demonstrated strong activity against malaria in chickens.[7] This study showed that doses of only 1 mg of bark extract per kg of body weight exhibited strong antimalarial activity. When new strains of malaria began to develop with resistance to our existing antimalarial drugs, scientists began studying simarouba once again.

Studies published between 1988 and 1997 demonstrated that simarouba and/or its three potent quassinoids were effective against malaria *in vitro* as well as *in vivo*.[5,8–13] More importantly, the research indicated that the plant and its chemicals were effective against the new drug-resistant strains *in vivo* and *in vitro*. While most people in North America will never be exposed to malaria, between 300 and 500 million cases of malaria occur each year in the world, leading to more than 1 million deaths annually. Having an easily grown tree in the tropics (where most malaria occurs) is an important resource for an effective natural remedy—it certainly has worked for the Indians in the Amazon for ages.

It will be interesting to see if North American scientists investigate simarouba as a possibility for North America's only malaria-like disease—the newest mosquito-borne threat, West Nile virus. It might be a good one to study because, in addition to its antimalarial properties, clinical research has shown good antiviral properties with simarouba bark. Researchers in 1978 and again in 1992 confirmed strong antiviral properties of the bark *in vitro* against herpes, influenza, polio, and vaccinia viruses.[14,15]

Another area of research on simarouba and its plant chemicals has focused on cancer and leukemia. The quassinoids responsible for the antiamebic and antimalarial properties have also shown in clinical research to possess active cancer-killing properties. Early cancer screening performed by the National Cancer Institute in 1976 indicated that an alcohol extract of simarouba root (and a water extract of its seeds) had toxic actions against cancer cells at very low dosages (less than 20 mcg/ml).[16] Following up on that initial screening, scientists discovered that several of the quassinoids in simarouba (glaucarubinone, alianthinone, and dehydroglaucarubinone) had antileukemic actions against lymphocytic leukemia *in vitro* and published several studies in 1977 and 1978.[17–19] Researchers found that yet another simarouba quassinoid, holacanthone, also possessed antileukemic and antitumorous actions in 1983.[20] Researchers in the United Kingdom cited the antitumorous activity of two of the quassinoids, ailanthinone and glaucarubinone, against human epidermoid carcinoma of the pharynx.[5] A later study in 1998 by U.S. researchers demonstrated the antitumorous activity of glaucarubinone against solid tumors (human and mouse cell lines), multi-drug-resistant mammary tumors in mice, and antileukemic activity against leukemia in mice.[21]

Simarouba is the subject of one U.S. patent so far and, surprisingly, it's not for its antimalarial, antiamebic, or even anticancerous actions. Rather, water extracts of simarouba were found to increase skin keratinocyte differentiation and to improve skin hydration and moisturization.[22] In 1997, a patent was filed on its use to produce a cosmetic or pharmaceutical skin product. The patent describes simarouba extract as having significant skin depigmentation activity (for liver spots), enhancing the protective function of the skin (which maintains better moisturization), and having a significant keratinocyte differentiation activity (which protects against scaly skin).[23]

CURRENT PRACTICAL USES

While at least one scientific research group attempts to synthesize one or more of simarouba's potent quassinoids for pharmaceutical use, the plant remains an important natural remedy in the herbal pharmacopoeias of many tropical countries, and in the rainforest shaman's arsenal of potent plant remedies. Natural health practitioners outside of South America are just beginning to learn about the properties and actions of this important rainforest medicinal plant and how to use it in their own natural health practices.

Simarouba bark tea is still the first line of defense for amebic dysentery and diarrhea among the natural products available. It is also a good natural remedy for viruses. Although not widely available in the U.S. today, it can be found in bulk supplies and in various natural multi-herb anti-parasite and antiviral formulas.

Traditional Preparation

For diarrhea or dysentery, the traditional remedy calls for preparing a standard decoction with the bark. A teacup full (about 6 ounces) is taken two to three times daily. If desired, 5–10 ml of a bark tincture twice daily can be substituted.

Contraindications

None reported. Reported side effects at high dosages (approximately three times the traditional remedy) include increased perspiration and urination, nausea, and/or vomiting.

Drug Interactions

None reported.

Worldwide Ethnomedical Uses

Region	Uses
Amazonia	for bleeding, constipation, dysentery, fever, malaria
Belize	for bowel disorders, diarrhea, dysentery, excessive menstruation, hemorrhages, internal bleeding, skin, sores, stomach disorders, wounds
Brazil	for anemia, anorexia, diarrhea, dysentery, dyspepsia, fever, hemorrhages, intestinal parasites, malaria, and as a bitter digestive aid
Cuba	for bleeding, colitis, diarrhea, digestive sluggishness, dysentery, malaria, menstrual disorders, parasites, sores, wounds
Dominican Republic	for colic, diarrhea, gonorrhea, malaria
El Salvador	for amebic infections, digestive stimulation
Haiti	for aches (body), anemia, dysentery, dyspepsia, fever, menstrual disorders, pain, rheumatism, skin problems, and to increase perspiration
Mexico	for amebic infections, dyspepsia, fever, malaria
Peru	for diarrhea, dysentery, fever, intestinal gas, malaria, stomach pains
Elsewhere	for bleeding, colds, diarrhea, dysentery, fever, malaria

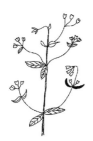

Family: Asteraceae

Genus: *Stevia*

Species: *rebaudiana*

Common Names: stevia, sweet leaf of Paraguay, caa-he-é, kaa jheé, ca-a-jhei, ca-a-yupi, azucacaa, eira-caa, capim doce, erva doce, sweet-herb, honey yerba, honey-leaf, yaa waan, candy leaf

Part Used: leaves

STEVIA
HERBAL PROPERTIES AND ACTIONS

Main Actions
- naturally sweetens
- lowers blood sugar
- increases urination
- lowers blood pressure
- dilates blood vessels

Other Actions
- kills bacteria
- kills fungi
- kills viruses
- reduces inflammation

Standard Dosage
Leaves

Ground leaves: $1/4$ tsp. substitutes 1 tsp. sugar

Infusion: 1 cup two to three times daily

Stevia is a perennial shrub that grows up to 1 m tall and has leaves 2–3 cm long. It belongs to the Aster family, which is indigenous to the northern regions of South America. Stevia is still found growing wild in the highlands of the Amambay and Iguacu districts (a border area between Brazil and Paraguay). It is estimated that as many as 200 species of Stevia are native to South America; however, no other *Stevia* plants have exhibited the same intensity of sweetness as *S. rebaudiana*.[1] It is grown commercially in many parts of Brazil, Paraguay, Uruguay, Central America, Israel, Thailand, and China.

TRIBAL AND HERBAL MEDICINE USES

For hundreds of years, indigenous peoples in Brazil and Paraguay have used the leaves of stevia as a sweetener. The Guarani Indians of Paraguay call it *kaa jheé* and have used it to sweeten their yerba mate tea for centuries. They have also used stevia to sweeten other teas and foods and have used it medicinally as a cardiotonic, for obesity, hypertension, and heartburn, and to help lower uric acid levels.

In addition to being a sweetener, stevia is considered (in Brazilian herbal medicine) to be hypoglycemic, hypotensive, diuretic, cardiotonic, and tonic. The leaf is used for diabetes, obesity, cavities, hypertension, fatigue, depression, sweet cravings, and infections. The leaf is employed in traditional medical systems in Paraguay for the same purposes as in Brazil.

Europeans first learned about stevia in the sixteenth century, when *conquistadores* sent word to Spain that the natives of South America were using the plant to sweeten herbal tea. Since then, stevia has been used widely throughout Europe and Asia. In the United States, herbalists use the leaf for diabetes, high blood pressure, infections, and as a sweetening agent. In Japan and Brazil, stevia is approved as a food additive and sugar substitute.

PLANT CHEMICALS

Western interest in stevia began around the turn of the nineteenth century, when researchers in Brazil started hearing about a plant with leaves so sweet that just one leaf would sweeten a whole gourd full of bitter yerba mate tea. It was first studied in 1899 by Paraguayan botanist Moises S. Bertoni, who wrote some of the earliest articles on stevia (in the early 1900s).

Over 100 phytochemicals have been discovered in stevia since. It is rich in terpenes and flavonoids. The constituents responsible for stevia's sweetness were documented in 1931, when eight novel plant chemicals called *glycosides* were discovered and named.[2] Of these eight glycosides, one called *stevioside* is considered the sweetest—and has been tested to be approximately 300 times sweeter than sugar.[3,4] Stevioside, comprising 6–18 percent of the stevia leaf, is also the most prevalent glycoside in the leaf. Other sweet constituents include steviolbioside, rebausiosides A–E, and dulcoside A.[2]

Chemicals in stevia are 300 times sweeter than sugar.

The main plant chemicals in stevia include apigenin, austroinulin, avicularin, beta-sitosterol, caffeic acid, campesterol, caryophyllene, centaureidin, chlorogenic acid, chlorophyll, cosmosiin, cynaroside, daucosterol, diterpene glycosides, dulcosides A–B, foeniculin, formic acid, gibberellic acid, gibberellin, indole-3-acetonitrile, isoquercitrin, isosteviol, jhanol, kaempferol, kaurene, lupeol, luteolin, polystachoside, quercetin, quercitrin, rebaudioside A–F, scopoletin, sterebin A–H, steviol, steviolbioside, steviolmonoside, stevioside, stevioside a-3, stigmasterol, umbelliferone, and xanthophylls.

BIOLOGICAL ACTIVITIES AND CLINICAL RESEARCH

The great interest in stevia as a non-caloric, natural sweetener has fueled many studies on it—including toxicological ones. The main sweet chemical, stevioside, has been found to be nontoxic in acute toxicity studies with rats, rabbits, guinea pigs, and birds.[4] It also has been shown not to cause cellular changes (mutagenic) or to have any effect on fertility.[4-6] The natural stevia leaf also has been found to be nontoxic[7] and has no mutagenic activity.[8] Studies conflict as to the effect of stevia leaf on fertility. The majority of clinical studies show stevia leaf to have no effect on fertility in both males and females.[9-12] In one study, however, a water extract of the leaf was shown to reduce testosterone levels and sperm count in male rats.[13]

Animal studies indicate that stevia can lower blood pressure and blood sugar levels.

Brazilian scientists recorded stevioside's ability to lower systemic blood pressure in rats in 1991.[14] Then, in 2000, a double-blind, placebo-controlled study was undertaken with 106 Chinese hypertensive men and women. Sixty subjects were given capsules containing stevioside (250 mg) or placebo thrice daily, and followed up at monthly intervals for one year. After three months, the systolic and diastolic blood pressure of the stevioside group decreased significantly and the effect persisted over the whole year.[15] The researchers concluded, "This study shows that oral stevioside is a well tolerated and effective modality that may be considered as an alternative or supplementary therapy for patients with hypertension."[15] Another team of scientists tested the hypoglycemic effects of the individual glycoside chemicals in stevia and attributed the effect on glucose production to the glycosides steviol, isosteviol, and glucosilsteviol.[16] The main sweetening glycoside, stevioside, did not produce this effect.[16] Researchers in Denmark published a study (in 2000) which demonstrated that the *in vitro* hypoglycemic actions of stevioside and steviol are a result of their ability to stimulate insulin secretion via a direct action on beta cells. They concluded, "Results indicate that the compounds may have a potential role as antihyperglycemic agents in the treatment of type 2 diabetes mellitus."[17]

Stevia's effects and uses as a heart tonic to normalize blood pressure levels, to regulate heartbeat, and for other cardiopulmonary indications first were reported in rat studies (in 1978).[18,19] Following these studies, a crude extract of stevia demonstrated hypotensive activity in a 1996 clinical study with rats, showing that "at dosages higher than used for sweetening purposes, [stevia extract] is a vasodilator agent in normo- and hypertensive animals."[20] In humans, a hot water extract of the leaf has been shown to lower both systolic and diastolic blood pressure.[21] Several earlier studies on both stevia extracts, as well as its isolated glycosides, demonstrated this hypotensive action (as well as a diuretic action).[22,23] In hypertensive rats, the leaf extract increased renal plasma flow, urinary flow, sodium excretion, and filtration rate.[20]

In addition to its studied hypotensive effects, a Brazilian research group demonstrated that water extracts of stevia leaves had a hypoglycemic effect and increased glucose tolerance in humans, reporting that it "significantly decreased plasma glucose levels during the test and after overnight fasting in all volunteers."[24] In another human study, blood sugar was reduced by 35 percent six to eight hours after oral ingestion of a hot water extract of the leaf.[25]

In other research, stevia has demonstrated antimicrobial,[26] antibacterial,[27,28] antiviral,[29] and anti-yeast activity.[30] A water extract was shown to help prevent dental cavities by inhibiting the bacteria *Streptococcus mutans* that stimulates plaque formation.[31] Additionally, a U.S. patent was filed in 1993 on an extract of stevia that claimed it to have vasodilatory activity and deemed it effective for various skin diseases (acne, heat rash, pruritis) and diseases caused by blood circulation insufficiency.[32]

CURRENT PRACTICAL USES

For nearly twenty years, millions of consumers in Japan and Brazil, where stevia is approved as a food additive, have been using stevia extracts as safe, natural, non-caloric sweeteners. Japan is the largest consumer of stevia leaves and extracts in the world, and there it is used to sweeten everything from soy sauce to pickles, confections, and soft drinks. Even multinational giants like Coca-Cola and Beatrice Foods use stevia extracts to sweeten foods (as a replacement for NutraSweet™ and saccharin) for sale in Japan, Brazil, and other countries where it is approved as a food additive. Not so in the United States, however, where stevia is specifically prohibited from use as a sweetener or as a food additive. Why? Many people believe that the national non-caloric sweetener giants have been successful in preventing this all-natural, inexpensive, and non-patentable sweetener from being used to replace their patented, synthetic, more expensive sweetener products.

Today, stevia leaves and leaf extracts are commonly found in most health food stores; however, they may only be sold in the United States as dietary/herbal supplements, not as food additives or sweeteners. In fact, in 1991 the Food and Drug Administration (FDA) even banned all imports of stevia into the country.[33] This political move was viewed by many to have monetary ties to the sweetener industry, which stood to lose a lot—and it created a huge public outcry in the natural products industry. The import ban was lifted in 1995 after much lobbying led by the American Herbal Products Association and other industry leaders. This allowed stevia to be sold as a dietary supplement under legislation called the Dietary Supplement Health and Education Act of 1994. The FDA, in one of its more politically incorrect debacles, has ruled that stevia is presumed safe as a dietary supplement but is considered unsafe as a food additive. This incongruity openly protects the profit margins of the "sweetener giants." In the words of Rob McCaleb, president of the Herb Research Foundation and member of the President's Commission on Dietary Supplements, "The FDA may have painted itself into a corner on this one. Its policy simply makes no sense."[34]

Traditional Preparation In the United States stevia is mostly employed as a sugar substitute. About ¼ teaspoon of the natural ground leaves (or one whole leaf) is the equivalent to about 1 teaspoon of sugar. In South America, a standard infusion is sometimes used as a natural aid for diabetes and hypertension; 1 cup is taken two to three times daily.

Contraindications Stevia leaf (at dosages higher than used for sweetening purposes) has been documented to have a hypoglycemic effect. Those with diabetes should use high amounts of stevia with caution and monitor their blood sugar levels, as medications may need adjusting.

Stevia leaf has been documented to have a hypotensive, or blood-pressure-lowering effect (at dosages higher than used for sweetening purposes). Persons with low blood pressure and those taking antihypertensive drugs should avoid using large amounts of stevia, and monitor their blood pressure levels accordingly for these possible effects.

Drug Interactions In large amounts, stevia may potentiate antihypertensive and antidiabetic medications.

Worldwide Ethnomedical Uses

Region	Uses
Brazil	for cavities, depression, diabetes, fatigue, heart support, hyperglycemia, hypertension, infections, obesity, sweet cravings, tonic, urinary insufficiency, wounds, and as a sweetener
Paraguay	for diabetes, and as a sweetener
South America	for diabetes, hypertension, infections, obesity, and as a sweetener
United States	for *Candida,* diabetes, hyperglycemia, hypertension, infections, and as a sweetener and vasodilator

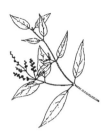

SUMA		
HERBAL PROPERTIES AND ACTIONS		
Main Actions	Other Actions	Standard Dosage
• supports hormones	• inhibits blood sickling	Root
• adaptogenic	• lowers cholesterol	**Decoction:** 1 cup twice daily
• relieves pain	• calms nerves	
• reduces inflammation	• inhibits tumor growth	**Tablets/Capsules:** 1–2 g twice daily
• inhibits cancer	• increases libido	
• kills leukemia cells	• oxygenates cells	
• enhances immunity		

Family: Amaranthaceae

Genus: *Pfaffia*

Species: *paniculata*

Common Names: suma, Brazilian ginseng, pfaffia, para toda, corango-acu

Part Used: root

TRIBAL AND HERBAL MEDICINE USES

In modern Brazilian herbal medicine practices, suma root is employed to increase oxygen to cells and taken to stimulate appetite and blood circulation, increase estrogen production, balance blood sugar levels, enhance the immune system, strengthen the muscular system, and enhance memory.

Suma is a large, rambling, shrubby ground vine with an intricate, deep, and extensive root system. It is indigenous to the Amazon basin and other tropical parts of (southern) Brazil, Ecuador, Panama, Paraguay, Peru, and Venezuela. Since its first botanical recording in 1826, it has been referred to by several botanical names, including *Pfaffia paniculata*, *Hebanthe paniculata*, and *Gomphrena paniculata*. The genus *Pfaffia* is well known in Central and South America, with over fifty species growing in the warmer tropical regions.

In South America, suma is known as *para toda* (which means "for all things") and as *Brazilian ginseng*, since it is widely used as an adaptogen with many applications (much as "regular" ginseng). The indigenous peoples of the Amazon region who named it *para toda* have used suma root for generations for a wide variety of health purposes, including as a general tonic; as an energy, rejuvenating, and sexual tonic; and as a general cure-all for many types of illnesses. Suma has been used as an aphrodisiac, a calming agent, and to treat ulcers for at least 300 years. It is an important herbal remedy in the folk medicine of several rainforest Indian tribes today.

In herbal medicine throughout the world today, suma is considered a tonic and an adaptogen. The herbal definition of an *adaptogen* is a plant that increases the body's resistance to adverse influences by a wide range of physical, chemical, and biochemical factors and has a normalizing or restorative effect on the body as a whole. In modern Brazilian herbal medicine practices, suma root is employed as a cellular oxygenator and taken to stimulate appetite and circulation, increase estrogen production, balance blood sugar levels, enhance the immune system, strengthen the muscular system, and enhance memory.

In North American herbal medicine, suma root is used as an adaptogenic and regenerative tonic regulating many systems of the body; as an immunostimulant; to treat exhaustion and chronic fatigue, impotence, arthritis, anemia, diabetes, cancer, tumors, mononucleosis, high blood pressure, PMS, menopause, hormonal disorders, and many types of stress. In herbal medicine in Ecuador today, suma is considered a tonic and "normalizer" for the cardiovascular system, the central nervous system, the reproductive system, and the digestive system; it is used to treat hormonal disorders, sexual dysfunction and sterility, arteriosclerosis, diabetes, circulatory and digestive disorders, rheumatism, and bronchitis. Thomas Bartram, in his book *Encyclopedia of Herbal Medicine*, reports that suma is used in Europe to restore nerve and glandular functions; to balance the endocrine system; to strengthen the immune system; for infertility; for menopausal and menstrual symptoms; to minimize the side effects of birth control medications; for high cholesterol; to neutralize toxins; and as a general restorative tonic after illness.

PLANT CHEMICALS

Nutritionally, suma root contains nineteen different amino acids, a large number of electrolytes, trace minerals, iron, magnesium, zinc, and vitamins A, B_1, B_2, E, K, and pantothenic acid.[2] Its high germanium content probably accounts for its properties as an oxygenator at the cellular level; its high iron content may account for its traditional use for anemia. The root also contains novel phytochemicals including saponins, pfaffic acids, glycosides, and nortriterpenes.

Suma has also been called "the Russian secret," as it has been taken by Russian Olympic athletes for many years and has been reported to increase muscle building and endurance, without the side effects associated with steroids. This action is attributed to an anabolic-type phytochemical called *beta-ecdysterone* and three novel ecdysteroid glycosides that are found in high amounts in suma.[1,2] Suma is such a rich source of beta-ecdysterone; the subject of a Japanese patent is for the extraction methods employed to obtain it from suma root (approximately 2.5 g of beta-ecdysterone can be extracted from 400 g of powdered suma root—or .63 percent).[3] These same Japanese researchers filed a U.S. patent in 1998 for a proprietary extract of suma (which extracted the ecdysterone and beta-ecdysterone); it claimed (through various *in vivo* and *in vitro* studies) that their compound maintained health, enhanced the immune system, and had a tonic and an anti-allergenic effect.[4] A French company also filed a U.S. patent on the topical use of these ecdysterone chemicals, claiming that their suma ecdysterone extract strengthened the water barrier function of the skin, increased skin keratinocyte differentiation (which would be helpful for psoriasis), gave the skin a smoother, softer appearance, and also improved hair appearance.

Suma root has a very high saponin content (up to 11 percent).[6] In phytochemistry, plant saponins are well known to have a wide spectrum of activities

> Suma has been called "the Russian secret," as it has been taken by Russian Olympic athletes for many years and has been reported to increase muscle building and endurance, without the side effects associated with steroids.

including lowering blood cholesterol, inhibiting cancer cell growth, and acting as antifungal and antibacterial agents. They are also known as natural detergent and foaming agents. Phytochemists report that saponins can act by binding with bile acids and cholesterol. It is thought that these chemicals "clean" or purge these fatty compounds from the body (thus lowering blood cholesterol levels). One of the most famous plant saponins is digitalis, derived from the common foxglove garden plant, which has been used as a heart drug for over 100 years.

The specific saponins found in the roots of suma include a group of novel phytochemicals that scientists have named *pfaffosides*. These saponins have clinically demonstrated the ability to inhibit cultured tumor cell melanomas (*in vitro*) and help to regulate blood sugar levels (*in vivo*).[7-9] The pfaffosides and pfaffic acid derivatives in suma were patented as anti-tumor compounds in several Japanese patents in the mid-1980s.[10-13] In a study described in one of the patents, researchers reported that an oral dosage of 100 mg/kg (of suma saponins) given to rats was active against abdominal cancer.[13] The other patents and Japanese research report that the pfaffic acids found in suma root had a strong *in vitro* activity against melanoma, liver carcinoma, and lung carcinoma cells at only 4–6 mcg of pfaffic acids.[9-11] However, it should be noted that this equates to taking 400–600 g (about 1 lb.) of natural suma root daily to achieve the therapeutic dosage of pfaffic acids reported to demonstrate toxic activity against these cancer cells. As such, it will probably be left up to the pharmaceutical companies to provide synthesized versions of these chemicals in therapeutic amounts.

Suma's main plant chemicals are allantoin, beta-ecdysterone, beta-sitosterol, daucosterol, germanium, iron, magnesium, nortriterpenoids, pantothenic acid, pfaffic acids, pfaffosides A–F, polypodine B, saponins, silica, stigmasterol, stigmasterol-3-o-beta-d-glucoside, and vitamins A, B_1, B_2, E, K, and zinc.

BIOLOGICAL ACTIVITIES AND CLINICAL RESEARCH

In addition to the pfaffic acids having anticancerous activity, research in Japan (in 2000) reported that natural suma root had anticancerous activity as well. In this *in vivo* study, an oral administration of powdered suma root (at a dosage of 750 mg/kg) was reported to inhibit the proliferation of lymphoma and leukemia in mice and, otherwise, delay mortality.[14] Notice, however, that this antiproliferative effect slowed the growth of these cancer cells—it did not eradicate them. These researchers postulated that the inhibitory effect evidenced might be due to the enhancement of the nonspecific and/or cellular immune systems.

In 1995, a U.S. patent was filed that detailed some beneficial effects of suma root against sickle-cell anemia. In a double-blind placebo human study, researchers reported that fifteen patients taking suma root for three months (1,000 mg three times daily) increased hemoglobin levels, inhibited red blood cell sickling, and generally improved their physical condition by reducing side effects during the treatment.[15] These results were statistically higher than the fifteen other patients on placebo. Unfortunately, once treatment was discontinued, symptoms and blood parameters returned to their pretreated state within three to six months. It was reported, however, that several patients in the study remained on the suma supplement for three years or longer. They reportedly maintained consistent improvement and a higher quality of life with no side effects. Other U.S. researchers (in 2000) studied suma root's actual mechanism of action in its ability to resickle blood cells and reported their findings—which again confirmed an anti-sickling effect and a rehydration effect of sickled cells (*in vitro*).[16]

Preliminary research with humans indicates that suma may be beneficial for people with sickle-cell anemia.

In other research, suma demonstrated analgesic and anti-inflammatory activities in various *in vivo* rat and mouse studies.[17,18] Another tested activity focused on its long history of use as a sexual stimulant and aphrodisiac. Researchers verified this traditional use, reporting in a 1999 clinical study that a suma root extract was able to increase the sexual performance in healthy, sexually sluggish and impotent rats.[19] In 2001, a U.S. patent was filed on a multi-plant combination containing suma for sexual enhancement in humans. The patent indicated that the suma extract tested increased sexual performance and function.[20]

Toxicity studies with humans indicated no toxicity at an oral dosage of 1.5 g of the root.[11] Another orally administered toxicity study with rats also reported no toxicity—even when suma root represented 50 percent of the rats' food supply for thirty days.[15] However, mice injected subcutaneously with the equivalent of 5 gm/kg (in an ethanol extract) evidenced sedation, drop in body temperature, and loss of motor coordination.[17] Mortality was observed at 10 g/kg (again, in an ethanol extract) when injected in mice.[18]

CURRENT PRACTICAL USES

Suma is another excellent example of a highly beneficial rainforest plant that has many activities and applications—with clinical research validating its traditional uses. No wonder it's called "for all things" throughout South America! With its varied applications—from cancer and sickle-cell anemia to its sexual stimulant and tonic qualities—it is finally becoming more popular and well known in North American herbal medicine practices as well. Suma root products are now more widely available in health food stores; several encapsulated, ground-root products (and root extracts in capsules and liquid extracts) are available on the shelves under various labels. There is also at least one standardized extract (standardized to the saponin content) that has made a recent appearance on the market.

Traditional Preparation The Brazilian traditional remedy calls for preparing a standard decoction with 10 g of suma root boiled in a liter of water; two cups of the decoction are generally taken daily. Herbalists and health practitioners also employ suma root powder in capsules (the decoction tastes quite bitter) with the reported dosage being 2–4 g daily depending on body weight and health condition. This daily dosage is usually taken in two or three divided dosages throughout the day. For standardized or liquid extract products, follow the labeled dosage instructions.

Contraindications Suma has been documented to contain a significant amount of plant sterols including a significant amount of beta-ecdysterone and small amounts of stigmasterol and beta-sitosterol. These sterols might have estrogenic properties or activities and/or cause an increase in estrogen production (although not clinically proven) as this plant has been used traditionally to regulate menstrual processes, as well as to treat menopause, PMS, and other hormonal disorders. Therefore, it is advisable for women with estrogen-positive cancers to avoid the use of this plant.

The root powder has been reported to cause asthmatic allergic reactions if inhaled.[21] When handling raw suma root powder or preparing decoctions with root powder, avoid inhalation of the root powder/dust.

Ingestion of large amounts of plant saponins in general (naturally occurring chemicals in suma) has shown to sometimes cause mild gastric disturbances, including nausea and stomach cramping. Reduce dosages if these side effects are noted.

Drug Interactions None reported.

Worldwide Ethnomedical Uses

Region	Uses
Brazil	for anemia, arthritis, asthma, cancer, chronic fatigue syndrome, circulation problems, diabetes, Epstein-Barr, hyperglycemia, hypertension, immune disorders, impotence, inflammation, leukemia, lymphatic diseases, mononucleosis, pain, rheumatism, skin problems, stress, tremors, tumors, ulcers; and as an antioxidant, aphrodisiac, appetite stimulant, rejuvenator, and tranquilizer
Ecuador	for arteriosclerosis, bronchitis, circulatory problems, diabetes, digestive disorders, hormonal problems, rheumatism, sexual dysfunction, sterility
Europe	for endocrine disorders, fertility, high cholesterol, immune disorders, menopause, menstrual disorders, nerve problems, stress
Japan	for cancer, steroid enhancement, tumors
Peru	for diarrhea, dysentery, fevers, flatulence, malaria, stomach pains
Russia	for muscle growth, steroid enhancement
United States	for chronic fatigue syndrome, diabetes, Epstein-Barr, hormonal disorders, hypertension, impotence, menopause, mononucleosis, nervousness, premenstrual syndrome (PMS), sickle-cell anemia, stress

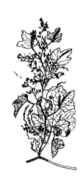

TAYUYA
HERBAL PROPERTIES AND ACTIONS

Main Actions	Other Actions	Standard Dosage
• relieves pain	• stimulates bile	Root
• reduces inflammation	• stimulates digestion	**Infusion:** 1 cup two to three times daily
• fights free radicals	• increases urination	
• reduces stress	• mildly laxative	**Tablets/Capsules:** 1–2 g two to three times daily
• calms nerves		
• cleanses blood		

Family: Cucurbitaceae

Genus: *Cayaponia*

Species: *tayuya, ficcifolia*

Common Names: tayuya, taiuiá, taioia, abobrinha-do-mato, anapinta, cabeca-de-negro, guardião, tomba

Part Used: root

Tayuya is a woody vine found in the Amazon rainforest predominantly in Brazil, Peru, and Bolivia. This important Amazon plant belongs to the Cucurbitaceae (gourd) family, which comprises over 100 genera and over 700 species—most of which are characterized by their long, tuberous roots. It is tayuya's long tap-root that is employed medicinally. Harvesting of it can only be performed during rainy season, when the ground is soft and wet; during dry season, the ground is too hard to extricate the root (which can extend to three feet long) from the dry clay soils in the Amazon. About fifty species of *Cayaponia* occur in the warmer parts of the Americas, West Africa, Madagascar, and Indonesia. Tayuya is known by several botanical names, which all refer to the same plant: *Cayaponia tayuya, C. ficcifolia, Trianosperma tayuya,* and *T. ficcifolia.* In Brazil, the plant is known as *taiuiá;* in Peru, it is called *tayuya.*

TRIBAL AND HERBAL MEDICINE USES

South American Indians have been using tayuya since prehistoric times, and the plant's value is well known. It has been used as a tonic and blood cleanser traditionally (and, usually, with a bit of honey or stevia added to tone down the strong, bitter taste). In the Amazon rainforest, Indians have used the root of tayuya for snakebite and rheumatism for centuries. Indians in Colombia use the plant for sore eyes; indigenous tribes of Peru use it for skin problems.

Tayuya has a long history in Brazilian herbal medicine; it was first recorded in the *Brazilian Pharmacopoeia* as an official herbal drug in 1929. Brazilian botanist J. Monteiro Silva reports tayuya is used for the treatment of all types of pain and recommends it as an anti-syphilitic agent. Monteiro also believes it helps to regulate metabolism. In Brazil today, tayuya is used as a pain-reliever, diuretic, anti-inflammatory, tonic, blood purifier and detoxifier; to treat diarrhea, epilepsy, metabolism disorders, backache, sciatic pain, headaches, gout, neuralgia, constipation, anemia, cholera, dyspepsia, stomach problems, fatigue and debility, skin disorders, arthritis and rheumatism, syphilis, tumors (especially in the joints); and as a general analgesic for many conditions.

Tayuya has a long history in Brazilian herbal medicine; it was first recorded in the *Brazilian Pharmacopoeia* as an official herbal drug in 1929.

Currently, tayuya is employed in North and South America for its pain-reducing properties, and more. Natural health practitioners in the United States are using tayuya to treat irritable bowel syndrome (IBS), dyspepsia and sluggish digestion, neuralgia, sciatica, gout, headaches, rheumatism, and as a metabolic regulator. Because of its reported effectiveness as a blood purifier and detoxifier, it is being used as a natural remedy for water retention, wounds, splotchiness on the face, eczema, herpes, severe acne, and other skin problems. In North America, it is also being used in athletic training and recovery to help remove lactic acid accumulation, to reduce swelling, and to relieve emotional fatigue and depression.

PLANT CHEMICALS

Tayuya is rich in flavones, glucosides, and cucurbitacin triterpenes. Almost every species in the huge Cucurbitaceae family is documented to contain cucurbitacin compounds—many of which evidence biological activity (and, often, the plant's medicinal activity is attributed to these chemicals). Novel cucurbitacins have been discovered in tayuya and named *cayaponosides* (twenty-four distinct cayaponosides have been discovered thus far). These phytochemicals have been documented to have antioxidant, anti-inflammatory and pain-relieving properties[1–3] and, more recently, to have anticancerous potential.

The National Cancer Center Research Institute in Tokyo, Japan reported (in 1995) that five cayaponosides in tayuya "exhibited significant anti-tumor-promoter activity in screening tests using an Epstein-Barr virus activating system" and that two other cayaponosides "also suppressed mouse skin tumor promotion in a two-stage carcinogenesis experiment."[4,5] Another cucurbitacin found in tayuya, *cucurbitacin R*, has been studied extensively in Russia. There it is cited as a powerful adaptogen, preventing stress-induced alterations in the body.[6–8] Other flavone phytochemicals in tayuya have been reported to act as potent scavengers of free radicals, providing an antioxidant effect[9] as well as protecting against damage induced by gamma-radiation.[10,11]

The main plant chemicals found in tayuya include alkaloids, cayaponosides, cucurbitacins, isoorientin, isovitexin, orientin, resins, saponins, spinosin, sterols, swertisin, vicenin 2, and vitexin.

BIOLOGICAL ACTIVITIES AND CLINICAL RESEARCH

While tayuya's compounds have come under some scientific scrutiny (and many of the documented uses in herbal medicine could be explained by some of the activities of its chemicals), very little research has been performed on the biological activity of the plant itself. Two animal studies (performed in the early 1990s) do verify that root extracts provide pain relieving and anti-inflammatory actions. One study documented that a root infusion given orally to mice had an analgesic action.[12] Another research group prepared the root in a methanol

Tayuya's traditional uses to relieve pain and inflammation have been confirmed in animal studies.

extract and reported mild anti-inflammatory actions when administered orally to mice.[13] The latter group reported no toxic effects in mice given 2 g/kg of body weight orally; however, toxicity was reported when 500 mg/kg was injected intraperitoneally. One *in vitro* study by Brazilian scientists reported that tayuya did not evidence any antimicrobial properties (against several common bacteria, fungi, and yeast microbes they tested).[14]

CURRENT PRACTICAL USES

In 2003, a widely publicized marketing campaign was started in Europe regarding tayuya that is, at best, unscrupulous—if not outright fraudulent. It makes unsupported claims that the plant can cure many diseases including arthritis, impotence, and gout, and was discovered through the "Tayuyis" Indians in Brazil (who never existed). Other easily recognized fallacies in their literature are that tayuya is "rare" (as it, supposedly, makes the soil sterile for fifteen to twenty years!), and that the leaf is used indigenously (rather than the root, which is well-documented in literature dating back a century). Consumers should be aware that no clinical studies exist to support any of these wild claims, and that tayuya will *not* provide the benefits advertised. While tayuya has a long history of traditional use by herbalists in the United States and South America for all types pain and joint aches, it is at best a good pain-reliever; it will *not* cure arthritis (nor any of the other diseases claimed in the marketing literature). It is unfortunate that a handful of unethical companies can affect the entire herbal products industry negatively with such scurrilous practices, but it continues to happen.

Although not widely available, tayuya is being employed by several companies as an ingredient in various herbal formulas (typically for pain, arthritis, and detoxification). Generally, it is employed by South American herbalists in combination with other plants, and not as a single therapy. Consumers and manufacturers should stick with reputable harvesters and importers for sourcing this particular tropical plant. The official plant that is sold as tayuya should be *Cayaponia tayuya*. One independent published survey in Brazil (the main exporter of the root), however, reported that almost any species of *Cayaponia* (of which about forty different species exist in South America) is harvested, marketed, and sold as *taiuiá* in Brazil.[15] They also reported that another completely different plant, *Wilbrandia ebracteata*, frequently has been found among the "taiuiá roots" sold in Brazilian herbal commerce.

Traditional Preparation

Tayuya root is traditionally prepared in infusions and taken in 1 cup dosages two to three times daily. Alternatively, 1–2 g of the powdered root is stirred into juice, water, or food and taken two to three times daily.

Contraindications

None known.

Drug Interactions   None known.

Worldwide Ethnomedical Uses

Region	Uses
Amazonia	for depression, edema, eye disorders, fatigue, swelling
Brazil	for arthritis, backache, blood cleansing, boils, cholera, constipation, detoxification, diarrhea, digestive disorders, dyspepsia, edema, eczema, epilepsy, fatigue, gout, headaches, inflammation, leprosy, menstrual disorders, metabolism regulation, neuralgia, pain, rabies, rheumatism, sciatica, scrofula, skin diseases, snakebite, stomach (dilated), syphilis, tumors (joint), ulcers, urinary insufficiency; and as a bitter digestive stimulant
Colombia	for sore eyes
Peru	for rheumatism, skin disorders, snakebite
United States	for acne, arthritis, backache, blood cleansing, depression, detoxification, digestion disorders, dyspepsia, eczema, edema, epilepsy, gout, headaches, herpes, irritable bowel syndrome, lactic acid excess, liver problems, metabolism disorders, nerve pain, pain, rheumatism, sciatica, skin disorders, spleen inflammation, ulcers, wounds

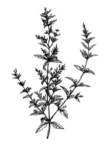

Family: Scrophulariceae

Genus: *Scoparia*

Species: *dulcis*

Common Names: vassourinha, ñuñco pichana, anisillo, bitterbroom, boroemia, broomweed, brum sirpi, escobilla, licorice weed, mastuerzo, piqui pichana, pottipooli, sweet broom, tapixava, tupixaba

Parts Used: leaves, bark, roots

VASSOURINHA
HERBAL PROPERTIES AND ACTIONS

Main Actions
- kills viruses
- kills leukemia cells
- inhibits tumors
- kills germs
- reduces inflammation
- relieves pain
- reduces spasms
- expels phlegm
- promotes menstruation
- reduces blood pressure
- strengthens heartbeat
- supports heart

Other Actions
- kills bacteria
- kills fungi
- reduces fever
- heals wounds
- lowers blood sugar
- lowers body temperature

Standard Dosage
Whole herb
Infusion: 1 cup twice daily
Tablets/Capsules: 2–3 g
   twice daily

Vassourinha is an erect annual herb in the foxglove family that grows up to 1/2 m high. It produces serrated leaves and many small, white flowers. It is widely distributed in many tropical countries in the world and is found in abundance in South America and the Amazon rainforest. It can be found as far north as the Southern United States, including Texas, Florida, and Louisiana. The plant is called *escobilla* in Peru, *vassourinha* in Brazil, and in the U.S. the plant is known as *sweet broomweed* or *licorice weed*. In many areas, the plant is considered an invasive weed.

TRIBAL
AND HERBAL
MEDICINE USES

Vassourinha has long held a place in herbal medicine in every tropical country where it grows, and its use by indigenous peoples is well documented. Indigenous tribes in Ecuador brew a tea of the entire plant to reduce swellings, aches, and pains. The Tikuna Indians make a decoction for washing wounds, and women drink the same decoction for three days each month during menstruation as a contraceptive and/or to induce abortions. In the rainforests of Guyana, indigenous tribes use a leaf decoction as an antiseptic wash for wounds, as an anti-nausea aid for infants, as a soothing bath to treat fever, and in poultices for migraine headaches. Indigenous peoples in Brazil use the leaf juice to wash infected wounds, and place it in the eyes for eye problems; they make an infusion of the entire plant to use as an expectorant and to soothe and soften the skin. Indigenous tribes in Nicaragua use a hot water infusion and/or decoction of vassourinha leaves (or the whole plant) for stomach pain, for menstrual disorders, as an aid in childbirth, as a blood purifier, for insect bites, fevers, heart problems, liver and stomach disorders, malaria, sexually transmitted diseases, and as a general tonic.

In Brazil, a vassourinha tea is prepared from the leaves or aerial parts of the plant for fevers and urinary tract diseases, upper respiratory disorders, bronchitis, coughs, menstrual disorders, and hypertension.

Vassourinha is still employed in herbal medicine throughout the tropics. In Peru, a decoction of the entire plant is recommended for upper respiratory problems, biliary colic or congestion, menstrual disorders, and fever; the leaf juice is still employed externally for wounds and hemorrhoids. In Brazilian herbal medicine, the plant is used to reduce fever, lower blood sugar and blood pressure, and as an expectorant for coughs and lung congestion. A tea is prepared from the leaves or aerial parts of the plant for fevers and urinary tract diseases, upper respiratory disorders, bronchitis, coughs, menstrual disorders, and hypertension. The leaf juice or a decoction of the leaves is also employed topically for skin ulcers and erysipelas. In Ayurvedic herbal medicine systems in India, a leaf tea is widely used for diabetes.

PLANT
CHEMICALS

Chemical screening of vassourinha has shown that it is a source of novel phytochemicals in the flavone and terpene classification, some of which have not been seen in science before.[1,2] Many of vassourinha's active biological properties, including its anticancerous properties, are attributed to these phytochemicals. The main chemicals being studied are scopadulcic acids A and B, scopadiol, scopadulciol, scopadulin, scoparic acids A, B, and C, and betulinic acid.[3–7]

The antitumorous activity of scopadulcic acid B was demonstrated in a 1993 study,[8] and anti-tumor activity against various human cancer cell lines was reported again in 2001.[9] This chemical and another compound named *sco-padulin* demonstrated antiviral properties in several studies, including against herpes simplex I, in hamsters.[10–12] Betulinic acid is another phytochemical that has been the subject of much independent cancer research (beginning in the late 1990s). Many studies report that this phytochemical has powerful anticancerous, antitumorous, antileukemic, and antiviral (including HIV) properties.[13–16] This potent phytochemical has displayed selective cytotoxic activity against malignant brain tumors, bone cancer, and melanomas (without harming healthy cells).[17–19]

> Plant chemicals found in vassourinha have evidenced anticancerous and antiviral actions in the laboratory.

Vassourinha's main plant chemicals include acacetin, amyrin, apigenin, benzoxazin, benzoxazolin, benzoxazolinone, betulinic acid, cirsimarin, cirsitakaoside, coixol, coumaric acid, cynaroside, daucosterol, dulcinol, dulcioic acid, friedelin, gentisic acid, glutinol, hymenoxin, ifflaionic acid, linarin, luteolin, mannitol, scopadiol, scopadulcic acid A and B, scopadulciol, scopadulin, scoparic acid A through C, scoparinol, scutellarein, scutellarin, sitosterol, stigmasterol, taraxerol, vicenin, and vitexin.

BIOLOGICAL ACTIVITIES AND CLINICAL RESEARCH

In addition to its tested anticancerous chemicals, a methanol extract of vassourinha leaves also showed toxic actions against cancer cells (with a 66 percent inhibition rate) by Japanese researchers.[20,21] These findings fueled more research on the chemicals in this plant and their activities, which is still ongoing today.

Some of vassourinha's other uses in herbal medicine have also been validated by western research. In early research, vassourinha demonstrated a cardiotonic effect in animals.[22] More than forty years later, researchers reconfirmed its blood-pressure-lowering properties in rats and dogs (while increasing the strength of the heartbeat).[23] Vassourinha also demonstrated anti-inflammatory, antispasmodic, and pain-relieving activity in animal studies with rats, mice, and guinea pigs.[23–25] A single chemical called *scoparinol* was identified by scientists as being responsible for the pain-relieving effects.[25] Another researcher, in a 2001 study, again documented significant pain-relieving and anti-inflammatory effects in laboratory animals—and also indicated that scoparinol demonstrated diuretic and barbiturate potentiation activity.[26] These documented actions could certainly explain its traditional use as a natural remedy for pain of all types (including menstrual pain and cramps, as well as during childbirth). In 2002, researchers in India verified vassourinha's antidiabetic and blood-sugar-lowering effects in rats.[27] In other *in vitro* laboratory tests, vassourinha demonstrated antioxidant actions,[28] as well as active properties against bacteria and fungi (which could explain its sustained use for respiratory and urinary tract infections).[29,30]

> In addition to its documented anti-cancerous activity, other animal studies reveal that vassourinha reduces pain, inflammation, and spasms.

CURRENT PRACTICAL USES

Scientists have been trying since the mid-1990s to synthesize several plant chemicals found in vassourinha, including scopadulcic acid B and betulinic acid, for their use in the pharmaceutical industry. Herbalists and natural health practitioners have used, and will continue to use, the plant as an effective natural remedy for upper respiratory problems and viruses, for menstrual problems, and as a natural pain-reliever and antispasmodic remedy when needed. Water and ethanol extracts given to mice at up to 2 g per kg of body weight showed no toxicity.[24]

Traditional Preparation

The reported therapeutic dosage generally used in South America is 2–3 g twice daily or 1 cup of a standard infusion twice daily.

Contraindications

None documented by clinical studies; however, the traditional use as an abortive and/or childbirth aid warrants that vassourinha should not be taken during pregnancy.

Avoid combining with antidepressants or barbiturates unless under the supervision of a qualified health care practitioner (see drug interactions below).

A vassourinha extract recently demonstrated hypoglycemic activity, significantly lowering blood sugar levels in rats. This plant is probably contraindicated in people with hypoglycemia. Diabetics should check their blood glucose levels closely if they use vassourinha to monitor these possible effects.

Drug Interactions

One human study documented that an ethanol extract of vassourinha inhibited radioligand binding to dopamine and seratonin.[31] Another study reported that a water extract given intragastrically to rats potentiated the effects of barbiturates.[24] As such, it is possible that vassourinha may enhance the effect of barbiturates and selective serotonin reuptake inhibitor antidepressants.

Worldwide Ethnomedical Uses

Region	Uses
Amazonia	for abortions, aches, bronchitis, contraception, coughs, diarrhea, erysipelas, eye infections, fever, hemorrhoids, kidney disease, liver problems, nausea, pain, sores (gonorrhea), stomach disorders, swelling, wounds
Brazil	for abortions, bronchitis, cardiopulmonary disorders, coughs, diabetes, earache, excessive phlegm, eye problems, fever, gastric disorders, hemorrhoids, hyperglycemia, hypertension, insect bites, jaundice, liver disorders, malaria, menstrual disorders, menstrual promotion, pain, skin problems, upper respiratory disorders, worms, wounds
Central America	for bruises, constipation, diarrhea, fever, flu, gonorrhea, kidney stones, liver disorders, menstrual disorders, menstrual promotion, skin infections, sore throat, stomach disease, stomach pain, wounds, and as an insecticide

Dominican Republic	for diabetes, sore throat
Haiti	for coughs, diabetes, earache, gonorrhea, headaches, inflammation, menstrual disorders, nerves, pain, piles, skin sores, sore throat, spasms, toothache, tumors; and as an antiseptic, astringent, and diuretic
India	for diabetes, dysentery, earache, fever, gonorrhea, headaches, jaundice, snakebite, stomach problems, toothache, warts
Nicaragua	for anemia, childbirth, blood cleansing, burns, cough, diarrhea, fever, headache, heart conditions, infections, insect bites and stings, itch, liver disorders, malaria, menstrual disorders, sexually transmitted diseases, snakebite, stomach disorders
Peru	for abortions, colic, contraception, diarrhea, excessive mucus, fever, hemorrhoids, kidney diseases, menstrual disorders, upper respiratory disorders, wounds (infected)
Suriname	for bronchitis, coughs, diabetes, fever, jaundice, rash
Trinidad	for blood cleansing, diabetes, eczema, eye problems, jaundice, malabsorption, mange, menstrual disorders, rashes, sores, wounds
Venezuela	for diarrhea, gonorrhea, menstrual disorders
West Indies	for diabetes, diarrhea, menstrual disorders
Elsewhere	for abortions, aches, albuminuria, anemia, bronchitis, cancer, childbirth, conjunctivitis, contraception, cough, detoxification, diabetes, diarrhea, dysentery, earache, fever, headache, hyperglycemia, hypertension, kidney disorders, kidney stones, leprosy, liver disease, menstrual disorders, migraine, nausea, pains, retinitis, sexually transmitted diseases, snakebite, stomachache, swellings, syphilis, toothache, worms, wounds; and as an antiseptic, aphrodisiac, diuretic, expectorant, and laxative

Xingu River near the Parakaná Indian village of the Brazilian Amazon.

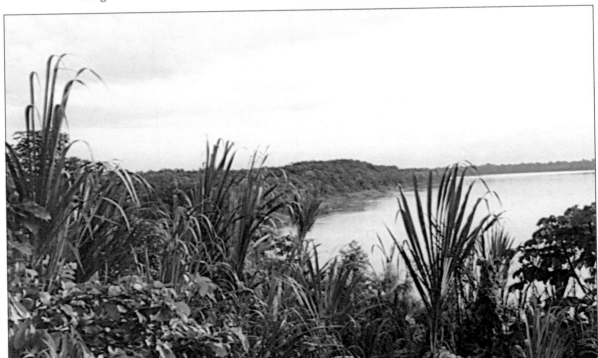

VELVET BEAN
HERBAL PROPERTIES AND ACTIONS

Main Actions
- is L-Dopa alternative
- increases testosterone
- increases libido
- reduces spasms
- lowers blood sugar
- lowers blood pressure
- increases urination

Other Actions
- relieves pain
- reduces inflammation
- kills parasites
- calms nerves
- reduces fever
- lowers cholesterol

Standard Dosage
Seed

Decoction: $\frac{1}{2}$–1 cup twice daily

Capsules/Tablets: 1–2 g twice daily

Standardized Extracts: Follow label instructions

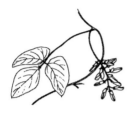

Family: Fabaceae

Genus: *Mucuna*

Species: *pruriens*

Common Names: velvet bean, nescafé, mucuna, pó de mico, fava-coceira, cabeca-de-frade, cowage, cowhage, cow-itch, bengal bean, mauritius bean, itchy bean, krame, picapica, chiporro, buffalobean

Part Used: seeds

TRIBAL AND HERBAL MEDICINE USES

In Brazil, velvet bean seeds have been used for Parkinson's disease, edema, impotence, intestinal gas, and worms.

PLANT CHEMICALS

Velvet bean is an annual climbing vine that grows 3–18 m in height. It is indigenous to tropical regions, especially Africa, India, and the West Indies. Its flowers are white-to-dark purple and hang in long clusters. The plant also produces clusters of pods, which contain seeds known as *mucuna beans*. The seed-pods are covered with reddish-orange hairs that are readily dislodged and can cause intense irritation to the skin. The species name *"pruriens"* (from the Latin, "itching sensation") refers to the results to be had from contact with the seed-pod hairs.

In Central America, mucuna beans have been roasted and ground to make a coffee substitute for decades; the plant has been widely known as *nescafé* for this reason. It is still grown as a food crop by the Ketchi indigenous people in Guatemala; the bean is cooked as a vegetable. In Brazil the seed has been used internally for Parkinson's disease, edema, impotence, intestinal gas, and worms. It is considered a diuretic, nerve tonic, and aphrodisiac. Externally it is applied to ulcers. Velvet bean has a long history of use in Indian Ayurvedic medicine, where it is used for worms, dysentery, diarrhea, snakebite, sexual debility, cough, tuberculosis, impotence, rheumatic disorders, muscular pain, sterility, gout, menstrual disorders, diabetes, and cancer. In India, it is considered an aphrodisiac, menstrual promoter, uterine stimulant, nerve tonic, diuretic, and blood purifier.

The seeds of velvet bean are high in protein, carbohydrates, lipids, fiber, and minerals. They are also rich in novel alkaloids, saponins, and sterols. The seeds of all *mucuna* species contain a high concentration of L-dopa; velvet bean seeds contain 7–10 percent L-dopa.[1-3] Concentrations of serotonin also have been found in the pod, leaf, and fruit.[4-5] The stinging hairs of the seed-pods contain the phytochemical mucunain, which is responsible for causing skin irritation and itch.

Velvet bean seeds contain up to 10 percent natural L-dopa, which is why the plant is used in herbal medicine systems to treat Parkinson's disease.

The main plant chemicals found in velvet bean include alkaloids, alkylamines, arachidic acid, behenic acid, betacarboline, beta-sitosterol, bufotenine, cystine, dopamine, fatty acids, flavones, galactose d, gallic acid, genistein, glutamic acid, glutathione, glycine, histidine, hydroxygenistein, 5-hydroxytryptamine, isoleucine, l-dopa, linoleic acid, linolenic acid, lysine, mannose d, methionine, 6-methoxyharman, mucunadine, mucunain, mucunine, myristic acid, niacin, nicotine, oleic acid, palmitic acid, palmitoleic acid, phenylalanine, prurienidine, prurienine, riboflavin, saponins, serine, serotonin, stearic acid, stizolamine, threonine, trypsin, tryptamine, tyrosine, valine, and vernolic acid.

BIOLOGICAL ACTIVITIES AND CLINICAL RESEARCH

Velvet bean has demonstrated little toxicity; however, it has been documented in animal studies to cause birth defects and should not be used during pregnancy.[6] Traditionally, velvet bean has been used as a nerve tonic for nervous system disorders. Due to the high concentration of L-dopa in the seeds, it has been studied for its possible use in Parkinson's disease. Parkinson's disease is a common age-related neurodegenerative disorder affecting more than four million people worldwide. It is associated with progressive degeneration of dopaminergic neurons in specific areas in the brain. Dopamine does not cross the blood-brain barrier and therefore cannot be used directly as a treatment. However, L-dopa (levodopa) does gain access to the brain—where it is converted to dopamine. There are two controversies surrounding side effects of the current pharmaceutical supplementation of L-dopa. Over the long term, supplemented L-dopa appears to lose its effectiveness. A second area of controversy questions whether L-dopa is toxic to dopamine neurons; there is little evidence, though, to support this statement.[7]

Preliminary reports suggest that velvet bean can provide the same benefits to Parkinson's patients as the prescription drug, levodopa, with fewer side effects.

Velvet bean is now being considered as an alternative to the pharmaceutical medication levodopa. In one case study, it was given to a Parkinson's patient for twelve years instead of the pharmaceutical L-dopa medication. It was found to slow the progression of Parkinson's symptoms (such as tremors, rigidity, slurring, drooling, and imbalance), and to have none of the side effects of the current pharmaceutical L-dopa.[8] Numerous *in vivo* studies also have been conducted in rats and humans. In one human study, the bean powder was given to sixty patients (twenty-six previously treated with L-dopa and thirty-four had never taken L-dopa). There were statistically significant reductions of Parkinson's symptoms in all study subjects.[9] In addition, a (2002) U.S. patent was awarded on velvet bean citing its use "for the treatment of disorders of the nervous system, including Parkinson's disease."[8]

Several *in vivo* studies have been conducted on the blood-sugar-lowering effect of velvet bean. These studies all validate the traditional use of the plant for diabetes. An ethanol-water extract of the root, fruit, and seed dropped blood sugar levels in rats by more than 30 percent. At 200 mg, an ethanol extract produced a 40 percent fall in blood glucose within one month, and a 51 percent reduction at four months.[10,11] In other studies, a decoction of the leaf reduced total cholesterol in rats;[12] the seed had the same effect.[13]

The root, fruit, leaf, and seed have shown significant *in vivo* antispasmodic,[14,15] anti-inflammatory,[16,17] pain relieving,[16] and fever-reducing activities[16] in various clinical research with animals. Traditionally, the seed has been used by indigenous peoples throughout the world for snakebite and several *in vivo* studies validate this traditional use.[18–21] In rats, a water extract of the seed inhibited venom-induced blood and coagulation alterations, and reduced lethality of the venom.[19] The antivenin effect of velvet bean is thought to be due to an immune mechanism, as proteins in the seed were documented to raise antibodies against the venom.[21]

Velvet bean has a long history of traditional use in Brazil and India as an aphrodisiac. Clinical studies in India have validated that the plant does indeed have aphrodisiac activity.[22,23] It also has been reported as having anabolic and growth hormone-stimulant properties.[24,25] The anabolic effect of the seed is due to its ability to increase testosterone.[26] In 2002, a U.S. patent was filed on the use of velvet bean to stimulate the release of growth hormone in humans.[25] Research cited in the patent indicated that the high levels of L-dopa in mucuna seed were converted to dopamine, which stimulated the release of growth hormone by the pituitary gland.[25] L-dopa and dopamine are also effective inhibitors of prolactin. Prolactin is a hormone released by the pituitary gland; increased levels are considered to cause erection failure in males. In one study, oral intake of the seeds in fifty-six human males was able to improve erection, duration of coitus, and post-coital satisfaction after only four weeks of treatment.[27] The seed also has documented fertility promoting and sperm producing effects in human males (being able to improve sperm count and motility).[28,29]

CURRENT PRACTICAL USES

Velvet bean has been gaining in popularity over the last few years in the natural products market—especially the sports nutrition industry. With its documented ability to increase testosterone and stimulate growth hormone (thereby increasing muscle mass), several companies have launched new products using mucuna beans, including several which are standardized to the L-dopa content. It is also showing up as an ingredient in various weight loss, libido, brain/memory, anti-aging, and body builder formulas.

Consumers should be aware however, altering the levels of brain chemicals like dopamine and serotonin also affect many other hormones, enzymes, and other chemicals that keep the body in balance. The long-term impacts on healthy humans taking high levels of L-dopa are unclear and warrant further research. It is best to proceed with caution when taking mucuna extracts and to follow the labeled dosages. It is a powerful plant with many biological actions that should be respected. In other words, the belief system of some people taking herbals supplements, "if some is good, more is better," does not apply with velvet bean.

Traditional Preparation

Traditionally, ½–1 cup of a seed decoction is taken twice daily. Alternatively, 1–2 g twice daily of seed powder (tablets or capsules) can be substituted. For standardized extract products, follow the labeled dosages provided.

Contraindications

The seed may cause birth defects and has uterine stimulant activity. It should not be used during pregnancy.

Velvet bean has shown to lower blood sugar. Those with hypoglycemia or diabetes should only use velvet bean under the supervision of a qualified healthcare practitioner.

Velvet bean is contraindicated in combination with M.A.O. inhibitors.

Velvet bean has androgenic activity, increasing testosterone levels. Persons with excessive androgen syndromes should avoid using velvet bean.

Velvet bean inhibits prolactin. If you have a medical condition resulting in inadequate levels of prolactin in the body, do not use velvet bean unless under the direction of your healthcare practitioner.

The seed contains high quantities of L-dopa. Levodopa is the pharmaceutical medication used for Parkinson's disease. Those with Parkinson's should only use velvet bean under the supervision of a qualified healthcare practitioner.

Drug Interactions

Velvet bean may potentiate androgenic, insulin, and antidiabetic medications. It will potentiate levodopa medications.

Worldwide Ethnomedical Uses

Region	Uses
Brazil	as an aphrodisiac, diuretic, and nerve tonic, and for edema and intestinal worms
Germany	for diabetes, high blood pressure, high cholesterol, intestinal gas, muscle pain, rheumatism, worms
India	for abortions, cancer, catarrh, cholera, cough, debility, delerium, diabetes, diarrhea, dysentery, edema, fertility, gout, impotency, kidney stones, menstrual disorders, nervousness, scorpion sting, snakebite, sterility, tuberculosis, worms; and as an aphrodisiac, diuretic, and uterine stimulant
Elsewhere	for asthma, burns, cancer, cholera, cough, cuts, diabetes, diarrhea, dog bite, edema, insanity, intestinal parasites, menstrual problems, mumps, nerves, pain, paralysis, pleurisy, ringworm, snakebite, sores, syphilis, tumors, wind-burns, worms, and as an aphrodisiac

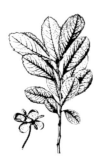

Family: Aquifoliaceae

Genus: *Ilex*

Species: *paraguariensis,
paraguayensis*

Common Names:
yerba maté, maté, erva
mate, congonha, erveira,
Paraguay cayi, Paraguay
tea, South American
holly, matéteestrauch,
erva-verdadeira,
St. Bartholomew's tea,
Jesuit's tea, hervea,
caminú, kkiro, kali chaye

Part Used: leaves

TRIBAL AND HERBAL MEDICINE USES

YERBA MATE		
HERBAL PROPERTIES AND ACTIONS		
Main Actions	**Other Actions**	**Standard Dosage**
• increases energy	relieves pain	Leaves
• burns fat	• increases bile	**Infusion:** 1 cup two to three
• suppresses appetite	• mildly laxative	times daily
• cleanses blood	• promotes perspiration	**Tablets/Capsules:** 1–2 g
• stimulates digestion	• enhances immunity	twice daily
• cleanses bowels		
• stimulates heart		
• fights free radicals		
• enhances memory		

Yerba mate is a widely cultivated, medium-sized evergreen tree that can grow to 20 m high in the wild. Commonly, when cultivated, it is pruned into a shrubby, 4–8 m tall tree to make harvesting easier. Yerba mate is in the holly family, and bears holly-like leaves that are quite stiff and leathery. In the wild it grows near streams, and thrives at 1,500–2,000 feet above sea level. It has graceful, full-leafed branches, and white flowers that produce small red, black, or yellow berries. It is yerba mate's tough, leathery leaves that are used medicinally and as a natural, refreshing tea beverage throughout South America. Yerba mate is indigenous to Paraguay, Brazil, Argentina, and Uruguay; however, it is now cultivated in many tropical countries to supply the world's demand for its leaves.

Yerba mate has been used as a beverage since the time of the ancient Indians of Brazil and Paraguay. In the early sixteenth century, Juan de Solís, a Spanish explorer of South America's famed La Plata River, reported that the Guarani Indians of Paraguay brewed a leaf tea that "produced exhilaration and relief from fatigue." The Spaniards tried the beverage and liked it. Their subsequent demand for the tea led the Jesuits to develop plantations of the wild species in Paraguay and yerba mate became known as "Jesuits' tea" or "Paraguay tea."

Methods of leaf preparation for the traditional tea beverage vary. In one method, the branches are cut, then held over an open fire (to fire-cure the leaves). This deactivates the enzymes in the leaves (making them more brittle) and the green color of the leaves is retained in the subsequent drying process (with charred bits often found in the resulting tea product, which lends to a smoky flavor). Other methods include a brief par-blanching of the leaves in boiling water (to deactivate the leaf enzymes and soften its leathery texture).

Yerba mate is considered a national drink in several countries. In addition, yerba mate is used as a tonic, diuretic, and as a stimulant to reduce fatigue, suppress appetite, and aid gastric function in herbal medicine systems throughout South America.

They then are toasted dry in large pans over a fire or inside a brick oven—resulting in a finished brown-leaf tea.

The wild plant has a distinct aroma and taste that has not been matched by plantation cultivation. In South America, yerba mate is considered a national drink in several countries; in Europe, it is called "the green gold of the Indios." In Brazil and Paraguay (leading exporters of mate), some production still comes from wild stands—most of which is found in the humid depressions of the foothills. It is not unusual for one wild tree to yield 30–40 kg of dried leaves annually. In wild harvesting, mate gatherers, called *tarrafeiros* or *yebateros,* travel through the jungle searching for a stand of trees (called a *mancha*). Harvesting is done between May and October, when the tree is in full leaf. Leaves are picked from the same tree only every third year, which protects it for subsequent crops. Most of the mate in commerce today, however, comes from large cultivation projects in Paraguay and Uruguay.

The word *mate* is Spanish for "gourd," and refers to the small gourd cup in which the tea beverage traditionally is served throughout South America. It is also served with a metal drinking straw or tube, called a *bombilla,* which has a filter attached to the lower end to strain out leaf fragments. The bottom third of the gourd is filled with fire-burned or toasted leaves, and hot water is added. Burnt sugar, lemon juice, and/or milk often are used to flavor the refreshing tea, which occupies a position rivaling that of coffee in the United States. Mate bars are as prevalent in South America as coffee bars are in North America and Europe; mate drinking has deep cultural roots.

In addition to its standing as a popular beverage, yerba mate is used as a tonic, diuretic, and as a stimulant to reduce fatigue, suppress appetite, and aid gastric function in herbal medicine systems throughout South America. It also has been used as a depurative (to promote cleansing and excretion of waste). In Brazil, mate is said to stimulate the nervous and muscular systems and is used for digestive problems, renal colic, nerve pain, depression, fatigue, and obesity. A poultice of the leaves also is applied topically to anthrax skin ulcers (for which mate's tannin content—highly astringent—may be the reasoning behind this use).

Yerba mate also has a long history of use worldwide. In Europe, it is used for weight loss, physical and mental fatigue, nervous depression, rheumatic pains, and psychogenic- and fatigue-related headaches. In Germany, it has become popular as a weight-loss aid. Yerba mate is the subject of a German monograph that lists its approved uses for mental and physical fatigue.[1] In France, yerba mate is approved for the treatment of asthenia (weakness or lack of energy), as an aid in weight-loss programs, and as a diuretic. It also appears in the *British Herbal Phamacopoeia* (1996) and is indicated for the treatment of fatigue, weight loss, and headaches. Yerba mate now is cultivated in India, and the Indian *Ayurvedic Phamacopoeia* lists mate for the treatment of psychogenic headaches, nervous depression, fatigue, and rheumatic pains.

PLANT CHEMICALS   The primary active chemical constituency of yerba mate comprises xanthine alkaloids (caffeine, theobromine, and theophylline), saponins, and 10 percent chlorogenic acid.[2,3] Sterols resembling ergosterol and cholesterol are also present in yerba mate, and novel saponins have been discovered in the leaf (and named *matesaponins*).[4,5] Saponins are plant chemicals with known pharmacological activities, including, as recent research shows, stimulating the immune system.[5-7] In addition, yerba mate leaf is a rich source of vitamins, minerals, and fifteen amino acids.[8]

In recent U.S. campaigns, yerba mate marketers claim that yerba mate contains no caffeine—rather, a chemical similar to caffeine called *mateine*. Mateine, they say, possesses all the benefits of caffeine and none of its negative effects (or so they would have consumers believe). Fact: yerba mate *does* contain caffeine. It has been chemically and scientifically identified, documented, verified, and validated to contain caffeine for many years by independent chemists and scientists around the world ("independent" being the operative term here). This fact continues to be confirmed by independent research every year. The caffeine content of yerba mate has been assayed to contain between .7 and 2 percent, with the average leaf yielding about 1 percent caffeine.[9] In living plants, xanthines (such as caffeine) are bound to sugars, phenols, and tannins, and are set free or unbound during the roasting and/or fermenting processes used to process yerba mate leaves, coffee beans, and even cacao beans. The mateine chemical "discovered" is probably just caffeine bound to a tannin or phenol in the raw leaf. The table below compares the caffeine content of yerba mate to other popular beverage products.

Caffeine Content Comparison
Common Beverage Products [9-12]

Plant Beverage	Caffeine Content	Avg. Caffeine (6 oz. serving)*
Yerba mate leaves	0.7–2%	50–100 mg
Coffee beans (*Coffea sp*)	1–2.5%	100–250 mg
Black tea (*Camellia sinensis*)	2.5–4.5%	10–60 mg
Guaraná seed (*Paullinia cupana*)	4–8%	200–400 mg
Chocolate (Cacao seed)	0.25%	13 mg

*Based on quantities used in standard preparation methods.

The traditional use of yerba mate for fatigue is explained by its primary active chemical: caffeine. Caffeine is a known stimulant, even documented with the ability to enhance athletic and cognitive performance after sleep deprivation and stress.[13,14] Yerba mate's traditional use for the heart may be due to the phytochemical theophylline, also known as a pharmaceutical medication used to stimulate the heart muscle.[15] All three xanthines (theobromine, caffeine, and theophylline) have diuretic properties, which may validate the traditional use of the plant as a diuretic.[10] These substances have several other documented pharmacological actions including central nervous system stimulation, relaxation of smooth muscle (especially bronchial muscle), myocardial stimulation, and peripheral vasoconstriction.

The main plant chemicals found in yerba mate include alpha-amyrin, alpha-terpineol, arachidic acid, beta-amyrin, butyric acid, caffeic acid, caffeine, 5-o-caffeoylquinic acid, calcium, carotene, chlorogenic acid, choline, chlorophyll, chrysanthemin, cyanidin-3-o-xylosyl-glucoside, cyanidin-3-glucoside, essential oil, eugenol, geraniol, geranyl acetone, guaiacin b, indole, inositol, ionone, iso-butyric acid, iso-capronic acid, iso-chlorogenic acid, iso-valeric acid, kaempferol, lauric acid, levulose, linalool, linoleic acid, matesaponins, neochlorogenic acid, nerolidol, nicotinic acid, nudicaucin c, octan-1-ol, octanoic acid, oleic acid, palmitic acid, palmitoleic acid, pyridoxine, quercetin, raffinose, safrole, stearic acid, tannins, theobromine, theophylline, trigonelline, and ursolic acid.

BIOLOGICAL ACTIVITIES AND CLINICAL RESEARCH

Researchers in Switzerland performed a study on human subjects (in 1999) that indicated yerba mate could be beneficial as a weight-loss aid. They noticed a thermogenic effect in healthy individuals, indicating a rise in the proportion of fat burned as energy.[16] In another study, yerba mate was given in combination with the plants guaraná and damiana. This combination prolonged gastric emptying (which made the subjects feel "fuller" longer) and reduced body weight.[17] Clinical studies indicate yerba mate leaf inhibits lipoxygenase, an enzyme involved in inflammation and inflammatory diseases.[18–20] Yerba mate extracts also have been shown to relax smooth muscle,[21] to increase bile flow,[22] and inhibit vasoconstriction.[23] A 2002 U.S. patent cites yerba mate for inhibiting monoamine oxidase (MAO) activity by 40–50 percent *in vitro*, reporting that it might be useful for a variety of such disorders as "depression, disorders of attention and focus, mood and emotional disorders, Parkinson's disease, extrapyramidal disorders, hypertension, substance abuse, eating disorders, withdrawal syndromes and the cessation of smoking."[24]

Clinical research reveals that yerba mate is a good weight-loss aid.

Yerba mate has significant antioxidant activity, demonstrated in numerous studies.[25–27] Its high antioxidant values are linked to rapid absorption of known antioxidant plant chemicals found in mate leaves.[28,29] An infusion of the leaf has been demonstrated to inhibit lipid peroxidation—particularly LDL (low-density lipoprotein) oxidation.[26,29] Oxidation of LDL is considered to be the initiating factor in the pathogenesis of atherosclerosis.[30,31] Another study *in vitro* has shown yerba mate to inhibit the formation of advanced glycation end products (AGEs), with an effect comparable to that of two pharmaceutical AGE inhibitor drugs.[32] The formation of AGEs play a part in the development of diabetic complications.[33]

CURRENT PRACTICAL USES

Yerba mate has long been a part of South American culture where it is more heavily consumed than coffee and tea. The average person in Uruguay will consume 9–10 kg annually! However—like many things—too much of a good thing can be harmful. Heavy drinkers of mate in South America were documented with an increased risk of upper-aerodigestive tract cancers (a 1.6- to 4-fold increase for heavy drinkers).[34–38] It was speculated that this risk was caused by the tannins in the leaf (mate contains 7–14 percent tannins) consumed at a high temperature. Despite several studies published in Uruguay reporting this increased cancer risk (and where some of the heaviest mate drinkers are found), it has done little to change the mate-drinking culture there. One interesting change was that more drinkers began adding milk to their mate—it was suggested that the milk would bind to the tannins in the brew, reduce the temperature, and mitigate much of their (possibly) negative effects.

Yerba mate has become more popular and available in the U.S. in recent years. Various mate products now can be widely found in health food stores: cut-leaf green and brown teas and tea bags, ground-leaf capsules, and standardized extracts (standardized to the caffeine content) are sold in capsules. It is also appearing as an ingredient in many more U.S.-manufactured herbal formulas designed for energy gain and/or weight-loss. There have been some sporadic problems in product quality—mostly involving other leaves (cheaper fillers) added as adulterants. Mango leaves are a common adulterant in South America but, in at least one documented case, a yerba mate commercial product sold in Scotland was adulterated with a plant (in the belladonna family) containing pyrrolizidine alkaloids—which caused negative side effects in one consumer. True yerba mate, however, is considered a safe supplement and is on the FDA's GRAS list (generally regarded as safe). Consumers should stick with reputable manufacturers who regularly test and control their imported plant ingredients to avoid such issues as adulterants.

Traditional Preparation

A leaf tea or infusion is the standard preparation, utilizing 2–4 g of cut leaves in 150 ml of hot water. Powdered leaf and leaf extracts with standardized caffeine content are being used in capsules and formulas in herbal products as well. General dosages recommended are the equivalent of 2 g once or twice daily, or follow the labeled dosage information.

Contraindications

Yerba mate is not to be used during pregnancy or while breastfeeding.

Yerba mate contains caffeine and should not be used by those who are sensitive or allergic to caffeine. Excessive consumption of caffeine is contraindicated for persons with high blood pressure, diabetes, ulcers, and other diseases.

Yerba mate should not be consumed excessively and chronically (as it has been documented to increase the risk of certain cancers such as oral and esophageal cancer).

Yerba mate has been reported to have MAO-inhibitor activity in one *in vitro* study. Those persons taking MAO-inhibitor drugs should use yerba mate with caution to monitor these possible effects.

Drug Interactions

None documented, however; it may potentiate monoamine oxidase inhibitor drugs (MAOIs).

Worldwide Ethnomedical Uses

Region	Uses
Brazil	for anthrax ulcers (topical), appetite suppression, asthenia, central nervous system stimulant, digestion stimulant, fatigue, heart support, hypertension, muscle weakness, nerve pain, obesity, renal colic, rheumatism, urinary insufficiency, and as a common beverage and stimulant
Europe	for asthenia, central nervous system disorders, depression, fatigue, gout, headache, heart regulation, obesity, rheumatism, spasms, ulcers, urinary insufficiency, weight loss
India	for fatigue, headache, nervous depression, rheumatic pains
South America	for appetite suppression, debility, energy, exhaustion, fatigue, gout, headache, heart regulation, memory enhancement, muscle weakness, neurasthenia, obesity, rheumatism, scurvy, spasms, stress, sweat promotion, wounds; and as a common beverage, diuretic, laxative, stimulant, tonic
Turkey	as a beverage, diuretic, laxative, stimulant, sweat promoter, and for scurvy
United States	for allergies, anti-aging, appetite suppression, arthritis, constipation, edema, endurance, fatigue, hay fever, headache, heart support, hemorrhoids, nervous system disorders, obesity, stamina, stress, urinary insufficiency, and as a stimulant
Elsewhere	as a cardiotonic, diuretic, stimulant, tonic

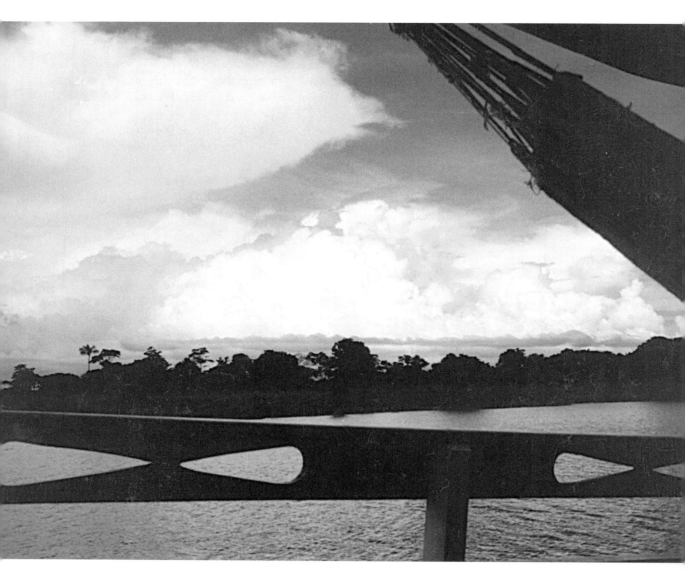

Sunset from a boat on the Amazon.

CONCLUSION

sincerely appreciate the opportunity to share my knowledge and passion about the Amazon rainforest, and its wealth of beneficial medicinal plants, within these pages. I truly do believe that providing knowledge about these plants will help teach people how to use them effectively, and thus, create profitable markets for them, which makes the rainforest more valuable than harvesting timber, grazing cows, or growing soybeans.

I would also feel remiss in not warning readers that there may come a time in the near future when medicinal plants like those found in this book might be out of their reach and simply unavailable to them. This possibility will not necessarily stem from the continued destruction of our tropical rainforests, rather, the erosion and destruction of our health freedom rights to choose alternative therapies.

The complementary and alternative health care (CAM) industry has been growing at an unprecedented rate. This is largely due to the failure of our current medical system and model to provide anything other than expensive long-term treatment of diseases and conditions, rather than any effective cures. Our current health care expenditures are approximately 1.4 trillion dollars annually with an estimated one-third of that spent on drugs. Americans are actively seeking alternative and effective ways to prevent and solve their health issues rather than to just treat them—and at the benefit of the very profitable world drug industry. Americans have spent more out-of-pocket expense for CAM treatments in the last five years than they have spent out of pocket for conventional health services. And it's rocking some boats in the world.

The international drug industry, which stands to lose billions of dollars if cheaper and more effective alternatives are more widely available, has beefed up its political ties and contributions on federal, state, and international levels in an effort to stymie the access to such alternatives. These efforts to suppress access to these alternatives have not escaped notice, however. A Harris Poll survey in July 2004 reported that only 13 percent of Americans believe that the pharmaceutical companies are "generally honest and trustworthy," putting the drug industry on par with tobacco, oil, and managed care companies. The survey indicated that public confidence in drug companies has plunged harder and faster than for any other industry.

Throughout this book I've warned readers that they must educate themselves about available natural products and the effective use of them for their own health and wellness. I now must also warn readers that they need to take the time and effort to research the legal and political issues surrounding their continued availability and regulation. In the words of Thomas Jefferson, "The price of freedom is eternal vigilance." We must always be on guard to ensure our health freedoms are not taken away. For example, some will be shocked to learn that effective August 2005, no one living in any country in the European Union will be able to buy any medicinal plant featured in this book unless they obtain a prescription from a doctor. None of these plants can be harvested in South America and imported into Europe unless they are sold to pharmaceutical companies for their manufacture of drugs.

Everything in Europe is about to change due to the EU Food Supplements Directive (FSD), which will soon go into full effect. As a result, around 5,000 safe formulas and nutrients that have been on the market for decades will be banned in fifteen European countries. This directive regulates that if a plant or herb is medicinal or effects physiological function in any way, it is a medicine and it is to be sold as a drug. This new regulation adversely effects all nutritional supplements, not just herbs. Banned items will include natural vitamins such as mixed tocopherols (natural vitamin E), carotenoids (natural vitamin A) and B_{12}; all forms of sulphur, boron, vanadium, silicon and most trace elements; the most readily absorbed and safest forms of calcium, magnesium, zinc, selenium, chromium and molybdenum; and other popular supplements such as CoQ_{10}, MSM, fatty acids, amino acids, and enzymes. It will severely limit the doses of vitamins and will remove all "high-dose" (in excess of recommended daily allowances [RDA]) products from the market. The directive will dramatically limit future innovation in the supplements industry, and seriously impact retail outlets, complementary practitioners, and consumers who choose to take responsibility for their own health and let food be their medicine. It will also greatly contribute to the profit margins of the European drug industry who will now be the only companies that can manufacture these products.

Why should you be worried about this new European legislation? Simply put, this new directive was the European Union's methodology of accepting and adopting a global harmonization of guidelines effecting nutritional supplements worldwide called "CODEX" which the U.S. is taking part in and is in the process of determining how it will be adopted and implemented here. The Codex Alimentarius Commission (CODEX) was set up in 1962 as a joint body of the Food and Agriculture Organization of the United Nations and the World Health Organization (WHO) under the heavy influence of the European drug industry. The United States signed up for CODEX in the 1990s, when we became members of the World Trade Organization (WTO).

According to the Congressional Research Service: "As a member of the World Trade Organization, the United States does commit to act in accordance with the rules of the multilateral body. The United States is legally obligated to ensure national laws do not conflict with World Trade Organization rules" including laws such as these new ones being adopted in the EU regulating our freedom to nutritional supplements. Therefore, as a member of the WTO, the U.S. will be bound by any finalized standards put forth in the EU directive. If we choose to ignore the regulations that this affiliation binds us to, we could face severe trade sanctions with other WTO countries, and damage part of our economy in our ability to export our goods overseas. Already U.S.-based nutritional manufacturers' ability to export their vitamin, mineral, and herbal products to countries in the European Union has disappeared.

Other countries have already adopted either full or partial CODEX regulations concerning nutritional supplements. The results? In Germany, until 1996, one could freely purchase 500 mg vitamin-C tablets, the way you can here. Now the highest dosage available to Germans is 200 mg; anything higher is sold through pharmacists at extremely high prices and only with a prescription. All herbs are regulated as drugs and manufactured only by German pharmaceutical companies, available to consumers only by prescription. In Norway, all vitamin and mineral supplements that exceed RDA levels are considered drugs. Many natural substances are available in

Norway only through very costly prescriptions, if they're available at all. A black market for supplements has emerged in Norway as a result. Closer to home, in Canada, herbs with medicinal effects (any herb for which claims are made that it improves health) are now classified as drugs. The supplements tryptophan and L-carnitine were once available in Canadian health food stores for $14 per 100 capsules. Now they are available only by prescription for about $120–$190 per 100 capsules.

Surely not in America, you say! Think again. Some form of CODEX can and will become part of our law and order regulations here. Do some research, do your homework, and educate yourself on the issues. It is much too involved and complex an issue to handle efficiently here in the conclusion of this book, but one which all Americans need to be aware of. I have provided some information and internet websites in the Rainforest Resources section, where you can begin your research. Once you have a grasp on the issues, take action! Call, write, or email your state's senators and congresspeople, and tell them of your opinions and how you want them to represent you and your freedom to health care and nutritional supplements. As I said in the introduction to this book—you, as a consumer, have power and can use it effectively to help preserve the rainforest through your consumer dollars. As a voter, you also have power to protect your freedom to choose the right health care services and products—use it effectively by getting informed and participating in the political process!

There's one more thing to do politically as well. (My, isn't it hard being a responsible consumer and participating American!) Before calling your local politicians about CODEX, do some additional research on how your state regulates the access and delivery of complementary and alternative health care services; you may have even more to discuss with your local political representatives. Many people are simply unaware that the provision of health care services related to naturopathy, herbalism, nutrition, and many other effective CAM disciplines are actually illegal in their states.

Many licensed practitioners, such as doctors, nurses, and others, desire to offer alternative health care approaches and CAM services to their patients. However, these healing methods are not the "acceptable and prevailing" conventional standards of care. As a result, practitioners who use CAM therapies may be disciplined by their state medical licensing boards, even if there has been no consumer harm. Licensed providers of alternative therapies nationwide have suffered loss of license, or been forced out of the state to practice, or incurred great legal expenses. As a result, many practitioners who would like to offer their patients CAM services choose not to do so. Others offer the services but do not advertise to that effect. Many consumers are therefore not aware of alternative options.

In reaction to the growing and profitable CAM industry, many state health departments have increased their harassment of licensed health providers practicing CAM in their states. It still has not reduced the popularity of CAM or the number of persons seeking CAM health services. As a result, patients' grassroots campaigns have mobilized to protect freedom of treatment choice and to offset pervasive health department tactics. And they have been effective—after all, these are voters making demands to politicians. Since 1990, thirteen states have passed new laws that protect medical doctors' use of alternative therapies, and three others have promulgated regulations to the same end. These new laws were designed to protect already licensed medical practitioners (medical doctors, osteopaths, etc.) from harassment from aggressive State health departments.

Is it working to protect the delivery of CAM therapy by doctors? Sometimes. Today, about fifty doctors in the U.S. are being investigated and persecuted for using effective alternative approaches to attention deficit hyperactivity disorder (ADHD), Lyme disease, allergies, diabetes, cancer, and other complex syndromes causing pain and misery. While many of these physicians—good reputable doctors—are struggling to rescue their reputations, incomes, and professional lives, their very public ordeals erode the status and practice of alternative medicine. These public cases go a long way in promoting fear and avoidance of doctors regarding the adoption of CAM into their existing practices. It usually depends on the state health department's view, policy, and motivation in administering these laws.

For example, in the state of New York, complementary and alternative physicians remain targets for harassing investigations, despite the 1994 law passed by legislators in response to voter's demands. At least nine New York physicians are currently facing charges of misconduct (and subsequent loss of medical license) simply for using non-conventional therapies like herbs, and have been subjected to questionable tactics employed by the health department. In response, state legislators introduced a new bill to specifically reform and strengthen the language of the original bill and to address the health department's ongoing prosecution of doctors for providing CAM services. This new health care reform bill was aimed directly at reforming the practices and prosecution authority of the New York health department (OPMC), and passed the Senate in July 2004 by unanimous vote.

While inroads are being made on the state level to allow doctors and physicians the ability to offer CAM services to their patients, many professions are not addressed by any state licensing program. Most of these practitioners (naturopaths, herbalists, aromatherapists, nutritionists, and the like) are considered by most state governments as "unlicensed health practitioners" and still subject to civil and criminal prosecution for practicing medicine without a license.

The state of Minnesota is a perfect example of how grassroots organizations of regular citizens are changing laws in regard to demanding free access to CAM services and the lawful provision of these services by unlicensed health practitioners. In 1996, a St. Paul naturopath, Helen Healy, was issued an injunction by the Minnesota Attorney General's office to close her practice; the charge was "practicing medicine without a license." Despite her educational degree (a doctorate in naturopathy) and national board certification, no medical licensing board existed in the state of Minnesota for the licensing of naturopaths (only twelve states currently provide state licensing for naturopaths). The news of the injunction spread quickly throughout the Minnesota natural health community, and they rose with one voice to protest what seemed to be an arbitrary action by the Minnesota Board of Medical Practice to shut down a natural health practitioner. Helen Healy, a graduate of National College of Naturopathic Medicine, had a successful practice in St. Paul for twelve years with no patient complaints or allegations of harm or misconduct.

The state departments backed off from Dr. Healy only after thousands of citizens led marches through the streets and conducted phone campaigns to their government representatives. The realization that all unlicensed CAM practitioners were still subject to legal prosecution at any time fueled the ongoing movement in Minnesota, despite the fact the authorities had backed down from closing Healy's practice. The health freedom campaign gained momentum (and became incorporated as the Minnesota Natural Health Coalition Action Network) and continued to apply a great deal of pressure on state politicians to address the legal problems and issues of unlicensed health practitioners providing much needed and much wanted services. The result? In direct response to voter's demands, the local politicians drafted and passed The Minnesota Complementary Health Practitioner Bill on May 11, 2000. This landmark health freedom law is the first of its kind in the U.S. and grants a virtually unlimited right of practice for unlicensed complementary health care providers without removing consequences for untoward outcomes. Its purpose was stated: "To protect the freedom of the individual to choose and receive the healing treatment that the individual desires and deems to correspond with his/her own view of health and disease, and which the individual deems to be effective in securing his/her own wellness; and to encourage and promote the practice of all healing methods; and to protect the right of health practitioners to practice complementary and alternative health care."

Where does your state and your state's politicians stand on keeping CAM products and services available to you? Find out! Many health codes on the books today were adopted in the 1950s and are very similar and rather standardized, especially within accepted definitions used in these health codes. The medical statute in Minnesota (which allowed the state to act against Helen Healy) is much like that found in every state health code. It states that a person is engaged in the practice of medicine (which requires a license from the state health department and/or state medical board) if she/he does the following: "offers or undertakes to prevent, diagnose, correct, or treat in any manner or by any means, methods, devices, or instrumentalities, any disease, illness, pain, wound, fracture, infirmity, deformity or defect of any person." This is the standard language found in most state health laws and that which is normally used by health departments to censure, regulate, and prosecute CAM practitioners.

What does this mean for CAM practitioners who do not have a state-sanctioned medical license? It means that they are clearly guilty of practicing medicine without a license, and could be prosecuted at any time. Again, it was evidenced in the Healy case that when a state government agency chooses to prosecute an unlicensed practitioner, the practitioner could not introduce evidence of the effectiveness of therapy/modality, the testimony of grateful clients attesting to efficacious and beneficial service, or the fact that no one had been injured. All of these things would be legally irrelevant and inadmissible, and the only point to be considered in a court of law is this: did this person actually practice medicine, as defined by the statute? Absolutely. Case closed. And in most state's health codes, it is a criminal offense to practice medicine without a license, therefore the delivery of most standard CAM services in the majority of states in this country is illegal and subjects the practitioner to civil and criminal penalties.

So far, only four states have written new legislation or amended their health code to correct these technical violations to old codes. In this, California joins Wisconsin, Idaho, and Rhode Island as the fourth state in the country to pass such legislation liberalizing and decriminalizing alternative and complementary medicine. A grassroots organization in North Carolina is lobbying for a similar bill.

Is there a grassroots organization in your state trying to preserve your freedom to complementary health care and medicinal plants like those found in this book? Take the time to find out, and if so—join! If not, at least take the time to talk to your local politicians and tell them what you want them to do. Try faxing or mailing them the landmark Minnesota legislation that effectively protected the rights of residents in that state and suggest the need for the same type of legislation.

My favorite quote of all time comes from Margaret Mead. Years ago she said, "Never doubt that a small group of thoughtful committed citizens can change the world; indeed, it's the only thing that ever has." I know from experience the value and truth in those words. Whether I am a member of citizens fighting for the preservation of the rainforest, the protection of indigenous peoples' land rights or intellectual property rights, or the preservation of my health freedom choices—I know I have to be an active member and join the fight with others. For together, we truly can change the world.

RAINFOREST RESOURCES

The growth and health of our economy today is defined by the intensive exploitation of natural resources. Our present economic model ignores environmental degradation when assessing profits. If we are to survive, principles of sustainability must become integrated into our system. Sustainability means that the functions and processes of an ecosystem can be maintained (or sustained) and the needs of the present can be met—all without compromising the needs of future generations.

Many factors must be taken into consideration, but two are key. The first step is to support the land and resource rights and economies of indigenous peoples. Preserving indigenous cultures is essential to saving the rainforest. These knowledgeable people and their ancestors have inhabited rainforests for millennia without destroying them. We need them to teach us how to use forests without damaging them. Medicines, foods, and other unknown treasures can be harvested without jeopardizing the future. People from developed countries have much to learn from indigenous peoples in terms of our relationship with the Earth. By respecting and allowing them to lead the way toward a true, stable utilization of the bountiful resources of the rainforest (it they choose to use it in any commercial way at all) we have the potential of achieving true sustainability.

The second step is to be a knowledgeable and responsible consumer—and that's hard work. How can you tell if a product has been sustainably harvested? Ask questions. Where do products really come from? Where are your dollars really going? Who is benefiting from the profit? Is any of the profit returned to the people who are supplying rainforest products or raw materials? How much? Who receives the funds there? As a consumer, you are directly affecting the economy and ecology of the globe.

SUSTAINABLE RAINFOREST PRODUCTS

As we support and utilize products like those listed below, we must also be aware that only a limited amount can be consumed. The concept of sustainability transcends the traditional rules of "supply and demand" as each ecosystem determines the ceiling of its productivity. The primary question for us must not be, "Which herbal supplement, backpack, or body lotion should I buy?" but, "Do I need to buy this?"

Aloha Tropicals

P.O. Box 6042
Oceanside, CA 92054
Phone: 760-631-2880
Email: alohatrop@aol.com
Website: www.alohatropicals.com/

The company sells tropical plants and seeds to grow, including several of the rainforest plants featured in this book.

Aveda Corporation

4999 Pheasant Ridge Drive
Blaine, MN 55449
Phone: 866-823-1425
Website: www.aveda.com

Aveda produces hair- and body-care products utilizing sustainably harvested rainforest ingredients (oils, butters, herbal extracts). Many of their harvesting programs for these rainforest resources support indigenous communities. Their products are distributed in salons, spas, and body-care product stores worldwide.

Bolsa Amazonia

Campus Universitário do Guama - Setor Profissional
Casa do Poema - CEP: 66075-900
Belém, Pará
Brazil
Phone: 011-55-91-3183-1686 · 011-55-91-3183-2027
Website: www.bolsaamazonia.com

A sustainable source of paper produced in the Amazon. Amazon Paper does not compete in the conventional paper market or the recycled paper market. Being manually produced from natural fibers through craftsmanship of the region, sheet by sheet, it is classified as "art paper."

Couro Vegetal da Amazônia

Rua Flack 144 Riachuelo
Rio de Janeiro
20960-160
Brazil
Phone: 011-55-21-241-1276
Website: http://treetap.amazonlife.com.br

Manufactures and sells a sustainable alternative to leather from tree-tapped rubber latex. Products include totebags, purses, backpacks, clothing, etc.

Forests of the World

607 Ellis Road, Bldg. 53-A1
Durham, NC 27703
Phone: 919-957-1500
Website: www.forestsoftheworld.com

This company is an importer, distributor, and retailer of educational products, fair trade crafts, and non-timber forest and food products made by indigenous groups and from rainforests, conservation and development projects, parks, protected areas, and hotspots of high biodiversity.

GreenDealer Exotic Seeds

P.O. Box 37328
Louisville, KY 40233
Phone: 502-459-9054
Website: www.greendealer-exotic-seeds.com

Sells tropical plants and seeds to grow, including several of the rainforest plants featured in this book.

Guayakí Sustainable Rainforest Products

P.O. Box 14730
San Luis Obispo, CA 93406
Phone: 888-482-9254 · 805-546-8111
Fax: 805-545-8111
Email: info@guayaki.com
Website: www.guayaki.com

Harvests, imports, and sells yerba mate from Paraguay. Guayakí's mission is to cultivate sustainability by working in harmony with indigenous cultures and their environment to produce products that promote market-driven conservation.

Jatun Sacha Foundation

Pasaje Eugenio de Santillán
N34-248 y Maurián
Quito
Ecuador

Phone: 011-59-32-2432-240/173/246
Email: jatunsacha@jatunsacha.org
Website: www.jatunsacha.org
A private, non-profit Ecuadorian foundation offering arts, crafts, and jewelry made from sustainable forest-gathered materials and resources.

Kallari Rainforest Originals
N39-188 Bermejo y Shushufindi
Urbanización Petrolera
Sector Monteserrín
Quito
Ecuador
Phone: 011-593-22-432-240 · 011-593-22-453-583
Website: www.kallari.com
Cooperative in Ecuador selling handmade fair trade jewelry, purses and bags, canoes and paddles, dishes, hats, and more in an effort to conserve Ecuadorian rainforests.

Moonshine Trading Co.
P.O. Box 896
Winters, CA 95694
Phone: 916-753-0601
Produces gourmet nut butters, spreads, and honey from sustainably cultivated and harvested rainforest nuts and wild collected honey.

One World Projects, Inc.
21 Ellicott Avenue
Batavia, NY 14020-2010
Phone: 585-343-4490
Fax: 585-344-3551
Email: sales@oneworldprojects.com
Website: www.oneworldprojects.com
This company is perhaps the largest distributor and importer of rainforest products in terms of the types of products and number of producer groups they support. Their mission is to develop markets for products made from renewable forest resources that can be harvested in a sustainable manner without damage to the forest ecosystem, while providing rainforest inhabitants with a just means of economic subsistence.

PatagonBird
353 East 72nd Street #24-B
New York, NY 10021
Phone: 212-717-4805
Email: info@patagonbird.com
Website: www.patagonbird.com
PatagonBird is a New York-based family-run company started in 1998 with a commitment to help indigenous people from Argentina, not by way of charity but helping them find new markets for their beautiful arts and crafts. They work with large communities of Indians in the Northwest of Argentina, such as the Wichi people from Mision Chaqueña, Salta, and the Chiriguano Indians from Salta and Formosa provinces.

Rainforest Seed Company Canada
207 Howard Park Avenue
Toronto, Ontario M6R-1V9
Canada
Phone: 416-767-0649
Email: rainseed@interlog.com
Website: www.interlog.com/~rainseed/
Operates a 1,500 acre protected rainforest situated in Northern Costa Rica, where most of their plant seeds are harvested and collected by hand.

RainSeed Company
P.O. Box 658
Elberta, AL 36530
Phone: 800-965-4299
Fax: 251-943-1716
Website: www.rainseed.com
Sells tropical plants and rainforest plant seeds to grow, including several of the rainforest plants featured in this book.

Raintree Nutrition, Inc.
3579 Hwy 50 East
P.O. Box 369
Carson City, NV 89701
Phone: 800-780-5902 · 775-841-4142
Email: info@rain-tree.com
Website: www.rain-tree.com

Harvests, imports, and distributes sustainably harvested rainforest medicinal plants. Manufactures a line of retail herbal supplements and another line of professional herbal products for practitioners of the healing arts. Many of the plants featured in this book are available through this company.

Rainforest Remedies

Distributed by: Lotus Brands, Inc.
P.O. Box 325
Twin Lakes, WI 53181
Phone: 800-824-6396

Rainforest Remedies is a product line of herbal extracts that come from the Central American rainforest of Belize. Produced by the Ix Chel Foundation, these formulas utilize the healing herbs used by the traditional healers of the area. These products can be found in most American health food stores and can be ordered online at www.internatural.com.

Samba, Inc.

927 Calle Negocio, Suite J
San Clemente, CA 92673
Phone: 949-574-0080 · 877-726-2296
Email: info@sambazon.com
Website: www.sambazon.com

Markets "Sambazon," a combination of three rainforest fruits: acai, acerola, and cupuacu, which is sustainably harvested in the Brazilian Amazon.

SmartWood

Goodwin-Baker Building
65 Millet Street, Suite 201
Richmond, VT 05477
Phone: 802-434-5491
Email: info@smartwood.org
Website: www.smartwood.org

SmartWood is a program of the Rainforest Alliance, an international non-profit environmental group based in New York City. SmartWood certifies forest products that come from "well-managed" forests ("sources"). Contact them or see their website to obtain a list of companies offering certified wood products.

Stokes Tropicals

4806 E Old Spanish Trail
Jeanerette, LA 7054
Phone: 800-624-9706
Email: info@stokestropicals.com
Website: www.stokestropicals.com

Sells tropical plants and seeds to grow, including several of the rainforest plants featured in this book.

Top Tropicals

11351 Orange Drive
Davie, FL 33330
Phone: 866-897-7957
Website: http://toptropicals.com

Sells tropical plants and seeds to grow, including several of the rainforest plants featured in this book.

Tropilab, Inc.

8240 Ulmerton Road
Largo, FL 33771
Phone: 888-613-4446
Website: www.tropilab.com

Exporter and wholesaler of medicinal plants, herbs, tropical seeds, and cut flowers from the Amazon in Suriname.

Yachana Gourmet

Distributed by: One World Projects
21 Ellicott Avenue
Batavia, NY 14020-2010
Phone: 800-637-7614
Email: yachana@oneworldprojects.com ·
   orders@yachanagourmet.com
Website: www.yachanagourmet.com

Yachana Gourmet™ and the people along the Napo River work together to bring exotic rainforest products to your table. Their product line includes tropical fruit spreads and chocolates and provides an alternative source of income for families who live in the rainforest. Yachana Gourmet supports fair trade practices while protecting rainforest resources.

NON-PROFIT RAINFOREST ORGANIZATIONS

The following organizations are actively involved with rainforest conservation projects and are deserving of support. Most provide extensive information about conservation problems and solutions on their websites and provide a method to donate to their organizations online.

ACEER Foundation

P.O. Box 2549
West Chester, PA 19383
Phone: 610-738-0477
Website: www.aceer.org

The Amazon Center for Environmental Education and Research supports its education and research programs in the Peruvian Amazon with classrooms, a field lab, demonstration gardens, interpreted trails, and a nature interpretation center for researchers, students, and others.

Amazon Conservation Association

1834 Jefferson Place NW
Washington, DC 20036
Phone: 202-452-0752
Email: info@amazonconservation.org
Website: www.amazonconservation.org

The Amazon Conservation Association envisions a network of state, community, and private lands managed for conservation and sustainable resource use so that the biological diversity of the southwest Amazon basin is conserved.

Amazon Conservation Team

4211 N. Fairfax Drive
Arlington, VA 22203
Phone: 703-522-4684
Website: www.ethnobotany.org

The Amazon Conservation Team works in partnership with indigenous people in conserving biodiversity, health, and culture in tropical America. They achieve these goals by the establishment of Shamans and Apprentices programs, the support of comprehensive mapping projects, and the building of Traditional Clinics.

Amazon Watch

1 Haight Street, Suite B
San Francisco, CA 94102
Phone: 415-487-9600
Email: amazon@amazonwatch.org
Website: www.amazonwatch.org

Works with indigenous and environmental organizations in the Amazon Basin to defend the environment and advance indigenous peoples' rights in the face of large-scale industrial development such as oil and gas pipelines, power lines, roads, and other mega-projects.

Ceiba Foundation for Tropical Conservation

2319 North Cleveland
Chicago, IL 60614
Fax: 773-871-3798
Website: www.ceiba.org

A non-profit organization founded in 1997, dedicated to the preservation and rehabilitation of tropical habitats, and the conservation of their plants and animals through scientific research, public education, and community-based actions.

Greenpeace International

702 H Street NW, Suite 300
Washington, DC 20001
Phone: 202-462 1177
Email: greenpeace.usa@wdc.greenpeace.org
Website: www.greenpeace.org

An independent campaigning organization that uses non-violent, creative confrontation to expose global environmental problems, including in the Amazon.

The Nature Conservancy

4245 North Fairfax Drive, Suite 100
Arlington, VA 22203-1606
Phone: 800-628-6860
Website: www.nature.org

A national non-profit organization with a mission to preserve the plants, animals, and natural communities that represent the diversity of life on Earth by protecting the lands and waters they need to survive.

Rainforest Action Network

221 Pine Street, Suite 500
San Francisco, CA 94104
Phone: 415-398-4404
Email: rainforest@ran.org
Website: www.ran.org

Rainforest Action Network works to protect the Earth's rainforests and support the rights of their inhabitants through education, grassroots organizing, and non-violent direct action. Since it was founded in 1985, the Rainforest Action Network has been working to protect rainforests and the human rights of those living in and around those forests.

The Rainforest Alliance

665 Broadway, Suite 500
New York, NY 10012
Phone: 212-677-1900 · 888-MY-EARTH
Website: www.rainforest-alliance.org

Rainforest Alliance is a leading international conservation organization. Their mission is to protect ecosystems and the people and wildlife that live within them by implementing better business practices for biodiversity, conservation, and sustainability through their certification programs.

The Rainforest Foundation UK

Suite A5, City Cloisters
196 Old Street
London EC1V 9FR
United Kingdom
Phone: 011-44-20-7251-6345
Email: rainforestuk@rainforestuk.com
Website: www.rainforestuk.com

The mission of the Rainforest Foundation is to support indigenous people and traditional populations of the world's rainforests in their efforts to protect their environment and fulfill their rights.

Survival International

6 Charterhouse Buildings
London EC1M 7ET
United Kingdom

Phone: 011-44-20-7687-8700
Email: info@survival-international.org
Website: www.survival-international.org

Survival International is a non-profit worldwide organization supporting tribal peoples and founded in 1969. It stands for their right to decide their own future and helps them protect their lives, lands, and human rights. They also offer a mail order catalog and online shopping of various gift items.

World Rainforest Movement

Maldonado 1858
11200 Montevideo
Uruguay
Phone: 011-598-2-413-2989
Email: wrm@wrm.org.uy
Website: www.wrm.org.uy

The World Rainforest Movement was established in 1986. It works to secure the lands and livelihoods of forest peoples and supports their efforts to defend the forests from commercial logging, dams, mining, plantations, shrimp farms, colonization and settlement, and other projects that threaten them.

INTERNET RESOURCES

The following websites are good places to start to learn more about medicinal plants, traditional herbal medicine, and alternative health.

The Raintree Tropical Plant Database

www.rain-tree.com/plants.htm

A comprehensive searchable database about the medicinal plants of the Amazon and other tropical medicinal plants (about 130 tropical plant files available). Contains color pictures of the plants, their history of uses, chemistry, and the research performed on them.

PubMed

www.ncbi.nlm.nih.gov/entrez/query.fcgi?db=PubMed

National Library of Medicine's search interface to access the 10 million citations in MEDLINE, and Pre-MEDLINE, and other related databases. Look up and access the journal abstracts of most of the published research cited in this book at this searchable database. Usually, using the plant's Latin genus and species name as search words will access most of the publications available on that plant.

Plants for a Future Database

www.scs.leeds.ac.uk/pfaf/index.html

From Leeds University, UK, the Species Database contains approximately 7,000 plants with edible or medicinal uses. There are links to three websites for searching, and downloadable versions.

HerbMed® Database

www.herbmed.org

An interactive, electronic herbal database that provides links to the scientific data underlying the use of herbs for health. It is an evidence-based information resource for professionals, researchers, and the general public.

The American Botanical Council

www.herbalgram.org

The American Botanical Council is the leading non-profit education and research organization disseminating science-based information promoting the safe and effective use of medicinal plants and phytomedicines. Several searchable databases are offered on their website.

Medicinal Plants Database

www.pl.barc.usda.gov/

From the USDA Beltsville Agricultural Research Center and the Beltsville Human Nutrition Research Center.

Dr. Duke's Phytochemical and Ethnobotanical Databases

www.ars-grin.gov/duke/

Several searchable databases from the US Agricultural Research Database covering ethnobotanical uses for plants and plant chemical constituents.

American Indian Ethnobotany Database

http://herb.umd.umich.edu/

Dr. Moerman's database of foods, drugs, dyes, and fibers of Native American Peoples, derived from plants. It is based at the University of Michigan.

TROPICOS Database

http://mobot.mobot.org/W3T/Search/vast.html

Not sure of a tropical plant's proper Latin name? This site provides access to the Missouri Botanical Garden's VAST (VAScular Tropicos) nomenclature database and associated authority files.

Southwest School of Botanical Medicine

www.swsbm.com/homepage/

The site offers tons of information, pictures, and educational materials about medicinal plants.

National Center for Complementary and Alternative Medicine (NCCAM)

http://nccam.nih.gov/

NCCAM, at the National Institutes of Health, is dedicated to exploring complementary and alternative healing practices in the context of rigorous science, training CAM researchers, and disseminating authoritative information.

IBIDS

http://ods.od.nih.gov/showpage.aspx?pageid=48

The database, International Bibliographic Information on Dietary Supplements, from the Office of Dietary Supplements, NIH, covers vitamins, minerals, and herbs.

Office of Cancer Complementary and Alternative Medicine (OCCAM)

www3.cancer.gov/occam/

This government agency was established to coordinate and enhance the activities of the National Cancer Institute in the arena of complementary and alternative medicine.

DATADIWAN

www.datadiwan.de/index_e.htm

The German, Patienteninformation fur Naturheilkunde, (Patient information for natural therapies) has a searchable database online, much of it in English, providing information on holistic medicine and a network linking research institutions and organizations worldwide. There are over 5,000 bibliographic entries and 1,000 addresses.

USPTO Database

www.uspto.gov/patft/index.html

The U.S. Patent and Trademark Office is an important and relatively unexplored source of information and often unpublished research data relevant to studies in alternative and complementary medicine, and plants with medicinal uses. Full text of the patents cited in this book are accessible at this website.

SUGGESTED READING

Rainforest Conservation and Sustainability Issues

To explore the complex issues of rainforest destruction, sustainable use of these valuable ecosystems, and possible methods of conservation, the following books offer some unique perspectives.

The Brazilian Amazon Rainforest

Luiz C. Barbosa. University Press of America; 2000.

Provides a global, world-systemic analysis of the problem of deforestation of the Brazilian Amazon rainforest. He shows how changes in global ecopolitics demanding sustainable development, coupled with the onset of democracy in Brazil, substantially altered the battle over the future of Amazonia.

Tropical Forest Conservation

Douglas Dewitt Southgate. Oxford University Press; 1998.

This book assesses the viability of conservation strategies predicated on the adoption of environmentally sound enterprises in and around threatened habitats. Drawing on research in Brazil, Costa Rica, Ecuador, and Peru, the author contends that human capital formation and related productivity-enhancing investment is the only sure path to economic progress and habitat conservation.

Medicinal Resources of the Tropical Forest

Michael J. Balick, et al. Columbia University Press; 1996.

This books targets the enormous resources of the Earth's rainforests and the potential impact of their destruction in terms of human health to inhabitants of both the developing and developed world.

Tropical Forests and the Human Spirit

Roger D. Stonea and Claudia D'Andrea. University of California Press; 2001.

This book, based on extensive international field research, highlights one solution for preserving this precious resource: empowering local people who depend on the forest for survival.

Conservation of Neotropical Forests

Christine Padoch and Kent H. Redford. Columbia University Press; 1999.

This provides important information for understanding the interactions of forest peoples and forest resources in the lowland tropics of Central and South America. This interdisciplinary study features experts from both the natural and social sciences to illuminate the present dilemma of conserving neotropical resources.

Quantifying Sustainable Development

Charles A. S. Hall, Gregoire Leclerc, and Carlos Leon Perez. Academic Press; 2000.

This interdisciplinary book covers the conditions of the developing tropics, the resistance of some of their problems to earlier attempts at solutions, and the use of new tools to develop a much more comprehensive and empirical framework for conservation and sustainability.

POLITICAL AND HEALTH FREEDOM RESOURCES

Alliance for Natural Health

Mount Manor House
16 The Mount
Guildford
Surrey GU2 4HS
United Kingdom
Phone/Fax: 011-44-1252-371-275
Email: info@alliance-natural-health.org
Website: www.alliance-natural-health.org

American Holistic Health Association
P.O. Box 17400
Anaheim, CA 92817-7400
Phone: 714-779-6152
Email: mail@ahha.org
Website: www.ahha.org/

The Coalition for Natural Health
Website: www.naturalhealth.org/

CODEX
Website: www.codexalimentarius.net/

The Friends of Freedom Inc.
Website: www.friendsoffreedom.org ·
      www.friendsoffreedominternational.org

Health Freedom Foundation
9912 Georgetown Pike, Suite D-2
Great Falls, VA 22066
Phone: 800-230-2762 · 703-759-0662
Email: healthfreedom2000@yahoo.com
Website: www.apma.net/

Institute for Health Freedom
1825 Eye Street NW, Suite 400
Washington, DC 20006
Phone: 202-429-6610
Website: www.forhealthfreedom.org/

International Advocates for Health Freedom
P.O. Box 625
Floyd, VA 24091
Phone: 800-333-2553 · 540-745-6534
Email: jham@iahf.com
Website: www.iahf.com

International Council for Health Freedom
5580 La Jolla Boulevard
PMB 429
La Jolla, CA 92037
Phone: 619-661-7488
Website: www.ichf.info

Minnesota Natural Health Coalition
Phone: 651-322-4542
Email: mnhc1@earthlink.net
Website: www.minnesotanaturalhealth.org/

Natural Health Freedom Coalition
PMB 218
2136 Ford Parkway
St. Paul, MN 55116-1863
Phone: 651-690-0732
Website: www.nationalhealthfreedom.org

Dr. Rath Health Foundation
The Hague Zurich Tower
Muzenstraat 89
NL-2511 WB
The Hague
Netherlands
Website: www.dr-rath-foundation.org

REFERENCES FOR PART THREE

Abuta

1. Anwer, F., et al. "Studies in medicinal plants 3. Protoberberine alkaloids from the roots of *Cissampelos pareira* Linn." *Experientia* 1968; 15.

2. Bhatnagar, A. K., et al. "Chemical examination of the roots of *Cissampelos pareira* Linn. V. Structure and stereochemistry of hayatidin." *Experientia* 1967; 15.

3. Bruneton, J. *Pharmaognosy, Phytochemistry, Medicinal Plants*. Andover, England: Intercept Limited, 1995.

4. Werbach, M. R., et al. *Botanical Influences on Illness—A Sourcebook of Clinical Research*. Tarzana, CA: Third Line Press, 1994.

5. Blumenthal, M. "Plant medicines from the New World." *Whole Foods Magazine*, April 1997.

6. Feng, P. C., et al. "Pharmacological screening of some West Indian medicinal plants." *J. Pharm. Pharmacol.* 1962; 14: 556–561.

7. Mokkhasmit, M., et al. "Pharmacological evaluation of Thai medicinal plants continued." *J. Med. Ass. Thailand* 1971; 54(7): 490–504.

8. Bork, P. M., et al. "Sesquiterpene lactone containing Mexican Indian medicinal plants and pure sesquiterpene lactones as potent inhibitors of transcription factor NF-KB." *Febs. Lett.* 1997; 402(1): 85–90.

9. Caceres, A., et al. "Diuretic activity of plants used for the treatment of urinary ailments in Guatemala." *J. Ethnopharmacol.* 1987; 19(3): 233–245.

10. Akah, P. A., et al. "Studies on anti-ulcer properties of *Cissampelos mucronata* leaf extract." *Indian J. Exp. Biol.* 1999; 37(9): 936–938.

11. Tripathi, S. N., et al. "Screening of hypoglycemic action in certain indigenous drugs." *J. Res. Indian Med. Yoga Homeopathy* 1979; 14(3): 159–169.

12. Adesina, S. K. "Studies on some plants used as anticonvulsants in Amerindian and African traditional medicine." *Fitoterapia* 1982; 53: 147–162.

13. Sanchez Medina, A., et al. "Evaluation of biological activity of crude extracts from plants used in Yucatecan traditional medicine part l. Antioxidant, antimicrobial and beta-glucosidase inhibition activities." *Phytomedicine* 2001; 8(2): 144–151.

14. George, M. and K. M. Pandalai. "Investigations on plant antibiotics. Part IV. Further search for antibiotic substances in Indian medicinal plants." *Indian J. Med. Res.* 1949; 37: 169–181.

15. Gessler, M. C., et al. "Screening of Tanzanian medicinal plants for antimalarial activity." *Acta. Tropica.* 1994; 56(1): 65–77.

16. Gessler, M. C., et al. "Tanzanian medicinal plants used traditionally for the treatment of malaria: *in vivo* antimalarial and *in vitro* cytotoxic activities." *Phytother. Res.* 1995; 9(7): 504–508.

17. Mokkhasmit, M., et al. "Study on toxicity of Thai medicinal plants." *Dept. Med. Sci.* 1971; 12 2/4: 36–65.

Acerola

1. Lung, A., and S. Foster. *Encyclopedia of Common Natural Ingredients*. New York: John Wiley & Sons, 1996.

2. Leme, J. Jr., et al. "Variation of ascorbic acid and beta-carotene content in lyophilized cherry from the West Indies (*Malpighia punicifolia* L.)." *Arch. Latinoam. Nutr.* 1973; 23(2): 207–215.

3. de Medeiros, R. B. "Proportion of ascorbic, dehydroascorbic and diketogulonic acids in green or ripe acerola (*Malpighia punicifolia*)." *Rev. Bras. Med.* 1969; 26(7): 398–400.

4. Pino, J. A., et al. "Volatile flavor constituents of acerola (*Malpighia emarginata* DC.) fruit." *J. Agric. Food Chem.* 2001; 49(12): 5880–5882.

5. Caceres, A. "Plants used in Guatemala for the treatment of dermatophytic infections 2. Evaluation of antifungal activity of seven American plants." *J. Ethnopharmacol.* 1993; 40: 3.

6. Hwang, J., et al. "Soy and alfalfa phytoestrogen extracts become potent low-density lipoprotein antioxidants in the presence of acerola cherry extract." *J. Agric. Food Chem.* 2001; 49(1): 308–314.

7. Raulf-Heimsoth, M., et al. "Anyphylactic reaction to apple juice containing acerola: Cross-reactivity to latex due to prohevein." *J. Aller. and Clin. Immunol.* 2002; 109(4).

Amargo

1. Hoffman, David. 1991. The New Holistic Herbal, Element Books, Inc.: Rockport, MA.

2. Duke, J. A. *CRC Handbook of Medicinal Herbs*. CRC Press: Boca Raton, FL, 1985.

3. Samuelsson, G. *Drugs of Natural Origin*. Swedish Pharmaceutical Press: Stockholm, Sweden, 1992.

4. Lueng, A. and S. Foster. *Encyclopedia of Common Natural Ingredients*. Wiley and Sons: New York, 1996.

5. Kupchan, S. M. "Quassimarin, a new antileukemic quassinoid from *Quassia amara*." *J. Org. Chem.* 1976; 41(21): 3481–3482.

5. Xu, Z., et al. "Anti-HIV agents 45(1) and antitumor agents 205. (2) Two new sesquiterpenes, leitneridanins A and B, and the cytotoxic and anti-HIV principles from *Leitneria floridana*." *J. Nat. Prod.* 2000; 63(12): 1712–1715.

7. O'Neill, M. J., et al. "Plants as sources of antimalarial drugs: *in vitro* antimalarial ac-

tivities of some quassinoids." *Antimicrob. Agents Chemother.* 1986; 30(1): 101–104.

8. Trager, W., et al. "Antimalarial activity of quassinoids against chloroquine-resistant *Plasmodium falciparum in vitro.*" *Am. J. Trop. Med. Hyg.* 1981; 30(3): 531–537.

9. Apers, S., et al. "Antiviral activity of simalikalactone D, a quassinoid from *Quassia africana.*" *Planta Med.* 2002; 25(9): 1151–1155.

10. Garcia Gonzalez, M., et al. "Pharmacologic activity of the aqueous wood extract from *Quassia amara* (Simarubaceae) on albino rats and mice." *Rev. Biol. Trop.* 1997; 44–45: 47–50.

11. Jensen, O. "Treatment of head lice with Quassia tincture." *Ugeskr. Laeger.* 1979; 141(4): 225–126.

12. Jensen, O. "*Pediculosis capitis* treated with Quassia tincture." *Acta. Derm. Venereol.* 1978; 58(6): 557–559.

13. Ninci, M. E. "Prophylaxis and treatment of pediculosis with *Quassia amarga.*" *Rev. Fac. Cien. Med. Univ. Nac. Cordoba* 1991; 49(2): 27–31.

14. Roark, R. C. "Some promising insecticidal plants." *Econ. Bot.* 1947; 1: 437–445.

15. Evans, D. A., et al. "Extracts of Indian plants as mosquito larvicides." *Indian J. Med. Res.* 1988; 88(1): 38–41.

16. Ajaiyeoba, E. O., et al. "*In vivo* antimalarial activities of *Quassia amara* and *Quassia undulata* plant extracts in mice." *J. Ethnopharmacol.* 1999; 67(3): 321–325.

17. Abdel-Malek, S., et al. "Drug leads from the Kallaway herbalists of Bolivia. 1. Background, rationale, protocol and anti-HIV activity." *J. Ethnopharmacol.* 1996; 50: 157–166.

18. Toma, W., et al. "Antiulcerogenic activity of four extracts obtained from the bark wood of *Quassia amara* L. (Simaroubaceae)." *Planta Med.* 2002; 68(1): 20–24.

19. Tada, H., et al. "Novel anti-ulcer agents and quassinoids." United States Patent 4,731,459; 1988.

20. Toma, W., et al. "Evaluation of the analgesic and antiedematogenic activities of *Quassia amara* bark extract." *J. Ethnopharmacol.* 2003; 85(1): 19–23.

21. Parveen, S., et al. "A comprehensive evaluation of the reproductive toxicity of *Quassia amara* in male rats." *Reprod. Toxicol.* 2003; 17(1): 45–50.

Amor Seco

1. Brandao, M., et al. "Survey of medicinal plants used as antimalarials in the Amazon." *J. Ethnopharmacol.* 1992; 36(2): 175–182.

2. Boye, G. and O. Ampopo. "Plants and traditional medicine in Ghana." *Economic and Medicinal Plant Research* 4 1990. Devon, England: Academic Press Ltd.: 33–34.

3. Ampopo, O. "Plants that heal." *World Health 1977.* 1977: 26–30.

4. Addy, M. E., et al. "Effects of the extracts of *Desmodium adscendens* on anaphylaxis." *J. Ethnopharmacol.* 1984; 11(3): 283–292.

5. Addy, M. E., et al. "Effect of *Desmodium adscendens* fraction F1 (DAFL) on tone and agonist-induced contractions of guinea pig airway smooth muscle." *Phytother. Res.* 1989; 3(3): 85–90.

6. Addy, M. E., et al. "Effect of *Desmodium adscendens* fractions on antigen- and arachidonic acid-induced contractions of guinea pig airways." *Can. J. Physiol. Pharmacol.* 1987; 66(6): 820–825.

7. Addy, M. E., et al. "Dose-response effect of one subfraction of *Desmodium adscendens* aqueous extract on antigen- and arachidonic acid-induced contractions of guinea pig airways." *Phytother. Res.* 1987; 1(4): 180–186.

8. Addy, M. E., et al. "Effect of *Desmodium adscendens* fraction 3 on contractions of respiratory smooth muscle." *J. Ethnopharmacol.* 1990; 29(3): 325–335.

9. Addy, M. E., et al. "Dose-response effects of *Desmodium adscendens* aqueous extract on histamine response, content and anaphylactic reactions in the guinea pig." *J. Ethnopharmacol.* 1996; 18(1): 13–20.

10. Addy, M. E., et al. "Several chromatographically distinct fractions of *Desmodium adscendens* inhibit smooth muscle contractions." *Int. J. Crude Drug Res.* 1989; 27(2): 81–91.

11. Addy, M. E., et al. "An extract of *Desmodium adscendens* activates cyclooxygenase and increases prostaglandin synthesis by ram seminal vesicle microsomes." *Phytother. Res.* 1995; 9(4): 287–293.

12. Addy, M. E., et al. "Some secondary plant metabolites in *Desmodium adscendens* and their effects on arachidonic acid metabolism." *Prostaglandins Leukotrienes Essent. Fatty Acids* 1992; 47(1): 85–91.

13. Hallstrand, T. S., et al. "Leukotriene modifiers." *Med. Clin. North. Am.* 2002; 86(5): 1009–1033.

14. Coffey, M., et al. "Extending the understanding of leukotrienes in asthma." *Curr. Opin. Allergy Clin. Immunol.* 2003; 3(1): 57–63.

15. Barreto, G. S. "Effect of butanolic fraction of *Desmodium adscendens* on the anococcygeus of the rat." *Braz. J. Biol.* 2002; 62(2): 223–230.

16. McManus, O. B., et al. "An activator of calcium-dependent potassium channels isolated from a medicinal herb." *Biochemistry* 1993; 32(24): 6128–6133.

17. N'Gouemo, P., et al. "Effects of an ethanolic extract of *Desmodium adscendens* on central nervous system in rodents." *J. Ethnopharmacol.* 1996; 52(2): 77–83.

Anamu

1. Mata-Greenwood, E., et al. "Discovery of novel inducers of cellular differentiation using HL-60 promyelocytic cells." *Anticancer Res.* 2001; 21(3B): 1763–1770.

2. Yan, R., et al. "Astilbin selectively facilitates the apoptosis of interleukin-2-dependent phytohemaglutinin-activated Jurkat cells." *Pharmacol. Res.* 2001; 44(2): 135–139.

3. Weber, U. S., et al. "Antitumor activities of coumarin, 7-hydroxy-coumarin and its glucuronide in several human tumor cell lines." *Res. Commun. Mol. Pathol. Pharmacol.* 1998; 99(2): 193–206.

4. Bassi, A. M., et al. "Comparative evaluation of cytotoxicity and metabolism of four aldehydes in two hepatoma cell lines." *Drug Chem. Toxicol.* 1997 Aug.; 20(3): 173–187.

5. Rossi, V., et al. "Antiproliferative effects of *Petiveria alliacea* on several tumor cell lines." *Pharmacol. Res. Suppl.* 1990; 22(2): 434.

6. Jovicevic, L., et al. "*In vitro* antiproliferative activity of *Petiveria alliacea L.* on several tumor cell lines." *Pharmacol. Res.* 1993; 27(1): 105–106.

7. Ruffa, M. J., et al. "Cytotoxic effect of Argentine medicinal plant extracts on human hepatocellular carcinoma cell line." *J. Ethnopharmacol.* 2002; 79(3): 335–339.

8. Rosner, H., et al. "Disassembly of microtubules and inhibition of neurite outgrowth, neuroblastoma cell proliferation, and MAP kinase tyrosine dephosphorylation by dibenzyl trisulphide." *Biochem. Biophys. Acta* 2001; 1540(2): 166–177.

9. Rossi, V., "Effects of *Petiveria alliacea L.* on cell immunity." *Pharmacol. Res.* 1993; 27(1): 111–112.

10. Marini, S., "Effects of *Petiveria alliacea L.* on cytokine production and natural killer cell activity." *Pharmacol. Res.* 1993; 27(1): 107–108.

11. Quadros, M. R., et al., "*Petiveria alliacea L.* extract protects mice against *Listeria monocytogenes* infection—effects on bone marrow progenitor cells." *Immunopharmacol. Immunotoxicol.* 1999 Feb; 21(1): 109–124.

12. Queiroz, M. L., et al., "Cytokine profile and natural killer cell activity in *Listeria monocytogenes* infected mice treated orally with *Petiveria alliacea* extract." *Immunopharmacol. Immunotoxicol.* 2000 Aug.; 22(3): 501–518.

13. Williams, L., et al. "Immunomodulatory activities of *Petiveria alliaceae L.*" *Phytother. Res.* 1997; 11(3): 251–253.

14. Dunstan, C. A., et al. "Evaluation of some Samoan and Peruvian medicinal plants by prostaglandin biosynthesis and rat ear oedema assays." *J. Ethnopharmacol.* 1997 Jun; 57(1): 35–56.

15. Germano, D., et al. "Pharmacological assay of *Petiveria alliaceae*. Oral anti-inflammatory activity and gastrotoxicity of a hydro alcoholic root extract." *Fitoterapia* 1993; 64(5): 459–467.

16. Di Stasi, L. C., et al. "Screening in mice of some medicinal plants used for analgesic purposes in the state of São Paulo." *J. Ethnopharmacol.* 1988; 24(2/3): 205–211.

17. de Lima, T. C., et al. "Evaluation of antinociceptive effect of *Petiveria alliacea* (Guine) in animals." *Mem. Inst. Oswaldo Cruz.* 1991; 86 Suppl 2: 153–158.

18. Lopes-Martins, R.A., et al. "The anti-inflammatory and analgesic effects of a crude extract of *Petiveria alliacea L.* (Phytolaccaceae)." *Phytomedicine* 2002; 9(3): 245–248.

19. Germano, D. H., et al. "Topical anti-inflammatory activity and toxicity of *Petiveria alliaceae*." *Fitoterapia* 1993; 64(5): 459–467.

20. Ruffa, M. J., et al. "Antiviral activity of *Petiveria alliacea* against the bovine diarrhea virus." *Chemotherapy* 2002; 48(3): 144–147.

21. Misas, C.A.J., et al. "The biological assessment of Cuban plants. III." *Rev. Cub. Med. Trop.* 1979; 31(1): 21–27.

22. Von Szczepanski, C., et al. "Isolation, structure elucidation and synthesis of an antimicrobial substance from *Petiveria alliacea*." *Arzneim-Forsch* 1972; 22: 1975.

23. Caceres, A., et al. "Plants used in Guatemala for the treatment of dermatophytic infections. I. Screening for antimycotic activity of 44 plant extracts." *J. Ethnopharmacol.* 1991; 31(3): 263–276.

24. Benevides, P. J., et al. "Antifungal polysulphides from *Petiveria alliacea L.*" *Phytochemistry* 2001; 57(5): 743–747.

25. Caceres, A., et al. "Plants used in Guatemala for the treatment of protozoal infections. I. Screening of activity to bacteria, fungi and American trypanosomes of 13 native plants." *J. Ethnopharmacol.* 1998 Oct; 62(2): 195–202.

26. Berger I., et al. "Plants used in Guatemala for the treatment of protozoal infections: II. Activity of extracts and fractions of five Guatemalan plants against *Trypanosoma cruzi*." *J. Ethnopharmacol.* 1998 Sep; 62(2): 107–115.

27. Lores, R. I., et al. "*Petiveria alliaceae L.* (anamu). Study of the hypoglycemic effect." *Med. Interne.* 1990; 28(4): 347–352.

28. Hoyos, L., et al. "Evaluation of the genotoxic effects of a folk medicine, *Petiveria alliaceae* (Anamu)." *Mutat. Res.* 1992; 280(1): 29–34.

29. Caceres, A., et al. "Plants used in Guatemala for the treatment of protozoal infections. I. Screening of activity to bacteria, fungi and American trypanosomes of 13 native plants." *J. Ethnopharmacol.* 1998 Oct; 62(3): 195–202.

30. Feng, P., et al. "Further pharmacological screening of some West Indian medicinal plants." *J. Pharm. Pharmacol.* 1964; 16: 115.

Andiroba

1. Bickii, J., et al. "In vitro antimalarial activity of liminoids from *Khaya grandifoliola* C.D.C. (Meliaceae)." *J. Ethnopharmacol.* 2000; 69(1): 27–33.

2. MacKinnon, S., et al. "Antimalarial activity of tropical Meliaceae extracts and gedunin derivatives." *J. Nat. Prod.* 1997; 60(4): 336–341.

3. Cohen, E., et al. "Cytotoxicity of nibolide, epoxyazadiradione and other liminoids from neem insecticide." *Life Sci.* 1996; 58(13): 1075–81.

4. Hammer, M. L., et al. "Tapping an Amazonian plethora: four medicinal plants of Marajó Island, Pará (Brazil)." *J. Ethnopharmacol.* 1993 Sep; 40(1): 53–75.

5. Nakanishi, K., et al. "Phytochemical survey of Malaysian plants." *Chem. Pharm. Bull.* 1965; 13(7): 882–890.

6. Titanji, J.P., et al. "Novel onchocerca volvulus filaricides from Carapa procera, Polyathia suaveolens and Pachypodanthium staudtii." *Acta Leiden.* 1990; 59:(1-2) 377–382.

7. Mikolajczak, K.L., et al. "A limonoid antifeedant from seed of Carapa procera." *J. Nat. Prod.* 1988; 51(3): 606–610

8. Gilbert, B., et al. "Activities of the Pharmaceutical Technology Institute of the Oswaldo Cruz Foundation with medicinal, insecticidal and insect repellent plants." *An. Acad. Bras. Cienc.* 1999; 71(2): 265–271.

9. Rouillard, F., et al. *Cosmetic or pharmaceutical composition containing an andiroba extract.* United States Patent 5,958,421; September 28, 1999.

10. Moura, M. D., et al. "Natural products reported as potential inhibitors of uterine cervical neoplasia." *Acta. Farm. Bonaerense.* 2002; 21(1): 67–74.

Annatto

1. Bressani, R., et al. "Chemical composition, amino acid content and nutritive value of the protein of the annatto seed (*Bixa orellana* L.)." *Arch. Latinoam. Nutr.* 33(2): 356–76.

2. Scita, G. "Retinoic acid and beta-carotene inhibit fibronectin synthesis and release by fibroblasts; antagonism to phorbol ester." *Carcinogenesis* 15 (1994): 1043–1048.

3. Zhang, L. X. "Carotenoids up-regulate connexin43 gene expression independent of their provitanin A or antioxidant properties." *Cancer Res.* 52 (1992): 5707–5712.

4. Di Mascio, P. "Carotenoids, tocopherols and thiols as biological singlet molecular oxygen quenchers." *Biochem. Soc. Trans.* 18 (1990): 1054–1056.

5. Hirose, S. "Energized state of mitochondria as revealed by the spectral change of bound bixin." *Arch. Biochem. Biophys.* 152 (1972): 36–43.

6. Inada, Y. "Spectral changes of bixin upon interaction with respiring rat liver mitochondria." *Arch. Biochem. Biophys.* 146 (1971): 366–367.

7. Campelo, C. R. "Contribuicao ao estudo das plantas medicinais no estado de alagoas III, VII." Simposio de Plantas Medicinais do Brasil, 1–3 de Setembro, 1982, Belo Horizonte-MG, 85m.

8. Dunham, N. W. et al. "A preliminary pharmacologic investigation of the roots of *Bixa orellana*." *J. Amer. Pharm. Ass. Sci. Ed.* 1960; 49: 218.

9. Morrison, E. Y., et al. "Extraction of an hyperglycaemic principle from the annatto (*Bixa orellana*), a medicinal plant in the West Indies." *Trop. Georg. Med.* 1991; 43(2): 184–188.

10. Morrison, E. Y., et al. "Toxicity of the hyperglycaemic-inducing extract of the annatto (*Bixa orellana*) in the dog." *West Indian Med. J.* 1985; 34(1): 38–42.

11. Morrison, E. Y., et al. "The effect of *Bixa orellana* (annatto) on blood sugar levels in the anaesthetized dog." *West Indian Med. J.* March 1985.

12. Terashima, S., et al. "Studies on aldose reductase inhibitors from natural products. IV. Constituents and aldose reductase inhibitory effect of *Chrysanthemum morifolium*, *Bixa orellana* and *Ipomoea batatas*." *Chem. Pharm. Bull.* 1991; 39(12): 3346–3347.

13. Otero, R., et al. "Snakebites and ethnobotany in the northwest region of Colombia. Part III: neutralization of lethal and enzymatic effects of *Bothrops atrox* venom." *J. Ethnopharmacol.* 2000; 71(3): 505–511.

14. Cáceres A., et al. "Antigonorrhoeal activity of plants used in Guatemala for the treatment of sexually transmitted diseases." *J. Ethnopharmacol.* October 1995.

15. George, M., et al. "Investigations on plant antibiotics. Part IV. Further search for antibiotic substances in Indian medicinal plants." *Indian J. Med. Res.* 1949; 37: 169–181.

16. Campelo, C. R. "Contribuicao ao estudo das plantas medicinais no estado de alagoas III, VII." Simposio de Plantas Medicinais do Brasil, 1–3 de Setembro, 1982, Belo Horizonte-MG, 85m.

17. Nish, W. A., et al. "Anaphylaxis to annatto dye: a case report." *Ann. Allergy* 1991; 66(2): 129–131.

Artichoke

1. Grogan, J. L., et al. "Potential hypocholesterolemic agents: dicinnamoyl esters as analogs of cynarin." *J. Pharm. Sci.* 1972; 61(5): 802–803.

2. Bobnis, W., et al. "Case of primary hyperlipemia treated with cynarin." *Wiad. Lek.* 1973; 26(13): 1267–1270.

3. Pristautz, H., et al. "Cynarin in the modern management of hyperlipemia." *Wien Med. Wochenschr.* 1975; 125(49): 705–709.

4. Montini, M., et al. "Controlled application of cynarin in the treatment of hyperlipemic syndrome. Observations in 60 cases." *Arzneimittelforschung* 1975; 25(8): 1311–1314.

5. Englisch, W., et al. "Efficacy of artichoke dry extract in patients with hyperlipoproteinemia." *Arzneimittelforschung* 2000; 40 (3): 260–265.

6. Gebhardt, R. "Inhibition of cholesterol biosynthesis in HepG2 cells by artichoke extracts is reinforced by glucosidase pretreatment." *Phytother. Res.* 2002; 16(4): 368–372.

7. Shimoda, H., et al. "Anti-hyperlipidemic sesquiterpenes and new sesquiterpene glycosides from the leaves of artichoke (*Cynara scolymus* L.): structure requirement and mode of action." *Bioorg. Med. Chem. Lett.* 2003; 13(2): 223–228.

8. Maros, T., et al. "Effects of *Cynara scolymus* extracts on the regeneration of rat liver. 1." *Arzneimittelforschung* 1966; 16(2): 127–129.

9. Adzet, T., et al. "Hepatoprotective activity of polyphenolic compounds from *Cynara scolymus* against CCl4 toxicity in isolated rat hepatocytes." *J. Nat. Prod.* 1987; 50(4): 612–617.

10. Gebhardt, R. "Prevention of taurolithate-induced hepatic bile canalicular distortions by HPLC-characterized extracts of artichoke (*Cynara scolymus*) leaves." *Planta Med.* 2002; 68(9): 776–779.

11. Gebhardt, R. "Anticholestatic activity of flavonoids from artichoke (*Cynara scolymus* L.) and of their metabolites." *Med. Sci. Monit.* 2001; (7) Suppl. 1: 316–20.

12. Gebhardt, R. "Inhibition of cholesterol biosynthesis in primary cultured rat hepatocytes by artichoke (*Cynara scolymus* L.) extracts." *J. Pharmacol. Exp. Ther.* 1998; 286(3): 1122–1128.

13. Gebhardt, R., et al. "Antioxidative and protective properties of extracts from leaves of the artichoke (*Cynara scolymus* L.) against hydroperoxide-induced oxidative stress in cultured rat hepatocytes." *Toxicol. Appl. Pharmacol.* 1997; 144(2): 279–286.

14. Brown, J. E. and C. A. Rice-Evans. "Luteolin-rich artichoke extract protects low density lipoprotein from oxidation *in vitro*." *Free Radic. Res.* 1990; 29(3): 247–255.

15. Zapolska-Downar, D., et al. "Protective properties of artichoke (*Cynara scolymus*) against oxidative stress induced in cultured endothelial cells and monocytes." *Life Sci.* 2002; 71(24): 2897.

16. Perez-Garcia, F., et al. "Activity of artichoke leaf extract on reactive oxygen in human leukocytes." *Free Rad. Res.* 2000; 33(5): 661–665.

17. Wegener, T., et al. "Pharmacological properties and therapeutic profile of arti-

choke (*Cynara scolymus* L.)." *Wien Med. Wochenschr.* 1999; 149 (8–10): 241–247.

18. Walker, A. F., et al. "Artichoke leaf extract reduces symptoms of irritable bowel syndrome in a post-marketing surveillance study." *Phytother. Res.* 2001; 15(1): 58–61.

Aveloz

1. Duke, J. *Euphorbia tirucalli L. Handbook of Energy Crops.* Unpublished. 1983. Available through Purdue University Center for New Crops & Plants Products.

2. Cataluna, P., et al. "The traditional use of the latex from *Euphorbia tirucalli* Linnaeus (Euphorbiaceae) in the treatment of cancer in South Brazil." ISHS Acta Horticulture 501: II WOCMAP Congress Medicinal and Aromatic Plants, Part 2: Pharmacognosy, Pharmacology, Phytomedicine, Toxicology.

3. Khan, A. Q., et al. "Euphorcinol: a new pentacyclic triterpene from *Euphorbia tirucalli.*" *Planta Medica* 1989; 55: 290–291.

4. Kinghorn, A. D. "Characterization of an irritant 4-deoxy-phorbol diester from *Euphorbia tirucalli.*" *J. Nat. Prod.* 1979; 42(1): 112–115.

5. Furstenberger, G., et al. "On the active principles of the Euphorbiaceae XII. Highly unsaturated irritant diterpene esters form *Euphorbia tirucalli* originating from Madagascar." *J. Nat. Prod.* 1986; 49(3): 386–397.

6. Imai, S., et al. "African Burkitt's lymphoma: a plant, *Euphorbia tirucalli,* reduces Epstein-Barr virus-specific cellular immunity." *Anticancer Res.* 1994; 14(3A): 933–936.

7. Aya, T., et al. "Chromosome translocation and c-MYC activation by Epstein-Barr virus and *Euphorbia tirucalli* in B lymphocytes." *Lancet* 1991; 337(8751): 1190.

8. Sugiura, M., et al. "Cryptic dysfunction of cellular immunity in asymptomatic human immunodeficiency virus (HIV) carriers and its actualization by an environmental immunosuppressive factor." *In Vivo* 1994; 8(6): 1019–1022.

9. Epstein-Barr Virus and Infectious Mononucleosis. National Center for Infectious Diseases. CDC. www.cdc.gov

10. MacNeil, A., et al. "Activation of Ep-

stein-Barr virus lytic cycle by the latex of the plant *Euphorbia tirucalli.*" *Br. J. Cancer.* 2003; 88(10): 1566–1569.

11. van den Bosch, C., et al. "Are plant factors a missing link in the evolution of endemic Burkitt's lymphoma?" *Br. J. Cancer* 1993; 68(6): 1232–1235.

12. Mizuno, F., et al. "Epstein-Barr virus-enhancing plant promoters in east Africa." *AIDS Res.* 1986; 2 Suppl 1: S151–155.

13. Prince, S., et al. "Latent membrane protein 1 inhibits Epstein-Barr virus lytic cycle induction and progress via different mechanisms." *J. Virol.* 2003; 77(8): 5000–5007.

Avenca

1. Murti, S. "Post coital anti-implantation activity of Indian medicinal plants." *Abstr. 32nd Indian Pharmaceutical Cong. Nagpur.* 1981; Abstract D14: 23–25.

2. Murthy, R. S. R., et al. "Anti-implantation activity of isoadiantone." *Indian Drugs* 1984; 21(4): 141–144.

3. Mahmoud, M. J., et al. "*In vitro* antimicrobial activity of *Salsola rosmarinus* and *Adiantum capillus-veneris.*" *Int. J. Crude Drug Res.* 1989; 27(1): 14–16.

4. Husson, G. P., et al. "Research into antiviral properties of a few natural extracts." *Ann. Pharm. Fr.* 1986; 44(1): 41–48.

5. Jain, S. R., et al. "Hypoglycaemic drugs of Indian indigenous origin." *Planta Med.* 1967; 15(4): 439–442.

6. Neef, H., et al. "Hypoglycemic activity of selected European plants." *Pharm. World & Sci.* 1993; 15(6): H11.

7. Neef, H., et al. "Hypoglycaemic activity of selected European plants." *Phytother. Res.* 1995; 9(1): 45–48.

Balsam of Peru/Balsam of Tolu

1. Lueng A., & Foster, S. *Encylcopedia of Common Natural Ingredients.* Ed. New York: John Wiley & Sons, 1996.

2. Monograph *Balsamum peruvianum, Bundesanzeiger,* no 173 (Sept. 18, 1986).

3. Duke, James. *Handbook of legumes of world economic importance.* New York: Plenum Press, pp. 173–177. 1981.

4. Ohsaki, A., et al. "Microanalysis of a selective potent anti-Helicobacter pylori

compound in a Brazilian medicinal plant, *Myroxylon peruiferum* and the activity of analogues." *Bioorg. Med. Chem. Lett.* 1999; 9(8): 1109–1112.

Bitter Melon

1. Takemoto, D. J., et al. "Guanylate cyclase activity in human leukemic and normal lymphocytes. Enzyme inhibition and cytotoxicity of plant extracts." *Enzyme* 1982; 27(3): 179–188.

2. Takemoto, D. J. "Purification and characterization of a cytostatic factor with antiviral activity from the bitter melon." *Prep. Biochem.* 1983; 13(4): 371–393.

3. Takemoto D. J., et al. "Purification and characterization of a cytostatic factor with anti-viral activity from the bitter melon. Part 2." *Prep Biochem.* 1983; 13(5): 397–421.

4. Takemoto, D. J., et al. "Purification and characterization of a cytostatic factor from the bitter melon Momordica charantia." *Prep Biochem.* 1982; 12(4): 355–375.

5. Takemoto, D. J., et al. "Partial purification and characterization of a guanylate cyclase inhibitor with cytotoxic properties from the bitter melon (*Momordica charantia*)." *Biochem. Biophys. Res. Commun.* 1980; 94(1): 332–339.

6. Claflin, A. J., et al. "Inhibition of growth and guanylate cyclase activity of an undifferentiated prostate adenocarcinoma by an extract of the balsam pear (*Momordica charantia* abbreviata)." *Proc. Natl. Acad. Sci.* 1978; 75(2): 989–993.

7. Vesely, D. L., et al. "Isolation of a guanylate cyclase inhibitor from the balsam pear (*Momordica charantia* abbreviata)." *Biochem. Biophys. Res. Commun.* 1977; 77(4): 1294–1299.

8. Terenzi, A., et al. "Anti-CD30 (BER=H2) immunotoxins containing the type-1 ribosome-inactivating proteins momordin and PAP-S (pokeweed antiviral protein from seeds) display powerful antitumor activity against CD30+ tumor cells *in vitro* and in SCID mice." *Br. J. Haematol.* 1996; 92(4): 872–879.

9. Lee-Huang, S., et al. "Plant proteins useful for treating tumors and HIV infection." 1-28-1996 United States Patent 5484889.

10. Lee-Huang, S., et al. "Inhibition of the

integrase of human immunodeficiency virus (HIV) type 1 by anti-HIV plant proteins MAP30 and GAP31." *Proc. Natl. Acad. Sci.* 1995; 92(19): 8818–8822.

11. Lee-Huang, S., et al. "Anti-HIV and anti-tumor activities of recombinant MAP30 from bitter melon." *Gene.* 1995; 161(2): 151–156.

12. Lee-Huang, S., "MAP 30: A new inhibitor of HIV-1 infection and replication." *FEBS Lett.* 1990; 272(1–2): 12–18.

13. Lifson, J. D., et al. "Method of inhibiting HIV." 1-28-1989 United States Patent 4795739.

14. Bourinbaiar, A. S., et al. "The activity of plant-derived antiretroviral proteins MAP30 and GAP31 against *Herpes simplex virus in vitro*." *Biochem. Biophys. Res. Commun.* 1996; 219(3): 923–929.

15. Raza, H., et al. "Modulation of xenobiotic metabolism and oxidative stress in chronic streptozotocin-induced diabetic rats fed with *Momordica charantia* fruit extract." *J. Biochem. Mol. Toxicol.* 2000; 14(3): 131–139.

16. Ahmad, N., et al. "Effect of *Momordica charantia* (Karolla) extracts on fasting and postprandial serum glucose levels in NIDDM patients." *Bangladesh Med. Res. Counc. Bull.* 1999; 25(1): 11–13.

17. Akhtar, M. S. "Trial of *Momordica charantia* Linn (Karela) powder in patients with maturity-onset diabetes." *J. Pak. Med. Assoc.* 1982; 32(4): 106–107.

18. Matsuda, H., et al. "Inhibition of gastric emptying by triterpene saponin, momordin Ic, in mice: Roles of blood glucose, capsaicin-sensitive sensory nerves, and central nervous system." *J. Pharmacol. Exp. Ther.* 1999; 289(2): 729–734.

19. Matsuda, H., et al. "Antidiabetic principles of natural medicines. III. Structure-related inhibitory activity and action mode of oleanolic acid glycosides on hypoglycemic activity." *Chem. Pharm. Bull.* (Tokyo)1998; 46(9): 1399–1403.

20. Ahmed, I., et al. "Effects of *Momordica charantia* fruit juice on islet morphology in the pancreas of the streptozotocin-diabetic rat." *Diabetes Res. Clin. Pract.* 1998; 40(3): 145–151.

21. Matsuda, H., et al. "Inhibitory mechanisms of oleanolic acid 3-O-monodesmosides on glucose absorption in rats." *Biol. Pharm. Bull.* 1997; 20(6): 717–719.

22. Platel, K., et al. "Plant foods in the management of *Diabetes mellitus*: Vegetables as potential hypoglycaemic agents." *Nahrung.* 1997; 41(2): 68–74.

23. Zhang, Q. C. "Preliminary report on the use of *Momordica charantia* extract by HIV patients." *J. Naturopath. Med.* 1992; 3: 65–69.

24. Sarkar, S., et al. "Demonstration of the hypoglycemic action of *Momordica charantia* in a validated animal model of diabetes." *Pharmacol. Res.* 1996; 33(1): 1–4.

25. Miura, T., et al. "Hypoglycemic activity of the fruit of the *Momordica charantia* in type 2 diabetic mice." *J. Nutr. Sci. Vitaminol.* 2001; 47(5): 340–344.

26. Ali, L., et al. "Studies on hypoglycemic effects of fruit pulp, seed and whole plant of *Momordica charantia* on normal and diabetic model rats." *Planta Med.* 1993; 59(5): 408–412.

27. Vikrant, V., et al. "Treatment with extracts of *Momordica charantia* and *Eugenia jambolana* prevents hyperglycemia and hyperinsulinemia in fructose fed rats." *J. Ethnopharmacol.* 2001; 76(2): 139–143.

28. Jayasooriya, A. P., et al. "Effects of *Momordica charantia* powder on serum glucose levels and various lipid parameters in rats fed with cholesterol-free and cholesterol-enriched diets." *J. Ethnopharmacol.* 2000; 72 (1–2): 331–336.

29. Ahmed, I., et al. "Hypotriglyceridemic and hypocholesterolemic effects of anti-diabetic *Momordica charantia* (Karela) fruit extract in streptozotocin-induced diabetic rats." *Diabetes Res. Clin. Pract.* 2001; 51(3): 155–161.

30. Nagasawa, H., et al. "Effects of bitter melon (*Momordica charantia*) or ginger rhizome (*Zingiber offiinale* Rosc.) on spontaneous mammary tumorigenesis in SHN mice." *Am. J. Clin. Med.* 2002; 30(2–3): 195–205.

31. West, M. E., et al. "The anti-growth properties of extracts from *Momordica charantia*." *West Indian Med. J.* 1971; 20(1): 25–34.

32. Takemoto, D. J., et al. "The cytotoxic and cytostatic effects of the bitter melon (*Momordica charantia*) on human lymphocytes." *Toxicon.* 1982; 20: 593–599.

33. Zhu, Z. J., et al. "Studies on the active constituents of *Momordica charantia* L." *Yao. Hsueh. Hsueh. Pao.* 1990; 25(12): 898–903.

34. Frame, A. D., et al. "Plants from Puerto Rico with anti-*Mycobacterium tuberculosis* properties." *P. R. Health Sci. J.* 1998; 17(3): 243–252.

35. Huang, T. M., et al. "Studies on antiviral activity of the extract of *Momordica charantia* and its active principle." *Virologica.* 1990; 5(4): 367–373.

36. George, M., et al. "Investigations on plant antibiotics. Part IV. Further search for antibiotic substances in Indian medicinal plants." *Indian J. Med. Res.* 1949; (37): 169–181.

37. Khan, M. R., et al. "*Momordica charantia* and *Allium sativum*: Broad spectrum antibacterial activity." *Korean J. Pharmacog.* 1998; 29(3): 155–158.

38 Omoregbe, R. E., et al. "Antimicrobial activity of some medicinal plants' extracts on *Escherichia coli, Salmonella paratyphi* and *Shigella dysenteriae*." *Afr. J. Med. Med. Sci.* 1996; 25(4): 373–375.

39. Hussain, H. S. N., et al. "Plants in Kano ethomedicine: Screening for antimicrobial activity and alkaloids." *Int. J. Pharmacog.* 1991; 29(1): 51–56.

40. Bhakuni, D. S., et al. "Screening of Indian plants for biological activity: Part XIII." *Indian J. Exp. Biol.* 1988; 26(11): 883RY–904.

41. Yesilada, E., et al. "Screening of Turkish anti-ulcerogenic folk remedies for anti-*Helicobacter pylori* activity." *J. Ethnopharmacol.* 1999; 66(3): 289–93.

42. Sharma, V. N., et al. "Some observations on hypoglycaemic activity of *Momordica charantia*." *Indian J. Med. Res.* 1960; 48(4): 471–547.

43. Dhawan, B. N., et al. "Screening of Indian plants for biological activity. Part IX." *Indian J. Exp. Biol.* 1980; 18: 594–606.

44. Prakash, A. O., et al. "Screening of In-

dian plants for antifertility activity." *Indian J. Exp. Biol.* 1976; 14: 623–626.

45. Shum, L. K. W., et al. "Effects of *Mordica charantia* seed extract on the rat mid-term placenta." Abstract 78. Abstract International Symposium on Chinese Medicinal Material Research. 1984; 12–14.

46. Dong, T. X., et al. "Ribosome inactivating protein-like activity in seeds of diverse Cucurbitaceae plants." *Indian J. Exp. Biol.* 1993; 25(3): 415–419.

47. Ng, T. B., et al. "Investigation of ribosome inactivating protein-like activity in tissues of Cucurbitaceae plants." *Indian J. Exp. Biol.* 1989; 21(12): 1353–1358.

48. Jamwal, K. S., et al. "Preliminary screening of some reputed abortifacient indigenous plants." *Indian J. Pharmacy* 1962; 24: 218–220.

49. Stepka, W., et al. "Antifertility investigation on *Momordica*." *Lloydia.* 1974; 37(4): 645c.

50. Koentjoro-Soehadi, T., et al. "Perspectives of male contraception with regards to Indonesian traditional drugs." Proc. Second National Congress of Indonesian Society of Andrology. 1982; Aug. 2–6: 12.

51. Dixit, V. P., et al. "Effects of *Momordica charantia* fruit extract on the testicular function of dog." *Planta Med.* 1978; 34: 280–286.

Boldo

1. Rueggett, A. Helv. *Chim. Acta.* 1959; 42: 754.

2. Hansel, R. *Phytopharmaka*, 2d ed. Berlin: Springer-Verlag, 1991: 186–191.

3. Hughes, D. W., et al. "Alkaloids of *Peumus boldus.* Isolation of (+) reticuline and isoboldine." *J. Pharm. Sci.* 1968; 57: 1023.

4. Hughes, D. W., et al. "Alkaloids of *Peumus boldus.* Isolation of laurotetanine and laurolitsine." *J. Pharm. Sci.* 1968.

5. Vanhaelen, M. "Spectrophotometric microdetermination of alkaloids in *Peumus boldus.*" *J. Pharm. Belg.* May–June 1973.

6. Jang, Y. Y., et al. "Protective effect of boldine on oxidative mitochondrial damage in streptozotocin-induced diabetic rats." *Pharmacol. Res.* 2000; 42(4): 361–371.

7. Kringstein, P., et al. "Boldine prevents human liver microsomal lipid peroxidation and inactivation of cytochrome P4502E1." *Free Radic. Biol. Med.* 1995; 18(3): 559–563.

8. Krug, H., et al. "New flavonol glycosides from the leaves of *Peumus boldus* Molina." *Pharmazie*, Novemeber 1965.

9. Speisky, H, et al. "Boldo and boldine: an emerging case of natural drug development." *Pharmacol. Res.* January–February, 1994.

10. Tavares, D. C., et al. "Evaluation of the genotoxic potential of the alkaloid boldine in mammalian cell systems *in vitro* and *in vivo.*" *Mutat. Res.* 1994; 321(3): 139–145.

11. Lanhers, M. C., et al. "Hepatoprotective and anti-inflammatory effects of a traditional medicinal plant of Chile, *Peumus boldus.*" *Planta Med.* 1991; 57(2): 110–115.

12. Lévy-Appert-Collin, M. C., et al. "Galenic preparations from *Peumus boldus* leaves (Monimiacea)." *J. Pharm. Belg.* 1977; 32: 13.

13. Backhouse N., et al. "Anti-inflammatory and antipyretic effects of boldine." *Agents Actions* 1994; 42(3–4): 114–117.

14. Kang, J. J., et al. "Studies on neuromuscular blockade by boldine in the mouse phrenic nerve diaphragm." *Planta Med.* 1999; 65(2): 178–179.

15. Kang, J. J., et al. "Effects of boldine on mouse diaphragm and sarcoplasmic reticulum vesicles isolated from skeletal muscle." *Planta Med.* 1998; 64(1): 18–21.

16. Gotteland, M., et al. "Protective effect of boldine in experimental colitis." *Planta Med.* 1997; 63(4): 311–315.

17. Jimenez, I., et al. "Protective effects of boldine against free radical-induced erythrocyte lysis." *Phytother. Res.* 2000; 14(5): 339–343.

18. Teng, C. M., et al. "Antiplatelet effects of some aporphine and phenanthrene alkaloids in rabbits and man." *J. Pharm. Pharmacol.* 1997; 49(7): 706–711.

19. Chen, K. S., et al. "Antiplatelet and vasorelaxing actions of some aporphinoids." *Planta Med.* 1996; 62(2): 133–136.

20. Eltze, M., et al. "Affinity profile at alpha(1)- and alpha(2) - adrenoceptor subtypes and in vitro cardiovascular actions of (+) - boldine." *Eur. J. Pharmacol.* 2002; 443(1-3): 151–168.

21. Schindler, H. *Arzneim. Forsch.* 1957; 7: 747.

22. Bombardelli, E., et al. *Fitoterapia* 1976; 47: 3.

23. Gotteland, M., et al. "Effect of a dry boldo extract on oro-cecal intestinal transit in healthy volunteers." *Rev. Med. Chil.* 1995; 123(8): 955–960.

24. Hirosue, T., et al. *Chem. Abstr.* 1988; 109: 229018d.

25. The Lawrence Review of Natural Products. *Boldo.* St Louis, MO, 1991; Facts and Comparisons, Inc.

26. Johnson, M. A., et al. "Biosynthesis of ascaridole: iodide peroxidase-catalyzed synthesis of a monoterpene endoperoxide in soluble extracts of *Chenopodium ambrosioides* fruit." *Arch. Biochem. Biophys.* 1984; 235(1): 254.

27. Duke, J. A. *CRC Handbook of Medicinal Herbs.* Boca Raton, FL, 1985; CRC Press.

28. Ivorra, M. D., et al. "Different mechanism of relaxation induced by aporphine alkaloids in rat uterus." *J. Pharm. Pharmacol.* 1993; 45(5): 439–443.

29. Almeida, E. R., et al. "Toxicological evaluation of the hydro-alcohol extract of the dry leaves of *Peumus boldus* and boldine in rats." *Phytother. Res.* 2000; 14(2): 99–102.

30. Kubinova, R., et al. "Chemoprotective activity of boldine: modulation of drug-metabolizing enzymes." *Pharmazie* 2001; 56(3): 242–243.

Brazil Nut

1. Vonderheide, I. P., et. al. "Characterization of selenium species in Brazil Nuts by HPLC-ICP-MS and ES-MS." *J. Agric. Food Chem.* 2002; 50(20): 5722–5728.

2. Ampe, C., et al. "The amino-acid sequence of the 2S sulfur-rich proteins from seeds of Brazil nut (*Bertholletia excelsa* H.B.K.)." *Eur. J. Biochem.* 1986 Sep 15; 159(3): 597–604.

3. Sun, S., et al. "Properties, biosynthesis and processing of a sulfur-rich protein in Brazil nut (*Bertholletia excelsa* H.B.K.)." *Eur. J. Biochem.* 1987 Feb 2; 162(3): 477–483.

4. Thorn, J., et al. "Trace nutrients. Selenium in British food." *Br. J. Nutr.* 1978 Mar; 39(2): 391–396.

5. Chang, J. C., et al. "Selenium content of Brazil nuts from two geographic locations in Brazil." *Chemosphere.* 1995 Feb; 30(4): 801–802.

6. Klein, E. A., et al. "The selenium and vitamin e cancer prevention trial." *World J. Urol.* 2003 May; 21(1): 21–27.

7. Ip, C., et al. "Bioactivity of selenium from Brazil nut for cancer prevention and selenoenzyme maintenance." *Nutr Cancer.* 1994; 21(3): 203–212.

8. Ip C, et al. "Characterization of tissue selenium profiles and anticarcinogenic responses in rats fed natural sources of selenium-rich products." *Carcinogenesis.* 1994 Apr; 15(4): 573–576.

Brazilian Peppertree

1. Terhune, S., et al. "B-spathulene: A new sesquiterpene in *Schinus molle* oil." *Phytochemistry* 1973; 13: 865.

2. Dominguez, X., et al. "A chemical survey of seventeen medicinal Mexican plants." *Planta Med.* 1970; 18: 51.

3. Pozzo-Balbi, T., et al. "The triterpenoid acids of *Schinus molle.*" *Phytochemistry* 1978; 17: 2107–2110.

4. Quiroga, E. N., et al. "Screening antifungal activities of selected medicinal plants." *J. Ethnopharmacol.* 2001; 74(1): 89–96.

5. Gundidza, M., et al. "Antimicrobial activity of essential oil from *Schinus molle* Linn." *Central African J. Med.* 1993; 39(11): 231–234.

6. Dikshit, A. "*Schinus molle*: a new source of natural fungitoxicant." *Appl. Environ. Microbiol.* 1986; 51(5): 1085–1088.

7. El-Keltawi, N., et al. "Antimicrobial activity of some Egyptian aromatic plants." *Herba Pol.* 1980; 26(4): 245–250.

8. Ross, S., et al. "Antimicrobial activity of some Egyptian aromatic plants." *Fitoterapia* 1980; 51: 201–205.

9. de Melo, Jr., E. J., et al. "Medicinal plants in the healing of dry socket in rats: Microbiological and microscopic analysis." *Phytomedicine* 2002; 9(2): 109–116.

10. Martinez, M. J., et al. "Screening of some Cuban medicinal plants for antimicrobial activity." *J. Ethnopharmacol.* 1996; 52(3): 171–174.

11. Camano, R., Method for treating bacterial infections. United States Patent 5,512,284; April 30, 1996.

12. Camano, R., Essential oil composition with bactericide activity. United States Patent 5,635,184; June 3, 1997.

13. Simons, J., et al. "Succulent-type as sources of plant virus inhibitors." *Phytopathology* 1963; 53: 677–683.

14. Bhakuni, D., et al. "Screening of Chilean plants for anticancer activity. I." *Lloydia* 1976; 39(4): 225–243.

15. Ruffa, M. J., et al. "Cytotoxic effect of Argentine medicinal plant extracts on human hepatocellular carcinoma cell line." *J. Ethnopharmacol.* 2002; 79(3): 335–339.

16. Bello, R., et al. "Effects on arterial blood pressure of the methanol and dichloromethanol extracts from *Schinus molle L.* in rats." *Phytother. Res.* 1996; 10(7): 634–635.

17. Zaidi, S., et al. "Some preliminary studies of the pharmacological activities of *Schinus molle.*" *Pak. J. Sci. Ind. Res.* 1970; 13: 53.

18. Moreno, M. S. F., "Action of several popular medicaments on the isolated uterus." *C. R. Seances. Soc. Biol. Ses. Fil.* 1922; 87: 563–564.

19. Barrachina, M. "Analgesic and central depressor effects of the dichloromethanol extract from *Schinus molle L.*" *Phytother. Res.* 1997; 11(4): 317–319.

20. Bello, R., et al. "In vitro pharmacological evaluation of the dichloromethanol extract from *Schinus molle L.*" *Phytother. Res.* 1998; 12(7): 523–525.

21. Carneiro, Wanick M., et al. "Anti-inflammatory and wound healing action of *Schinus aroeira* Vell in patients with cervicitis and cervico-vaginitis." *Rev. Inst. Antibiot.* 1974; 14(1–2): 105–106.

22. Jain, M. K., et al. "Specific competitive inhibitor of secreted phospholipase A2 from berries of *Schinus terebinthifolius.*" *Phytochemistry* 1995; 39(3): 537–547.

23. Okuyama, T., et al. "Studies on cancer bio-chemoprevention of natural resources. X. Inhibitory effect of spices on TPA-enhanced 3H-choline incorporation in phospholipid of C3H10T cells and on TPA-induced ear edema." *Zhonghua Yao Xue Zazhi* 1995; 47(5): 421–430.

24. Cuella, M. J., et al. "Two fungal lanostane derivatives as phospholipase A2 inhibitors." *J. Nat. Prod.* 1996; 59(10): 977–979.

25. Opdyke, D. L. J., "Monographs on fragrance raw materials. *Schinus molle* oil."

26. *Food Cosmet. Toxicol.* 1976; 14: 861.

Camu-Camu

1. Beckstrom-Sternberg, S., and J. A. Duke. *Ethnobotany and Phytochemical Databases,* U.S. Dept. of Agriculture, Agricultural Research Service, USDA.

2. Zapata, S. M., et al. "Camu-camu *Myrciaria dubia* (HBK) McVaugh: chemical composition of fruit." *J. Sci. Food Agric.,* 1993; 61(3): 349–351.

3. Franco, M. R., and T. Shibamoto. "Volatile composition of some Brazilian fruits: umbu-caja (*Spondias citherea*), camu-camu (*Myrciaria dubia*), araca-boi (*Eugenia stipitala*), and cupuacu (*Theobroma grandiflorum*)." *J. Agric. Food Chem.* 2000 Apr.; 48(4): 1263–1265.

4. Justi, K. C., et al. "Nutritional composition and vitamin C stability in stored camu-camu (*Myrciaria dubia*) pulp." *Arch. Latinoam. Nutr.* 2000 Dec.; 50(4): 405–408.

Carqueja

1. Sosa, M. E., et al. "Insect antifeedant activity of clerodane diterpenoids." *J. Nat. Prod.* 1994; 57(9): 1262–1265.

2. Soicke, H., et al. "Characterisation of flavonoids from *Baccharis trimera* and their antihepatotoxic properties." *Planta Medica* 1987; 53(1): 37–39.

3. Gamberini, M. T., et al. "Açoes antiúlcera e antiácida do extracto aquoso e das fraçoes da *Baccharis trimera.*" Anais XII Simposio de Plantas Medicinais do Brasil. UFP: Curitiba, Paraná, 15–17 September 1992.

4. Sousa, B., et al., "Avaliaçao da atividade antiulcera do extrato bruto e fraçoes de *Baccharis trimera.*" Anais XII Simposio de Plantas Medicinais do Brasil. UFP: Curitiba, Paraná, 15–17 September 1992.

5. Gamberini, M. T., et al. "Inhibition of gastric secretion by a water extract from *Baccharis triptera*. Mart." *Mem. Inst. Oswaldo Cruz.* 1991; 86(Suppl. 2): 137–139.

6. Gonzales, E., et al. "Gastric cytoprotection of Bolivian medicinal plants." *J. Ethnopharmacol.* 2000; 70(3): 329–333.

7. Gene, R. M., et al. "Anti-inflammatory and analgesic activity of *Baccharis trimera*: Identification of its active constituents." *Planta Med.* 1996; 62(3): 232–235.

8. Hossen, S., et al. "Evaluacion *in vivo* de la actividad hipoglucemiante de plantas medicinales de los valles altos y bajos de Cochabamba." Ed. Universidad Mayor De San Simón Instituto de Investigaciones Bioquímico-Farmacéuticas-Programa 2001; Cochabamba, Bolivia.

9. Xavier, A. A., et al. "Effect of an extract of *Baccharis genistelloides* on the glucose level of the blood." *C. R. Seances Soc. Biol. Fil.* 1967; 16(4): 972–974.

10. Alonso, P. E., et al. "Uso racional de las plantas medicinales." Ed. Fin De Siglo Facultad de Química 1992; Montevideo, Uruguay.

11. Abad, M. J., et al. "Antiviral activity of Bolivian plant extracts." *Gen. Pharmacol.* 1999; 32(4): 499–503.

12. Abdel-Malek, S., et al. "Drug leads from the Kallawaya herbalists of Bolivia. 1. Background, rationale, protocol and anti-HIV activity." *J. Ethnopharmacol.*. 1996; 50(3): 157–166.

13. Robinson, W. E., et al. "Inhibitors of HIV-1 replication that inhibit HIV Integrase." *Proc. Natl. Acad. Sci.* 1996; 93(13): 6326–6331.

Cashew

1. Bicalho, B., et al. "Volatile compounds of cashew apple (*Anacardium occidentale L.*)." *Z. Naturforsch.* 2001; 56(1–2): 35–39.

2. Mota, M. L., et al. "Anti-inflammatory actions of tannins isolated from the bark of *Anacardium occidentale L.*" *J. Ethnopharmacol.* 1985; 13(3): 289–300.

3. Jurberg, P., et al. "Effect of Niclosamide (Bayluscide WP 70), *Anacardium occidentale* hexane extract and *Euphorbia splendens* latex on behavior of *Biomphalaria glabrata* (Say, 1818), under laboratory conditions."

Mem. Inst. Oswaldo Cruz 1995; 90(2): 191–194.

4. Laurens, A., et al. "Molluscacidal activity of *Anacardium occidentale* L. (Anacardiaceae)." *Ann. Pharm. Fr.* 1987; 45(6): 471–473.

5. Mendes, N. M., et al. "Molluscacide activity of a mixture of 6-n-alkyl salicylic acids (anacardic acid) and 2 of its complexes with copper (II) and lead (II)." *Rev. Soc. Bras. Med. Trop.* 1990; 23(4): 217–224.

6. de Souza, C. P., et al. "The use of the shell of the cashew nut, *Anacardium occidentale*, as an alternative molluscacide." *Rev. Inst. Med. Trop.*, São Paulo, Brazil 1992; 34(5): 459–466.

7. Kubo, J., et al. "Tyrosinase inhibitors from *Anacardium occidentale* fruits." *J. Nat. Prod.* 1994; 57(4): 545–551.

8. Laurens, A., et al. "Study of antimicrobial activity of *Anacardium occidentale L.*" *Ann. Pharm. Fr.* 1982; 40(2): 143–146.

9. Kudi, A. C., et al. "Screening of some Nigerian medicinal plants for antibacterial activity." *J. Ethnopharmacol.* 1999; 67(2): 225–228.

10. Akinpelu, D. A., "Antimicrobial activity of *Anacardium occidentale* bark." *Fitoterapia* 2001; 72(3): 286–287.

11. Kubo, J., et al. "Anti-Helicobacter pylori agents from the cashew apple." *J Agric Food Chem* 1999; 47(2): 533–537.

12. França, F., et al. "An evaluation of the effect of a bark extract from the cashew (*Anacardium occidentale L.*) on infection by *Leishmania* (*Viannia*) *braziliensis*." *Rev. Soc. Bras. Med. Trop.* 1993; 26(3): 151–155.

13. França. F., et al. "Plants used in the treatment of leishmanial ulcers due to *Leishmania* (*Viannia*) *braziliensis* in an endemic area of Bahia, Brazil." *Rev. Soc. Bras. Med. Trop.* 1996; 29(3): 229–232.

14. Swanston-Flatt, S. K., et al. "Glycaemic effects of traditional European plant treatments for diabetes. Studies in normal and streptozotocin diabetic mice." *Diabetes Res.* 1989; 10(2): 69–73.

15. Kamtchouing, P., et al. "Protective role of *Anacardium occidentale* extract against streptozotocin-induced diabetes in rats." *J. Ethnopharmacol.* 1998; 62(2): 95–99.

Cat's Claw

1. Cabieses, Fernando. *The Saga of the Cat's Claw.* Lima: Via Lactera Editores, 1994.

2. Immodal Pharmaka, GmbH., "Krallendorn(r) *Uncaria tomentosa* (Willd.) DC Root Extract. Information for Physicians, and Dispensing Chemists. 3d rev. ed." Volders, Austria: September 1995, 20 pages.

3. Keplinger, U. M. "Einfluss von Krallendorn extrakt auf Retrovirale Infektioned," Zurcher AIDS Kongress. Zurich, Switzerland, October 16 and 17, 1992, program and abstracts.

4. Keplinger, U. M., "Therapy of HIV-infected individuals in the pathological categories CDC Al and CDC B2 with a preparation containing IMM-207," IV. Osterreichicher AIDS-Kongress, Vienna, Austria, September 17 and 18, 1993, abstracts: 45.

5. Keplinger, H., et al. "Oxindole alkaloids having properties stimulating the immunologic system and preparation containing same." United States Patent 5,302,611; April 12, 1994.

6. Keplinger, H., et al. "Oxindole alkaloids having properties stimulating the immunologic system and preparation containing the same." United States Patent 4,940,725; July 10, 1990.

7. Keplinger, H., et al. "Oxindole alkaloids having properties stimulating the immunologic system and preparation containing the same." United States Patent 4,844,901; July 4, 1989.

8. Keplinger, H., et al. "Process for the production of specific isomer mixtures from oxindole alkaloids." United States Patent 5,723,625; March 3, 1998.

9. Montenegro de Matta, S., et al. "Alkaloids and procyanidins of an *Uncaria* sp. from Peru." *Il. Farmaco. Ed. Sc.* 1976; 31: 527–535.

10. Ozaki, Y., et al. "Pharmacological studies on Uncaria and Amsonia alkaloids." *Japanese Journal of Pharmacology* (suppl.) 1980; 30: 137pp.

11. Kreutzkamp, B. "Niedermolekulare Inhalstoffe mit Immunstimulierenden Eigenschaften aus Uncaria tomentosa, Okoubaka aubrevillei und anderen Drogen."

Dissertation of the faculty of chemistry and pharmacy of Ludwig Maximilians University, Munich, May 1984.

12. Stuppner, H., et al. "HPLC analysis of the main oxindole alkaloids from *Uncaria tomentosa.*" *Chromatographia* 1992; 34 (11/12): 597–600.

13. Wagner, H., et al. "Die Alkaloide von *Uncaria tomentosa* und ihre Phagozytosesteigernde Wirkung." *Planta Medica* 1985; 51: 419–423.

14. Laus, G., et al. "Separation of sterioisomeric oxindole alkaloids from *Uncaria tomentosa* by high performance liquid chromatography." *J. of Chromatography* 1994; 662: 243–249.

15. Lavault, M., et al. "Alcaloides de l'*Uncaria guianensis.*" *Planta Medica* 1983; 47: 244–245.

16. Hemingway, S. R. and J. D. Phillipson. "Alkaloids from South American species of *Uncaria* (Rubiaceae)." *J. Pharm. Pharmacol.* 1974 suppl.; 26: 113pp.

17. Lemaire, I., et al. "Stimulation of interleukin-1 and -6 production in alveolar macrophages by the neotropical liana, *Uncaria tomentosa* (uña de gato)." *J. Ethnopharmacol.* 1999; 64(2): 109–115.

18. Marina, M. D., "Evaluacion de la actividal immunoestimulante de *Uncaria tomentosa* (Willd.) DC. Uña de gato en ratones albinos." *Biodiversidad Salud* 1998; 1(1): 16–19.

19. Sheng Y, et al., "Treatment of chemotherapy-induced leukopenia in a rat model with aqueous extract from *Uncaria tomentosa.*" *Phytomedicine* 2000; 7(2): 137–143.

20. Sheng, Y., et al., "Enhanced DNA repair, immune function and reduced toxicity of C-Med-100, a novel aqueous extract from *Uncaria tomentosa.*" *J. Ethnopharmacol.* 2000; 69(2): 115–126.

21. Sheng, Y., et al., "DNA repair enhancement of aqueous extracts of *Uncaria tomentosa* in a human volunteer study." *Phytomedicine* 2001; 8(4): 275–282.

22. Lamm, S., et al, "Persistent response to pneumococcal vaccine in individuals supplemented with a novel water soluble extract of *Uncaria tomentosa,* C-Med-100." *Phytomedicine* 2001; 8(4): 267–274.

23. Gotuzzo, E., et al. "En marcha seria investigacion: Uña de gato y pacientes con el VIH." *De Ciencia y Tecnologia* 1993; 34.

24. Inchaustegui and Gonzales, R. "Estudio preliminar sobre. CAS y SIDA." Utilizando Plantas Medicinales, Anos 1989–1994, Hospital IPSS, Iquitos, Peru. Iquitos, Peru: Hospital del Instituto Peruano de Seguridad Social Iquitos Comite ETS-SIDA, February 1993, 24 pp.

25. Stuppner, H., et al. "A differential sensitivity of oxindole alkaloids to normal and leukemic cell lines." *Planta Medica* (1993 suppl.); 59: A583.

26. Peluso, G., et al. "Effetto antiproliferativo su cellule tumorali di estrattie metaboliti da Uncaria tomentosa. Studi in vitro sulla loro azione DNA polimerasi." 11 Congreso Italo-Peruano de Etnomedicina Andina, Lima, Peru, October 27–30, 1993, 21–22.

27. Rizzi, R., et al. "Mutagenic and antimutagenic activities of Uncaria tomentosa and its extracts." Premiere Colloque Européan d'Ethnopharmacologie, Metz, France, March 22–24, 1990.

28. Rizzi, R., et al. "Bacterial cytotoxicity, mutagenicity and antimutagenicity of *Uncaria tomentosa* and its extracts. Antimutagenic activity of *Uncaria tomentosa* in humans." Premiere Colloque Européan d'Ethnopharmacologie, Metz, France, March 22–24, 1990.

29. Rizzi, R., et al. "Mutagenic and antimutagenic activities of *Uncaria tomentosa* and its extracts." *J. Ethnopharmacol.* 1993; 38: 63–77.

30. Muhammad, I., et al. "Investigation of Uña de Gato I. 7-Deoxyloganic acid and 15N NMR spectroscopic studies on pentacyclic oxindole alkaloids from *Uncaria tomentosa.*" *Phytochemistry.* 2001; 57(5): 781–785.

31. Riva, L., et al. "The antiproliferative effects of *Uncaria tomentosa* extracts and fractions on the growth of breast cancer cell line." *Anticancer Res.* 2001; 21(4A): 2457–2461.

32. Salazar, E. L., et al. "Depletion of specific binding sites for estrogen receptor by

Uncaria tomentosa." *Proc. West. Pharmacol. Soc.* 1998; 41(1): 123–124.

33. Sheng, Y., et al. "Induction of apoptosis and inhibition of proliferation in human tumor cells treated with extracts of *Uncaria tomentosa.*" *Anticancer Res.* 1998; 18(5A): 3363–3368.

34. Yepez, A. M., et al. "Quinovic acid glycosides from *Uncaria guianensis.*" *Phytochemisty* 1991; 30: 1635–1637.

35. Aquino, R., et al. "Plant metabolites. New compounds and anti-inflammatory activity of *Uncaria tomentosa.*" *J. Nat. Prod.* 1991; 54: 453–459.

36. Aquino, R., et al. "New polyhydroxylated triterpenes from *Uncaria tomentosa.*" *J. Nat. Prod.* 1990: 559–564.

37. Cerri, R., et al. "New quinovic acid glycosides from *Uncaria tomentosa.*" *J. Nat. Prod.* 1988; 51: 257–261.

38. Yasukawa, K., et al. "Effect of chemical constituents from plants on 12-O-tetradecanoylphorbol-13-acetate-induced inflammation in mice." *Chemical and Pharmaceutical Bulletin* 1989; 37: 1071–1073.

39. Recio, M. C., et al. "Structural requirements for the anti-inflammatory activity of natural triterpenoids." *Planta Medica* 1995; 61(2): 182–185.

40. Sandoval-Chacon, M., et al. "Anti-inflammatory actions of cat's claw: the role of NF-kappaB." *Aliment. Pharmacol. Ther.* 1998; 12(12): 1279–1289.

41. Aguilar, J. L., et al. "Anti-inflammatory activity of two different extracts of *Uncaria tomentosa* (Rubiaceae)." *J. Ethnopharmacol.* 2002; 81(2): 271–276.

42. Fazzi, Marco A. Costa. "Evaluation de l'*Uncaria tomentosa* (Uña de gato) en lan prevencion de ulceras gastricas de stress producidas experimentalmente en rats." Dissertation of the faculty of medicine, University Peruana Cayetano Heredia, Lima, Peru, 1989.

43. Desmarchelier, C., et al. "Evaluation of the *in vitro* antioxidant activity in extracts of *Uncaria tomentosa* (Willd.) DC." *Phytother. Res.* 1997; 11(3): 254–256.

44. Sandoval, M., et al. "Cat's claw inhibits TNFalpha production and scavenges free

radicals: role in cytoprotection." *Free Radic. Biol. Med.* 2000; 29(1): 71–78.

45. Sandoval, M., et al., "Anti-inflammatory and antioxidant activities of cat's claw (*Uncaria tomentosa* and *Uncaria guianensis*) are independent of their alkaloid content." *Phytomedicine* 2002; 9(4): 325–337.

46. Mur, E., et al. "Randomized double blind trial of an extract from the pentacyclic alkaloid-chemotype of *Uncaria tomentosa* for the treatment of rheumatoid arthritis." *J. Rheumatol.* 2002 Apr; 29(4): 678–681.

47. Aquino, R., et al. "Plant metabolites. Structure and *in vitro* antiviral activity of quinovic acid glycosides from *Uncaria tomentosa* and *Guettarda platypoda*." *J. Nat. Prod.* 1989; 4(52): 679–685.

48. Yano, S., et al. "Ca2, channel-blocking effects of hirsutine, an indole alkaloid from *Uncaria* genus, in the isolated rat aorta." *Planta Medica* 1991; 57: 403–405.

49. Chan-Xun, C., et al. "Inhibitory effect of rhynchophylline on platelet aggregation and thrombosis." *Acta Pharmacologica Sinica* 1992; 13(2): 126–30.

50. Jin, R. M., et al. "Effect of rhynchophylline on platelet aggregation and experimental thrombosis." *Acta Pharmacologica Sinica* 1991; 25: 246–249.

51. Mohamed, A. F., et al. "Effects of *Uncaria tomentosa* total alkaloid and its components on experimental amnesia in mice: elucidation using the passive avoidance test." *J. Pharm. Pharmacol.* 2001; 52(12): 1553–1561.

52. Castillo, G., et al. "Pharmaceutical compositions containing *Uncaria tomentosa* extract for treating Alzheimer's disease and other amyloidoses." *Patent-Pct. Int. Paol.* 1998; 00 33,659: 67pp.

53. Kang, T. H., et al. "Pteropodine and isopteropodine positively modulate the function of rat muscarinic M(1) and 5-HT(2) receptors expressed in Xenopus oocyte." *Eur. J. Pharmacol.* 2002 May 24; 444(1-2): 39–45.

54. Roth, B. L., et al. "Insights into the structure and function of 5-HT(2) family serotonin receptors reveal novel strategies for therapeutic target development." *Expert Opin. Ther. Targets* 2001 Dec; 5(6): 685–695

Catuaba

1. Chian, Sing. *Cura com Yoga e Plantas Medicinais*. Rio de Janeiro: Freitas Bastos, 1979.

2. van Straten, Michael. *Guarana: The Energy Seeds and Herbs of the Amazon Rainforest*. Essex, England: C. W. Daniel Company, Ltd., 1994.

3. Altman, R. F. A. "Presenca de ioimbina na catuaba." *Ser. Quim. Publ.* 1958; 1.

4. Maia, J. G., et al. *Estudos Integrados de Plantas da Amazonia*. V Simposio de Plantas Medicinais do Brasil, São Paulo, Brazil, Sep. 6, 1978: 7.

5. Garcez, W. S., et al. "Sesquiterpenes from *Trichilia catigua*." *Fitoterapia* 1997; 68(1): 87–88.

6. Satoh, M., et al. "Cytotoxic constituents from *Erythroxylum catuaba*. Isolation and cytotoxic activities of cinchonain." *Natural Med.* 2000; 54(2): 97–100.

7. Pizzolatti, M. G., et al. "Two epimeric flavalignans from *Trichilia catigua* (Meliaceae) with antimicrobial activity." *Z. Naturforsch* 2002; 57(5–6): 483–888.

8. Manabe, H., et al. "Effects of catuaba extracts on microbial and HIV infection." *In Vivo* 1992; 6(2): 161–165.

9. Sander, P. C., et al. "Pharmaceutical formulations comprising vegetal material selected from trichilia." U.S. Patent no. 6335039; Jan 1, 2002.

10. Vaz, Z. R., et al. "Analgesic effect of the herbal medicine Catuaba in thermal and chemical models of nociception in mice." *Phytother. Res.* 1997; 11(2): 101–106.

Chá de Bugre

1. Saito, M. L., et al. "Morfodiagnose e identificacao cromatografica em camada delgada de chá de bugre — *Cordia ecalyculata* Vell." *Rev. Bras. Farm.* 1986; 67: 1–16.

2. Hayashi K., et al. "Antiviral activity of an extract of *Cordia salicifolia* on herpes simplex virus type 1." *Planta Med.* 1990; 56(5): 439–443.

3. Arisawa, M., et al. "Cell growth inhibition of KB Cells by Plant Extracts." *Natural Medicines* 1994; 48(4): 338–347.

4. Matsunaga, K., et al. "Excitatory and inhibitory effects of paraguayan medicinal plants *Equisetum giganteum*, *Acanthpspermum australe*, *Allophylus edlis* and *Cordia salicifolia* on contraction of rabbit aorta and giunea-pig left atrium." *Natural Medicines* 1997; 51: 478–481.

Chanca Piedra

1. Santos, D. R. *Cha de "quebra-pedra" (Phyllanthus niruri) na litiase urinaria em humanos e ratos*. Thesis, 1990. Escola Paulista de Medicina (São Paulo, Brazil).

2. Campos, A.H., et al. "*Phyllanthus niruri* inhibits calcium oxalate endocytosis by renal tubular cells: its role in urolithiasis." *Nephron.* 1999; 81(4): 393–397.

3. Freitas, A. M., et al. "The effect of *Phyllanthus niruri* on urinary inhibitors of calcium oxalate crystallization and other factors associated with renal stone formation." *B. J. U. Int.* 2002; 89(9): 829–834.

4. Barros ME, et al. "Effects of an aqueous extract from *Phyllantus niruri* on calcium oxalate crystallization in vitro." *Urol Res.* 2003 Feb; 30(6): 374–379.

5. Calixto, J. B. "Antispasmodic effects of an alkaloid extracted from *Phyllanthus sellowianus*: a comparative study with papaverine." *Braz. J. Med. Biol. Res.* 1984; 17(3–4): 313–321.

6. Dhar, M. L., et al. "Screening of Indian plants for biological activity: Part I." *Indian J. Exp. Biol.* 1968; 6: 232–247.

7. Kitisin, T., et al. "Pharmacological studies. 3. *Phyllanthus niruri*." *Sirriaj. Hosp. Gaz.* 1952; 4: 641–649.

8. Maxwell, N. *A Witch-Doctor's Apprentice, Hunting for Medicinal Plants in the Amazon*. Citadel Press, 1990.

9. Khanna, A. K., et al. "Lipid lowering activity of *Phyllanthus niruri* in hyperlipemic rats." *J. Ethnopharmacol.* 2002; 82(1): 19–22.

10. Umarani, D., et al. "Ethanol induced metabolic alterations and the effect of *Phyllanthus niruri* in their reversal." *Ancient Sci. Life* 1985; 4(3): 174–180.

11. Ueno, H., et al. "Chemical and pharmaceutical studies on medicinal plants in

Paraguay. Geraniin, an angiotensin-converting enzyme inhibitor from 'paraparai mi,' *Phyllanthus niruri.*" *J. Nat. Prod.* 1988; 51(2): 357–359.

12. Srividya, N., et al. "Diuretic, hypotensive and hypoglycaemic effect of *Phyllanthus amarus.*" *Indian J. Exp. Biol.* 1995; 33(11): 861–864.

13. Arauio, A. *On Diuresis and its Medications Under the Influence of Various Fluid Extracts of Brazilian Plants.* Thesis, 1929. University of São Paulo, Brazil.

14. Devi, M. V., et al. "Effect of *Phyllanthus niruri* on the diuretic activity of Punarnava tablets." *J. Res. Edu. Ind. Med.* 1986; 5(1): 11–12.

15. Ramakrishnan, P. N., et al. "Oral hypoglycaemic effect of *Phyllanthus niruri* (Linn.) leaves." *Indian J. Pharm. Sci.* 1982; 44(1): 10–12.

16. Hukeri, V. I., et al. "Hypoglycemic activity of flavonoids of *Phyllanthus fraternus* in rats." *Fitoterapia* 1988; 59(1): 68–70.

17. Shimizu, M., et al. "Studies on aldose reductase inhibitors from natural products. II. Active components of a Paraguayan crude drug, 'paraparai mi,' *Phyllanthus niruri.*" *Chem. Pharm. Bull.* (Tokyo) 1989; 37(9): 2531–32.

18. Santos, A. R., et al. "Analgesic effects of callus culture extracts from selected species of *Phyllanthus* in mice." *J. Pharm. Pharmacol.* 1994; 46(9): 755–759.

19. Santos, A. R., et al. "Further studies on the antinociceptive action of the hydroalcohlic extracts from plants of the genus *Phyllanthus.*" *J. Pharm. Pharmacol.* 1995; 47(1): 66–71.

20. Santos, A. R., et al. "Analysis of the mechanisms underlying the antinociceptive effect of the extracts of plants from the genus *Phyllanthus.*" *Gen. Pharmacol.* 1995; 26(7): 1499–1506.

21. Miguel, O. G., et al. "Chemical and preliminary analgesic evaluation of geraniin and furosin isolated from *Phyllanthus sellowianus.*" *Planta Med.* 1996; 62(2): 146–149.

22. Santos, A. R., et al. "Antinociceptive properties of extracts of new species of plants of the genus *Phyllanthus* (Euphor-

biaceae)." *J. Ethnopharmacol.* 2000; 72(1/2): 229–238.

23. Souza, C. R., et al. "Compounds extracted from *Phyllanthus* and *Jatropha elliptica* inhibit the binding of [3H]glutamate and [3H]GMP-PNP in rat cerebral cortex membrane." *Neurochem. Res.* 2000; 25(2): 211–215.

24. Hung, C. R., et al. "Prophylactic effects of sucralfate and geraniin on ethanol-induced gastric mucosal damage in rats." *Chin. J. Physiol.* 1995; 38(4): 211–217.

25. Syamasundar, K. V., et al. "Antihepatotoxic principles of *Phyllanthus niruri* herbs." *J. Ethnopharmacol.* 1985; 14(1): 41–44.

26. Padma, P., et al. "Protective effect of *Phyllanthus fraternus* against carbon tetrachloride-induced mitochondrial dysfunction." *Life Sci.* 1999; 64(25): 2411–2417.

27. Sreenivasa, R. Y., "Experimental production of liver damage and its protection with *Phyllanthus niruri* and *Capparis spinosa* (both ingredients of LIV52) in white albino rats." *Probe* 1985; 24(2): 117–119.

28. Prakash, A., et al. "Comparative hepatoprotective activity of three *Phyllanthus* species, *P. urinaria, P. niruri* and *P. simplex,* on carbon tetrachloride induced liver injury in the rat." *Phytother. Res.* 1995; 9(8): 594–596.

29. Bhumyamalaki , et al. "*Phyllanthus Niruri* and jaundice in children." *J. Natl. Integ. Med. Ass.* 1983; 25(8): 269–272.

30. Thabrew, M. R., et al. "Phytogenic agents in the therapy of liver disease." *Phytother. Res.* 1996; 10(6): 461–467.

31. Wang. M.X., et al. "Observations of the efficacy of *Phyllanthus* spp. in treating patients with chronic Hepatitis B." 1994; 19(12): 750–752.

32. Rajeshkumar, N. V., et al. "*Phyllanthus amarus* extract administration increases the life span of rats with hepatocellular carcinoma." *J. Ethnopharmacol.* 2000 Nov; 73(1–2): 215–219.

33. Jeena, K. J., et al. "Effect of *Emblica officinalis, Phyllanthus amarus* and *Picrorrhiza kurroa* on n-nitrosodiethylamine induced hepatocarcinogenesis." *Cancer Lett.* 1999; 136(1): 11–16.

34. Agarwa, K., et al. "The efficacy of two species of *Phyllanthus* in counteracting nickel clastogenicity." *Fitoterapia* 1992; 63(1): 49–54.

35. Raphael, K. R. "Anti-mutagenic activity of *Phyllanthus amarus* (Schum. & Thonn.) *in vitro* as well as *in vivo.*" *Teratog. Carcinog. Mutagen.* 2002; 22(4): 285–291.

36. Sripanidkulchai, B., et al. "Antimutagenic and anticarcinogenic effects of *Phyllanthus amarus.*" *Phytomedicine* 2002; 9(1): 26–32.

37. Rajeshkumar, N. V. "Antitumour and anticarcinogenic activity of *Phyllanthus amarus* extract." *J. Ethnopharmacol.* 2002; 81(1): 17–22.

38. Dhir, H., et al. "Protection afforded by aqueous extracts of *Phyllanthus* species against cytotoxicity induced by lead and aluminium salts." *Phytother. Res.* 1990; 4(5): 172–176.

39. Devi, P.U. "Radioprotective effect of *Phyllanthus niruri* on mouse chromosomes." *Curr. Sci.* 2000; 78(10): 1245–1247.

40. Thyagarajan, S. P., et al. "Effect of *Phyllanthus amarus* on chronic carriers of Hepatitis B virus." *Lancet* 1988; 2(8614): 764–766.

41. Thyagarajan, S. P., et al. "*In vitro* inactivation of HBsAG by *Eclipta alba* (Hassk.) and *Phyllanthus niruri* (Linn.)" *Indian J. Med. Res.* 1982; 76s: 124–130.

42. Venkateswaran, P. S., et al. "Effects of an extract from *Phyllanthus niruri* on Hepatitis B and wood chuck hepatitis viruses: *in vitro* and *in vivo* studies." *Proc. Nat. Acad. Sci.* (U.S.A.) 1987; 84(1): 274–278.

43. Venkateswaran, P. S., et al. "Composition, pharmaceutical preparation and method for treating viral hepatitis." U.S. Patent #4,673,575; June 16, 1987 (Filed April 26, 1985) (Assigned to Fox Chase Canc. Cent., Philadelphia, PA, U.S.A.).

44. Venkateswaran, P., et al. "Method of treating retrovirus infection." U.S. Patent #4,937,074; June 26, 1990 (Filed March 29, 1988) (Assigned to Fox Chase Canc. Cent., Philadelphia, PA, U.S.A.).

45. Thabrew, M. R., et al. "Phytogenic agents in the therapy of liver disease." *Phytother. Res.* 1996; 10(6): 461–467.

46. Wang, M. X., et al. "Herbs of the genus *Phyllanthus* in the treatment of chronic Hepatitis B: Observation with three preparations from different geographic sites." *J. Lab. Clin. Med.* 1995; 126(4): 350–352.

47. Xin-Hua , W., et al. "A comparative study of *Phyllanthus amarus* compound and interferon in the treatment of chronic viral Hepatitis B." *Southeast Asian J. Trop. Med. Public Health* 2001; 32(1): 140–142.

48. Huang, R.L., et al. "Screening of 25 compounds isolated from *Phyllanthus* species for anti-human hepatitis B virus in vitro." *Phytother Res.* 2003 May; 17(5): 449–453.

49. Liu, J., et al. "Genus *Phyllanthus* for chronic Hepatitis B virus infection: A systematic review." *Viral Hepat.* 2001; 8(5): 358–366.

50. Ogata, T., et al. "HIV-1 reverse transcriptase inhibitor from *Phyllanthus niruri.*" *AIDS Res. Hum. Retroviruses* 1992; 8(11): 1937–1944.

51. Qian-Cutrone, J. "Niruriside, a new HIV REV/RRE binding inhibitor from *Phyllanthus niruri.*" *J. Nat. Prod.* 1996; 59(2): 196–199.

52. Notka, F., et al. "Inhibition of wild-type human immunodeficiency virus and reverse transcriptase inhibitor-resistant variants by *Phyllanthus amarus.*" *Antiviral Res.* 2003 Apr; 58(2): 175–186.

53. Bork, P. M., et al. "Nahua Indian medicinal plants (Mexico): Inhibitory activity on NF-KB as anti-inflammatory model and antibacterial effects." *Phytomedicine* 1996; 3(3): 263–269.

54. Farouk, A., et al. "Antimicrobial activity of certain Sudanese plants used in folkloric medicine. Screening for antibacterial activity (I)." *Fitoterapia* 1983; 54(1): 3–7.

55. Mesia, L.T.K., et al. "*In-vitro* antimalarial activity of Cassia occidentalis, *Morinda morindoides* and *Phyllanthus niruri.*" *Ann. Trop. Med. Parasitol.* 2001; 95(1): 47–57.

56. Tona, L., et al. "Antimalarial activity of 20 crude extracts from nine African medicinal plants used in Kinshasa, Congo." *J. Ethnopharmacol.* 1999; 68(1/3): 193–203.

57. Rao, M. V., and K. M. Alice. "Contraceptive effects of *Phyllanthus amarus* in female mice." *Phytother. Res.* 2001; 15(3): 265–267.

Chuchuhuasi

1. Itokawa, H., et al. "Isolation, structural elucidation and conformational analysis of sesquiterpene pyridine alkaloids from *Maytenus ebenifolia* Reiss. X-ray molecular structure of ebenifoline W-1." *J. Chem. Soc. Perkin. Trans. I* 1993; 11: 1247–1254.

2. Morita, H., et al. "Triterpenes from Brazilian medicinal plant "chuchuhuasi" (*Maytenus krukovii*)." *J. Nat. Prod.* 1996; 59(11): 1072–1075.

3. Honda, T., et al. "Partial synthesis of krukovines A and B, triterpene ketones isolated from the Brazilian medicinal plant *Maytenus krukovii.*" *J. Nat. Prod.* 1997; 60(11): 1174–1177.

4. DiCarlo, F. J., et al. "Reticuloendothelial system stimulants of botanical origin." *Journal of the Reticuloendothelial Society* 1964: 224–232.

5. Moya, S., et al. "Phytochemical and pharmacological studies on the antiarthritics of plant origin." *Rev. Colomb. Cienc. Quim. Farm.* 1977; 3(2): 5.

6. Gonzalez, J. G., et al. "Chuchuhuasha—a drug used in folk medicine in the Amazonian and Andean areas. A chemical study of *Maytenus laevis.*" *J Ethnopharm.* 1982; 5: 73–77.

7. Itokawa, H., et al. "Oligo-nicotinated sesquiterpene polyesters from *Maytenus ilicifolia.*" *J. Nat. Prod.* 1993; 56: 1479–1485.

8. Sekar, K. V., et al. "Mayteine and 6-benzoyl-6-deacetyl-mayteine from *Maytenus krukovii.*" *Planta Medica* 1995; 61: 390.

9. Bradshaw, D., et al. "Therapeutic potential of protein kinase C inhibitors." *Agents and Actions* 1993; 38: 135–147.

10. Chavez, H., et al. "Friedelane triterpenoids from *Maytenus macrocarpa.*" *J. Nat. Prod.* 1998; 61(1): 82–85.

11. Martinod, P., et al. "Isolation of tingenone and pristimerin from *Maytenus chuchuhuasha.*" *Phytochemistry* 1976; 15: 562–563.

12. Piacente, S., et al. "Laevisines A and B: two new sesquiterpene-pyridine alkaloids from *Maytenus laevis.*" *J. Nat. Prod.* 1999; 62(1): 161–163.

13. Perez-Victoria, et al. "New natural sesquiterpenes as modulators of daunomycin resistance in a multidrug-resistant *Leishmania tropica* line." *J. Med. Chem.* 1999; 42(1): 4388–4393.

14. Chavez, H., et al. "Sesquiterpene polyol esters from the leaves of *Maytenus macrocarpa.*" *J. Nat. Prod.* 1999; 62(11): 1576–1577.

15. Chavez, H., et al. "Macrocarpins A–D, new cytotoxic nor-triterpenes from *Maytenus macrocarpa.*" *Bioorg. Med. Chem. Lett.* 2000; 10(8): 759–762.

Cipó Cabeludo

1. Muradian, J. M., et al. "Flavonols and (-) karu-16-en-19-oic acid from *Mikania hirsutissima.*" *Rev. Latinam. Quim.* 1977; 8: 88–89.

2. Davino, S. C., et al. "Antimicrobial activity of kaurenoic acid derivatives substituted on carbon-15." *Braz. J. Med. Biol. Res.* 1989; 22(9): 1127–1129.

3. Wilkins, M., et al. "Characterization of the bactericidal activity of the natural diterpene kaurenoic acid." *Planta Med.* 2002; 68(5): 452–454.

4. de Oliveira, F. "Contribution to the botanical study of *Mikania hirsutissima* DC. var. *hirsutissima*. II. External morphology and anatomy of the leaf, flower, fruit and seed." *Rev. Farm. Bioquim.* (Univ. São Paulo) 1972; 10(1): 15–36.

5. de Oliveira, F. "Contribution to the botanical study of *Mikania hirsutissima* DC. var. *hirsutissima*. I. External morphology and anatomy of the axophyte." *Rev. Farm. Bioquim.* (Univ. São Paulo) 1971; 9(1): 79–100.

6. de Souza, C. P., et al. "Chemoprophylaxis of schistosomiasis: molluscacidal activity of natural products—assays with adult snails and oviposition." *An. Acad Bras Cienc.* 1984; 56(3): 333–338.

7. Ohkoshi, E., et al. "Studies on the constituents of *Mikania hirsutissima* (Compositae)." *Chem. Pharm. Bull.* (Tokyo) 1999; 47(10): 1436–1438.

8. Ohkoshi, E., et al. "A novel bisnorditerpenelactone from *Mikania hirsutissima.*"

Chem. Pharm. Bull. (Tokyo) 2000; 48(11): 1774–1775.

9. Suyenaga, E. S., et al. "Antiinflammatory investigation of some species of *Mikania.*" *Phytother. Res.* 2002; 16(6): 519–523.

Clavillia

1. Habuka, N., et al. "Antiviral protein." United States Patent 5,340,732; 1994.

2. Wong, R. N. S., et al. "Characterization of *Mirabilis* antiviral protein—a ribosome inactivating protein from *Mirabilis jalapa* L." *Biochem. Int.* 1992; 28(4): 585–593.

3. Vivanco, J. M., et al. "Characterization of two novel type 1 ribosome-inactivating proteins from the storage roots of the Andean crop *Mirabilis expansa.*" *Plant Physiol.* 1999; 119(4): 1447–1456.

4. Kataoka, J., et al. "Adenine depurination and inactivation of plant ribosomes by an antiviral protein of *Mirabilis jalapa* (MAP)." *Plant Mol. Biol.* 1992; 20(6): 111–119.

5. Bolognesi, A. et al. "Ribosome-inactivating and adenine polynucleotide glycosylase activities in *Mirabilis jalapa* L. tissues." *J. Biol. Chem.* 2002; 277(16) 13709–13716.

6. Cordeiro, N., et al. "The purification and amino acid sequences of four Tx2 neurotoxins from the venom of the Brazilian 'armed' spider *Phoneutria nigriventer* (Keyes)." *FEBBS Lett.* 1992; 310(2): 153–156.

7. Cammue, B. P. A., et al. "Isolation and characterization of a novel class of plant antimicrobial peptides from *Mirabilis jalapa* L. seeds." *J. Biol. Chem.* 1992; 267(4): 2228–2233.

8. De Bolle, M. F. C., et al. "Antimicrobial peptides from *Mirabilis jalapa* and *Amarantus caudatus*: expression, processing, localization and biological activity in transgenic tobacco." *Plant Mol. Biol.* 1996; 31(5): 993–1008.

9. Kusamba, C., et al. "Antibacterial activity of *Mirabilis jalapa* seed powder." *J. Ethnopharmacol.* 1991; 35(2): 197–199.

10. Yang, S.W., et al. "Three new phenolic compounds from a manipulated plant cell culture, *Mirabilis jalapa.*" *J. Nat. Prod.* 2001; 64(3): 313–317.

11. Caceres, A., et al. "Plants used in Guatemala for the treatment of dermato-

phytic infections. Screening for antimycotic activity of 44 plant extracts." *J. Ethnophamacol.* 1991; 31(3): 263–276.

12. Dimayuga, R. E.., et al. "Antimicrobial activity of medicinal plants from Baja California Sur (Mexico)." *Pharmaceutical Biol.* 1998; 36(1): 33–43.

13. Caceres, A., et al. "Screening of antimicrobial activity of plants popularly used in Guatemala for the treatment of dermatomucosal diseases." *J. Ethnopharmacol.* 1987; 20(3): 223–237.

14. Dhar, M. L., et al. "Screening of Indian plants for biological activity: Part I." *Indian J. Exp. Biol.* 1968; 6: 232–247.

Clavo Huasca

There are no studies published on this plant.

Copaiba

1. Wenninger, J. A., et al. "Sequiterpene hydrocarbons of commercial copaiba and American cedarwood oils." *J. Amer. Oil Chemists Soc.* 1967; 50: 1201–1312.

2. Mahajam, J. R., et al. "New diterpenoids from copaiba oil." *An. Acad. Bras. Cienc.* 1971; 43: 611–613.

3. Paiva, L. A., et al. "Investigation on the wound healing activity of oleo-resin from *Copaifera langsdorfii* in rats." *Phytother. Res.* 2002; 16(8): 737–739.

4. Fernandes, R. M., *Contribuicao para o conhecimento do efito antiinflamatorio e analgesico do balsamo de copaiba e alguns de seus constituintes quimicos.* Thesis, 1986. Federal University of Rio de Janeiro.

5. Basile, A. C., et al. "Anti-inflammatory activity of oleoresin from Brazilian *Copaifera.*" *J. Ethnopharmacol.* 1988; 22: 101–109.

6. Cascon, V., et al. "Characterization of the chemical composition of oleoresins of *Copaifera guianensis* Desf., *Copaifera duckei* Dwyer and *Copaifera multijuna* Hayne." *Phytochemistry* 2000; 55(7): 773–778.

7. Veiga, V. F., et al. "Phytochemical and antioedematogenic studies of commercial copaiba oils available in Brazil." *Phytother. Res.* 2001; 15(6): 476–480.

8. Ghelardini, C., et al. "Local anaesthetic

activity of beta-caryophyllene." *Farmaco* 2001; 56(5–7): 387–389.

9. Yang, D., et al. "Use of caryophyllene oxide as an antifungal agent in an *in vitro* experimental model of onychomycosis." *Mycopathologia* 1999; 148(2): 79–82.

10. Tambe, Y., et al. "Gastric cytoprotection of the non-steroidal anti-inflammatory sesquiterpene, beta-caryophyllene." *Planta Med.* 1996; 62(5): 469–470.

11. Paiva, L. A., et al. "Gastroprotective effect of *Copifera langsdorffii* oleo-resin on experimental gastric ulcer models in rats." *J. Ethnopharmacol.* 1998; 62(1): 73–78.

12. Opdyke, D. L. "Monographs on Fragrance Raw Materials." *Food Cosmet. Toxicol.* 1973; 11: 1075.

13. Maruzzella, J. C., et al. "Antibacterial activity of essential oil vapors." *J. Am. Pharm. Assoc.* 1960; 49: 692–694.

14. Tincusi, B. M., et al. "Antimicrobial terpenoids from the oleoresin of the Peruvian medicinal plant *Copaifera paupera.*" *Planta Med.* 2002; 68(9): 808–812.

15. de Almeida Alves, T. M., et al. "Biological screening of Brazilian medicinal plants." *Mem. Inst. Oswaldo Cruz* 2000; 95(3): 367–373.

16. Wilkins, M., et al. "Characterization of the bactericidal activity of the natural diterpene kaurenoic acid." *Planta Med.* 2002 68(5): 452–454.

17. Davino, S. C., et al. "Antimicrobial activity of kaurenoic acid derivatives substituted on carbon-15." *Braz. J. Med. Biol. Res.* 1989; 22(9): 1127–1129.

18. Ohsaki, A., et al. "The isolation and *in vivo* potent antitumor activity of clerodane diterpenoids from the oleoresin of Brazilian medicinal plant *Copaifera langsdorffii* Desfon." *Bioorg. Med. Chem. Lett.* 1994; 4: 2889–2892.

19. Costa-Lotufo, L. V., et al. "The cytotoxic and embryotoxic effects of kaurenoic acid, a diterpene isolated from *Copaifera langsdorffi.*" *Toxicon* 2002; 40(8): 1231–1234.

20. Richard, M. A. "Copahic erythema." *Ann. Dermatol. Venereol.* 2001; 128(4): 580.

21. Leung, A. and S. Foster. *Encyclopedia of Common Natural Ingredients.* New York: John Wiley & Sons, 1996.

Curare

1. Lee, C., et al. "Conformation, action, and mechanism of action of neuromuscular blocking muscle relaxants." *Pharmacol. Ther.* 2003; 98(2): 143–169.

2. Tuba, Z., et al. "Synthesis and structure-activity relationships of neuromuscular blocking agents." *Curr. Med. Chem.* 2002; 9(16): 1507–1536.

3. Farthing, M. J. G. "5-Hydroxytryptamine and 5-hydroxytryptamine-3 receptor antagonists." *Scand. J. Gastroenterol.* 1991; 26(suppl 188): 92–100.

4. Perez, E. A. "Review of the preclinical pharmacology and comparative efficacy of 5-hydroxytryptamine-3 receptor antagonists for chemotherapy-induced emesis." *J. Clin. Oncol.* 1995; 13(4): 1036–1043.

5. Breitinger, H. G., et al. "Inhibition of the serotonin 5-HT3 receptor by nicotine, cocaine, and fluoxetine investigated by rapid chemical kinetic techniques." *Biochemistry* 2001; 40(28): 8419–8429.

6. Seth, P., et al. "Nicotinic-serotonergic interactions in brain and behaviour." *Pharmacol. Biochem. Behav.* 2002; 71(4): 795–805.

7. Costall, B., et al. "Anxiolytic potential of 5-HT3 receptor antagonists." *Pharmacol. Toxicol.* 1992; 70(3): 157–162.

8. Hardman, J. G., et al. *The pharmacological basis of therapeutics.* 9th ed. Goodman and Gilman's; 1996.

Damiana

1. Anonymous. New York Alumni Association of the Philadelphia College of Pharmacy: Meeting Minutes—August 3, 1875. *Am. J. Pharm.* 1875; 47: 426.

2. Steinmetz, E. F. *Acta Phytother.* 1960; 7(1)

3. Domínguez. X. A. and M. Hinojosa. "Mexican medicinal plants. XXVIII. Isolation of 5-hydroxy-7,3′,4′-trimethoxy-flavone from *Turnera diffusa.*" *Planta Med.* 1976; 30(1): 68–71.

4. Piacente, S., et al. "Flavonoids and arbutin from *Turnera diffusa.*" *Z. Naturforsch.* 2002; 57c: 983–985.

5. Committee for veterinary medicinal products *Turnera diffusa* summary report. The European agency for the evaluation of medicinal products veterinary medicines evaluation unit. August 1999.

6. Arletti, R., et al. "Stimulating property of *Turnera diffusa* and *Pfaffia paniculata* extracts on the sexual-behavior of male rats." *Psychopharmacology* (Berl). 1999; 143(1): 15–19.

7. Heleen, P. A. "Herbal composition for enhancing sexual response." United States Patent 6,444,237; 2002.

8. Morrow, T. "Herbal compound for relief of PMS through menopausal symptoms." United States Patent 5,707,630; 1998.

9. Zava, D. T., et al. "Estrogen and progestin bioactivity of foods, herbs and spices." *Proc. Soc. Exp. Biol. Med.* 1998; 217(3): 369–378.

10. Jiu, J. "A survey of some medicinal plants of Mexico for selected biological activity." *Lloydia.* 1966; 29: 250–259.

11. Andersen, T., et al. "Weight loss and delayed gastric emptying following a South American herbal preparation in overweight patients." *J. Hum. Nutr. Diet.* 2001; 14(3): 243–250.

12. Mann, M. A., et al. "Appetite suppressant composition and method relating thereto." United States Patent 5,273,754; 1993.

13. Hessel, L. L., et al. "Compositions and methods for weight reduction." United States Patent 5,945,107; 1999.

14. Perez, R. M., et al. "A study of the hypoglycemic effect of some Mexican plants." *J. Ethnopharmacol.* 1984; 12(3): 253–262.

15. Alarcon-Aguilara, F. J., et al. "Study of the anti-hyperglycemic effect of plants used as antidiabetics." *J. Ethnopharmacol.* 1998; 61(2): 101–110.

16. Alarcon-Aguilara, F. J., et al. "Investigation on the hypoglycaemic effects of extracts of four Mexican medicinal plants in normal and alloxan-diabetic mice." *Phythother. Res.* 2002; 16(4): 383–386.

Embauba

1. Paulo, G., et al. "Utilization of an extract of a plant of the *Cecropia* genus." United States Patent 6,403,125; 2002.

2. Lacaille-Dubois., et al. "Search for potential angiotensin converting enzyme (ACE)-inhibitors from plants." *Phytomedicine* 2001; 8(1): 47–52.

3. Perea Guerrero, C., et al. "A pharmacological study of *Cecropia obtusifolia* Bertol. aqueous extract." *J. Ethnopharmacol.* 2001; 76(3): 279–284.

4. Feng, P. C., et al. "Pharmacological screening of some West Indian medicinal plants." *J. Pharm. Pharmacol.* 1962; 14: 556–561.

5. Carbajal, D., et al. "Pharmacological screening of plant decoctions commonly used in Cuban folk medicine." *J. Ethnopharmacol.* 1991; 33: 21–24.

6. Vargas Howell, R., et al. "Diuretic effect of *Cecropia obtusifolia* (Moraceae) on albino rats." *Rev. Biol. Trop.* 1996; 44(1): 93–96.

7. Vidrio, H., et al. "Hypotensive activity of *Cecropia obtusifolia.*" *J. Pharm. Sci.* 1982; 71(4): 475–476.

8. Salas, I., et al. "Antihypertensive effect of *Cecropia obtusifolia* (Moraceae) leaf extract on rats." *Rev. Biol. Trop.* 1987; 35(1): 127–130.

9. Andrade-Cetto, A., et al. "Hypoglycemic effect of *Cecropia obtusifolia* on streptozotocin diabetic rats." *J. Ethnopharmacol.* 2001; 78(2–3): 145–149.

10. Perez, R. M., et al. "A study of the hypoglycemic effect of some Mexican plants." *J. Ethnopharmacol.* 1984; 12(3): 253–262.

11. Raman-Ramos, R., et al. "Experimental study of hypoglycemic activity of some antidiabetic plants." *Arch. Invest. Med.* (Mex). 1991; 22(1): 87–93.

12. Mellado, V., et al. "Effect of the aqueous extract of *Cecropia obtusifolia* on the blood sugar of normal and pancreatectomized dogs." *Int. J. Crude Drug Res.* 1984; 22(1): 11–16.

13. Misas, C. A. J., et al. "Contribution to the biological evaluation of Cuban plants. I." *Rev. Cub. Med. Trop.* 1979; 31: 5–12.

14. Zavala, M. A., et al. "Antimicrobial screening of some medicinal plants." *Phytother. Res.* 1997; 11(5): 368–371.

15. Lopez Abraham, A. N., et al. "Potential antineoplastic activity of Cuban plants." *Rev. Cubana Farm.* 1981; 15(1): 71–77.

16. Velazquez, E., et al. "Antioxidant activity of Paraguayan plant extracts." *Fitoterapia* 2003; 74 (1–2): 91–7.

Epazote

1. *PDR for Herbal Medicines*. 2nd Ed. Medical Economics Company; Montvale, New Jersey, 2000.

2. Johnson, M. A., et al. "Biosynthesis of ascaridole: iodide peroxidase-catalyzed synthesis of a monoterpene endoperoxide in soluble extracts of *Chenopodium ambrosioides* fruit." *Arch. Biochem. Biophys.* 1984; 235(1): 254–266.

3. Kiuchi, F., et al. "Monoterpene hydroperoxides with trypanocidal activity from *Chenopodium ambrosioides*." *J. Nat. Prod.* 2002; 65(4): 509–512.

4. Okuyama, E., et al. "Ascaridole as a pharmacologically active principle of "Paico," a medicinal Peruvian plant." *Chem. Pharm. Bull.* (Tokyo) 1993; 41(7): 1309–1311.

5. Kishore, N., et al. "Fungitoxicity of essential oils against dermatophytes." *Mycoses* 1993; 36(5-6): 211–215.

6. Pollack, Y., et al. "The effect of ascaridole on the in vitro development of *Plasmodium falciparum*." *Parasitol. Res.* 1990; 76(7): 570–572.

7. Morsy, T. A., et al. "The effect of the volatile oils of *Chenopodium ambrosioides* and *Thymus vulgaris* against the larvae of Lucilia sericata (Meigen)." *J. Egypt Soc. Parasitol.* 1998; 28(2): 503–510.

8. Gadano, A., et al. "In vitro genotoxic evaluation of the medicinal plant *Chenopodium ambrosioides* L." *J. Ethnopharmacol.* 2002; 81(1): 11–16.

9. Anon., WHO Chronicle, 1977; 31: 428.

10. Giove Nakazawa, R. A. "Traditional medicine in the treatment of enteroparasitosis." *Rev. Gastroenterol. Peru* 1996; 16(3): 197–202.

11. Lopez de Guimaraes, D., et al. "Ascariasis: comparison of the therapeutic efficacy between paico and albendazole in children from Huaraz." *Rev. Gastroenterol Peru* 2001; 21(3): 212–219.

12. Hmamouchi, M., et al. "Molluscicidal activity of some Moroccan medicinal plants." *Fitoterapia* 2000; 71(3): 308–314.

13. Lall, N., et al. "In vitro inhibition of drug-resistant and drug-sensitive strains of *Mycobacterium tuberculosis* by ethnobotanically selected South African plants." *J. Ethnopharmacol.* 1999; 66(3): 347–354.

14. Zhang, Y., et al. "Chinese drug composition for treatment of peptic ulcer and preparation thereof." United States Patent 6,344,219; 2003.

15. Ruffa, M. J., et al. "Cytotoxic effect of Argentine medicinal plant extracts on human hepatocellular carcinoma cell line." *J. Ethnopharmacol.* 2002; 79(3): 335–339.

16. Efferth, T., et al. "Activity of ascaridol from the anthelmintic herb *Chenopodium anthelminticum* L. against sensitive and multidrug-resistant tumor cells." *Anticancer Res.* 2002; 22(6C): 4221–4224.

Erva Tostão

1. Mungantiwarn, A. A., et al. "Studies on the immunomodulatory effects of Boerhaavia diffusa alkaloidal fraction." *J. Ethnopharmacol.* 1999 May; 65(2): 125–131.

2. Mehrotra, S., et al. "Immunomodulation by ethanolic extract of *Boerhaavia diffusa* roots." *Int. Immunopharmacol.* 2002; 7: 987–996.

3. Chowdhury, A., et al. "Boerhaavia diffusa—effect on diuresis and some renal enzymes." *Ann. Biochem. Exp. Med.* 1955; 15: 119–126.

4. Mudgal, V. "Studies on medicinal properties of *Convolvulus pluricaulis* and *Boerhaavia diffusa*." *Planta Med.* 1975; 28: 62.

5. Gaitonde, B. B., et al. "Diuretic activity of punarnava (Boerhaavia diffusa)." *Bull. Haffkine Inst.* 1974; 2: 24.

6. Singh, R. P., et al. "Recent approach in clinical and experimental evaluation of diuretic action of punarnava (*B. diffusa*) with special reference to nephrotic syndrome." *J. Res. Edu. Ind. Med.* 1955; 7(1): 29–35.

7. Devi, M. V., et al. "Effect of *Phyllanthus niruri* on the diuretic activity of punarnava tablets." *J. Res. Edu. Ind. Med.* 1986; 5(1): 11–12.

8. Mishra, J. P., et al. "Studies on the effect of indigenous drug *Boerhaavia diffusa* Rom. on kidney regeneration." *Indian J. Pharmacy* 1980; 12: 59.

9. Chandan, B. K., et al. "*Boerhaavia diffusa*: a study of its hepatoprotective activity." *J. Ethnopharmacol.* 1991; 31(3): 299–307.

10. Rawat, A. K., et al. "Hepatoprotective activity of *Boerhaavia diffusa* L. roots—a popular Indian ethnomedicine." *J. Ethnopharmacol.* 1997; 56(1): 61–66.

11. Ramabhimaiah, S., et al. "Pharmacological investigations on the water soluble fraction of methanol extract of *Boerhaavia diffusa* root." *Indian Drugs* 1984; 21(8): 343–344.

12. Dhar, M., et al. "Screening of Indian plants for biological activity: Part I." *Indian J. Exp. Biol.* 1968; 6: 232–247.

13. Hiruma-Lima, C. A., et al. "The juice of fresh leaves of *Boerhaavia diffusa* L. (Nyctaginaceae) markedly reduces pain in mice." *J. Ethnopharmacol.* 2000; 71(1–2): 267–274

14. Sohni, Y., et al. "The antiamoebic effect of a crude drug formulation of herbal extracts against *Entamoeba histolytica in vitro* and *in vivo*." *J. Ethnopharmacol.* 1995; 45(1): 43–52.

15. Barthwal, M., et al. "Management of IUD-associated menorrhagia in female rhesus monkeys (*Macaca mulatta*)." *Adv. Contracept.* 1991; 7(1): 67–76.

16. Barthwal, M., et al. "Histologic studies on endometrium of menstruating monkeys wearing IUDS: comparative evaluation of drugs." *Adv. Contracept.* 1990; 6(2): 113–124.

17. Adesina, S. "Anticonvulsant properties of the roots of *Boerhaavia diffusa*." *Q. J. Crude Drug Res.* 1979; 17: 84–86.

18. Akah, P., et al. "Nigerian plants with anti-convulsant property." *Fitoterapia* 1993; 64(1): 42–44.

19. Olukoya, D., et al. "Antibacterial activity of some medicinal plants from Nigeria." *J. Ethnopharmacol.* 1993; 39(1): 69–72.

20. Perumal, Samy R., et al. "Ethnomedicinal plants from India." *J. Ethnopharmacol.* 1999; 66(2): 235–240.

21. Aynehchi, Y. "Screening of Iranian plants for antimicrobial activity." *Acta Pharm. Suecica.* 1982; 19(4): 303–308.

22. Verma, H., et al. 1979. "Antiviral activity of *Boerhaavia diffusa* root extract and physical properties of the virus inhibitor." *Can. J. Bot.* 1979; 57: 926–932.

23. Singh, A., et al. "An experimental evaluation of possible teratogenic potential in *Boerhaavia diffusa* in albino rats." *Planta Med.* 1991; 57(4): 315–316.

24. Hansen, K., et al. "*In vitro* screening of traditional medicines for anti-hypertensive effect based on inhibition of the angiotensin converting enzyme (ACE)." *Ethnopharmacol.* 1995; 48(1): 43–51.

Espinheira Santa

1. Oliveira, M. G., et al. "Pharmacologic and toxicologic effects of two *Maytenus* species in laboratory animals." *J. Ethnopharmacol.*, 1991; 34(1): 29–41.

2. Dinari, Dr. H., Unpublished data from Buenos Aires, Argentina. Personal communication (1978) from the University of Illinois NAPRALERT report.

3. Bingel, A. S., et al. "Antifertility screening of selected plants in female rats." *Lloydia.* 1976: 39(6): 475C.

4. Montanari, T., et al. "Effect of *Maytenus ilicifolia* Mart. on pregnant mice." *Contraception* 2002 Feb; 65(2): 171–175.

5. Montanari, T., et al. "Effect of *Maytenus ilicifolia* Mart. Ex. Reiss on spermatogenesis." *Contraception* 1998; 57(5): 335–339.

6. de Lima, O. G., et al. "Substabcias antimicrobiano de plantas superiores. Comunicacao XXXI. Maitenina, novo antimicrobiano con acao antineoplastica, isolade de celastracea de pernambuco." *Revista do Instituto de Antibioticos* 1969; (9): 17–25.

7. de Lima, O. G., et al. "Antimicrobial substances from higher plants. XXXVI. On the presence of maytenin and pristimerine in the cortical part of the roots of *Maytenus ilicifolia* from the south of Brazil." *Rev. Inst. Antibiot.*, 1971 Jun.

8. Monache, F. D., et al., "Maitenin: A new antitumoral substance from *Maytenus* sp." *Gazetta Chimica Italiana* 1972; 102: 317–320.

9. Wolpert-Defillipes, M. K., et al., "Initial studies on the cytotoxic action of maytansine, a novel ansa macrolide." *Biochemical Pharmacology* 24 (1975): 751–754.

10. Anon. Unpublished data, National Cancer Institute (1976). From NAPRA LERT Files, University of Illinois, 1995.

11. de Santana, C. F., et al. "Primeiras observacoes sobre o emprego da maitenina em pacientes cancerosos." *Rev. Inst. Antibiot.* 1971; 11: 37–49.

12. Melo, A. M., et al. "First observations on the topical use of primin, plumbagin and maytenin in patients with skin cancer." *Rev. Inst. Antibiot.* 1974 Dec.

13. Chabner, B. A., et al., "Initial clinical trials of mayansine, an antitumor plant alkaloid." *Cancer Treatment Reports* 1978; (62): 429–433.

14. O'Connell, M. J., et al. "Phase II trial of maytansine in patients with advanced colorectal carcinoma." *Cancer Treatment Reports* 1978 (62); 1237–1238.

15. Cabanillas, F., et al. "Phase I study of maytansine using a 3-day schedule." *Cancer Treatment Reports* 1976; (60): 1127–1139.

16. Suffnes, M. J., et al. "Current status of the NCI plant and animal product program." *Journal of Natural Products* 1982; 45: 1–14.

17. Hartwell, J. L., "Plants used against cancer: A survey." *Lloydia* 1968; 31: 114.

18. Crovetto, P. M., *Las plantas utilizadas en medicina popular en el noroeste de corrientes.* Tucuman, Argentina: Ministeris de Cultura y Educacion, Foundacion Miguel Lillo; 1981.

19. Itokawa, H., et al. "New triterpene dimers from *Maytenus ilicifolia*." *Tetrahedron Lett.* 1990; 31(47): 6881–6882.

20. Itokawa, H., et al. "Triterpenes from *Maytenus ilicifolia*." *Phytochemistry* 1991; 30(11): 3713–3716.

21. Itokawa, H., et al. "Antitumor substances from South American plants." *Pharmacobio. Dyn.* 1992; 15(1): S-2.

22. Arisawa, M., et al. "Cell growth inhibition of KB cells by plant extracts." *Natural Med.* 1994; 48(4): 338–347.

23. Shirota, O., et al. "Cytotoxic aromatic triterpenes from *Maytenus ilicifolia* and *Maytenus chuchuhuasca*." *J. Nat. Prod.* 1994; 57(12): 1675–1681.

24. Miura, N. et al. "Protective effects of triterpene coupounds against the cytotoxicity of cadmium in HepG2 cells." *Mol. Pharm.* 1999; 56(6); 1324–1328.

25. Itokawa, H., et al. "Oligo-nicotinated sesquiterpene polyesters from *Maytenus ilicifolia*." *J. Nat. Prod.* 1993; 56(9); 1479–1485.

26. Itokawa, H., et al. "Cangorins F–J, five additional oligo-nicotinated sesquiterpene polyesters from *Maytenus ilicifolia*." *J. Nat. Prod.* 1994; 57(4): 460–470.

27. Souza-Formigoni, M. L., et al. "Antiulcerogenic effects of two *Maytenus* species in laboratory animals." *J. Ethnopharmacol.* August 1991.

28. Nakamura M., et al. Anti-ulcerative drug. Patent—Eur–O 776 667 A2. 1997: 1–7.

Fedegoso

1. Elujoba, A., et al. "Chemical and biological analyses of Nigerian *Cassia* species for laxative activity." *J. Pharm. Biomed. Anal.* 1989; 7(12): 1453–1457.

2. Sama, S., et al. "Efficacy of an indigenous compound preparation (LIV-52) in acute viral hepatitis—A double blind study." *Indian J. Med. Res.* 1976; 64: 738.

3. Subbarao, V. V., et al. "Changes in serum transaminases due to hepatotoxicity and the role of an indigenous hepatotonic, LIV-52." *Probe* 1978; 17(2): 175–178.

4. Sethi, J. P., et al. "Clinical management of severe acute hepatic failure with special reference to LIV-52 in therapy." *Probe* 1978; 17(2): 155–158.

5. Sharma, N., et al. "Protective effect of *Cassia occidentalis* extract on chemical-induced chromosomal aberrations in mice." *Drug Chem. Toxicol.* 1999; 22(4): 643–653.

6. Saraf, S., et al. "Antiheptatotoxic activity of *Cassia occidentalis*." *Int. J. Pharmacog.* 1994; 32(2): 178–183.

7. Jafri, M. A., et al. "Hepatoprotective activity of leaves of *Cassia occidentalis* against paracetamol and ethyl alcohol intoxication in rats." *J. Ethnopharmacol.* 1999; 66(3): 355–361.

8. Bin-Hafeez, B., et al. "Protective effect of *Cassia occidentalis* L. on cyclophosphamide-induced suppression of humoral

immunity in mice." *J. Ethnopharmacol.* 2001; 75(1): 13–18.

9. Sharma, N., et al. "*In vitro* inhibition of carcinogen-induced mutagenicity by *Cassia occidentalis* and *Emblica officinalis.*" *Drug Chem. Toxicol.* 2000; 23(3): 477–484.

10. Sadique, J., et al. "Biochemical modes of action of *Cassia occidentalis* and *Cardiospermum halicacabum* in inflammation." *J. Ethnopharmacol.* 1987; 19(2): 201–212.

11. Feng, P., et al. "Pharmacological screening of some West Indian medicinal plants." *J. Pharm. Pharmacol.* 1962; 14: 556–561.

12. Gasquet, M., et al. "Evaluation *in vitro* and *in vivo* of a traditional antimalarial, 'Malarial 5.'" *Fitoterapia* 1993; 64(5): 423.

13. Schmeda-Hirschmann, G., et al. "A screening method for natural products on triatomine bugs." *Phytother. Res.* 1989; 6(2): 68–73.

14. Hussain, H., et al. "Plants in Kano ethomedicine: screening for antimicrobial activity and alkaloids." *Int. J. Pharmacog.* 1991; 29(1): 51–56.

16. Caceres, A., et al. "Plants used in Guatemala for the treatment of dermatophytic infections. 1. Screening for antimycotic activity of 44 plant extracts." *J. Ethnopharmacol.* 1991; 31(3): 263–276.

16. Anesini, C., et al. "Screening of plants used in Argentine folk medicine for antimicrobial activity." *J. Ethnopharmacol.* 1993; 39(2): 119–128.

17. Gaind, K. N., et al. "Antibiotic activity of *Cassia occidentalis.*" *Indian J. Pharmacy* 1966; 28(9): 248–250.

18. Samy, R. P., et al. "Antibacterial activity of some folklore medicinal plants used by tribals in Western Ghats of India." *J. Ethnopharmacol.* 2000; 69(1): 63–71.

19. Tona, L., et al. "In-vivo antimalarial activity of *Cassia occidentalis*, *Morinda morindoides* and *Phyllanthus niruri.*" *Ann. Trop. Med. Parasitol.* 2001; 95(1): 47–57.

Gervâo

1. Sheng, G. Q., et al. "Protective effect of verbascoside on 1-methyl-4-phenylpyridinium ion-induced neurotoxicity in PC12 cells." *Eur. J. Pharmacol.* 2002; 451(2): 119–124.

2. Bermejo, P., et al. "Antiviral activity of seven iridoids, three saikosaponins and one phenylpropanoid glycoside extracted from *Bupleurum rigidum* and *Scrophularia scorodonia.*" *Planta Med.* 2002; 68(2): 106–110.

3. Didry, N., et al. "Isolation and antibacterial activity of phenylpropanoid derivatives from *Ballota nigra.*" *J. Ethnopharmacol.* 1999; 67(2): 197–202.

4. Xiong, Q., et al. "Acteoside inhibits apoptosis in D-galactosamine and lipopolysaccharide-induced liver injury." *Life Sci.* 1999; 65(4): 421–430.

5. Xiong, Q., et al. "Hepatoprotective activity of phenylethanoids from *Cistanche deserticola.*" *Planta Med.* 1998; 64(2): 120–125.

6. Pennacchio, M., et al. "Mechanism of action of verbascoside on the isolated rat heart: increases in level of prostacyclin." *Phytother. Res.* 1999; 13(3): 254–255.

7. Li, J., et al. "Differentiation of human gastric adenocarcinoma cell line MGc80-3 induced by verbascoside." *Planta Med.* 1997; 63(6): 499–502.

8. Zhou, J., et al. "Ventricular remodeling by Scutellarein treatment in spontaneously hypertensive rats." *Chin Med. J.* (Engl.) 2002; 115(3): 375–377.

9. Gil, B., et al. "Effects of flavonoids on Naja Naja and human recombinant synovial phospholipases A2 and inflammatory responses in mice." *Life Sci.* 1994; 54(20): PL333–338.

10. Spedding, G., et al. "Inhibition of reverse transcriptases by flavonoids." *Antiviral Res.* 1989; 12(2): 99–110.

11. Hazekamp, A., et al. "Isolation of a bronchodilator flavonoid from the Thai medicinal plant *Clerodendrum petasites.*" *J. Ethnopharmacol.* 2001; 78(1): 45–49.

12. Ferrandiz, M. L., et al. "Hispidulin protection against hepatotoxicity induced by bromobenzene in mice." *Life Sci.* 1994; 55(8): PL145–150.

13. Bourdillat, B., et al. "Hispidulin, a natural flavone, inhibits human platelet aggregation by increasing cAMP levels." *Eur. J. Pharmacol.* 1988; 147(1): 1–6.

14. Feng, P. C., et al. "Pharmacological screening of some West Indian medicinal plants." *J. Pharm. Pharmacol.* 1962; 14: 556–561.

15. Robinson, R. D., et al. "Investigations of *Strongyloides stercoralis* filariform larvae *in vitro* by six commercial Jamaican plant extracts and three anthelmintics." *West Indian Med. J.* 1990; 39(4): 213–217.

16. Evans, D. A., et al. "Extracts of Indian plants as mosquito larvicides." *Indian J. Med. Res.* 1988; 88(1): 38–41.

17. Schapoval, E. E., et al. "Anti-inflammatory and antinociceptive activities of extracts and isolated compounds from *Stachytarpheta cayennensis.*" *J. Ethnopharmacol.* 1998; 60(1): 53–59.

18. Almeida, C. E., et al. "Analysis of antidiarrhoeic effect of plants used in popular medicine." *Rev. Saude. Publica.* 1995; 29(6): 428–433.

19. Vela, S. M., et al. "Inhibition of gastric acid secretion by the aqueous extract and purified extracts of *Stachytarpheta cayennensis.*" *Planta Med.* 1997; 63(1): 36–39.

20. Melita, Rodriguez S., et al. "Pharmacological and chemical evaluation of *Stachytarpheta jamaicensis* (Verbenaceae)." *Rev. Biol. Trop.* 1996; 44(2A): 353–359.

Graviola

1. Zeng, L., et al. "Five new monotetrahydrofuran ring acetogenins from the leaves of *Annona muricata.*" *J. Nat. Prod.* 1996; 59(11): 1035–1042.

2. Rieser, M. J., et al. "Five novel monotetrahydrofuran ring acetogenins from the seeds of *Annona muricata.*" *J. Nat. Prod.* 1996; 59(2): 100–108.

3. Wu, F. E., et al. "Additional bioactive acetogenins, annomutacin and (2,4-trans and cis)-10R-annonacin-A-ones, from the leaves of *Annona muricata.*" *J. Nat. Prod.* 1995; 58(9): 1430–1437.

4. Wu, F. E., et al. "New bioactive monotetrahydrofuran Annonaceous acetogenins, annomuricin C and muricatocin C, from the leaves of *Annona muricata.*" *J. Nat. Prod.* 1995; 58(6): 909–915.

5. Wu, F. E., et al. "Muricatocins A and B, two new bioactive monotetrahydrofuran

Annonaceous acetogenins from the leaves of *Annona muricata*." *J. Nat. Prod.* 1995; 58(6): 902–908.

6. Wu, F. E., et al. "Two new cytotoxic monotetrahydrofuran Annonaceous acetogenins, annomuricins A and B, from the leaves of *Annona muricata*." *J. Nat. Prod.* 1995; 58(6): 830–836.

7. Rieser, M. J., et al. "Bioactive single-ring acetogenins from seed extracts of *Annona muricata*." *Planta Med.* 1993; 59(1): 91–92.

8. Rieser, M. J., et al. "Muricatacin: a simple biologically active acetogenin derivative from the seeds of *Annona muricata* (Annonaceae)" *Tetrahedron Lett.* 1991; 32(9): 1137–1140.

9. Kim, G. S., et al. "Muricoreacin and murihexocin C, mono-tetrahydrofuran acetogenins, from the leaves of *Annona muricata*." *Phytochemistry* 1998; 49(2): 565–571.

10. Padma, P., et al. "Effect of the extract of *Annona muricata* and *Petunia nyctaginiflora* on *Herpes simplex* virus." *J. Ethnopharmacol.* 1998; 61(1): 81–83.

11. Gleye, C., et al. "Cis-monotetrahydrofuran acetogenins from the roots of *Annona muricata* 1. *J. Nat. Prod.* 1998; 61(5): 576–579.

12. Kim, G. S., et al. "Two new monotetrahydrofuran ring acetogenins, annomuricin E and muricapentocin, from the leaves of *Annona muricata*." *J. Nat. Prod.* 1998; 61(4): 432–436.

13. Keinan, E., et al. "Antibody-catalyzed organic and organometallic transformations and chemical libraries of Annonaceous acetogenins." *The Skaggs Institute for Chemical Biology Scientific Report* 1997–1998.

14. Anon., *Purdue News* September 1997; Purdue University, West Lafayette, IN. http://www.purdue.edu/UNS/newsandphotos.html

15. Feras, Q., et al. "Annonaceous acetogenins: Recent progress." *J. Nat. Prod.* 1999; 62(3): 504–540.

16. Anon. Unpublished data, National Cancer Institute. Nat Cancer Inst Central Files (1976). From NAPRALERT Files, University of Illinois, 1995.

17. Liaw, C. C., et al. "New cytotoxic monotetrahydrofuran Annonaceous acetogenins from *Annona muricata*." *J. Nat. Prod.* 2002; 65(4): 470–75.

18. Chang, F. R., et al. "Novel cytotoxic annonaceous acetogenins from *Annona muricata*." *J. Nat. Prod.* 2001; 64(7): 925–931.

19. Betancur-Galvis, L., et al. "Antitumor and antiviral activity of Colombian medicinal plant extracts." *Mem. Inst. Oswaldo Cruz* 1999; 94(4): 531–535.

20. Chang, F. R., et al. "New Adjacent Bis-Tetrahydrofuran Annonaceous Acetogenins from *Annona muricata*." *Planta Med.* 2003; 69(3): 241–246.

21. Jaramillo, M. C., et al. "Cytotoxicity and antileishmanial activity of *Annona muricata* pericarp." *Fitoterapia* 2000; 71(2): 183–186.

22. Nicolas, H., et al. "Structure-activity relationships of diverse Annonaceous acetogenins against multidrug resistant human mammary adenocarcinoma (MCF-7/Adr) cells." *J. Med. Chem.* 1997; 40(13): 2102–2106.

23. Yuan, S. S., et al. "Annonacin, a monotetrahydrofuran acetogenin, arrests cancer cells at the G1 phase and causes cytotoxicity in a Bax- and caspase-3-related pathway." *Life Sci.* 2003 May 9; 72(25): 2853–2861.

24. Wang, L. Q., et al. "Annonaceous acetogenins from the leaves of *Annona montana*." *Bioorg. Med. Chem.* 2002; 10(3): 561–565.

25. Feng, P. C., et al. "Pharmacological screening of some West Indian medicinal plants." *J. Pharm. Pharmacol.* 1962; 14: 556–561.

26. Meyer, T. M. "The alkaloids of *Annona muricata*." *Ing. Ned. Indie.* 1941; 8(6): 64.

27. Carbajal, D., et al. "Pharmacological screening of plant decoctions commonly used in Cuban folk medicine." *J. Ethnopharmacol.* 1991; 33(1/2): 21–24.

28. Misas, C. A. J., et al. "Contribution to the biological evaluation of Cuban plants. IV." *Rev. Cubana Med. Trop.* 1979; 31(1): 29–35.

29. Sundarrao, K., et al. "Preliminary screening of antibacterial and antitumor activities of Papua New Guinean native medicinal plants." *Int. J. Pharmacog.* 1993; 31(1): 3–6.

30. Heinrich, M., et al. "Parasitological and microbiological evaluation of Mixe Indian medicinal plants (Mexico)." *J. Ethnopharmacol.* 1992; 36(1): 81–85.

31. Lopez, Abraham A. M. "Plant extracts with cytostatic properties growing in Cuba. I." *Rev. Cubana Med. Trop.* 1979; 31(2): 97–104.

32. Bories, C., et al. "Antiparasitic activity of *Annona muricata* and *Annona cherimolia* seeds." *Planta Med.* 1991; 57(5): 434–436.

33. Antoun, M. D., et al. "Screening of the flora of Puerto Rico for potential antimalarial bioactives." *Int. J. Pharmacog.* 1993; 31(4): 255–258.

34. Gbeassor, M., et al. "*In vitro* antimalarial activity of six medicinal plants." *Phytother. Res.* 1990; 4(3): 115–117.

35. Tattersfield, F., et al. "The insecticidal properties of certain species of *Annona* and an Indian strain of *Mundulea sericea* (Supli)." *Ann. Appl. Biol.* 1940; 27: 262–273.

36. Hasrat, J. A., et al. "Isoquinoline derivatives isolated from the fruit of *Annona muricata* as 5-HTergic 5-HT1A receptor agonists in rats: unexploited antidepressive (lead) products." *J. Pharm. Pharmacol.* 1997; 49(11): 1145–1149.

37. Lannuzel, A., et al. "Toxicity of Annonaceae for dopaminergic neurons: potential role in atypical parkinsonism in Guadeloupe." *Mov. Disord.* 2002; 1: 84–90.

38. Caparros-Lefebvre, D., et al. "Possible relation of atypical parkinsonism in the French West Indies with consumption of tropical plants: a case-control study. Caribbean Parkinsonism Study Group." *Lancet.* 1999 Jul 24; 354(9175): 281–286.

39. Padma, P., et al. "Effect of *Annona muricata* and *Polyalthia cerasoides* on brain neurotransmitters and enzyme monoamine oxidase following cold immobilization stress." *J. Natural Remedies* 2001; 1(2): 144–146.

40. N'gouemo, P., et al. "Effects of ethanol extract of *Annona muricata* on pentylenetetrazol-induced convulsive seizures in mice." *Phytother. Res.* 1997; 11(3): 243–245.

Guacatonga

1. Borges, M., et al. "Neutralization of proteases from Bothrops snake venoms by the aqueous extract from *Casearia sylvestris* (*Flacourtiaceae*)." *Toxicon* 2001; 39(12): 1863–1869.

2. Borges, M., et al. "Effects of aqueous extract of *Casearia sylvestris* (*Flacourtiaceae*) on actions of snake and bee venoms and on activity of phospholipases A(2)." *Comp. Biochem. Physiol. B.* 2000 Sep 1; 127(1): 21–30.

3. Borges, M., et al. "Partial purification of *Casearia sylvestris* Sa. extract and its anti-PLA2 Action." *Comp. Biochem. Physiol. Ser. B.* 2000; 127b(1): 21–30.

4. Itokawa, H., et al. "Antitumor principles from *Casearia sylvestris* Sw. (*Flacourtiaceae*), structure elucidation of new clerodane diterpenes by 2-D NMR spectroscopy." *Chem. Pharm. Bull.* (Tokyo) 1988 March; 36(4): 1585–1588.

5. Itokawa, H., et al. "Isolation of diterpenes as antitumor agents from plants." Patent—Japan *Kokai Tokyo Koho–01* 1989; 149, 779: 6pp.

6. Itokawa, H., et al. "New antitumor principles, casearins A–F, for *Casearia sylvestris* Sw. (*Flacourtiaceae*)" *Chem. Pharm. Bull.* (Tokyo) 1990; 38(12): 3384–3388.

7. Morita, H., et al. "Structures and cytotoxic activity relationship of casearins, new clerodane diterpenes from *Casearia sylvestris* Sw." *Chem. Pharm. Bull.* (Tokyo) 1991 Dec; 39(3): 693–697.

8. Itokawa, H., et al. "Antitumor substances from South American plants." *J. Pharmacobio. Dyn.* 1992; 15(1): S-2.

9. Oberlies, N. H., et al. "Novel bioactive clerodane diterpenoids from the leaves and twigs of *Casearia sylvestris*." *J. Nat. Prod.* 2002; 65(2): 95–99.

10. Beutler, J. A., "Novel cytotoxic diterpenes from Casearia arborea." *J. Nat. Prod.* 2000 63 (5): 657–661.

11. Sai Prakash, C. V., et al. "Structure and stereochemistry of new cytotoxic clerodane diterpenoids from the bark of Casearia lucida from the Madagascar rainforest." *J. Nat. Prod.* 2002 65 (2): 100–107.

12. Basile, A. C., et al. "Pharmacological assay of *Casearia sylvestris*. I: Preventive anti-ulcer activity and toxicity of the leaf crude extract." *J. Ethnopharmacol.* 1990; 30(2):185–197.

13. Sertie, J. A., et al. "Antiulcer activity of the crude extract from the leaves of *Casearia slyvestris*." *Pharmaceutical Biol.* 2000; 38(2): 112–119.

14. Ruppelt, B. M., et al. "Pharmacological screening of plants recommended by folk medicine as antisnake venom—I. Analgesic and anti-inflammatory activities." *Mem. Inst. Oswaldo Cruz* 1991; 86: 203–205.

15. Almeida, A. (Dissertation, 4/02/99) "Antitumor and anti-inflammatory effects of extract from *Casearia sylvestris*: comparative study with Piroxicam and Meloxicam." Instituto de Ciencias Biomedicas, University of São Paulo.

16. Chiappeta, A. D., et al. "Higher plants with biological activity—plants of Pernambuco. I." *Rev. Inst. Antibiot.* 1983; 21 (1/2): 43–50.

17. de Almeida Alves, T. M., "Biological screening of Brazilian medicinal plants." *Mem. Inst. Oswaldo Cruz.* May/Jun. 2000; 95(3): 367–373.

Guaco

1. Cabral, L. M., et al. "Development of a profitable procedure for the extraction of 2-H-1- benzopyran-2-one (coumarin) from *Mikania glomerata*." *Drug. Dev. Ind. Pharm.* 2001; 27 (1): 103–106.

2. Rungeler, P., et al. "Germacranolides from *Mikania guaco*." *Phytochemistry* 2001; 56(5): 475–489.

3. Peluso, G., et al. "Studies on the inhibitory effects of caffeoylquinic acids on monocyte migration and superoxide ion production." *J. Nat. Prod.* 1995; 58(5): 639–646.

4. Davino, S. C., et al. "Antimicrobial activity of kaurenoic acid derivatives substituted on carbon-15." *Braz. J. Med. Biol. Res.* 1989; 22(9): 1127–1129.

5. Coimbra, R., "Guaco: formas farmaceuticas, usos e posologia." *Notas de fitoterapia.* Rio de Janeiro: L.C.S.A., 1942, p. 130.

6. Lima, D. R. A., *Famacologia Clinica de Planta Medicinais*, VIII Simposio de Plantas Medicinais do Brazil. p. 29. 4–6 September, Manaus-AM, 1984

7. Leite, M. G. R., et al. "Actividade bronchodilatora de *Mikania glomerata*, *Justicia pectoralis* e *Torresea cearensis*." *Simposio de Plantas Medicinais do Brazil.* December 1992. Curitiba. Resumos. p. 21

8. Oliveira, F., et al. "Caraterizacao cromatograpfica do extracto fluido de *Mikania glomerata* Sprengel." *Simposio de Plantas Medicinais do Brazil.* December 1992. Curitiba. Resumos. p. 96

9. Oliveira, F., et al. "Isolation and identification of chemical components of *Mikania glomerata* Sprengel and *Mikania laevigata* Schultz Bib ex Baker." *Rev. Rarm. Bioquim.* 1984; 20(2): 169–183.

10. Soares de Moura, R., et al. "Bronchodilator activity of *Mikania glomerata* Sprengel on human bronchi and guinea-pig trachea." *J. Pharm. Pharmacol.* 2002; 54(2): 249–256.

11. Ruppelt, B. M., et al. "Pharmacological screening of plants recommended by folk medicine as anti-snake venom—I. Analgesic and anti-inflammatory activities." *Mem. Inst. Oswaldo Cruz.* 1991; 86 Suppl 2: 203–205.

12. Fierro, I. M., et al. "Studies on the anti-allergic activity of *Mikania glomerata*." *J. Ethnopharmacol.* 1999; 66(1): 19–24.

13. Suyenaga, E. S., et al. "Antiinflammatory investigation of some species of *Mikania*." *Phytother Res.* 2002; 16(6): 519–523.

14. Rojas de Arias A., et al. "Mutagenicity, insecticidal and trypanocidal activity of some Paraguayan Asteraceae." *J. Ethnopharmacol.* 1995; 45(1): 35–41.

15. Muelas-Serrano, S., "In vitro screening of American plant extracts on *Trypanosoma cruzi* and *Trichomonas vaginalis*." *J. Ethnopharmacol.* 2000; 71(1–2): 101–107.

16. Holetz, F. B., "Screening of some plants used in the Brazilian folk medicine for the treatment of infectious diseases." *Mem. Inst. Oswaldo Cruz.* 2002 Oct; 97(7): 1027–31.

17. de Cassia da Silveira e Sa, R., et al. "Evaluation of long-term exposure to Mikania glomerata (Sprengel) extract on male Wistar rats' reproductive organs,

sperm production and testosterone level."
Contraception. 2003; 67(4): 327–331.

Guaraná

1. Henman, A. R. "Guaraná (*Paullinia cupana* var. sorbilis): ecological and social perspectives on an economic plant of the central Amazon basin." *J. Ethnopharmacol.* 1982; 6: 311–338.

2. Latoxan (www.latoxan.com): Ion Channel and Receptor Ligands, Toxins and Alkaloids. "Caffeine."

3. ChemFinder (www.chemfinder.com). "Caffeine."

4. Bertrand, G., et al. "Guaraná paste." *Bull. Soc. Chim.* 1931; 49: 1093–1096.

5. Belliardo, F., et al. "HPLC determination of caffeine and theophylline in *Paullinia cupana* Kunth (guaraná) and Cola spp. samples." *Z. Lebensm. Unters. Forsch.*1985; 180(5): 398–401.

6. Marx, F., et al. "Analysis of guaraná (*Paullinia cupana* var. sorbilis). Part 1. HPLC determination of caffeine, theobromine and theophylline in guaraná seeds." *Dtsch. Lebenstm. Tundsch.* 1985; 81(12): 390–392.

7. Duke, J. A. *Handbook of Phytochemical Constituents of GRAS Herbs and Other Economic Plants.* Boca Raton, FL: CRC Press, 1992.

8. National Toxicology Program. "NTP toxicology and carcinogenesis studies of theophylline (Cas No. 58-55-9) in F344/N rats and B6C3F1 mice (feed and gavage studies)." *Natl. Toxicol. Program Tec. Rep. Ser.* 1998; 478: 1–326.

9. Bruneton, J. *Pharmacognosy, Phytochemistry, Medicinal Plants.* Hampshire, England: Intercept, Ltd., 1995.

10. Kuhrts, E. H. "Methods and compositions for producing weight loss." United States Patent 6,475,530; 2002.

11. Fleischner, A. M. "Weight loss product." United States Patent 6,420,350; 2002.

12. Mattei, R., et al. "Guaraná (*Paullinia cupana*): Toxic behavioral effects in laboratory animals and antioxidant activity in vitro." *J. Ethnopharmacol.* 1998; 60(2): 111–116.

13. Cannon, M. E., et al. "Caffeine-induced cardiac arrhythmia: an unrecognised danger of healthfood products." *Med. J. Aust.* 2001; 174(10): 520–521.

14. Subbiah, M. T. Ravi. "Guaraná seed extract and method of preparation." United States Patent 4,861,594; 1989.

15. Bydlowski, S. P., et al. "A novel property of an aqueous guaraná extract (*Paullinia cupana*): inhibition of platelet aggregation *in vitro* and *in vivo.*" *Braz. J. Med. Biol Res.* 1988; 21(3): 535–538.

16. Bydlowski, S. P., et al. "An aqueous extract of guaraná (*Paullinia cupana*) decreases platelet thromboxane synthesis." *Braz. J. Med. Biol. Res.* 1991; 24(4): 421–424.

17. Espinola, E. B., et al. "Pharmacological activity of guaraná (*Paullinia cupana* Mart.) in laboratory animals." *J. Ethnopharmacol.* 1997; 55(3): 223–229.

18. Galduróz, J. C., et al. "Acute effects of the *Paulinia cupana*, 'guaraná,' on the cognition of normal volunteers." *Rev. Paul. Med.* 1994; 112(3): 607–611.

19. Galduróz, J. C. , et al. "The effects of long-term administration of guaraná on the cognition of normal, elderly volunteers." *Rev. Paul. Med.* 1996; 114(1): 1073–1078.

20. Benoni, H., et al. "Studies on the essential oil from guaraná ." *Z. Lebensm. Unters. Forsch.* 1996; 203(1): 95–98.

21. Weber, R. B., et al. "Compositions, kits and methods for providing and maintaining energy and mental alertness." United States Patent 6,413,558; 2002.

22. Barreca, J. "Center-filled supplement gum." United States Patent 6,491,540; 2002.

23. Andersen, T., et al. "Weight loss and delayed gastric emptying following a South American herbal preparation in overweight patients." *J. Hum. Nutr. Diet.* 2001; 14(3): 243–250.

24. Vaz, Z. R., et al. "Analgesic effect of the herbal medicine Catuama in thermal and chemical models of nociception in mice." *Phytother. Res.* 1997; 11(2): 101–106.

25. Kelly, G. J., et al. "Herbal composition to relieve pain." United States Patent 6,312,736; 2001.

26. da Fonseca, C. A., et al. "Genotoxic and mutagenic effects of guaraná (*Paullinia cupana*) in prokaryotic organisms." *Mutat. Res.* 1994; 321(3): 165–173.

27. Miura, T., et al. "Effect of guaraná on exercise in normal and epinephrine-induced glycogenolytic mice." *Biol. Pharm. Bull.* 1998; 21(6): 646–648.

28. Carlson, M., et al. "Liquid chromatographic determination of methylxanthines and catechins in herbal preparations containing guaraná." *J. AOAC Int.* 1998; 81(4): 691–701.

Guava

1. Conde Garcia, E. A., et al. "Inotropic effects of extracts of *Psidium guajava* L. (guava) leaves on the guinea pig atrium." *Braz. J. of Med. & Biol. Res.* 2003; 36: 661–668.

2. Suntornsuk, L., et al. "Quantitation of vitamin C content in herbal juice using direct titration." *J. Pharm. Biomed. Anal.* 2002; 28(5): 849–855.

3. Beckstrom-Sternberg, S. M., et al. "The phytochemical database." (ACEDB version 4.3-Data version July 1994.) National Germplasm Resources Laboratory (NGRL), Agricultural Research Service (ARS), U.S. Department of Agriculture.

4. Jimenez-Escrig, A., et al. "Guava fruit (*Psidium guajava* L.) as a new source of antioxidant dietary fiber." *J. Agric. Food Chem.* 2001; 49(11): 5489–5493.

5. Smith, Nigel J. H., et al. *Tropical Forests and their Crops.* London: Cornell University Press. 1992.

6. Arima, H., et al. "Isolation of antimicrobial compounds from guava (*Psidium guajava* L.) and their structural elucidation." *Biosci. Biotechnol. Biochem.* 2002; 66(8): 1727–1730.

7. Morales, M. A., et al. "Calcium-antagonist effect of quercetin and its relation with the spasmolytic properties of *Psidium guajava* L." *Arch. Med. Res.* 1994; 25(1): 17–21.

8. Lozoya, X., et al. "Quercetin glycosides in *Psidium guajava* L. leaves and determination of a spasmolytic principle." *Arch. Med. Res.* 1994; 25(1): 11–15.

9. Begum, S., et al. "Triterpenoids from the leaves of *Psidium guajava.*" *Phytochemistry* 2002; 61(4): 399–403.

10. Lozoya, X., et al. "Intestinal anti-spas-

modic effect of a phytodrug of *Psidium guajava* folia in the treatment of acute diarrheic disease." *J. Ethnopharmacol.* 2002; 83(1-2): 19–24.

11. Wei, L., et al. "Clinical study on treatment of infantile rotaviral enteritis with *Psidium guajava L." Zhongguo Zhong Xi Yi Jie He Za Zhi* 2000; 20(12): 893–895.

12. Tona, L., et al. "Biological screening of traditional preparations from some medicinal plants used as antidiarrhoeal in Kinshasa, Congo." *Phytomedicine* 1999; 6(1): 59–66.

13. Lozoya, X., et al. "Model of intraluminal perfusion of the guinea pig ileum in vitro in the study of the antidiarrheal properties of the guava (*Psidium guajava*)." *Arch. Invest. Med.* (Mex). 1990; 21(2): 155–162.

14. Almeida, C. E., et al. "Analysis of antidiarrhoeic effect of plants used in popular medicine." *Rev. Saude Publica.* 1995; 29(6): 428–433.

15. Lin, J., et al. "Anti-diarrhoeal evaluation of some medicinal plants used by Zulu traditional healers." *J. Ethnopharmacol.* 2002; 79(1): 53–56.

16. Lutterodt, G. D. "Inhibition of Microlax-induced experimental diarrhea with narcotic-like extracts of *Psidium guajava* leaf in rats." *J. Ethnopharmacol.* 1992; 37(2): 151–157.

17. Lutterodt, G. D. "Inhibition of gastrointestinal release of acetylcholine by quercetin as a possible mode of action of *Psidium guajava* leaf extracts in the treatment of acute diarrhoeal disease." *J. Ethnopharmcol.* 1989; 25(3): 235–247.

18. Coutino-Rodriguez, R., et al, "Lectins in fruits having gastrointestinal activity: their participation in the hemagglutinating property of *Escherichia coli* O157:H7." *Arch. Med. Res.* 2001; 32(4): 251–257.

19. Abdelrahim, S. I., et al. "Antimicrobial activity of *Psidium guajava L." Fitoterapia* 2002; 73(7-8): 713–715.

20. Holetz, F. B., et al. "Screening of some plants used in the Brazilian folk medicine for the treatment of infectious diseases." *Mem. Inst. Oswaldo Cruz* 2002; 97(7): 1027–1031.

21. Caceres, A., et al. "Plants used in Guatemala for the treatment of gastrointestinal disorders. 1. Screening of 84 plants against enterobacteria." *J. Ethnopharmacol.* 1990; 30(1): 55–73.

22. Garcia, S., et al, "Inhibition of growth, enterotoxin production, and spore formation of *Clostridium perfringens* by extracts of medicinal plants." *J. Food Prot.* 2002; 65(10): 1667–1669.

23. Tona, L., et al. "Antiamoebic and spasmolytic activities of extracts from some antidiarrhoeal traditional preparations used in Kinshasa, Congo." *Phytomedicine* 2000; 7(1): 31–38.

24. Tona, L., et al. "Antiamoebic and phytochemical screening of some Congolese medicinal plants." *J. Ethnopharmacol.* 1998; 61(1): 57–65.

25. Nundkumar, N., et al. "Studies on the antiplasmodial properties of some South African medicinal plants used as antimalarial remedies in Zulu folk medicine." *Methods Find Exp. Clin. Pharmacol.* 2002; 24(7): 397–401.

26. Yamashiro, S., et al. "Cardioprotective effects of extracts from *Psidium guajava L.* and *Limonium wrigth* II, Okinawan medicinal plants, against ischemia-reperfusion injury in perfused rat hearts." *Pharmacology* 2003; 67(3): 128–135.

27. Singh, R. B., et al. "Can guava fruit intake decrease blood pressure and blood lipids?" *J. Hum Hypertens.* 1993; 7(1): 33–38.

28. Singh, R. B., et al. "Effects of guava intake on serum total and high-density lipoprotein cholesterol levels and on systemic blood pressure." *Am. J. Cardiol.* 1992; 70(15): 1287–1291.

29. Shaheen, H. M., et al. "Effect of *Psidium guajava* leaves on some aspects of the central nervous system in mice." *Phytother. Res.* 2000; 14(2): 107–111.

30. Lutterodt, G. D., et al. "Effects on mice locomotor activity of a narcotic-like principle from *Psidium guajava* leaves." *J. Ethnopharmacol.* 1988; 24(2-3): 219–231.

31. Jaiarj, P., et al. "Anticough and antimicrobial activities of *Psidium guajava* Linn. leaf extract." *J. Ethnopharmacol.* 1999; 67(2): 203–212.

32. Cheng, J. T., et al. "Hypoglycemic effect of guava juice in mice and human subjects." *Am. J. Clin. Med.* 1983; 11(1-4): 74–76.

33. Roman-Ramos, R., et al. "Anti-hyperglycemic effect of some edible plants." *J. Ethnopharmacol.* 1995.

Iporuru

1. Ogungbamila, F. O., et al. "Smooth muscle–relaxing flavonoids from *Alchornea cordifolia." Acta Pharm. Nord.* 1990; 2(6): 421–422.

2. Dunstan, C. A., et al. "Evaluation of some Samoan and Peruvian medicinal plants by prostaglandin biosynthesis and rat ear oedema assays." *J. Ethnopharmacol.* 1997; 57: 35–56.

3. Persinos-Perdue, G., et al. "Evaluation of Peruvian folk medicine by the natural products research laboratories." *Abstra. Joint Meeting American Society of Pharmacognosy and Society for Economic Botany,* Boston, 1981; (5): 13–17.

4. Macrae, W. D., et al. "Studies on the pharmacological activity of Amazonian Euphorbiaceae." *J. Ethnopharmacol.* 1988; 22(2): 143–172.

Jaborandi

1. Ringold, S., et al. "On Jaborandi." *The Lancet* 1875; 30: 157–159.

2. Holmstedt, B., et al. "Jaborandi: An Interdisciplinary Approach." *J. Ethnopharmacology* 1979; 1(1): 3–21.

3. Merck Index. *An encyclopedia of chemicals, drugs and biologicals.* Rahway, New Jersey: Merck & Co., 1983.

4. Distelhorst, J. S., et al. "Open-angle glaucoma." *Am. Fam. Physician* 2003; 67(9): 1937–1944.

5. Kaneyuki, H., et al. "Enhanced miotic response to topical dilute pilocarpine in patients with Alzheimer's disease." *Neurology* 1998; 50(3): 802–804.

6. Hawthorne, M., et al. "Pilocarpine for radiation-induced xerostomia in head and neck cancer." *Int. J. Palliat. Nurs.* 2000; 6(5): 228–232.

7. "Oral pilocarpine: new preparation. Xerostomia after radiation therapy: moder-

ately effective but costly." *Prescribe. Int.* 2002; 11(60): 99–101.

8. LeVeque, F. G., et al. "A multicenter, randomized, double-blind, placebo-controlled, dose-titration study of oral pilocarpine for treatment of radiation-induced xerostomia in head and neck cancer patients." *J. Clin. Oncology* 1993; 11(6): 1124–1131.

9. *PDR for Herbal Medicines.* 2nd Edition. Montvale, New Jersey: Medical Economics Company.

10. Pinheiro, C. U. B. "Jaborandi (*Pilocarpus sp., Rutaceae*): A wild species and its rapid transformation into a crop." *Econ. Bot.* 1997; 51(1): 49–58.

Jatobá

1. Damar, A. N., et al. "Contact allergy to manilla resin. Nomenclauture and physico-chemistry of *Manilla kauri.*" *Contact Dermatitis* 1989; 21(4): 228–238.

2. Muroi, H., et al. "Combination effects of antibacterial compounds in green tea flavor against *Streptococcus mutans.*" *J. Agric. Food Chem.* 1993; 41: 1102–1105.

3. Denyer, C. V., et al. "Isolation of antirhinoviral sesquiterpenes from ginger (*Zingiber officinale*)." *J. Nat. Prod.* 1994; 57(5): 658–662.

4. Tincusi, B. M., et al. "Antimicrobial terpenoids from the oleoresin of the peruvian medicinal plant *Copaifera paupera.*" *Planta Med.* 2002; 68(9): 808–812.

5. Abdel-Kader, M., et al. "Isolation and absolute configuration of ent-halimane diterpenoids from *Hymenaea courbaril* from the Suriname rain forest." *J. Nat. Prod.* 2002; 65(1): 11–15.

6. Yang, D., et al. "Use of caryophyllene oxide as an antifungal agent in an *in vitro* experimental model of onychomycosis." *Mycopathologia* 1999; 148(2): 79–82.

7. Lopez, J. A. "Isolation of astilbin and sitosterol from *Hymenaea courbaril.*" *Phytochemistry* 1976; 15: 2027F.

8. Closa, D., et al. "Prostanoids and free radicals in CCl4-induced hepatotoxicity in rats: effect of astilbin." *Prostaglandins Leukot. Essent. Fatty Acids.* 1997; 56(4): 331–334.

9. Arrhenius, S.P., et al. *Phytochemistry* 1983; 22: 471.

10. Arrhenius, S.P., et al. "Inhibitory effects of *Hymenaea* and *Copaifera* leaf resins on the leaf fungus, *Pestalotia subcuticulari.*" *Biochem. Syst. Ecol.* 1983; 11(4): 361–366.

11. Marsaioli, A. J., et al. "Diterpenes in the bark of *Hymenaea courbaril.*" *Phytochemistry* 1975; 14: 1882–1883.

12. Giral, F., et al. "Ethnopharmacognostic observation on Panamanian medicinal plants. Part 1." *Q. J. Crude Drug Res.* 1979; 167(3/4): 115–130.

13. Pinheiro de Sousa, M., et al. "Molluscicidal activity of plants from Northeast Brazil." *Rev. Bras. Pesq. Med. Biol.* 1974; 7(4): 389–394.

14. Rahalison, L., et al. "Screening for antifungal activity of Panamanian plants." *Inst. J. Pharmacog.* 1993; 31(1): 68–76.

15. Hostettmann, K., et al. "Phytochemistry of plants used in traditional medicine." *Proceedings of the Phytochemical Society of Europe.* Clarendon Press, Oxford. 1995.

16. Rouquayrol, M. Z., et al. "Molluscicidal activity of essential oils from Northeastern Brazilian plants." *Rev. Brasil Pesq. Med. Biol.* 1980; 13: 135–143.

17. Verpoorte, R., et al. "Medicinal plants of Surinam. IV. Antimicrobial activity of some medicinal plants." *J. Ethnopharmacol.* 1987; 21(3): 315–318.

18. Caceres, A., et al. "Plants used in Guatemala for the treatment of dermatomucosal infections. 1: Screening of 38 plant extracts." *J. Ethnopharmacol.* 1991; 33(3): 277–283.

19. Gupta, M. P. "Plants and Traditional Medicine in Panama." Vol 4., *Economic and Medicinal Plant Research.* Academic Press Ltd., London. 1990.

Jergón Sacha

There are no studies published on this plant.

Juazeiro

1. Schühly, W., et al. "New triterpenoids with antibacterial activity from *Zizyphus joazeiro.*" *Planta Med.* 1999; 65(8): 740–743.

2. Schühly, W., et al., Novel triterpene saponins from *Ziziphus joazeiro.*" *Helv. Chim. Acta* 2000; 83: 1509–1516.

3. Pisha, E., et al. "Discovery of betulinic acid as a selective inhibitor of human melanoma that functions by induction of apoptosis." *Nat. Med.* 1995; 1(10): 1046–1051.

4. Kim, D. S., et al. "Synthesis of betulinic acid derivatives with activity against human melanoma." *Bioorg. Med. Chem. Lett.* 1998; 8(13): 1707–1712.

5. Nunes, P. H., et al. "Antipyretic activity of an aqueous extract of *Zizyphus joazeiro* Mart. (Rhamnaceae)." *Braz. J. Med. Biol. Res.* 1987; 20(5): 599–601.

6. Jesus, T. P. *Cienc. Cult.* 1983; 35(7): 82–83.

7. Fabiyi, J. P., et al. "Traditional therapy of dracunculiasis in the state of Bauchi — Nigeria." *Dakar Med.* 1993; 38(2): 193–195.

Jurubeba

1. Ripperger, H. "Structure of paniculonin A and B, two new spirostane glycosides from *Solanum paniculatum* L." *Chem. Ber.* 1968; 101(7): 2450–2458.

2. Ripperger, H. "Isolation of neochlorogenin and painculogenin from *Solanum paniculatum* L." *Chem. Ber.* 1967; 100(5): 1741–1752.

3. Ripperger, H. "Jurubin, a nitrogen containing steroidsaponin of a new structural type from *Solanum paniculatum* L; concerning the structure of paniculidin." *Chem. Ber.* 1967; 100(5): 1725–1740.

4. Meyer, K. F. and M. Bernoulli. *Pharmac. Acta. Helvetiae.* 1961; 36: 80–96.

5. Leekning, M. E. and M. A. Rocca. *Rev. Fac. Farm. Adont. Araraquara* 1968; 2(2): 299–300.

6. Siqueira, N. S. and A. Macan. *Trib. Farm. Curitiba.* 1976; 44(1–2): 101–104.

7. Braga, F. T., et al. *Jurubeba.* Centro Universitário de Lavras, Lavras-MG Brazil, 2002.

8. Cambiachi, S., et al. *Ann. Chim.* (Rome) 1971; 61(1): 99–111.

9. Coimbra, R. *Manual de Fitoterapia,* 2nd ed. São Paulo, Brazil: Dados Internacionais de Catalogacao na Pulicacao, 1994.

10. Mesia-Vela, S., et al. "*Solanum panicula-*

tum L. (Jurubeba): Potent inhibitor of gastric acid secretion in mice." *Phytomedicine* 2002; 9(6): 508–514.

11. Barros, G. S. G., et al. "Pharmacological screening of some Brazlian northeasern plants." *Rev. Bras. Farm.* 1970; 48: 195–204.

12. Barros, G. S. G., et al. "Phamacological screening of some Brazilian plants." *J. Pharm. Pharmac.* 1969; 22: 116–122.

13. Nishie, K., et al. "Positive inotropic action of Solanaceae glycoalkaloids." *Res. Commun. Chem. Pathol. Pharmacol.* 1976; 15(3): 601–607.

Kalanchoe

1. Supratman, U., et al. "Anti-tumor promoting activity of bufadienolides from *Kalanchoe pinnata* and *K. daigremontiana* x tubiflora." *Biosci. Biotechnol. Biochem.* 2001; 65(4): 947–949.

2. Supratman, U., et al. "New insecticidal bufadienolide, bryophyllin C, from *Kalanchoe pinnata.*" *Biosci. Biotechnol. Biochem.* 2000; 64(6): 1310–1312.

3. Yamagishi, T., et al. "Antitumor agents, 110. Bryophyllin B, a novel potent cytotoxic bufadienolide from *Bryophyllum pinnatum.*" *J. Nat. Prod.* 1989 Sep–Oct; 52(5): 1071–1079.

4. Yamagishi, T., et al. "Structure and stereochemistry of bryophyllin-A, a novel potent cytotoxic bufadienolide orthoacetate from *Bryophyllum pinnatum.*" *Chem. Pharm. Bull.* (Tokyo). 1988; 36(4): 1615–1617.

5. Shirobokov, V. P., et al. "Antiviral activity of representatives of the family Crassulaceae." *Antibiotiki* 1981; 26(12): 897–900.

6. Rai, M. K., et al. "Screening of medicinal plants of Chindwara district against *Trichophyton mentagrophytes*: a causal organism of *Tinea pedis.*" Hindustan Antibiot. Bull. 1988; 30(1/2): 33–36.

7. Ogungbamila, F. O., et al. "A new acylated flavan-3-ol from *Bryophyllum pinnatum.*" *Nat. Prod. Lett.* 1997; 10(3): 201–203.

8. Akinpelu, D. A. "Antimicrobial activity of *Bryophyllum pinnatum* leaves." *Fitoterapia* 2000; 71(2): 193–194.

9. Obaseiki-Ebor, E. E. "Preliminary report on the in vitro antibacterial activity of *Bryophyllum pinnatum* leaf juice." *Afr. J. Med. Med. Sci.* 1985; 14(3–4): 199–202.

10. Rossi-Bergmann, B., et al. "Treatment of cutaneous Leishmaniasis with *Kalanchoe pinnata*: experimental and clinical data." *Phytomedicine Suppl.* 2000; 7(2): SL115.

11. Da-Silva, S. A. G., et al. "The anti-leishmanial effect of Kalanchoe is mediated by nitric oxide intermediates." *Parasitology* 1999; 118(6): 575–582.

12. Nassis, C. Z., et al. "Antihistamine activity of *Bryophyllum calycinum.*" *Braz. J. Med. Biol. Res.* 1992; 25(9): 929–936.

13. Pal, S., et al. "Studies on the anti-ulcer activity of a *Bryophyllum pinnatum* leaf extract in experimental animals." *J. Ethnopharmacol.* 1991; 33(1 / 2): 97–102.

14. Olajide, O. A., et al. "Analgesic, anti-inflammatory and antipyretic effects of *Bryophyllum pinnatum.*" *Fitoterapia* 1998; 69(3): 249–252.

15. Siddharta, P., et al. "Further studies on the anti-inflammatory profile of the methanolic fraction of the fresh leaf extract of *Bryophyllum pinnatum.*" *Fitoterapia* 1992; 63(5): 451–459.

16. Pal, S., et al. "Neuropsychopharmacological profile of the methanolic fraction of *Bryophyllum pinnatum* leaf extract." *J. Pharm. Pharmacol.* 1999; 51(3): 313–318.

17. Mourao, R. H., et al. "Anti-inflammatory activity and acute toxicity (LD50) of the juice of *Kalanchoe brasiliensis* (comb.) leaves picked before and during blooming." *Phytother. Res.* 1999; 13(4): 352–354.

18. Siddhartha, P., et al. "Anti-inflammatory action of *Bryophyllum pinnatum* leaf extract." *Fitoterapia* 1990; 61(6): 527–533.

19. Rossi-Bergmann, B., et al. "Immunosuppressive effect of the aqueous extract of *Kalanchoe pinnata* in mice." *Phytother. Res.* 1994; 8(7): 399–402.

20. Gaind, K. N., et al. "Flavonoid glycosides from *Kalanchoe pinnata.*" *Planta Med.* 1971; 20(4): 368–373.

21. Moraes, V. L. G., et al. "Inhibition of lymphocyte activation by extracts and fractions of *Kalanchoe, Alternathera, Paullinia* and *Mikania* species." *Phytomedicine* 1994; 1(3): 199–204.

22. Pal, S., et al. "Neuropsychopharmacological profile of the methanolic fraction of *Bryophyllum pinnatum* leaf extract." *J. Pharm. Pharmacol.* 1999; 51(3): 313–318.

23. Reppas, G. P. "*Bryophyllum pinnatum* poisoning of cattle." *Aust. Vet. J.* 1995; 72(11): 425–427.

24. McKenzie, R. A., et al. "The toxicity to cattle and bufadienolide content of six *Bryophyllum* species." *Aust. Vet. J.* 1987; 64(10): 298–301.

Maca

1. Quiros, C., et al. "Physiological studies and determination of chromosome number in maca, *Lepidium meyenii.*" *Econ. Bot.* 1996; 50(2): 216–223.

2. Report of an ad hoc panel of the Advisory Committee on Technical Innovation, Board on Science and Technology for International Development, National Research Council, *Lost Crops of the Incas: Little-Known Plants of the Andes with Promise for Worldwide Cultivation*; 1989.

3. Dini, A., et al. "Chemical composition of *Lepidium meyenii.*" *Food Chem.* 1994; 49: 347–349.

4. Johns, T. "The anu and the maca." *J. Ethnobio.* 1981; 1: 208–212.

5. Li, Genyl and Carlos F. Quiros. "Glucosinolate contents in Maca (*Lepidium peruvianum* Chacón) seeds, sprouts, mature plants and several derived commercial products." *Econ. Bot.* 2001; 55(22): 255–262.

6. Chacón, R. C. "Estudio fitoquimico de *Lepidium meyenii.*" Dissertation, Univ., Nac. Mayo de San Marcos, Peru, 1986.

7. Zheng, B. L., et al. "Effect of a lipidic extract from *Lepidium meyenii* on sexual behavior in mice and rats." *Urology* 2000; 55(4): 598–602.

8. Cicero, A. F., et al. "*Lepidium meyenii* Walp. improves sexual behaviour in male rats independently from its action on spontaneous locomotor activity." *J. Ethnopharmacol.* 2001; 75(2–3): 225–229.

9. Gonzales, G. F., et al. "Effect of *Lepidium meyenii* (maca) roots on spermatogenesis of male rats." *Asian J. Androl.* 2001; 3(3): 231–233.

10. Gonzales, G. F., et al. "*Lepidium meyenii* (maca) improved semen parameters in

adult men." *Asian J. Androl.* 2001; 3(4): 301–303.

11. Cicero, A. F., et al. "Hexanic maca extract improves rat sexual performance more effectively than methanolic and chloroformic maca extracts." *Andrologia* 2002; 34(3): 177–179.

12. Gonzales, G. F., et al. "Effect of *Lepidium meyenii* (maca) on sexual desire and its absent relationship with serum testosterone levels in adult healthy men." *Andrologia* 2002; 34(6): 367–372.

13. Scibona, M., et al. "L-arginine and male infertility." *Minerva Urol. Nefrol.* 1994; 46(4): 251–253.

14. Cara, A. M., et al. "The role of histamine in human penile erection." *Br. J. Urol.* 1995; 75(2): 220–224.

15. Gonzales, G. F., et al. "Effect of *Lepidium meyenii* (maca), a root with aphrodisiac and fertility-enhancing properties, on serum reproductive hormone levels in adult healthy men." *J. Endocrinol.* 2003; 176(1): 163–168.

16. *ETC group briefing Peruvian farmers and indigenous people denounce maca patents.* Contact details: In UK: Hannah Crabtree, ActionAid, tel: + 44 (0)20 7561 7627 or +44 (0)77539 73486. In the U.S.: Hope Shand, ETC group (Action Group on Erosion, Technology and Concentration, formerly RAFI), tel: (919) 960-5223.

Macela

1. Hirschmann, G. S. "The constituents of *Achyrocline satureoides* D.C." *Rev. Latinoamer. Quim.* 1984; 15(3): 134–135.

2. Mesquita, A., et al. "Flavonoids from four Compositae species." *Phytochemistry* 1986; 25(5): 1255–1256.

3. Simoes, C. M., et al. 1988. "Pharmacological investigations on *Achyrocline satureoides* (Lam). D.C., Compositae." *J. Ethnopharmacol.* 1988; 22(3): 281–293.

4. Simoes, C. M., 1988. "Anti-inflammatory action of *Achyrocline satureoides* extracts applied topically." *Fitoterapia* 1988; 59(5): 419–421.

5. Vargas, V., et al. "Genotoxicity of plant extracts." *Mem. Inst. Oswaldo Cruz* 1991; 86(11): 67–70.

6. de Souza, C. P., et al. "Chemoprophylaxis of schistosomiasis: molluscicidal activity of natural products." *An. Acad. Brasil. Cienc.* 1984; 56(3): 333–338.

7. Vargas, V. M. F., et al. "Mutagenic and genotoxic effects of aqueous extracts of *Achyrocline satureoides* in prokaryotic organisms." *Mutat. Res.* 1990; 240(1): 13–18.

8. Anesini, C., et al. "Screening of plants used in Argentine folk medicine for antimicrobial activity." *J. Ethnopharmacol.* 1993; 39(2): 119–128.

9. Desmarchelier, C., et al. "Antioxidant and free radical scavenging effects in extracts of the medicinal herb *Achyrocline satureioides* (Lam.) D.C. (marcela)." *Braz. J. Med. Biol. Res.* 1998; 31(9): 163–170.

10. Desmarchelier, C., et al. "Antioxidant and prooxidant activities in aqueous extracts of Argentine Plants." *Int. J. Pharmacog.* 1997; 35(2): 116–120.

11. Kadarian, C., et al. "Hepatoprotective activity of *Achyrocline satureioides* (Lam.) D.C." *Pharmacol. Res.* 2002; 45(1): 57–61.

12. Gugliucci, A., et al. "Three different pathways for human LDL oxidation are inhibited *in vitro* by water extracts of the medicinal herb *Achyrocline satureoides*." *Life Sci.* 2002; 71(6): 693–705.

13. Carney, J. R., et al. "Achyrofuran, a new antihyperglycemic dibenzofuran from the South American medicinal plant *Achyrocline satureioides*." *J. Nat. Prod.* 2002; 65(2): 203–205.

14. Gonzalez, A., et al. "Biological screening of Uruguayan medicinal plants." *J. Ethnopharmacol.* 1993; 39(3): 217–220.

15. Rojas De Arias, A., et al. "Mutagenicity, insecticidal and trypanocidal activity of some Paraguayan Asteraceae." *J. Ethnopharmacol.* 1995; 45(1): 35–41.

16. Santos, A. L. G., et al. "Immunomodulatory effect of *Achyrocline satureioides* (Lam.) D.C. aqueous extracts." *Phytother. Res.* 1999; 13(1):65–66.

17. Arisawa, M. "Cell growth inhibition of KB cells by plant extracts." *Nat. Med.* 1994; 48(4): 338–347.

18. Ruffa, M. J., et al. "Cytotoxic effect of Argentine medicinal plant extracts on human hepatocellular carcinoma cell line." *J. Ethnopharmacol.* 2002; 79(3): 335–339.

19. Wagner, H., et al. "Immunostimulating polysaccharides (heteroglycanes) of higher plants." *Arzneimforsch.* 1985; 35(7): 1069–1075.

20. Wagner, H., et al. "Immunostimulating polysaccharides (heteroglycanes) of higher plants/preliminary communication." *Arzneimforsch.* 1984; 34(6): 659–661.

21. Abdel-Malek, S., et al. "Drug leads from the Kallawaya herbalists of Bolivia. 1. Background, rationale, protocol and anti-HIV activity." *J. Ethnopharmacol.* 1996; 50: 157.

22. Zanon, S. M., et al. "Search for antiviral activity of certain medicinal plants from Cordoba, Argentina." *Rev. Latinoamer. Microbiol.* 1999; 41(2): 59–62.

Manacá

1. Castioni, P., et al. "Volatile constituents from *Brunfelsia grandiflora* sp.: Qualitative analysis by GM-MS." *Sci. Pharm.* 1996; 64(1): 83–91.

2. de Costa, A. O. "A pharmacologic study of manacá (*Brunfelsia hopeana*)." *Bol. Assoc. Bras. Pharm.* 1933; 14: 295–299.

3. Ichiki, H., et al. "Studies on the constituents of *Brunfelsia hopeana* Benth." *Natural Med.* 1994; 48(4): 314–316.

4. Gellert, E., et al. "The alkaloids of *Brunfelsia hopeana* Benth." *Chem. Nat. Prod.* 1978; 2: 5–8.

5. Duke, J. A. *CRC Handbook of Medicinal Herbs.* Boca Raton, FL: CRC Press, 1985.

6. Oliveira, E. J., et al. "Intracellular calcium mobilization as a target for the spasmolytic action of scopoletin." *Planta Med.* 2001; 67: 605–608.

7. Muschietti, L., et al. "Phenolic compounds with anti-inflammatory activity from *Eupatorium buniifolium*." *Planta Med.* 2001; 67(8): 743–744.

8. Kang, S. Y., et al. "Hepatoprotective activity of scopoletin, a constituent of *Solanum lyratum*." *Arch. Pharm. Res.* 1998; 21(6): 718–722.

9. Liu, X. L., et al. "Effect of scopoletin on PC(3) cell proliferation and apoptosis." *Acta. Pharmacol. Sin.* 2001; 22(10): 929–933.

10. Kayser, O., et al. "Antibacterial activity of extracts and constituents of *Pelargonium*

sidoides and *Pelargonium reniforme." Planta Med.* 1997; 63(6): 508–510.

11. Jain, D. C., et al. "Process for the isolation of compound scopoletin useful as nitric oxide synthesis inhibitor." United States Patent 6,337,095; 2002.

12. Gentiloni, S. N., et al. "Nitric oxide. A general review about the different roles of this innocent radical." *Minerva Med.* 2001; 92(3): 167–171.

13. Chiou, L. C., et al. "Chinese herb constituent beta-eudesmol alleviated the electroshock seizures in mice and electrographic seizures in rat hippocampal slices." *Neurosci. Lett.* 1997; 231(3): 171–174.

14. Ruppelt, B. M., et al. "Pharmacological screening of plants recommended by folk medicine as anti-snake venom–I. Analgesic and anti-inflammatory activities." *Mem. Inst. Oswaldo Cruz* 1991; 86: 203–205.

15. Iyer, R. P., et al. "*Brunfelsia hopeana* I: Hippocratic screening and antiinflammatory evaluation." *Lloydia.* 1977; 40(4): 356–360.

16. Iyer, R. P., et al. "*Brunfelsia hopeana*—Pharmacologic screening: isolation and characterization of hoppeanine." *Diss. Abstr. Int. B.* 1978; 39: 761.

17. Heal, R. E., et al. "A survey of plants for insecticidal activity." *Lloydia* 1950; 13 1: 89–162.

18. Wall, M. E., et al. "Plant antimutagenic agents, 1. General bioassay and isolation procedures." *J. Nat. Prod.* 1988; 51(5): 866–873.

19. Yun, B. S., et al. "Coumarins with monoamine oxidase inhibitory activity and antioxidative coumarino-lignans from *Hibiscus syriacus." J. Nat. Prod.* 2001; 64 9: 1238–1240.

Muira Puama

1. Anselmino, Elisabeth. "Ancestral sources of Muira-puama." *Ach. Pharm.* 1933; 271: 296–314.

2. Brazilian Pharmacopeia. "Muira puama. *Ptychopetalum olacoides.*" Rio de Janeiro, Brazil, 1956.

3. British Herbal Pharmacopoeia. "Muira

puama." West York, England: British Herbal Medicine Association, 1983; 132–133.

4. Youngken, H. W. "Observations on Muira puama." *J. Am. Pharm. Assoc.* 1921; 10: 690–692.

5. Olofsson, Eric. "Action of extract of *Liriosma ovata* on the blood pressure, vessels and respiration of the rabbit." *Compt. Rend. Soc. Biol.* 1927; 97: 1639–1640.

6. Gaebler, H. "Revival of the drug Muira puama." *Deut. Apoth.* 1979; 22(3): 94–96.

7. Dias Da Silva, Rodolpho. "Medicinal plants of Brazil. Botanical and pharmacognostic studies. Muira puama." *Rev. Bras. Med. Pharm.* 1925; 1(1): 37–41.

8. Iwasa, J., et al. "Constituents of Muira puama." *Yakungaka Zasshi* (Japan) 1969; 89(8): 1172–1174.

9. Auterhoff, H., et al. "Components of Muira puama." *Arch. Pharm. Ber. Dtsch. Pharm. Ges.* 1968; 301(7): 481–489.

10. Auterhoff, H., et al. "Components of Muira puama II." *Arch. Pharm. Ber. Dtsch. Pharm. Ges.* 1969; 302(3): 209–212.

11. Auterhoff, H., et al. "Lipophilic constituents of Muira puama." *Arch. Pharm. Ber. Dtsch. Pharm. Ges.* 1971; 304(3): 223–228.

12. Steinmetz, E. "Muira puama." *Quart. J. Crude Drug Res.* 1971; 11(3): 1787–1789.

13. Ninomiya, Ruriko, et al. "Studies of Brazilian crude drugs." *Shoyakugaku Zasshi* (Japan) 1979; 33(2): 57–64.

14. Bucek, E., et al. "Volatile constituents of *Ptychopetalum olacoides* root oil." *Planta Med.* 1989; 53(2): 231.

15. Penna, M. *Notas Sobre Plantas Brasileriras.* Rio de Janeiro: Araujo Penn & Cia., 1930, 258.

16. Waynberg, J. "Contributions to the clinical validation of the traditional use of *Ptychopetalum guyanna.*" Presented at the First International Congress on Ethnopharmacology, Strasbourg, France, June 5–9, 1990.

17. Waynberg, J. "Male sexual asthenia—interest in a traditional plant-derived medication." *Ethnopharmacology*; 1995.

18. Hanawa., et al. "Composition containing an extract from Muira puama root and

plant worm extract." Taisho Pharmacuetical Co., Ltd., Tokyo, United States Patent 6024984; 2000.

19. Paiva, Laf, et al. "Effects of *Ptychocepalum olacoides* extract on mouse behaviour in forced swimming and open field tests." *Phytother. Res.* 1998; 12(4): 294–296.

20. Siqueira, I. R., et al. "Psychopharamcological properties of *Ptychopetalum olachoides* Bentham (Olacaceae)." *Pharmaceutical Biol.* 1998; 36(5): 327–334.

21. Elisabetsky, E., et al. *Propriedades Psicofarmacologicas de Oleaceas,* IX Simposio de Plantas Medicinais do Brazil, Rio de Janeiro, 1–3 September 1986, 32.

22. Asano, T., et al. "Oral compositions containing Muira purama for gastric mucosal lesions." Japan Kokai Tokyo Hoho, Patent 11343244; 1999.

23. Vaz, Z. R., et al. "Analgesic effect of the herbal medicine Catuama in thermal and chemical models of nociception in mice." *Phytother. Res.* 1997; 11(2): 101–106.

24. Cherksey, B. D. "Method of preparing Muira puama extract and its use for decreasing body fat percentage and increasing lean muscle mass." United States Patent 5516516; 1996.

25. Siqueira, I.R., et al. "*Ptychopetalum olacoides,* a traditional Amazonian "nerve tonic", possesses anticholinesterase activity." *Pharmacol. Biochem. Behav.* 2003; Jun; 75 (3): 645–650.

26. Siqueira, I.R., et al. "Neuroprotective effects *of Ptychopetalum olacoides* Bentham (Olacaceae) on oxygen and glucose deprivation induced damage in rat hippocampal slices." *Life Sci.* 2004; Aug. 75(15): 1897–1906.

27. Forgacs, P., et al. "Phytochemical and biological activity studies on 18 plants from French Guyana." *Plant Med. Phytother.* 1983; 17(1): 22–32.

Mulateiro

1. Lopes, Reinaldo Jose. Rede de bioprospeccao ja pensa em patente. Folha Online. 12/08/2002 www1.folha.uol.com.br/folha/ciencia/

2. Portillo, A., et al. "Antifungal activity of Paraguayan plants used in traditional

medicine." *J. Ethnopharmacol.* 2001; 76(1): 93–98.

Mullaca

1. Vasina, O. E., et al. "Withasteroids of Physalis. VII. 14-alpha-hydroxyixocarpanolide and 24,25-epoxywithanolide D." *Chem. Nat. Comp.* 1987; 22(5): 560–565.

2. Chen, C. M., et al. "Withangulatin A, a new withanolide from *Physalis angulata.*" *Heterocycles* 1990; 31(7): 1371–1375.

3. Shingu, K., et al. "Physagulin C, a new withanolide from *Physalis angulata L.*" *Pharm. Bull.* 1991; 39(6): 1591–1593.

4. Shingu, K., et al. "Three new withanolides, physagulins A, B and D from *Physalis angulata L.*" *Chem. Pharm. Bull.* 1992; 40(8): 2088–2091.

5. Shingu, K., et al. "Three new withanolides, physagulins E, F and G from *Physalis angulata L.*" *Chem. Pharm. Bull.* 1992; 40(9): 2448–2451.

6. Basey, K., et al. "Phygrine, an alkaloid from *Physalis* species." *Phytochemistry* 1992; 31(12): 4173–4176.

7. Anon. "Biological assay of antitumor agents from natural products." Abstr.: Seminar on the Development of Drugs from Medicinal Plants Organized by the Department of Medical Science Department at Thai Farmer Bank, Bangkok, Thailand 1982; 129.

8. Antoun, M. D., et al. "Potential antitumor agents. XVII. physalin B and 25,26-epidihydrophysalin C from *Witheringia coccoloboides.*" *J. Nat. Prod.* 1981; 44(5): 579–585.

9. Chiang, H., et al. "Antitumor agent, physalin F from *Physalis angulata L.*" *Anticancer Res.* 1992; 12(3): 837–843.

10. Ismail, N., et al. "A novel cytotoxic flavonoid glycoside from *Physalis angulata.*" *Fitoterapia* 2001 Aug. 72(6): 676–679.

11. Chiang, H. et al. "Inhibitory effects of physalin B and physalin F on various human leukemia cells *in vitro.*" *Anticancer Res.* 1992; 12(4): 1155–1162.

12. Kawai, M., et al. "Cytotoxic activity of physalins and related compounds against HeLa cells." *Pharmazie* 2002; 57(5): 348–350.

13. Lin, Y. S. et al. "Immunomodulatory activity of various fractions derived from Physalis angulata L. extract." *Amer. J. Chinese Med.* 1992; 20(3/4): 233–243.

14. Sakhibov, A. D. et al. "Immunosuppressive properties of vitasteroids." *Dokl. Akad. Nauk. Uzb. SSR.* 1990; 1: 43–45.

15. Soares, M. B., et al. "Inhibition of macrophage activation and lipopolysaccaride-induced death by seco-steroids purified from Physalis angulata L." *Eur. J. Pharmacol.* 2003; 459(1): 107–112.

16. Lee, W. C., et al. "Induction of heatshock response and alterations of protein phosphorylation by a novel topoisomerase II inhibitor, withangulatin A, in 9L rat brain tumor cells." *Cell Physiol.* 1991; 149(1): 66–67.

17. Juang, J. K., et al. "A new compound, withangulatin A, promotes type II DNA topoisomerasemediated DNA damage." *Biochem. Biophys. Res. Commun.* 1989; 159(3): 1128–1134.

18. Lee, Y. C., et al. "Integrity of intermediate filaments is associated with the development of acquired thermotolerance in 9L rat brain tumor cells." *J. Cell. Biochem.* 1995; 57(1): 150–162.

19. Perng, M. D., et al. "Induction of aggregation and augmentation of protein kinase-mediated phosphorylation of purified vimentin intermediate filaments by withangulatin A." *Mol. Pharmacol.* 1994; 46(4): 612–617.

20. Januario, A. H., et al. "Antimycobacterial physalins from *Physalis angulata L.* (Solanaceae)." *Phytother. Res.* 2002; 16(5): 445–448.

21. Pietro, R. C., et al. "*In vitro* antimycobacterial activities of *Physalis angulata L.*" *Phytomedicine* 2000; 7(4): 335–338.

22. Hussain, H., et al. "Plants in Kano ethnomedicine; screening for antimicrobial activity and alkaloids." *Int. J. Pharmacol.* 1991; 29(1): 51–56.

22. Ogunlana, E. O., et al. "Investigations into the antibacterial activities of local plants." *Planta Med.* 1975; 27: 354.

24. Otake, T., et al. "Screening of Indonesian plant extracts for anti-Human Immunodeficiency Virus- Type 1 (HIV-1) Activity." *Phytother. Res.* 1995; 9(1): 6–10.

25. Kusumoto, I. T., et al. "Screening of some Indonesian medicinal plants for inhibitory effects on HIV-1 protease." *Shoyakugaku Zasshi* 1992; 46(2): 190–193.

26. Kusumoto, I., et al. "Inhibitory effect of Indonesian plant extracts on reverse transcriptase of an RNA tumour virus (I)." *Phytother. Res.* 1992; 6(5): 241–244.

27. Kurokawa, M. et al. "Antiviral traditional medicines against *Herpes simplex* virus (HSV-1), polio virus, and measles virus *in vitro* and their therapeutic efficacies for HSV-1 infection in mice." *Antiviral Res.* 1993; 22(2/3): 175–188.

28. Cox, P. A. "Pharmacological activity of the Samoan ethnopharacopoeia." *Econ. Bot.* 1989; 43(4): 487–497.

29. Cesario De Mello, A., et al. "Presence of acetylcholine in the fruit of *Physalis angulata* (Solanaceae)." *Cienc. Cult.* (São Paulo) 1985; 37(5): 799–805.

30. Kone-Bamba, D., et al. "Hemostatic activity of 216 plants used in traditional medicine in the Ivory Coast." *Plant Med. Phytother.* 1987; 21(2): 122–130.

31. Richter, R. K., et al. "Reporting biological assay results on tropical medicinal plants to host country collaborators." *J. Ethnopharmacol.* 1998; 62(1): 85–88.

Mulungu

1. Pohill, R. M., et al. *Advances in Legume Systematics.* Part 2. Kew, England: Royal Botanic Gardens, 1981.

2. Sanzen, T., et al. "Expression of glycoconjugates during intrahepatic bile duct development in the rat: an immunohistochemical and lectin-histochemical study." *Hepatology* 1995; 3: 944–951.

3. Lee, R. F., et al. "The metabolism of glyceryl (35 S) sulfoquinovoside by the coral tree, *Erythrina crista-galli* and alfalfa, *Medicago sativa.*" *Biochim. Biophys. Acta.* 1972; 261(1): 35–37.

4. Santos, W. O., et al. "Pesquisas de substancias cardioativas em plantas xerofilas medicinais." IX Simposio de Plantas Medicinais do Brasil, Rio de Janeiro, 1986; 45: 1–3.

5. Mansbach, R. S., et al. "Effects of the competitive nicotinic antagonist erysodine on behavior occasioned or maintained by nicotine: comparison with mecamylamine." *Psychopharmacology* 2000; 148(3): 234–242.

6. Decker, M. W., et al. "Erysodine, a competitive antagonist at neuronal nicotinic acetylcholine receptors." *Eur. J. Pharmacol*. 1995; 280(1): 79–89.

7. Onusic, G. M., et al. "Effect of acute treatment with a water-alcohol extract of *Erythrina mulungu* on anxiety-related responses in rats." *Braz. J. Med. Biol. Res.* 2002; 35(4): 473–477.

8. Kittler, J. T., et al. "Mechanisms of GABA receptor assembly and trafficking: implications for the modulation of inhibitory neurotransmission." *Mol. Neurobiol.* 2002; 26(2–3): 251–268.

9. Mitscher, L. A., et al. "Erycristin, a new antimicrobial pterocarpan from *Erythrina crista-galli*." *Phytochemistry* 1988; 27(2): 381–385.

10. Mitscher, L. A., et al. "Antimicrobial agents from higher plants. Erycristagallin, a new petrocarpene from the roots of the Bolivian coral tree, *Erythrina crista-galli*." *Heterocycles* 1984; 22(8): 1673–1675.

Mutamba

1. Takahashi, T., et al. "Toxicological studies on procyanidin B-2 for external application as a hair growing agent." *Food Chem. Toxicol.* 1999; 37(5): 545–552.

2. Takahashi, T., et al. "Several selective protein kinase C inhibitors including procyanidins promote hair growth." *Skin Pharmacol. Appl. Skin Physiol.* 2000; 13(3–4): 133–142.

3. Takahashi, T., et al. "The first clinical trial of topical application of procyanidin B-2 to investigate its potential as a hair growing agent." *Phytother. Res.* 2001; 15(4): 331–336.

4. Kamimura, A., et al. "Procyanidin B-2, extracted from apples, promotes hair growth: A laboratory study." *Br. J. Dermatol.* 2002; 146(1): 41–51.

5. Hor, M., et al. "Proanthocyanidin polymers with antisecretory activity and proanthocyanidin oligomers from Guazuma ulmifolia bark." *Phytochemistry* 1996; 42(1): 109–119.

6. Kashiwada, Y., et al. "Antitumor agents, 129. Tannins and related compounds as selective cytotoxic agents." *J. Nat. Prod.* 1992; 55(8): 1033–1043.

7. Ito, H., et al. "Antitumor activity of compounds isolated from leaves of Eriobotrya japonica." *J. Agric. Food Chem.* 2002; 50(8): 2400–2403.

8. Vieira, J. E. V., et al. "Pharmacologic screening of plants from northeast Brazil. II." *Rev. Brasil. Farm.* 1968; 49: 67–75.

9. Barros, G. S. G., et al. "Pharmacological screening of some Brazilian plants." *J. Pharm. Pharmacol.* 1970; 22: 116.

10. Caceres, A., et al. "Plants used in Guatemala for the treatment of gastrointestinal disorders. 1. Screening of 84 plants against enterobacteria." *J. Ethnopharmacol.* 1990; 30(1): 55–73.

11. Heinrich, M., et al. "Parasitological and microbiological evaluation of Mixe Indian medicinal plants." (Mexico) *J. Ethnopharmacol.* 1992; 36(1): 81–85.

12. Caceres, A., et al. "Plants used in Guatemala for the treatment of respiratory diseases. 2: Evaluation of activity of 16 plants against gram-positive bacteria." *J. Ethnopharmacol.* 1993; 39(1): 77–82.

13. Caceres, A., et al. "Plants used in Guatemala for the treatment of gastrointestinal disorders. 3. Confirmation of activity against enterobacteria of 16 plants." *J. Ethnopharmacol.* 1993; 38(1): 31–38.

14. Caceres, A., et al. "Screening of antimicrobial activity of plants popularly used in Guatemala for the treatment of dermatomucosal diseases." *J. Ethnopharmacol.* 1987; 20(3): 223–237.

15. Caceres, A., et al. "Anti-gonorrhoeal activity of plants used in Guatemala for the treatment of sexually transmitted diseases." *J. Ethnopharmacol.* 1995; 48(2): 85–88.

16. Camporese, A., et al. "Screening of anti-bacterial activity of medicinal plants from Belize (Central America)." *J. Ethnopharmacol.* 2003 Jul;87(1):103–107.

17. Navarro, M. C., et al. "Antibacterial, antiprotozoal and antioxidant activity of five plants used in Izabal for infectious diseases." *Phytother. Res.* 2003 Apr; 17(4): 325–329.

18. Hattori, M., et al. "Inhibitory effects of various Ayurvedic and Panamania medicinal plants on the infection of Herpes simplex virus-1 in vitro and in vivo." *Phytother. Res.* 1995; 9(4): 270–276.

19. Tseng, C. F. "Inhibition of in vitro prostaglandin and leukotriene biosyntheses by cinnamoyl-beta-phenethylamine and N-acyldopamine derivatives." *Chem. Pharm. Bull.* 1992; 40(2): 396–400.

20. Hor, M., et al. "Inhibition of intestinal chloride secretion by proanthocyanidins from Guazuma ulmifolia." *Planta Med.* 1995; 61(3): 208–212.

21. Alarcon-Aguilara, F. J., et al. "Study of the anti-hyperglycemic effect of plants used as antidiabetics." *J. Ethnopharmacol.* 1998; 61(2): 101–110.

22. Nascimento, S. C., et al. "Antimicrobial and cytotoxic activities in plants from Pernambuco, Brazil." *Fitoterapia* 1990; 61(4): 353–355.

23. Caballero-George, C., et al. In vitro inhibition of [3H]-angiotensin II binding on the human AT1 receptor by proanthocyanidins from *Guazuma ulmifolia* bark. *Planta Med.* 2002; 68(12): 1066–1071.

Nettle

1. De Clercq., E. "Current lead natural products for the chemotherapy of human immunodeficiency virus (HIV) infection." *Med. Res. Rev.* 2000; 20(5): 323–349.

2. Balzarini, J., et al. "The mannose-specific plant lectins from *Cymbidium hybrid* and *Epipactis helleborine* and the (N-acetylglucosamine)n-specific plant lectin from *Urtica dioica* are potent and selective inhibitors of human immunodeficiency virus and cytomegalovirus replication in vitro." *Antiviral Res.* 1992; 18(2): 191–207.

3. Does, M. P., et al. "Characterization of *Urtica dioica* agglutinin isolectins and the encoding gene family." *Plant Mol. Biol.* 1999; 39(2): 335–347.

4. Le Moal, M. A., et al. "*Urtica dioica* agglutinin, a new mitogen for murine T lymphocytes: unaltered interleukin-1 production but late interleukin 2-mediated

proliferation." *Cell Immunol.* 1988; 115(1): 24–35.

5. Wagner, H., et al. "Biologically active compounds from the aqueous extract of *Urtica dioica.*" *Planta Med.* 1989; 55(5): 452–454.

6. Galelli, A., et a. "*Urtica dioica* agglutinin. A superantigenic lectin from stinging nettle rhizome." *J. Immunol.* 1993; 151(4): 1821–1831.

7. Akbay, P., et al. "In vitro immunomodulatory activity of flavonoid glycosides from *Urtica dioica* L." *Phytother. Res.* 2003; 17(1): 34–37.

8. Randall, C., et al. "Randomized controlled trial of nettle sting for treatment of base-of-thumb pain." *J. R. Soc. Med.* 2000; 93(6): 305–309.

9. Obertreis, B., et al. "Anti-inflammatory effect of *Urtica dioica folia* extract in comparison to caffeic malic acid." *Arzneimittelforschung* 1996; 46(1): 52–56.

10. Schulze-Tanzil, G., et al. "Effects of the antirheumatic remedy hox alpha–a new stinging nettle leaf extract–on matrix metalloproteinases in human chondrocytes in vitro." *Histol. Histopathol.* 2002; 17(2): 477–485.

11. Riehemann, K., et al. "Plant extracts from stinging nettle (*Urtica dioica*), an antirheumatic remedy, inhibit the proinflammatory transcription factor NF-kappaB." *FEBS Lett.* 1999; 442(1): 89–94.

12. Teucher, T., et al. "Cytokine secretion in whole blood of healthy subjects following oral administration of *Urtica dioica* L. plant extract." *Arzneimittelforschung* 1996; 46(9): 906–910.

13. Mittman, P. "Randomized, double-blind study of freeze-dried *Urtica dioica* in the treatment of allergic rhinitis." *Planta Med.* 1990; 56(1): 44-7.

14. Thornhill, S. M., et al. 'Natural treatment of perennial allergic rhinitis." *Altern. Med. Rev.* 2000; 5(5): 448–454.

15. Legssyer, A., et al. "Cardiovascular effects of *Urtica dioica* L. in the isolated rat heart and aorta." *Phytother. Res.* 2002; 16(6): 503–507.

16. Testai, L., et al. "Cardiovascular effects of *Urtica dioica* L. (Urticaceae) roots ex-

tracts: in vitro and in vivo pharmacological studies." *J. Ethnopharmacol.* 2002; 81(1): 105–109.

17. Tahri, A., et al. "Acute diuretic, natriuretic and hypotensive effects of a continuous perfusion of aqueous extract of *Urtica dioica* in the rat." *J. Ethnopharmacol.* 2000; 73(1–2): 95–100.

18. Lasheras, N., et al. "Etude pharmacologique preliminaire de *Prunus spinosa* L., *Amelanchier ovalis* medikus, *Juniperus communis* L, et *Urtica dioica* L." *Plant Med. Phyother.* 1986; 20: 219–226.

19. Brocano, F. J., et al. "Etude de l'effet sure le centre cardiovasulaire de quelques prepartions de l'*Urtica diocia* L." *Planta Med.* 1983; 17: 222–229.

20. Brocano, J., et al., "Estudio de diferentes preparados de *Urtica dioica* L. sobre SNC." *An. R. Acad. Farm.* 1987; 53: 284–291

21. Levine, A. C., et al. "The role of sex steroids in the pathogenesis and maintenance of benign prostatic hyperplasia." *Mt. Sinai J. Med.* 1997; 64(1): 20–25.

22. Carson, C., et al. "The role of dihydrotestosterone in benign prostatic hyperplasia." *Urology* 203; 61(4 Suppl 1): 2–7.

23. Sciarra, F., et al. "Role of estrogens in human benign prostatic hyperplasia." *Arch. Androl.* 2000; 44(3): 213–220.

24. Schottner, M., et al. "Lignans from the roots of *Urtica dioica* and their metabolites bind to human sex hormone binding globulin (SHBG)." *Planta Med.* 1997; 63(6): 529–532.

25. Hryb, D. J., et al. "The effect of extracts of the roots of the stinging nettle (*Urtica dioica*) on the interaction of SHBG with its receptor on human prostatic membranes." *Planta Med.* 1995; 61(1): 31–32.

26. Koch, E. "Extracts from fruits of saw palmetto (*Sabal serrulata*) and roots of stinging nettle (*Urtica dioica*): viable alternatives in the medical treatment of benign prostatic hyperplasia and associated lower urinary tracts symptoms." *Planta Med.* 2001; 67: 489–500.

27. Koch E. and A. Biber. "Pharmacological effects of saw palmetto and urtica extracts for benign prostatic hyperplasia." *Urologe* 1994; 34(2): 90–95.

28. Konrad, L., et al. "Antiproliferative effect on human prostate cancer cells by a stinging nettle root (*Urtica dioica*) extract." *Planta Med.* 2000; 66(1): 44–47.

29. Lichius, J. J., et al. "The inhibiting effects of *Urtica dioica* root extracts on experimentally induced prostatic hyperplasia in the mouse." *Planta Med.* 1997; 63(4): 307–310.

30. Krzeski, T., et al. "Combined extracts of *Urtica dioica* and *Pygeum africanum* in the treatment of benign prostatic hyperplasia: double-blind comparison of two doses." *Clin. Ther.* 1993; 15(6): 1011–1020.

31. Sokeland, J. "Combined sabal and urtica extract compared with finasteride in men with benign prostatic hyperplasia: analysis of prostate volume and therapeutic outcome." *BJU Int.* 2000; 86(4): 439–442.

32. Kaufman, K. D. "Androgens and alopecia." *Mol. Cell Endocrinol.* 2002; 198(1–2): 89–95.

33. Chizick, S., et al. "Natural preparation for treatment of male pattern hair loss." United States Patent 5,972,345; 1999.

Passionflower

1. Mowrey, Daniel. *The Scientific Validation of Herbal Medicine.* New Canaan, CT: Keats Publishing, Inc, 1986.

2. Lutomski, J. "Alkaloidy *Pasiflora incarnata* L." Dissertation, Institut for Medicinal Plant Research, Pozan, 1960.

3. Bruneton, J. *Pharmacognosy, Phytochemistry, Medicinal Plants.* Intercept, Ltd., Hampshire, England. 1995.

4. Flynn, R., and Roest, M. *Your Guide to Standardized Herbal Products.* One World Press, 1995.

5. Wolfman, C., et al. "Possible anxiolytic effects of chrysin, a central benzodiazepine receptor ligand isolated from Passiflora coerulea." *Pharmacol. Biochem. Behav.* 1994;47(1):1–4.

6. Zanoli, P., et al. "Behavioral characterisation of the flavonoids apigenin and chrysin." *Fitoterapia.* 2000; 71 Suppl 1: S117–23.

7. Mowrey, Daniel. *The Scientific Validation of Herbal Medicine.* New Canaan, CT: Keats Publishing, Inc, 1986.

8. Lutomski, J. "Alkaloidy *Pasiflora incarnata L.*" Dissertation, Institut for Medicinal Plant Research, Pozan, 1960.

9. Lueng. A., Foster, S. *Encyclopedia of Common Natural Ingredients.* New York: Wiley & Sons, 1996.

10. Yasukawa, K., et al. "Inhibitory effect of edible plant extracts on 12-o-tetradecanoylphorbol-13-acetate-induced ear oedema in mice." *Phytother. Res.* 1993;7(2): 185–189.

11. Lutomski, J., et al. "Pharmacochemical investigation of the raw materials from Passiflora genus. 2. The pharmacochemical estimation of juices from the fruits of *Passiflora edulis* and *Passiflora edulis* forma flavicarpa." *Planta Med.* 1975; 27: 112–121.

12. De a Ribeiro, R., et al. "Acute diuretic effects in conscious rats produced by some medicinal plants used in the state of São Paulo, Brasil." *J. Ethnopharmacol.* 1988;24 (1):19–29.

13. Dhawan, K., et al. "Aphrodisiac activity of methanol extract of leaves of *Passiflora incarnata* Linn. in mice." *Phytother. Res.* 2003; 17(4): 401–403.

14. Dhawan, K., et al. "Antitussive activity of the methanol extract of *Passiflora incarnata* leaves." *Fitoterapia.* 2002; 73(5): 397–399.

15. HerbClip: Passionflower., "An Herbalist's View of Passionflower" *American Botanical Council*, Austin, Texas, April 10, 1996.

Pata de Vaca

1. Yokozawa, T., et al. "Protective effects of some flavonoids on the renal cellular membrane." *Exp. Toxicol. Pathol.* 1999; 51(1): 9–14.

2. Hamzah, A. S., et al. "Kaempferitrin from the leaves of Hedyotis verticillata and its biological activity." *Planta Med.* 1994 Aug; 60(4): 388–389.

3. Juliane, C. "Acao hipoglicemiante da unha-de-vaca." *Rev. Med. Pharm. Chim. Phys.* 1929; 2(1): 165–169.

4. Juliane, C. "Acao hipoglicemiante de *Bauhinia forficata*. Novos estudos experimentails." *Rev. Sudam Endocrin. Immol. Quimiot.* 1931; 14: 326–334.

5. Juliani, C. "Hypoglycemic action of bauintrato (*Bauhinia forficata* preparation) new clinical and experimental study." *J. Clin.* 1941; 22: 17.

6. Costa, O. A. "Estudo farmacoquimico da unha-de-vaca." *Rev. Flora Medicinal* 1945; 9(4): 175–189.

7. Almeida, R., and Agra, M. F. "Levantamento da flora medicinal de uso no tratamento da diabete e alguns resultados experimentais." *VIII Simposio de Plantas Medicinais do Brasil*, Manaus-AM, Brazil. September 4–6, 1984, 23.

8. Miyake, E. T., et al. "Caracterizacao farmacognostica de pata-de-vaca (*Bauhinia fortificata*)." *Rev. Bras. Farmacogn.* 1986; 1(1): 56–68.

9. Lemus, I., et al. "Hypoglycemic activity of four plants used in Chilean popular medicine." *Phytother. Res.* 1999; 13(2): 91–94.

10. Silva, F. R., et al. "Acute effect of *Bauhinia forficata* on serum glucose levels in normal and alloxan-induced diabetic rats." *J. Ethnopharmacol.* 2002; 83(1–2): 33–37.

11. Pepato, M. T., et al. "Anti-diabetic activity of *Bauhinia forficata* decoction in streptozotocin-diabetic rats." *J. Ethnopharmacol.* 2002; 81(2): 191–197.

12. Lino, S., et al. "Antidiabetic activity of Bauhinia forficata extracts in alloxan-diabetic rats." *Biol. Pharm. Bull.* 2004 Jan; 27(1): 125–127.

13. de Sousa, E., et al. "Hypoglycemic effect and antioxidant potential of kaempferol-3,7-O-(alpha)-dirhamnoside from *Bauhinia forficata* leaves." *J. Nat. Prod.* 2004; 67(5): 829–832.

14. Pepato, M. T., et al. "Evaluation of toxicity after one-months treatment with *Bauhinia forficata* decoction in streptozotocin-induced diabetic rats." *BMC Complement Altern Med.* 2004 Jun 8; 4(1): 7.

15. Damasceno, D. C., et al. "Effect of *Bauhinia forficata* extract in diabetic pregnant rats: maternal repercussions." *Phytomedicine.* 2004; 11(2–3): 196–201.

Pau d' Arco

1. Rao, K. V., et al. "Recognition and evaluation of lapachol as an antitumor agent." *Canc. Res.* 1968; 28: 1952–1954.

2. Block, J. B., et al. "Early clinical studies with lapachol (NSC-11905)." *Cancer Chemother. Rep.* 1974; 4: 27–28.

3. Linardi, M. D. C., et al. "A lapachol derivative active against mouse lymphocyte leukemia P-388." *J. Med. Chem.* 1975; 18(11): 1159–1162.

4. Santana, C. F., et al. "Preliminary observation with the use of lapachol in human patients bearing malignant neoplasms." *Revista do Instituto de Antibioticos* 1971; 20: 61–68.

5. Beckstrom-Sternberg, Stephen M., and Duke, James A. "The Phytochemical Database." ACEDB version 5.3: July 1994. National Germplasm Resources Laboratory (NGRL), Agricultural Research Service (ARS), U.S. Department of Agriculture.

6. Murray, Michael T. *The Healing Power of Herbs.* Rocklin, CA: Prima Publishing, 1995.

7. Giuraud, P., et al. "Comparison of antibacterial and antifungal activities of lapachol and b-lapachone." *Planta Med.* 1994; 60: 373–374.

8. Li, C. J., et al. "Three inhibitors of type 1 human immunodeficiency virus long terminal repeat-directed gene expression and virus replication." *Proc. Nat'l. Acad. Sci. USA* 1993; 90(5): 1839–1842.

9. Pardee, A., et al. "Treatment of human prostate disease." United States Patent 6,245,807; June 12, 2001.

10. Muller, K., et al. "Potential antipsoriatic agents: lapacho compounds as potent inhibitors of HaCaT cell growth." *J. Nat. Prod.* 1999; 62(8): 1134–1136.

11. Jiang, Z., et al. "Synthesis of beta-lapachone and its intermediates." United States Patent 6,458, 974; October 1, 2002.

12. de Lima, O. G., et al. "Primeiras observacoes sobre a acao antimicrobiana do lapachol." *Anais da Sociedade de Biologica de Pernambuco* 1956; 14: 129–135.

13. de Lima, O. G., et al. "Una nova substancia antibiotica isolada do 'Pau d'Arco,' Tabebuia sp." *Anais da Sociedade de Biologica de Pernambuco* 1956; 14: 136–140.

14. Burnett, A. R., et al. "Naturally occurring quinones. The quinonoid constituents

of *Tabebuia avellanedae*." *J. Chem.* Soc. 1967: 2100–2104.

15. Gershon, H., et al. "Fungitoxicity of 1,4-naphthoquinonoes to *Candida albicans* and *Trichophyton menta* grophytes." *Can. J. Microbiol.* 1975; 21: 1317–1321.

16. Binutu, O. A., et al. "Antimicrobial potentials of some plant species of the *Bignoniaceae* family." *Afr. J. Med. Sci.* 1994; 23(3): 269–273.

17. Nagata, K., et al. "Antimicrobial activity of novel furanonaphthoquinone analogs." *Antimicrobial Agents Chemother.* 1998; 42(3): 700–702.

18. Anesini, C., et al. "Screening of plants used in Argentine folk medicine for antimicrobial activity." *J. Ethnopharmacol.* 1993; 39(2): 119–128.

19. Segelman, Alvin Burton. "Composition and method for treating and preventing *Helicobactor-pylori*-associated stomach gastritis, ulcers and cancer." United States Patent 6,187,313; February 13, 2001.

20. de Lima, O. G., et al. "A new antibiotic substance isolated from pau d'arco (*Tabebuia*)." *Anais. Soc. Biol. Pernambuco.* 1956; 14: 136–140.

21. Portillo, A., et al. "Antifungal activity of Paraguayan plants used in traditional medicine." *J. Ethnopharmacol.* 2001; 76(1): 93–98.

22. Linhares, M. S., et al. "Estudo sobre of efeito de substancias antibioticas obitdas de *Streptomyces* e vegatais superiores sobre o herpesvirus hominis." *Revista Instituto Antibioticos, Recife* 1975; 15: 25–32.

23. Lagrota, M., et al. "Antiviral activity of lapachol." *Rev. Microbiol.* 1983; 14: 21–26.

24. Schuerch, A. R., et al. "B-Lapachone, an inhibitor of oncornavirus reverse transcriptase and eukarotic DBA polymerase-a. Inhibitory effect, thiol dependency and specificity." *Eur. J. Biochem.* 1978; 84: 197–205.

25. Austin, F. R. "*Schistosoma mansoni* chemoprophylaxis with dietary lapachol." *Am. J. Trop. Med. Hyg.* 1979; 23: 412–419.

26. Gilbert, B., et al. "Schistosomiasis. Protection against infection by terpenoids." *An. Acad. Brasil. Cienc.* 1970; 42 (Suppl): 397–400.

27. Oga, S., et al. "Toxicidade e atividade anti-inflamatoria de *Tabebuia avellanedae* Lorentz ('Ipe Roxo')." *Rev. Fac. Farm. Bioquim.* 1969; 7: 4.

28. Taylor, Leslie. Personal observations in Manaus, Belem, and São Paulo, Brazil, 1996 to present.

29. Awang, D. V. C. "Commerical taheebo lacks active ingredient." Information Letter 726 (August 13, 1987). *Can. Pharm. J.* 1991; 121: 323–326.

Pedra Hume Caá

1. Yoshikawa, M., et al. "Antidiabetic principles of natural medicines. II. Aldose reductase and alpha-glucosidase inhibitors from Brazilian natural medicine, the leaves of *Myrcia multiflora* DC (myrtaceae): structures of myrciacitrins I and II and myrciaphenones A and B." *Chem. Pharm. Bull.* 1998; 46(1): 113–119.

2. Schmeda-Hirschmann, G., et al. "Preliminary pharmacological studies on *Eugenia uniflora* leaves: xanthine oxidase inhibitory activity." *J. Ethnopharmacol.* 1987; 21(2): 183–186.

3. Varma, S. D., et al. "Flavonoids as inhibitors of lens aldose reductase." *Science* 1975; 188(4194): 1215–1216.

4. Matsuda, H., et al. "Structural requirements of flavonoids and related compounds for aldose reductase inhibitory activity." *Chem. Pharm. Bull.* (Tokyo). 2002; 50(6): 788–795.

5. Chaudhry, P. S., et al. "Inhibition of human lens aldose reductase by flavonoids, sulindac and indomethacin." *Biochem. Pharmacol.* 1983; 32(13): 1995–1998.

6. Martins de Toledo, O. *Tese de Doutoramento.* Faculdade de Medicina de São Paulo. São Paulo, Brazil, 1929.

7. Coutinho, A. B. *Tese de Catedra.* Faculdade de Medicina de Recife. Recife, Brazil, 1938.

8. Mendes dos Reis Arruda, L., et al. "Efeito hipoglicemiante induzido pelo extracto das raizes de *Myrcia citrifolia* (pedra-hume-caá), esudo famacologico preliminar." *V Simposio de Plantas Medicinais do Brasil*, São Paulo-SP, Brazil, 1978; 74 (September 4–6).

9. Brune, U., et al. "*Myrcia spaerocarpa, D.C.*, planta diabetica." *V Simposio de Plantas Medicinais do Brasil*, São Paulo-SP, Brazil, 1978; 74 (September 4–6).

10. Grune, U., et al. "Sobre o principio antidiabetico da pedra-hume-caá, *Myrcia multiflora* (Lam)." Thesis 1979; Federal University of Rio de Janeiro.

11. Russo, E. M., et al. "Clinical trial of *Myrcia uniflora* and *Bauhinia forficata* leaf extracts in normal and diabetic patients." *Braz. J. Med. Biol. Res.* 1990; 23(1): 11–20.

12. Pepato, M. T., et al. "Assessment of the antidiabetic activity of *Myrcia uniflora* extracts in streptozotocin diabetic rats." *Diabetes Res.* 1993; 22(2): 49–57.

Picão Preto

1. Wat, C. K., et al. "Ultraviolet-mediated cytotoxic activity of phenylheptatriyne from *Bidens pilosa* L." *J. Nat. Prod.* 1979; 42(1): 103–111.

2. Arnason, T., et al. "Photosensitization of *Escherichia coli* and *Saccharomyces cerevisiae* by phenylheptatriyne from *Bidens pilosa*." *Can. J. Microbiol.* 1980; 26(6): 698–705.

3. Krettli, A. U., et al. "The search for new antimalarial drugs from plants used to treat fever and malaria or plants randomly selected; a review." *Mem. Inst. Oswaldo Cruz* 2001; 96(8): 1033–1042.

4. Geissberger, P., et al. "Constituents of *Bidens pilosa* L.: do the components found so far explain the use of this plant in traditional medicine?" *Acta Trop.* 1991; 48(4): 251–261.

5. Alvarez, L., et al. "Bioactive polyacetylenes from *Bidens pilosa*." *Planta Med.* 1996; 62(4): 355–357.

6. Chin, H. W., et al. "The hepatoprotective effects of Taiwan folk medicine 'hamhong-chho' in rats." *Am. J. Chin. Med.* 1996; 24(3–4): 231–240.

7. Chih, H. W., et al. "Anti-inflammatory activity of Taiwan folk medicine 'hamhong-chho' in rats." *Am. J. Chin. Med.* 1995; 23(3–4): 273–278.

8. Pereira, R. L., et al. "Immunosuppressive and anti-inflammatory effects of methanolic extract and the polyacetylene

isolated from *Bidens pilosa L.*" *Immunopharmacology* 1999; 43(1): 31–37.

9. Jager, A. K., et al. "Screening of Zulu medicinal plants for prostaglandin-synthesis inhibitors" *J. Ethnopharmacol.* 1996; 52(2): 95–100.

10. Alvarez, A., et al. "Gastric antisecretory and antiulcer activities of an ethanolic extract of *Bidens pilosa L.* var. *radiata* Schult. Bip." *J. Ethnopharmacol.* 1999; 67(3): 333–340.

11. Avalos, A. A., et al. "Influence of extracts from leaves and stem of *Bidens pilosa* on experimental ulcerogenesis in rats." *Rev. Cubana Farm.* 1984; 18(2): 143–150.

12. Tan, P. V., et al. "Effects of methanol, cyclohexane and methylene chloride extracts of *Bidens pilosa* on various gastric ulcer models in rats." *J. Ethnopharmacol.* 2000; 73(3): 415–421.

13. Alarcon-Aguilara, F. J., et al. "Study of the anti-hyperglycemic effect of plants used as antidiabetics." *J. Ethnopharmacol.* 1998; 61(2): 101–110.

14. Perez, R. M., et al. "A study of the hypoglycemic effect of some Mexican plants." *J. Ethnopharmacol.* 1984; 12(3): 253–262.

15. Alarcon-Aguilar, F. J., et al. "Investigation on the hypoglycaemic effects of extracts of four Mexican medicinal plants in normal and alloxan-diabetic mice." *Phytother. Res.* 2002; 16(4): 383–386.

16. Ubillas, R. P. "Antihyperglycemic acetylenic glucosides from *Bidens pilosa.*" *Planta Med.* 2000; 66(1): 82–83.

17. Dimo, T., et al. "Leaf methanol extract of *Bidens pilosa* prevents and attenuates the hypertension induced by high-fructose diet in Wister rats." *J. Ethnopharmacol.* 2002; 83(3): 183–191.

18. Dimo, T., et al. "Effects of the aqueous and methylene chloride extracts of *Bidens pilosa* leaf on fructose-hypertensive rats." *J. Ethnopharmacol.* 2001; 76(3): 215–221.

19. Dimo, T., et al. "Hypotensive effects of a methanol extract from *Bidens pilosa* Linn. on hypertensive rats." *C. R. Acad. Sci. Paris* 1999; 322(4): 323–329.

20. Dimo, T., et al. "Effects of leaf aqueous extract of *Bidens pilosa* (Asteraceae) on

KCL- and norepinephrine-induced contractions of rat aorta." *J. Ethnopharmacol.* 1998; 60(2): 179–182.

21. Rabe, T. "Antibacterial activity of South African plants used for medicinal purposes." *J. Ethnopharmacol.* 1997; 56(1): 81–87.

22. Chariandy, C. M., et al. "Screening of medicinal plants from Trinidad and Tobago for antimicrobial and insecticidal properties." *J. Ethnopharmacol.* 1999; 64(3): 265–270.

23. Desta, B. "Ethiopian traditional herbal drugs. Part II: Antimicrobial activity of 63 medicinal plants." *J. Ethnopharmacol.* 1993; 39(2): 129–139.

24. Sarg, T. M., et al. "Constituents and biological activity of *Bidens pilosa* l grown in Egypt." *Acta. Pharm. Hung.* 1991; 61(6): 317–323.

25. Khan, M. R., et al. "Anti-microbial activity of *Bidens pilosa, Bischofia javanica, Elmerillia papuana* and *Sigesbekia orientalis.*" *Fitoterapia* 2001; 72(6): 662–665.

26. Boily, Y., et al. "Screening of medicinal plants of Rwanda (central Africa) for antimicrobial activity." *J. Ethnopharmacol.* 1986; 16(1): 1–13.

27. van Puyvelde, L., et al. "*In vitro* inhibition of mycobacteria by Rwandese medicinal plants." *Phytother. Res.* 1994; 8(2): 65–69.

28. Bondarenko, A. S., et al. "The antimicrobial properties of the polyacetylene antibiotic phenylheptatriyne." *Mikrobiol. Zh.* 1985; 47(2): 81–83.

29. Hudson, J. B., et al. "Investigation of the antiviral action of the photoactive compound phenylheptatriyne." *Photochem. Photobiol.* 1986; 43(1): 27–33.

30. Hudson, J. B., et al. "Nature of the interaction between the photoactive compound phenylheptatriyne and animal viruses." *Photochem. Photobiol.* 1982; 36(2): 181–185.

31. Krettli, A. U., et al. "New antimalarial drugs: A search based on plants used in popular medicine to treat fever and malaria." *Folha. Med.* 2001; 120(2): 119–126.

32. Brandao, M. G. L., et al. "Antimalarial activity of extracts and fractions from

Bidens pilosa and other *Bidens* species (Asteraceae) correlated with the presence of acetylene and flavonoid compound." *Eur. J. Pharmacol.* 1997; 57(2): 131–138.

33. Chippaux, J. P., et al. "Drug or plant substances which antagonize venoms or potentiate antivenins." *Bull. Soc. Pathol. Exot.* 1997; 90(4): 282–285.

34. Gonzalez, A., et al. "Biological screening of Uruguayan medicinal plants." *J. Ethnopharmacol.* 1993; 39(3): 217–220.

35. Gupta, M. P., et al. "Screening of Panamanian medicinal plants for brine shrimp toxicity, crown gall tumor inhibition, cytotoxicity and DNA intercalation." *Int. J. Pharmacog.* 1996; 34(1): 19–27.

36. Hostettmann, K., et al. "Phytochemistry of plants used in traditional medicine." *Proceedings of the Phytochemical Society of Europe.* Clarendon Press: Oxford England, 1995.

37. Chang, J. S., et al. "Antileukemic activity of *Bidens pilosa L.* var. *minor* (Blume) Sherff. and *Houttuynia cordata* Thunb." *Amer. J. Chinese Med.* 2001; 29(2): 303–312.

38. Chagnon, M. "General pharmacologic inventory of medicinal plants of Rwanda." *J. Ethnopharmacol.* 1984; 12(3): 239–251.

Quinine

1. Aviado, D. M., et al. "Antimalarial and antiarrhythmic activity of plant extracts." *Medicina Experimentalis—International Journal of Experimental Medicine* 1969; 19(20): 79–94.

2. Man-Son-Hing, M., et al. "Quinine for nocturnal leg cramps: a meta-analysis including unpublished data." *J. Gen. Intern. Med.* 1998; 13(9): 600–606.

3. Diener, H. C., et al. "Effectiveness of quinine in treating muscle cramps: a double-blind, placebo-controlled, parallel-group, multicentre trial." *Int. J. Clin. Pract.* 2002; 56(4): 243–246.

4. Lung, A. and S. Foster. *Encyclopedia of Common Natural Ingredients* 1996. Wiley & Sons: New York.

Samambaia

1. Vasange, M., et al. "Sulpholipid composition and methods for treating skin dis-

orders." United States Patent 6,124, 266; 2000.

2. Valetas, J. "Method for preparing a substance having properties against collagen diseases and products obtained." United States Patent 4,206,222; 1980.

3. Pathak, M. A., et al. "*Polypodium* extract as photoprotectant." United States Patent 5,614,197; 1997.

4. Padilla, H. C. "A new agent (hydrophilic fraction of *Polypodium leucotomos*) for management of psoriasis." *Int. J. Dermatol.* 1974; 13(5): 276–282.

5. Mercadal Peyri, O., et al. "Preliminary communication on the treatment of psoriasis with anapsos." *Actas Dermosifiliogr.* 1981; 72(1–2): 65–68.

6. Capella Perez, M. C., et al. "Double-blind study using 'anapsos' 120 mg. in the treatment of psoriasis." *Actas Dermosifiliogr.* 1981; 72(9–10):487–494.

7. Del Pino Gamboa , J., et al. "Comparative study between 120 mg. of anapsos and a placebo in 37 psoriasis patients." *Med. Cutan. Ibero. Lat. Am.* 1982; 10(3): 203–208.

8. Pineiro Alvarez, B. "2 years personal experience in anapsos treatment of psoriasis in various clinical forms." *Med. Cutan. Ibero. Lat. Am.* 1983; 11(1): 65–72.

9. Vargas, J., et al. "Anapsos, an antipsoriatic drug which increases the proportion of suppressor cells in human peripheral blood." *Ann. Immunol.* (Paris) 1983; 134C (3): 393–400.

10. Jimenez, D., et al. "Anapsos modifies immunological parameters and improves the clinical course in atopic dermatitis." *Dermatologica* 1986; 173(3): 154–155.

11. Jimenez, D., et al. "Anapsos, an antipsoriatic drug, in atopic dermatitis." *Allergol. Immunopathol.* (Madrid) 1987; 15(4):185–189.

12. Mohammad A. "Vitiligo repigmentation with Anapsos (*Polypodium leucotomos*)." *Int. J. Dermatol.* 1989; 28(7): 479.

13. Vasange, M., et al. "The fern *Polypodium decumanum*, used in the treatment of psoriasis, and its fatty acid constituents as inhibitors of leukotriene B4 formation." *Prostaglandins Leukotrienes Essent. Fatty Acids* 1994; 50: 279–284.

14. Tuominen, M., et al. "Effects of calaguala and an active principle, adenosine, on platelet activating factor." *Planta Med.* 1992; 58(4): 306–310.

15. Vasange, M., et al. "A sulphonoglycolipid from the fern *Polypodium decumanum* and its effect on the platelet activating factor receptor in human neutrophils." *J. Pharm. Pharmacol.* 1997; 49(5): 562–617.

16. Vasange, M., et al. "Flavonoid constituents of two *Polypodium* species (Calaguala) and their effect on the elastase release in human neutrophils." *Planta Med.* 1997; 63(6): 511–517.

17. Sempere-Ortells , J. M., et al. "Effect of Anapsos (Polypodium leucotomos extract) on *in vitro* production of cytokines." *Br. J. Clin. Pharmacol.* 1997; 43(1): 85–89.

18. Gonzalez, S., et al. "An extract of the fern *Polypodium leucotomos* (Difur) modulates Th1/Th2 cytokines balance in vitro and appears to exhibit anti-angiogenic activities in vivo: Pathogenic relationships and therapeutic implications." *Anticancer Res.* 2000; 20(3a): 1567–1575.

19. Bernd, A., et al. "In vitro studies on the immunomodulating effects of *Polypodium leucotomos* extract on human leukocyte fractions." *Arzneimittelforschung.* 1995; 45(8): 901–904.

20. Sempere-Ortells, J. M., et al. "Anapsos (Polypodium leucotomos) modulates lymphoid cells and the expression of adhesion molecules." *Pharmacol. Res.* 2002; 46(2): 185–190.

21. Rayward, J. et al., *Polypodium leucotomos* (PL), an herbal extract, inhibits the proliferative response of T. lymphocytes to polyclonal mitogens." *Second Intl. Cong. on Biol. Response Modifiers,* San Diego, 1993.

22. Tuominen, M. et al., "Enhancing effect of extract *Polypodium leucotomos* on the prevention of rejection on skin transplants." *Phytotherapy Research* 1991; 5: 234–237.

23. Navarro-Blasco, F. J., et al. "Modification of the inflammatory activity of psoriatic arthritis in patients treated with extract of *Polypodium leucotomos* (Anapsos)." *Br. J. Rheumatol.* 1998; 37(8): 912.

24. Ferrer, M. Y., et al. "Water-soluble fractions of *Phlebodium decumanum* and its use as nutritional supplement in AIDS and cancer patients." United States Patent 6,228,366; 2001.

25. Quintanilla A. E., et al. "Pharmaceutical composition of activity in the treatment of cognitive and/or neuroimmune dysfunctions." United States Patent 5,601,829; 1997.

26. Fernandez-Novoa, L., et al. "Effects of Anapsos on the activity of the enzyme Cu-Zn-superoxide dismutase in an animal model of neuronal degeneration." *Methods Find. Exp. Clin. Pharmacol.* 1997; 19(2): 99–106.

27. Gomes, A. J., et al. "The antioxidant action of *Polypodium leucotomos* extract and Kojic acid: Reactions with reactive oxygen species." *Braz. J. Med. Biol. Res.* 2001; 34(11): 1487–1494.

28. Álvarez, X. A., et al. "Anapsos reverses interleukin-1 beta overexpression and behavioral deficits in nbM-lesioned rats." *Methods Find. Exp. Clin. Pharmacol.* 1997; 19(5): 299–309.

29. Álvarez, X. A., et al. "Anapsos improves learning and memory in rats with Beta-Amyloid (1-28) deposits in the hippocampus" in *Progress in Alzheimer's and Parkinson's diseases,* Ed. Fisher, A., Yoshida, M. and Hannin, I., Plenum Press, New York, pp. 699–703 (1998).

30. Álvarez, X. A., et al. "Double-blind, randomized, placebo-controlled pilot study with anapsos in senile dementia: effects on cognition, brain bioelectrical activity and cerebral hemodynamics." *Methods Find. Exp. Clin. Pharmacol.* 2000; 22(7): 585–594.

31. Cacabelos, R., et al. "A pharmacogenomic approach to Alzheimer's disease." *Acta Neurol. Scand. Suppl.* 2000; 176: 12–19.

32. Gonzalez, S., et al. "Inhibition of ultraviolet-induced formation of reactive oxygen species, lipid peroxidation, erythema and skin photosensitization by *Polypodium leucotomos.*" *Photodermatol. Photoimmunol. Photomed.* 1996; 12(2): 45–56.

33. Gonzalez, S., et al. "Topical or oral administration with an extract of *Polypodium leucotomos* prevents acute sunburn and psoralen-induced phototoxic reactions as well as depletion of Langerhans cells

in human skin." *Photodermatol. Photoimmunol. Photomed.* 1997; 13(1–2): 50–60.

34. Alcaraz, M. V., et al. "An extract of *Polypodium leucotomos* appears to minimize certain photoaging changes in a hairless albino mouse animal model. A pilot study." *Photodermatol. Photoimmunol. Photomed.* 1999; 15(3–4): 120–26.

35. Middelkamp-Hup, M. A., et al., "Orally administered *Polypodium leucotomos* extract decreases psoralen-UVA-induced phototoxicity, pigmentation, and damage of human skin." *J. Am. Acad. Dermatol.* 2004; 50(1): 41–49.

36. Philips, N., et al., "Predominant effects of *Polypodium leucotomos* on membrane integrity, lipid peroxidation, and expression of elastin and atrixmetalloproteinase-1 in ultraviolet radiation exposed fibroblasts, and keratinocytes." *J. Dermatol. Sci.* 2003 Jun; 32(1): 1–9.

37. Alonso-Lebrero, J. L., et al. "Photoprotective properties of a hydrophilic extract of the fern Polypodium leucotomos on human skin cells." *J. Photochem. Photobiol. B.* 2003 Apr; 70(1): 31–37.

38. Manna, S. K., et al. "Calagualine inhibits nuclear transcription factors-kappaB activated by various inflammatory and tumor promoting agents." *Cancer Lett.* 2003; 20; 190(2): 171–182.

Sangre de Grado

1. Duke, James A. "Added Comments on the Rainforest." *Whole Foods Magazine,* May 1997.

2. Perdue, G. P., et al. "South American plants II: Taspine isolation and anti-inflammatory activity." *J. Pharm. Sci.* 1979; 68(1): 124–126.

3. Vlietinck, A. J. and R. A. Dommisse, eds. *Advances in Medicinal Plant Research.* Stuttgart: Wiss. Verlag, 1985.

4. Vaisberg, A. J., et al. "Taspine is the cicatrizant principle in sangre de grado extracted from *Croton lechleri.*" *Planta Med.* 1989; 55(2): 140–143.

5. Porras-Reyes, B. H., et al. "Enhancement of wound healing by the alkaloid taspine defining mechanism of action." *Proc. Soc. Exp. Biol. Med.* 1993; 203(1): 18–25.

6. Itokawa, H., et al. "A cytotoxic substance from sangre de grado." *Chem. Pharm. Bull.* (Tokyo) 1991; 39(4): 1041–1042.

7. Pieters, L., et al. "Isolation of a dihydrobenzofuran lignan from South American dragon's blood (*Croton* sp.) as an inhibitor of cell proliferation." *J. Nat. Prod.* 1993; 56(6): 899–906.

8. Chen, Z. P., et al. "Studies on the anti-tumour, anti-bacterial, and wound-healing properties of dragon's blood." *Planta Med.* 1994; 60(6): 541–545.

9. Desmarchelier, C., et al. "Effects of sangre de drago from *Croton lechleri* Muell.-Arg. on the production of active oxygen radicals." *J. Ethnopharmacol.* 1997; 58: 103–108.

10. Macrae, W. D., et al. "Studies on the pharmacological activity of Amazonian Euphorbiaceae." *J. Ethnopharmacol.* 1988; 22(2): 143–172.

11. Miller, M. J., et al. "Treatment of gastric ulcers and diarrhea with the Amazonian herbal medicine sangre de grado." *Am. J. Physiol. Gastrointest. Liver Physiol.* 2000; 42: G192–200.

12. Sandoval, M., et al. "Sangre de grado *Croton palanostigma* induces apoptosis in human gastrointestinal cancer cells." *J. Ethnopharmacol.* 2002; 80(2–3): 121–129.

13. Rossi, D., et al. "Evaluation of the mutagenic, antimutagenic and antiproliferative potential of *Croton lechleri* (Muell. Arg.) latex." *Phytomedicine.* 2003 Mar; 10 (2–3):139–144.

14. Meza E. N., ed. *Desarrollando Nuestra Diversidad Biocultural: "Sangre de Grado" y el Reto de su Producción Sustentable en el Perú.* Lima: Universidad Nacional Mayor de San Marcos; 1999.

15. Sidwell R., et al. "Influenza virus-inhibitory effects of intraperitoneally and aerosol-administered SP-303, a plant flavonoid." *Chemotherapy* 1994; 40(1): 42–50.

16. Williams, J. E. "Review of antiviral and immunomodulating properties of plants of the Peruvian rainforest with a particular emphasis on Uña de Gato and Sangre de Grado." *Altern. Med. Rev.* 2001; 6(6): 567–579.

17. Miller, M. J., et al. "Inhibition of neuro-genic inflammation by the Amazonian herbal medicine sangre de grado." *J. Invest. Dermatol.* 2001; 117(3): 725–730.

Sarsaparilla

1. Hobbs, Christopher. "Sarsaparilla, a literature review." *HerbalGram* 17. 1988.

2. Lueng, Albert and Steven Foster. *Encyclopedia of Common Natural Ingredients.* New York: John Wiley & Sons, 1996.

3. Willard, Terry. *The Wild Rose Scientific Herbal.* Alberta: Wild Rose College of Natural Healing, 1991, 307.

4. Botanical Monograph, "Sarsaparilla (*Smilax sarsaparilla*)." *American Journal of Natural Medicine* 1996; 3(9).

5. Newal, Carol, Linda Anderson, and J. David. Phillipson. *Herbal Medicine: A Guide for Health-care Professionals.* Cambridge, England: The Pharmaceutical Press, 1996.

6. Santos, W. R., et al. "Haemolytic activities of plant saponins and adjuvants. Effect of *Periandra mediterranea* saponin on the humoral response to the FML antigen of *Leishmania donovani.*" *Vaccine* 1997; 15(9): 1024–1029.

7. Chen, T., et al. "A new flavanone isolated from *Rhizoma smilacis glabrae* and the structural requirements for its derivatives for preventing immunological hepatocyte damage." *Planta Med.* 1999; 65(1): 56–59.

8. Xu, Q., et al. "Immunosuppressive agents." United States Patent 6,531,505; 2003.

9. Xia, Z., et al. "Smilagenin and its use." United States Patent 6,258,386; 2001.

10. Thurman, F. M. "The treatment of psoriasis with sarsaparilla compound." *New England Journal of Medicine* 1942; 337: 128–133.

11. Juhlin, L., et al. "The influence of treatment and fibrin microclot generation in psoriasis." *Br. J. Dermatol.* 1983; 108: 33–37.

12. Rollier, R. "Treatment of lepromatous leprosy by a combination of DDS and sarsaparilla (*Smilax ornata*)." *Int. J. Leprosy* 1959; 27: 328–340.

13. Tanaka, M., et al. "Therapeutic agents for respiratory diseases." United States Patent 6,309,674; 2001.

14. D'Amico, M. L. "Ricerche sulla presen-

za di sostanze ad azione antibiotica nelle piante superiori." *Fitoterapia* 1950; 21(1): 77–79.

15. Fitzpatrick, F. K. "Plant substances active against mycobacterium tuberculosis." *Antibiotics and Chemotherapy* 1954; 4(5): 528–536.

16. Caceres, A., et al. "Plants used in Guatemala for the treatment of dermatophytic infections. 1. Screening for antimycotic activity of 44 plant extracts." *J. Ethnopharmacol.* 1991; 31(3): 263–276.

17. Tschesche, R. "Advances in the chemistry of antibiotic substances from higher plants." In H. Wagner and L. Horhammer, *Pharmacognosy and Phytochemisty.* New York: Springer Verlag, 1971. 274–276.

18. Ageel, A. M., et al. "Experimental studies on antirheumatic crude drugs used in Saudi traditional medicine." *Drugs Exp. Clin. Res.* 1989; 15(8): 369–372.

19. Jiang, J., et al. "Immunomodulatory activity of the aqueous extract from rhizome of *Smilax glabra* in the later phase of adjuvant-induced arthritis in rats." *J. Ethnopharmacol.* 2003; 85(1): 53–59.

20. Rafatullah, S., et al. "Hepatoprotective and safety evaluation studies on sarsaparilla." *Int. J. Pharmacognosy* 1991; 29: 296–301.

21. Harnischfeger, G., et al. "*Smilax* Species—Sarsaparille." In *Bewahrte Pflanzendrogen in Wissenschaft* und Medizin. Bad Homburg/Melsungen: Notamed Verlag, 1983. 216–225.

22. Humpert, F. "The effect of a sarsaparilla preparation (renotrat) in chronic nephritis, with particular reference to the uric acid content of the blood and urine." *Klin. Wochschr.* 1933; 12: 1696.

23. Rittmann, R., al. "A new agent in kidney therapy." *Klin. Wochschr.* 1930; 9: 401–408.

Scarlet Bush

1. Borges del Castilo, J., et al., "Salvadorian flora. 5. Study of alkaloids. From *Hamelia patens* Jacq." *An. Quim. Ser. C.* 1982; 78: 180–183.

2. Keplinger, K., et al. "Oxindole alkaloids having properties stimulating the immunologic system and preparation containing the same." United States Patent 5,302,611; 1994.

3. Kang, T. H., et al. "Pteropodine and isopteropodine positively modulate the function of rat muscarinic M(1) and 5-HT(2) receptors expressed in Xenopus oocyte." *Eur. J. Pharmacol.* 2002 May 24; 444 (1–2): 39–45.

4. Roth, B. L., et al. "Insights into the structure and function of 5-HT(2) family serotonin receptors reveal novel strategies for therapeutic target development." *Expert Opin. Ther. Targets* 2001 Dec; 5(6): 685–695

5. Borges del Castillo, J., et al. "Oxindole alkaloids from *Hamelia patents* Jacq." Proc. 1st Int. Conf. Chem. Biotechnol. Biol. Act. Nat. Prod. 1981.

6. Chaudhuri, P. K., et al. "*Hamelia patens*: a new source of ephedrine." *Planta Med.* 1991; 57(2): 199.

7. Aquino, R., et al. "A flavanone glycoside from *Hamelia patens*." *Phytochemistry* 1990; 29(7): 2358–2360.

8. Yun, S. Y., et al. "Synergistic immunosupressive effects of rosmarinic acid and rapamycin in vitro and in vivo." *Transplantation* 2003; 75(10): 1758–1760.

9. Takeda, H., et al. "Rosmarinic acid and caffeic acid produce antidepressive-like effect in the forced swimming test in mice." *Eur. J. Pharmacol.* 2002; 449(3): 261–267.

10. Esposito-Avella, M., et al. "Pharmacological screening of Panamanian medicinal plants. Part 1." *Int. J. Crude Drug Res.* 1985; 23(1): 17–25.

11. Sosa, S., et al. "Screening of the topical anti-inflammatory activity of some Central American plants." *J. Ethnopharmacol.* 2002; 81(2): 211–215.

12. Misas, C. A. J., et al. "Contribution of the biological evaluation of Cuban plants. VI." *Rev. Cub. Med. Trop.* 1979; 31: 45–51.

13. Camporese, A., et al. "Screening of anti-bacterial activity of medicinal plants from Belize (Central America)." *J. Ethnopharmacol.* 2003; 87(1): 103–107.

14. Lopez Abraham A., et al. "Potential antineoplastic activity of Cuban plants. IV." *Rev. Cubana Farm.* 1981; 15(1): 71–77.

15. Lopez Abraham A., et al. "Plant extracts with cytostatic properties growing in Cuba. II." *Rev. Cubana Med.* 1979; 21(2): 105–111.

Simarouba

1. Brendler, Thomas. *Heilpflanzen-Herbal Remedies.* CD-ROM. Berlin, Germany: Institut für Phytopharmaka, Gmbh., 1996.

2. Shepheard, S., et al. "Persistent carriers of *Entameba histolytica*." *Lancet* 1918: 501.

3. Cuckler, A. C., et al. "Efficacy and toxicity of simaroubidin in experimental amoebiasis." *Fed. Proc.* 1944; 8: 284.

4. Duriez, R., et al. "Glaucarubin in the treatment of amebiasis." *Presse Med.* 1962; 70: 1291.

5. Wright, C. W., et al. "Quassinoids exhibit greater selectivity against *Plasmodium falciparum* than against *Entameba histoyltica, Giardia intestinalis* or *Toxoplasma gondii* in vitro." *J. Eukaryot. Microbiol.* 1993; 40(3): 244–246.

6. Caceres, A. "Plants used in Guatemala for the treatment of gastrointestinal disorders. 1. Screening of 84 plants against enterobacteria." *J. Ethnopharmacol.* 1990; 30(1): 55–73.

7. Spencer, C. F., et al. "Survey of plants for antimalarial activity." *Lloydia* 1947; 10: 145–174.

8. Trager, W., et al. "Antimalarial activity of quassinoids against chloroquine-resistant *Plasmodium falciparum* in vitro." *Am. J. Trp. Med. Hyg.* 1981; 30(3): 531–537.

9. O'Neill, M. J., et al. "Plants as sources of antimalarial drugs, Part 6. Activities of *Simarouba amara* fruits." *J. Ethnopharmacol.* 1988; 22(2): 183–190.

10. O'Neill, M. J., et al. "The activity of *Simarouba amara* against chloroquine-resistant *Plasmodium falciparum* in-vitro." *J. Pharm. Pharmacol.* 1987; Suppl. 39: 80.

11. Kirby, G. C., et al. "In vitro studies on the mode of action of quassinoids with activity against chloroquine-resistant *Plasmodium falciparum*." *Biochem. Pharmacol.* 1989; 38(24): 4367–4374.

12. Franssen, F. F., et al. "In vivo and in vitro antiplasmodial activities of some plants traditionally used in Guatemala against malaria." *Antimicrob. Agents Chemother.* 1997; 41(7): 1500–1503.

13. Monjour, I., et al., "Therapeutic trials of experimental murine malaria with the quassinoid, glaucarubinone." *C. R. Acad. Sci. Ill.* 1987; 304(6): 129–132.

14. May, G., et al., "Antiviral activity of aqueous extracts from medicinal plants in tissue cultures." *Arzneim-Forsch* 1978; 28 (1): 1–7.

15. Kaif-A-Kamb, M., et al. "Search for new antiviral agents of plant origin." *Pharm. Acta Helv.* 1992; 67(5–6): 130–147.

16. Anon. Unpublished data, National Cancer Institute. Nat. Cancer Inst. central files 1976; from the NAPRALERT on Simarouba, University of Illinois.

17. Ghosh, P. C., et al. "Antitumor plants. IV. Constituents of *Simarouba versicolor.*" *Lloydia* 1977; 40(4): 364–369.

18. Polonsky, J. "The isolation and structure of 13,18-dehydroglaucarubinone, a new antineoplastic quassinoid from *Simarouba amara.*" *Experientia* 1978; 34(9): 1122–1123.

19. Ogura, M. et al. "Potential anticancer agents VI. Constituents of *Ailanthus excelsa* (Simaroubaceae)." *Lloydia* 1977; 40(6): 579–584.

20. Handa, S. S., et al. "Plant anticancer agents XXV. Constituents of *Soulamea soulameoides.*" *J. Nat. Prod.* 1983; 46(3): 359–364.

21. Valeriote, F. A., et al. "Anticancer activity of glaucarubinone analogues." *Oncol Res.* 1998; 10(4): 201–208.

22. Bonte, F., et al. "*Simarouba amara* extract increases human skin keratinocyte differentiation." *J. Ethnopharmacol.* 1996; 53(2): 65–74.

23. Bonte, F., et al. "Use of a simarouba extract for reducing patchy skin pigmentation." United States Patent 5,676,948; October 14, 1997.

Stevia

1. Soejarto, D. D., et al. "Potential sweetening agents of plant origin. III. Organoleptic evaluation of stevia leaf herbarium specimens for sweetness." *J. Nat. Prod.* 1982; 45(5): 590–599.

2. Bridel, M., et al. *J. Pharm. Chem.* 1931; 14: 99.

3. Samuelsson, Gunnar. *Drugs of Natural Origin.* Stockholm: Swedish Pharmaceutical Press, 1992.

4. Leung, A. and S. Foster. *Encyclopedia of Common Natural Ingredients.* New York: John Wiley & Sons, 1996.

5. Sekihashi, K., et al. "Genotoxicity studies of stevia extract and steviol by the comet assay." *J. Toxicol. Sci.* 2002; 27 (Suppl. 1): 1–8.

6. Matsui, M., et al. "Evaluation of the genotoxicity of stevioside and steviol using six in vitro and one in vivo mutagenicity assays." *Mutagenesis.* 1996; 11(6): 573–579.

7. Suzuki, H., et al. "Influence of the oral administration of stevioside on the levels of blood glucose and liver glycogen in intact rats." *Nogyo Kagaku Zasshi* 1977; 51(3): 45.

8. Naves, Y. R. "Volatile plant materials. XXV. Presence of matsutake's alcohol (oct-1-en-3-ol) and 3-menthylcyclohexanol in essential oil of European pennyroyal (*Mentha pulegium*)." *Helv. Chim. Acta.* 1943; 26: 1992–2001.

9. Aritajat, S., et al. "Dominant lethal test in rats treated with some plant extracts." *Southeast Asian J. Trop. Med. Public Health* 2000; 31 (Suppl. 1): 171–173.

10. Oliveira-Filho, R. M., et al. "Chronic administration of aqueous extract of *Stevia rebaudiana* (Bert.) Bertoni in rats: endocrine effects." *Gen. Pharmacol.* 1989; 20(2): 187–191.

11. von Czepanski, C. "Testing of selected plants for antifertility activity." Personal Communication 1977.

12. Felippe, G. M., et al. "*Stevia rebaudiana.* A review." *Cienc. Cult.* 1977; 29: 1240.

13. Melis, M. S. "Effects of chronic administration of *Stevia rebaudiana* on fertility in rats." *J. Ethnopharmacol.* 1999; 167(2): 157–161.

14. Melis, M.S., et al. "Effect of calcium and verapamil on renal function of rats during treatment with stevioside." *J. Ethnopharmacol.* 1991; 33(3): 257–262.

15. Chan, P., et al. "A double-blind placebo-controlled study of the effectiveness and tolerability of oral stevioside in human hypertension." *Br. J. Clin. Pharmacol.* 2000; 50(3): 215–220.

16. Yamamoto, N. S., et al. "Effect of steviol and its structural analogues on glucose production and oxygen uptake in rat renal tubules." *Experientia* 1985; 41(1): 55–57.

17. Jeppesen, P. B., et al. "Stevioside acts directly on pancreatic beta cells to secrete insulin: actions independent of cyclic adenosine monophosphate and adenosine triphosphate-sensitive K+-channel activity." *Metabolism* 2000; 49(2): 208–214.

18. Boeckh, E. M. A., et al. "Avaliacao Clinica do Efeito Cronico do Edulcorante Natural *Stevia rebaudiana* Bertoni Sobre o Teste de Tolerancia a Glicose, Parametros Clinicos e Eletrocardiograficos em Individuos Normais." *V Simposio de Plantas Medicinais do Brasil.* 1978; (4–6): 208.

19. Humbolt, G., et al. "Steviosideo: Efeitos Cardio-circulatorios em Ratos." *V Simposio de Plantas Medicinais do Brasil.* 1978; (4–6): 208.

20. Melis, M. S. "A crude extract of *Stevia rebaudiana* increase the renal plasma flow of normal and hypertensive rats." *Braz. J. Med. Biol. Res.* 1996; 29(5): 669–675.

21. Boeckh, E. M. A. "*Stevia rebaudiana* bertoni: Cardio-circulatory effects of total water extract in normal persons and of stevioside in rats and frogs." First Brazilian seminar on *Stevia rebaudiana,* Inst. Technol. Aliment. Campinas, Brazil, June 25–26, 1981.

22. Melis, M. S. "Chronic administration of aqueous extract of *Stevia rebaudiana* in rats: renal effects." *J. Ethnopharmacol.* 1995; 47(3): 129–134.

23. Melis, M. S. "Stevioside effect on renal function of normal and hypertensive rats." *J. Ethnopharmacol.* 1992; 36(3): 213–217.

24. Curi, R., et al. "Effect of *Stevia rebaudiana* on glucose tolerance in normal adult humans." *Braz. J. Med. Biol. Res.* 1986; 19(6): 771–774.

25. Oviedo, C. A., et al. "Hypoglycemic action of *Stevia rebaudiana.*" *Excerpta medica.* 1970; 209: 92.

26. Kinghorn, A. D., et al. *Economic and medicinal plant research.* Vol. 1. Academic Press: Orlando, FL. 1985.

27. Anon. "Stevia components as sweetening agents and antibiotics." *Japanese Patent* 8092,323; 1980.

28. Tomita, T., et al. "Bactericidal activity of a fermented hot-water extract from *Stevia rebaudiana* bertoni towards enterohemorrhagic *Escherichia coli* 0157:h7 and other food-borne pathogenic bacteria." *Microbiol. Immunol.* 1997; 41(12): 1005–1009.

29. Takahashi, K., et al. "Analysis of anti-rotavirus activity of extract from *Stevia rebaudiana.*" *Antiviral Res.* 2001; 49(1): 15–24.

30. Takaki, M., et al. "Antimicrobial activity in leaves extracts of *Stevia rebaudiana* bert." *Rev. Inst. Antibiot. Univ. Fed. Pernambuco. Recife* 1985; 22(1/2): 33–39.

31. Pinheiro, C. E., et al. "Effect of guarana and *Stevia rebaudiana* bertoni (leaves) extracts, and stevioside, on the fermentation and synthesis of extracellular insoluble polysaccharides of dental plaque." *Rev. Odont. Usp.* 1987; 1(4): 9–13.

32. Dozono, Fumio. "Stevia extract-containing medicine." *United States Patent* 5,262,161; 1993.

33. FDA Import Alert No. 45-06. May 17, 1991.

34. Blumenthal, Mark. "Perspectives on FDA's new stevia policy, after four years, the agency lifts its ban—but only partially." *Whole Foods Magazine,* February 1996.

Suma

1. Nishimoto, N., et al. "Constituents of 'Brazil ginseng' and some *Pfaffia* species." *Tennen Yuki Kagobutsu Toronkai Keon Yoshishu* 1988; 10: 17–24.

2. Nishimoto, N., et al. "Three ecdysteroid glycosides from *Pfaffia.*" *Phytochemistry* 1988; 27(6): 1665–1668.

3. Matsumoto, I., Beta-ecdysone from *Pfaffia paniculata.* Japanese Patent 82/118,422. January 20, 1984.

4. Shibuya, I. et al. Composition. United States Patent 6,224,872; July 20,1998.

5. Meybeck, A. et al. Use of an ecdysteroid for the preparation of cosmetic or dermatological compositions intended, in particular, for strengthening the water barrier function of the skin or for the preparation of a skin cell culture medium, as well as to the compositions. United States Patent 5,609,873; March 11, 1997.

6. de Oliveira, F. G., et al. "Contribution to the pharmacognostic study of Brazilian ginseng *Pfaffia paniculata.*" *An. Farm. Quim.* 1980; 20(1–2): 277–361.

7. Nakai, S., et al. "Pfaffosides. Part 2. Pfaffosides, nortriterpenoid saponins from *Pfaffia paniculata.*" *Phytochemistry* 1984; 23(8): 1703–1705.

8. Nishimoto, N., et al. "Pfaffosides and nortriterpenoid saponins from *Pfaffia paniculata*" *Phytochemistry* 1984; 23(1): 139–142.

9. Takemoto, T., et al. "Pfaffic acid, a novel nortriterpene from *Pfaffia paniculata* Kuntze." *Tetrahedron Lett.* 1983; 24(10): 1057–1060.

10. Takemoto, T., et al. Antitumor pfaffosides from Brazilian carrots. Japanese Patent 84/184,198; October 19, 1984.

11. Takemoto, T., et al. Pfaffic acids and its derivatives. Japanese Patent (SHO-WA)-118872; 1982. 16 pp.

12. Takemoto, T., et al. Pfaffic acids and its derivatives. Japanese Patent 84/10,548; January 20, 1984.

13. Takemoto, T., et al. Pfaffosides. Japanese Patent; (SHO-WA)-58-57547; 1983.

14. Watanabe, T., et al. "Effects of oral administration of *Pfaffia paniculata* (Brazilian ginseng) on incidence of spontaneous leukemia in AKR/J mice." *Cancer Detect. Prev.* 2000; 24(2): 173–178.

15. Araujo, J. T. Brazilian ginseng derivatives for treatment of sickle cell symptomatology. United States Patent 5,449,516; Sept. 12, 1995.

16. Ballas, S. K., et al. "Hydration of sickle erythrocytes using a herbal extract (*Pfaffia paniculata*) in vitro." *Brit. J. Hematol.* 2000; 111(1): 359–362.

17. Mazzanti, G., et al. "Anti-inflammatory activity of *Pfaffia paniculata* (Martius) Kuntze and *Pfaffia stenophylla* (Sprengel) Stuchl." *Pharmacol. Res.* 1993; 27(1): 91–92.

18. Mazzanti, G., et al. "Analgesic and anti-inflammatory action of *Pfaffia paniculata* (Martius) Kuntze." *Phytother. Res.* 1994; 8(7): 413–416.

19. Arletti, R., et al. "Stimulating property of *Turnera diffusa* and *Pfaffia paniculata* extracts on the sexual behavior of male rats." *Psychopharmacology* 1999; 143(1): 15–19.

20. Heleen, Pamela A. Herbal composition for enhancing sexual response. United States Patent 6,444,237; Sept 13, 2001.

21. Subiza, J., et al. "Occupational asthma caused by Brazil ginseng dust." *J. Allergy Clin. Immunol.* 1991; 88(5): 731–736.

Tayuya

1. Bauer, R. and H. Wagner. *Dtsch. Apoth. Ztg.* 1983; 123: 1313.

2. Bauer, R., et al. "Cucurbitacins and flavone C-glycosides from *Cayaponia tayuya.*" *Phytochemisty* 1984: 1587–1591.

3. Himeno, E., et al. "Structures of cayaponosides A, B, C and D, glucosides of new nor-cucurbitacins in the roots of *Cayaponia tayuya.*" *Chem. Pharm. Bull.* (Tokyo) 1992; 40(10): 2885–2887.

4. Konoshima, T., et al. "Inhibitory effects of cucurbitane triterpenoids on Epstein-Barr virus activation and two-stage carcinogenesis of skin tumor." *Biol. Pharm. Bull.* 1995; 18(2): 284–287.

5. Anon., "Anti-tumor-promoter activity of natural substances and related compounds." *Annual Report 1995.* National Cancer Center Research Institute, Tokyo, Japan, 1996.

6. Panosian, A., et al. "On the mechanism of action of plant adaptogens with particular reference to cucurbitacin R diglucoside." *Phytomedicine* 1999; 6(3): 147Q–155.

7. Panosian, A. G., et al. "Action of adaptogens: cucurbitacin R diglucoside as a stimulator of arachidonic acid metabolism in the rat adrenal gland." *Probl. Endokrinol.* (Mosk). 1989; 35(2): 70–74.

8. Panosian, A. G., et al. "Effect of stress and the adaptogen cucurbitacin R diglycoside on arachidonic acid metabolism." *Probl. Endokrinol.* (Mosk). 1989; 35(1): 58–61.

9. Huguet, A. I., et al. "Superoxide scavenging properties of flavonoids in a non-enzymic system." *Z. Natur. Forsch.* 1990; 45(1–2): 19–24.

10. Vrinda, B., et al. "Radiation protection

of human lymphocyte chromosomes *in vitro* by orientin and vicenin." *Mutat. Res.* 2001; 498 (1–2): 39–46.

11. Uma Devi, P., et al. "*In vivo* radioprotection by ocimum flavonoids: survival of mice." *Radiat. Res.* 1999; 151(1): 74–8.

12. Ruppelt, B. M., et al. "Pharmacological screening of plants recommended by folk medicine as anti-snake venom—I. Analgesic and anti-inflammatory activities." *Mem. Inst. Oswaldo Cruz* 1991; 86 (Suppl. 2): 203–205.

13. Rios, J. L., et al. "A study of the anti-inflammatory activity of *Cayaponia tayuya* root." *Fitoterapia* 1990; 61(3): 275–278.

14. Chiappeta, A. D. A., et al. "Higher plants with biological activity—Plants of Pernambuco. I." *Rev. Inst. Antibiot. Univ. Fed. Pernambuco Recife* 1983; 21 (1/2): 43–50.

15. Faria, M. R. and E. P. Schenkel. "Caracterizacao de cucurbitacinas em especies vegetais cohecidas popularmente como taiuiá." *Ciencia e Cultura* (São Paulo) 1987; 39: 970–973.

Vassourinha

1. Mahato, S., et al. "Triterpenoids of *Scoparia dulcis*." *Phytochemistry* 1981; 20: 171–173.

2. Hayashi, T., et al. "Scopadulcic acid-A and -B, new diterpenoids with a novel skeleton, from a Paraguayan crude drug 'typycha kuratu' (*Scoparia dulcis* L.)." *Tetrahedron Lett.* 1987; 28(32): 3693–3696.

3. Kawasaki, M. "Structure of scoparic acid A, a new labdane-type diterpenoid from a Paraguayan crude drug 'typycha kurata' (*Scoparia dulcis* L.)." *Chem. Pharm. Bull.* 1987; 35(9): 3963–3966.

4. Hayashi, T. "Structures of new diterpenoids from a Paraguayan crude drug 'typycha kuratu' (*Scoparia dulcis* L.)." *Tennen Yuki Kagobutsu Toronkai Koen Yoshishu* 1987; 29: 544–551.

5. Ahmed, M. "Diterpenoids from *Scoparia dulcis*." *Phytochemistry* 1990; 29(9): 3035–3037.

6. Hayashi, T. "Scopadulciol, an inhibitor of gastric H+, K+-atpase from *Scoparia dulcis,* and its structure-activity relationships." *J. Nat. Prod.* 1991; 54(3): 802–9.

7. Hayashi, T. "Scoparic acid A, a beta-glucuronidase inhibitor from *Scoparia dulcis*." *J. Nat. Prod.* 1992; 55(12): 1748–1755.

8. Nishino, H. "Antitumor-promoting activity of scopadulcic acid B, isolated from the medicinal plant *Scoparia dulcis* L." *Oncology* 1993; 50(2): 100–103.

9. Riel, M. A. "Efficacy of scopadulcic acid A against Plasmodium falciparum in vitro." *J. Nat. Prod.* 2002; 65(4): 614–615.

10. Hayashi, T. "Antiviral agents of plant origin. III. Scopadulin, a novel tetracyclic diterpene from *Scoparia dulcis* L." *Chem. Pharm. Bull.* 1990; 38(4): 945–947.

11. Hayashi, K. "In vitro and in vivo antiviral activity of scopadulcic acid B from *Scoparia dulcis*, Scrophulariaceae, against *Herpes simplex* virus type 1." *Antiviral Res.* 1988; 9(6): 345–354.

12. Hayashi, T., et al. "Antiviral agents of plant origin. II. Antiviral activity of scopadulcic acid B derivatives." *Chem. Pharm. Bull.* 1990; 38(1): 239–242.

13. Kanamoto, T., et al. "Anti-human immunodeficiency virus activity of YK-FH312 (a betulinic acid derivative), a novel compound blocking viral maturation." *Antimicrob. Agents Chemother.* 2001; 45(4): 1225–1230.

14. Noda, Y., et al. "Enhanced cytotoxicity of some triterpenes toward leukemia L1210 cells cultured in low pH media; possibility of a new mode of cell killing." *Chem. Pharm. Bull.* 1997; 45(10): 1665–1670.

15. Salti, G. I., et al. "Betulinic acid reduces ultraviolet-c-induced DNA breakage in congenital melanocytic naeval cells: evidence for a potential role as a chemopreventive agent." *Melanoma Res.* 2001; 11(2): 99–104.

16. Fulda, S., et al. "Betulinic acid induces apoptosis through a direct effect on mitochondria in neuroectodermal tumors." *Med. Pediatr. Oncol.* 2000; 35(6): 616–618.

17. Wachsberger, P. R., et al. "Betulinic acid sensitization of low pH adapted human melanoma cells to hyperthermia." *Int. J. Hyperthermia* 2002; 18(2): 153–164.

18. Zuco, V., et al. "Selective cytotoxicity of betulinic acid on tumor cell lines, but not on normal cells." *Cancer Lett.* 2002; 175(1): 17–25.

19. Fulda, S., et al. "Betulinic acid: A new cytotoxic agent against malignant brain-tumor cells." *Int. J. Cancer* 1999; 82(3): 435–441.

20. Arisawa, M. "Cell growth inhibition of KB cells by plant extracts." *Natural Med.* 1994; 48(4): 338–347.

21. Hayashi, R. J., et al. "A cytotoxic flavone from *Scoparia dulcis* L." *Chem. Pharm. Bull.* 1988; 36: 4849–4851.

22. Pereira, N. A. "Contribucao ao estudo da tapixava (*Scoparia dulcis* L.)" *Rev. Flora Med.* (Rio de Janeiro) 1949; 16: 363–381.

23. Freire, S., et al. "Analgesic and anti-inflammatory properties of *Scoparia dulcis* L. extracts and glutinol in rodents." *Phytother. Res.* 1993; 7: 408–414.

24. Freire, S., et al. "Sympathomimetic effects of *Scoparia dulcis* L. and catecholamines isolated from plant extracts." *J. Pharm. Pharmacol.* 1996; 48(6): 624–628.

25. Freire, S., et al. "Analgesic activity of a triterpene isolated from *Scoparia dulcis* (vassourinha)." *Mem. Inst. Oswaldo Cruz* 86 (Suppl. II): 149–151.

26. Ahmed, M., et al. "Analgesic, diuretic, and anti-inflammatory principle from *Scoparia dulcis*." *Pharmazie* 2001; 56(8): 657–660.

27. Pari, L., et al. "Hypoglycaemic activity of *Scoparia dulcis* L. extract in alloxan induced hyperglycaemic rats." *Phytother. Res.* 2002 Nov; 16(7): 662–664.

28. Babincova, M., et al. "Free radical scavenging activity of Scoparia dulcis extract." *J. Med. Food.* 2001; 4(3): 179–181.

29. Laurens, A., et al. "Antimicrobial activity of some medicinal species of Dakar markets." *Pharmazie* 1985; 40(7): 482–485.

30. Singh, J., et al. "Antifungal activity of *Mentha spicata*." *Int. J. Pharmacog.* 1994; 32(4): 314–319.

31. Hasrat, J., et al. "Medicinal plants in Suriname: Screening of plant extracts for receptor binding activity." *Phytomedicine* 1997; 4(1): 59–65.

Velvet Bean

1. Polhill, R. M., et al. "Advances in Legume systematics." Proceedings of the

International Legume Conference. Kew, England. July 24–29, 1978.

2. Vaidya, R. A., et al. "Activity of bromo-ergocryptine, *Mucuna pruriens* and l-dopa in the control of hyperprolactinemia." *Neurology.* 1978; 26: 179–182.

3. Lubis, I., et al. "L-dihydroxyphenylala-nine (l-dopa) in mucuna seeds." *Ann. Bogor.* 1981; 7(3): 107–114.

4. Ghosal, S., et al. "Alkaloids of *Mucuna pruriens*. Chemistry and pharmacology." *Planta Med.* 1971; 19: 279.

5. Smith, T. A. "Tryptamine and related compounds in plants." Review. *Phytochemistry.* 1977; 16: 171–175.

6. Nath, D., et al. "Commonly used Indian abortifacient plants with special reference to their teratologic effects in rats." *J. Ethnopharmacol.* 1992; 36(2): 147–154.

7. Olanow, W., et al. "Levodopa: Why the Controversy?" *CME* 2002; 23.

8. Pruthi, Som C., et al. "Ayurvedic composition for the treatment of disorders of the nervous system including Parkinson's disease." United States Patent 6,106,839; 2000.

9. Liebert, Mary Ann. "An alternative medicine treatment for Parkinson's disease: results of a multicenter clinical trial. HP-200 in parkinson's disease study group." *J. Altern. Complement. Med.* 1995; 1(3): 249–255.

10. Rathi, S. S., et al. "Prevention of experimental diabetic cataract by Indian Ayurvedic plant extracts." *Phytother. Res.* 2002; 16(8): 774–777.

11. Rathi, S. S., et al. "The effect of *Momordica charantia* and *Mucuna pruriens* in experimental diabetes and their effect on key metabolic enzymes involved in carbohydrate metabolism." *Phytother. Res.* 2002; 16(3): 236–243.

12. Iauk, L., et al. "*Mucuna pruriens* decoction lowers cholesterol and total lipid plasma levels in the rat." *Phytother. Res.* 1989; 3(6): 263–264.

13. Pant, M. C., et al. "Blood sugar and total cholesterol lowering effect of glycine soya (Sieb and Zucc.), *Mucuna pruriens* (D.C.) and *Dolichos biflorus* (Linn.) seed di-ets in normal fasting albino rats." *Indian J. Med. Res.* 1968; 56(12): 1808–1812.

14. Uguru, M. O., et al. "Mechanism of action of the aqueous seed extract of *Mucuna pruriens* on the guinea-pig ileum." *Phytother. Res.* 1997; 11(4): 328–329.

15. Dhar, M. L., et al. "Screening of Indian plants for biological activity. Part 1." *Indian J. Exp. Biol.* 1968; 6: 232–247.

16. Jauk, L., et al. "Analgesic and antipyretic effects of *Mucuna pruriens.*" *Int. J. Pharmacog.* 1993; 31(3): 213–216.

17. Dabral, P. K., et al. "Evaluation of the role of Rumalaya and Geriforte in chronic arthritis—a preliminary study." *Probe* 1983; 22(2): 120–127.

18. Aguiyi, J. C., et al. "Studies on possible protection against snake venom using *Mucuna pruriens* protein immunization." *Fitoterapia* 1999; 70(1): 21–24.

19. Aguiyi, J. C., et al. "Blood chemistry of rats pretreated with *Mucuna pruriens* seed aqueous extract MP101UJ after *Echis carinatus* venom challenge." *Phytother. Res.* 2001; 15(8): 712–714.

20. Guerranti, R., et al. "Effects of *Mucuna pruriens* extract on activation of prothrombin by *Echis carinatus* venom." *J. Ethnopharmacol.* 2001; 75(2/3): 175–180.

21. Guerranti, R., et al. "Proteins from *Mucuna pruriens* and enzymes from *Echis carinatus* venom: characterization and cross-reactions." *J. Biol. Chem.* 2002; 277(19).

22. Bhargava, N. C., et al. "Fortege, and indigenous drug in common sexual disorders in males." *Mediscope* 1978; 21(6): 140–144.

23. Jayatilak, P. G., et al. "Effect of an indigenous drug (speman) on human accessory reproductive function." *Indian J. Surg.* 1976; 38: 12–15.

24. Jayatilak, P. G., et al. "Effect of an indigenous drug (speman) on accessory reproductive functions in mice." *Indian J. Exp. Biol.* 1976; 14: 170.

25. Mesko, C. A. "Composition for potentiating a growth hormone and a method for preparation of said composition." United States Patent 6,340,474; 2002.

26. Mitra, S. K., et al. "Experimental assessment of relative efficacy of drugs of herbal origin on sexual performance and hormone levels in alcohol exposed and normal rats." *Phytother. Res.* 1996; 10(4): 296–299.

27. Sankaran, J. R. "Problem of male virility—an oriental therapy." *J. Natl. Integ. Med. Ass.* 1984; 26(11): 315–317.

28. Madaan, S. "Speman in oligospermia." *Probe* 1985; 115–117.

29. Solepure, A. B., et al. "The effect of 'speman' on quality of semen in relation to magnesium concentration." *Indian Practitioner.* 1979; 32: 663–668.

Yerba Mate

1. Blumenthal, M., et al. *The Complete German Commission E Monographs: Therapeutic Guide to Herbal Medicines.* 1st ed. Newton, MA: Integrative Medicine Communications, 1998.

2. Alikaridis, F. "Natural constituents of *Ilex* species." *J. Ethnopharmacol.* 1987; 20(2): 121–144.

3. Fossati, C. "On the virtue and therapeutic properties of 'yerba-maté' (*Ilex paraguayensis* or *paraguariensis* St. Hilaire 1838)." *Clin. Ter.* 1976; 78(3): 265–272.

4. Martine, A., et al. "NMR and lC-MS-N characterization of two minor saponins from *Ilex paraguariensis.*" *Phytochem. Anal.* 2001; 12(1): 48–52.

5. Gosmann, G. "Triterpenoid saponins from *Ilex paraguariensis.*" *J. Nat. Prod.* 1995; 58(3): 438.

6. Kraemer, K. H. "Matesaponin 5, a highly polar saponin from *Ilex paraguariensis.*" *Phytochemistry* 1996; 42(4): 1119–1122.

7. Schenkel, E. P. "Triterpene saponins from maté, *Ilex paraguariensis.*" *Adv. Exp. Med. Biol.* 1996; 405: 47–56.

8. Sanz, M. D., T. "Mineral elements in maté herb (*Ilex paraguariensis* St. H.)." *Arch. Latinoam. Nutr.* 1991; 41(3): 441–454.

9. Pomilio, A. B., et al. "High-performance capillary electrophoresis analysis of maté infusions prepared from stems and leaves of *Ilex paraguariensis* using automated micellar electrokinetic capillary chromatography." *Phytochem. Anal.* 2002; 13(4): 235–241.

10. Samuelsson, Gunnar. *Drugs of Natural*

Origin: A Textbook of Pharmacognosy, 3rd ed. Stockholm, Sweden: Swedish Pharmaceutical Press, 1992.

11. Duke, J. A. *Handbook of Phytochemical Constituents of GRAS Herbs and Other Economic Plants.* Boca Raton, FL: CRC Press, 1992.

12. Vasquez, A., et al. "Studies on maté drinking." *J. Ethnopharmacol.* 1986; 18: 267–272.

13. Collomp, K., et al. "Effects of salbutamol and caffeine ingestion on exercise metabolism and performance." *Int. J. Sports Med.* 2002; 23(8): 549–554.

14. Lieberman, H. R., et al. "Effects of caffeine, sleep loss, and stress on cognitive performance and mood during U.S. Navy SEAL training." *Psychopharmacology* (Berl). 2002; 164(3): 250–261.

15. National Toxicology Program. "NTP toxicology and carcinogenesis studies of theophylline (CAS No. 58-55-9) in F344/N rats and B6C3F1 mice (feed and gavage studies)." *Natl. Toxicol. Program Tech. Rep. Ser.* 1998; 478: 1–326.

16. Martinet, A., et al. "Thermogenic effects of commercially available plant preparations aimed at treating human obesity." *Phytomedicine* 1999; 6(4): 231–238.

17. Anderson, T., et al. "Weight loss and delayed gastric emptying following a South American herbal preparation in overweight patients." *J. Hum. Nutr. Diet.* 2001; 14(3): 243–250.

18. Matsunaga, K., et al. "Inhibitory action of Paraguayan medicinal plants on 5-lipoxygenase." *Natural Med.* 2000; 54(3): 151–154.

19. Marr, K., et al. "Pharmacokinetics and pharmacodynamics of fenleuton, a 5-lipoxygenase inhibitor, in ponies." *Res. Vet. Sci.* 1998; 64(2): 111–117.

20. Yasukawa, K., et al. "Inhibitory effect of edible plant extracts on 12-o-tetradecanoylphorbol-13-acetate-induced ear oedema in mice." *Phytother. Res.* 1993; 7(2): 185–189.

21. Matsunaga, K., et al. "Excitatory and inhibitory effects of Paraguayan medicinal plants *Equisetum giganteum, Acanthospermum australe, Allopylus edulis* and *Cordia*

salicifolia on contraction of rabbit aorta and guinea-pig left atrium." *Natural Med.* 1997; 51(5): 478–481.

22. Gorzalczany, S., et al. "Choleretic effect and intestinal propulsion of 'maté' (*Ilex paraguariensis*) and its substitutes of adulterants." *J. Ethnopharmacol.* 2001; 75(2–3): 291–294.

23. Muccillo Baisch, A. L., et al. "Endothelium-dependent vasorelaxing activity of aqueous extracts of *Ilex paraguariensis* on mesenteric arterial bed of rats." *J. Ethnopharmacol.* 1998; 60(2): 133–139.

24. Williams, J. R., et al. "Treating depression with alcohol extracts of tobacco." U.S. patent no. 6,350,479; 2002.

25. Filip, R., et al. "Antioxidant activity of *Ilex paraguariensis* and related species." *Nutr. Res.* 2000; 20(10): 1437–1446.

26. Schinella, G. R., et al. "Antioxidant effects of an aqueous extract of *Ilex paraguariensis.*" *Biochem. Biophys. Res. Commun.* 2000; 269(2): 357–60.

27. Actis-Goretta, L., et al. "Comparative study on the antioxidant capacity of wines and other plant-derived beverages." *Ann. N. Y. Acad. Sci.* 2002; 957: 279–83.

28. Gugliucci, A. "Antioxidant effects of *Ilex paraguariensis*: induction of decreased oxidability of human LDL *in vivo.*" *Biochem. Biophys. Res. Commun.* 1996; 224(2): 338–344.

29. Gugliucci, A. "Low-density lipoprotein oxidation is inhibited by extracts of *Ilex paraguariensis.*" *Biochem. Mol. Biol. Int.* 1995; 35(1): 47–56.

30. Heinecke, J. W. "Clinical trials of vitamin E in coronary artery disease: Is it time to reconsider the low-density lipoprotein oxidation hypothesis?" *Curr. Atheroscler. Rep.* 2003; 5(2): 83–87.

31. Leborgne, L., et al. "Oxidative stress, atherogenesis and cardiovascular risk factors." *Arch. Mal. Coeur. Vaiss.* 2002; 95(9): 805–814.

32. Gugliucci, A., et al. "The botanical extracts of *Achyrocline satureoides* and *Ilex paraguariensis* prevent methylglyoxal-induced inhibition of plasminogen and antithrombin III." *Life Sci.* 2002; 72(3): 279–292.

33. Kalousova, M., et al. "Advanced glycation end-products and advanced oxidation protein products in patients with diabetes mellitus." *Physiol. Res.* 2002; 51(6): 597–604.

34. De Stefani, E., et al. "Black tobacco, wine and maté in oropharyngeal cancer." *Rev. Epidemiol. Sante. Publique.* 1988; 36(6): 389–394.

35. De Stefani, E., et al. "Black tobacco, maté and bladder cancer. A case-control study from Uruguay." *Cancer* 1991; 67(2): 536–540.

36. De Stefani, E., et al. "Meat intake, 'maté' drinking and renal cell cancer in Uruguay: a case-control study." *Br. J. Cancer* 1998; 78(9): 1239–1243.

37. Castellsague, X., et al. "Influence of maté drinking, hot beverages and diet on esophageal cancer risk in South America." *Int. J. Cancer* 2000; 88(4): 658–664.

General References
Tribal/Herbal Medicine Uses

Acero, D. *Principales Plantas Utiles De La Amazonia Colombiana.* Bogata: Proyecto Radargrametrico Del Amazonas, 1979.

Agromídia Software. Plantas Medicinais (CD-ROM). São Paulo, Brazil, 2002.

Almeida, de, E. R. *Plantas Medicinais Brasileiras, Conhecimentos Populares E Cientificos.* São Paulo: Hemus Editora Ltda., 1993.

Alves, T. M. A, et al. "Biological Screening of Brazilian Medicinal Plants." *Mem. Inst. Oswaldo Cruz.* 2000; 95 (3): 369–373.

Arvigo, Rosita and Michael Balick. *Rainforest Remedies, One Hundred Healing Herbs of Belize.* Twin Lakes, WI: Lotus Press, 1993.

Asprey, G. F. and P. Thornton. "Medicinal Plants of Jamaica. III." *West Indian Med. J.* 1995 4: 69–92.

Ayensu, E. S. "Medicinal Plants of the West Indies." Unpublished Manuscript: 110 Pages. Washington, D.C: Office of Biological Conservation, Smithsonian Institution, 1978.

Balee, William. *Footprints of the Forest Ka'apor Ethnobotany—the Historical Ecology of*

Plant Utilization by an Amazonian People. New York: Columbia University Press, 1994.

Bartram, Thomas. *Encyclopedia of Herbal Medicine.* Dorset, England: Ed Grace Publishers, 1995.

Beckstrom-Sternberg, Stephen M., and James A. Duke. "The Phytochemical Database." (Acedb Version 4.3—data Version July 1994). National Germplasm Resources Laboratory (Ngrl), Agricultural Research Service (Ars), U.S. Department of Agriculture.

Beckstrom-Sternberg, Stephen M., James A. Duke, and K. K. Wain. "The Ethnobotany Database." (Acedb Version 4.3-data Version July 1994). National Germplasm Resources Laboratory (Ngrl), Agricultural Research Service (Ars), U.S. Department of Agriculture.

Bernardes, Antonio. *A Pocketbook of Brazilian Herbs.* Rio de Janeiro: a Shogun Editora E Arta Ltda, 1984.

Berry, Paul E., Bruce Holst, and Kay Yatskievych. *Flora of the Venezuelan Guayana.* Missouri Botanical Garden, 1995.

Branch, L. C. and I. M. F. Da Silva. "Folk Medicine of Alter Do Chao, Para, Brazil." *Acta Amazonica* 1983; 13 (5/6): 737–797.

Bruneton, J. *Pharmacognosy, Phytochemistry, Medicinal Plants.* Hampshire, England: Intercept, Ltd., 1995.

Caribé, Dr. José, and Dr. José Mariá Campos. *Plantas Que Ajudam O Homem: Guia Prático Para a Época Atual, 5th Ed.* São Paulo, Brazil: Editora Pensimento, Ltda., 1997.

Coee, F., et al. "Ethnobotany of the Garifuna of Eastern Nicaragua." *Econ. Bot.* 1996; 50 (1): 71–107.

Coimbra, Raul. *Manual de Fitoterapia,* 2nd Ed. São Paulo, Brazil: Dados Internacionais De Catalogacao Na Pulicacao, 1994.

Correa, Pio. *Dicionario De Plantas Uteis Do Brazil e Exoticas Cultivadas,* Vols. 1–6, Brazilia: IBDF, 1984.

Cruz, G. L. *Dicionario Das Plantas Uteis Do Brazil,* 5th Ed. Rio de Janeiro: Bertrand, 1995.

Cruz, G. L. *Livro Verde Das Plantas Medicinais E Industriais Do Brazil,* Vol. 2, 1st Ed. Brazil: Belo Horizonte, 1965.

Dennis, P. "Herbal Medicine Among the Miskito of Eastern Nicaragua." *Econ. Bot.* 1988; 42 (1): 16–28.

Duke, James. *Handbook of Phytochemical Constituents of Gras Herbs and Other Economic Plants.* Boca Raton, FL: CRC Press, 1992.

Duke, James. *CRC Handbook of Medicinal Herbs.* Boca Raton, FL: CRC Press, 1985.

Duke, James. *Handbook of Northeastern Indian Medicinal Plants.* Boston, MA: Quarterman Publications, 1986.

Duke, James and K. K. Wain. *Medicinal Plants of the World.* Computer Index with More than 85,000 Entries. 3 Vols., 1981, P. 1654.

Duke, James and Rudolfo Vasquez. *Amazonian Ethnobotanical Dictionary.* Boca Raton, FL: CRC Press Inc., 1994.

Elkins, Rita. *Medicinal Herbs of the Rain Forest.* Pleasant Grove, UT: Woodland Publishing, 1997.

Feo, de, V. "Medicinal and Magical Plants in the Northern Peruvian Andes." *Fitoterapia* 1992; 63: 417–440.

Flynn, Rebecca and Mark Roest. *Your Guide to Standardized Herbal Products.* Prescott, Az: One World Press, 1995.

Forero, P. L. "Ethnobotany of the Cuna and Waunana Indigenous Communities." *Cespedesia* 1980; (9) 33: 115–202.

Franco, Lelington. *As Sensacionais 50 Plantas Medicinais: Campe_ De Poder Curativo,* Vol. 1, 4th Ed. Brazil: Editora Naturista, 1999.

Valdizan, H. and A. Maldonado. *La Medicina Popular Peruana.* Lima, Peru: Imp. Torres Aquirre, 1982.

Garcia-Barriga, H. *Flora Medicinal De Colombia, Botanica-Medica.* 3 Vols. Bogata, Colombia: Ins. Cein. Nat. Bogota, 1974–1975.

Gentry, Alwyn H. *A Field Guide to the Families and Genera of Woody Plants of Northwest South America.* Chicago, IL: University of Chicago Press, 1993.

Gentry, Alwyn H. *Woody Plants of Northwest South America (Colombia, Ecuador, Peru).* Chicago, IL: University of Chicago Press, 1993.

Girón, L M., et al. "Ethnobotanical Survey of the Medicinal Flora Used by the Caribs of Guatemala." *J. Ethnopharmacol.* 1991: 9.

Grenand, P., C. Moretti, and H. Jacquemin. *Pharmacopées Traditionelles En Guyane: Créoles, Palikur, Waypi.* (Coll. Mem No. 108.) Paris, France: Editorial L-Orstrom, 1987.

Grieve, Maude. *A Modern Herbal.* New York, NY: Dover Publications, 1971.

Heinerman, John. *Heinerman's Encyclopedia of Healing Herbs & Spices.* New York, NY: Parker Publishing Co., 1996.

Hirschmann, G., et al. "A Survey of Medicinal Plants of Minas Gerais." *Brazil. J. Ethnopharmacol.* 1990; 29 (2): 159–172.

Hoffman, David. *The Herbal Handbook.* Rochester, VT: Healing Arts Press, 1987.

Hoffman, David. *The New Holistic Herbal.* Rockport, MA: Element Books, Inc., 1991.

Joyce, Christopher. *Earthly Goods: Medicine-Hunting in the Rainforest.* New York: Little, Brown, & Company, 1994.

Lawrence Review of Natural Products. St. Louis, Mo: Facts and Comparisons Inc.

Lecta Revista De Farmacia. E Biologia. Vol 11, No. 1. Universidade Sao Francisco. Editora Da. Jan-dez 1993.

Lewis, Walter H., and Memory Lewis. *Medical Botany.* New York: John Wiley & Sons, 1977.

List, P. H. and L. Horhammer. *Hager's Handbuch Der Pharmazeutischen Praxis,* Vols. 2–6. Berlin: Springer-Verlag, 1969–1979.

Los Productos Natureles. Anvario Naturista. 5th Ed. Ecuador: Internacional. Mundo Naturista, 1992.

Lucas, Richard. *Miracle Medicine Herbs.* West Nyak, NY: Parker Publishing, 1991.

Lung, A. and S. Foster. *Encyclopedia of Common Natural Ingredients.* New York: John Wiley & Sons, 1996.

Matos, F. J. Abreu. *Farmacias Vivas: Sistema De Utilizaco De Plantas Medicinais Projetado Para Pequenas Comunidades.* Fortaleza, Brazil: Edicoes UFC, 1994.

Maxwell, Nicole. *Witch Doctor's Apprentice: Hunting for Medicinal Plants in the Amazon*, 3d Ed. New York: Citadel Press, 1990.

Mejia, Kember and Elsa Rengifo. *Plantas Medicinales De Uso Popular En La Amazonía Peruana*. Lima: AECI and IIAP, 1995.

Mindell, Earl. *Earl Mindell's Herb Bible*. New York: Simon & Shuster, 1992.

Moreira, Frederico. *Plantas De Curam: Cudie Da Sua Saúde Através De Natureza*, 5th Ed. São Paulo, Brazil: Hemus Editora Ltda., 1996.

Mors, W. B. and C. T. Rizzini. *Useful Plants of Brazil*. San Francisco: Holden-Day, Inc., 1966.

Mors, W. B., C. T. Rizzini, and N. A. Pereira. *Medicinal Plants of Brazil*. Algonac, Michigan: Reference Publications, Inc., 2000.

Morton, J. F. *Major Medicinal Plants: Botany, Culture and Uses*. Springfield, IL: Charles C. Thomas Publishing, 1977.

Mowrey, Daniel. *Herbal Tonic Therapies*. New Canaan, CT: Keats Publishing, Inc., 1993.

Mowrey, Daniel. *The Scientific Validation of Herbal Medicine*. New Canaan, CT: Keats Publishing, Inc., 1986.

Murray, Michael. *The Healing Power of Herbs*. Rocklin, CA: Prima Publishing, 1995.

Panizza, Sylvio, and Cherio De Mato. *Plantas Que Curam:*, 11th Ed. São Paulo, Brazil: Ibrasa, 1997.

Plotkin, Mark, J. *Tales of a Shaman's Apprentice*. Middlesex, England: Penguin Books, 1993.

Ramirez, V., et al.. *Vegetales Empleados En Medicina Tradicional Norperuana*. Trujillo, Peru: Banco Agrario Del Peru and Nacional Universidad Trujillo, June, 1988.

Rios, De, Marlene Dubkin. *Amazon Healer: the Life and Times of an Urban Shaman*. Garden City Park, NY: Avery Publishing Group, 1992.

Robineau, L., Ed. *Towards a Caribbean Pharmacopoeia*. Enda Caribe, Santo Domingo: Tramil-4 Workshop, UNAH, 1991.

Rodrigues, V. E. G., et al., "Ethnobotanical Survey of the Medicinal Plants in the Dominion of Meadows in the Region of the Alto Rio Grande - Minas Gerais." *Cienc. Agrotec. Lavras.* 2001; 25 (1): 102–123.

Roig, J. T. *Plantas Medicinales, Aromaticas O Venenosas De Cuba*. Havana, Cuba: Cientifico-Tecnica, 1988.

Ruiz, Rodolfo B. *Plantas Utiles De La Amazonia Peruana: Caracteristicas, Usos, Y Posibilidades*. Trujillo, Peru: Editorial Liberdad E.I.R.L., 1994.

Rutter, R. A. *Catalogo De Plantas Utiles De La Amazonia Peruana*. Yarinacocha, Peru: Instituto Linguistico De Verano, 1990.

Samuelsson, Gunnar. *Drugs of Natural Origin*. Stockholm: Swedish Pharmaceutical Press, 1992.

Schauenberb, Paul, and Ferdinand Paris. *Guide to Medicinal Plants*. Cambridge, England: Keats Publishing, 1977.

Schultes, R. E. "Gifts of the Amazon Flora to the World." *Arnoldia* 1990; (2) 50: 21–34.

Schultes, R. E. and Raffauf. *The Healing Forest: Medicinal and Toxic Plants of the Northwest Amazonia*. Portland, OR: Dioscorides Press, 1990.

Schwontkowski, Donna. "Herbal Treasures from the Amazon," Parts 1, 2, and 3. *Healthy & Natural Journal* (1996).

Schwontkowski, Donna. *Herbs of the Amazon: Traditional and Common Uses*. Utah: Science Student Braintrust Publishing, 1993.

Silva, M. *Catalogo De Extractos Fluidos*. Rio de Janeiro: Araija E Cia, Ltd., 1930.

Smith, Nigel, J. Williams, Donald Plucknett, and Jennifer Talbot. *Tropical Forests and Their Crops*. New York: Comstock Publishing, 1992.

Soukup, J. *Vocabulary of the Common Names of the Peruvian Flora and Catalog of the Genera*. Lima: Editorial Salesiano, 1970.

Sousa, De, M. P., and F. J. Matos, et al. *Constituintes Quimicos Ativos De Planta Medicinais Brazileiras*. Fortaleza, Brazil: Laboratorio De Produtos Naturais, 1991.

Taylor, Leslie. Personal Field Notes from Interviews of Curanderos, Shamans, and Herbalists in Peru, Brazil, and Ecuador, 1994–2003.

Valdizan, H. and A. Maldonado. *La Medicina Popular Peruana*. Lima: Imp. Torres Aquirre, 1982.

Van Den Berg, E. *Plantas Medicinais Na Amazonia*. Belem: Museu Goeldi, 1983.

Vasquez, M. R. *Useful Plants of Amazonian Peru*. Second Draft. Filed with USDA's National Agricultural Library, 1990.

Werbach, Melvyn R., and Michael T. Murray. *Botanical Influences on Illness—A Sourcebook of Clinical Research*. Tarzana, CA: Third Line Press, 1994.

Wichtl, M. *Herbal Drugs and Phytopharmaceuticals*. Boca Raton, FL: CRC Press, 1994.

World Preservation Society. *Powerful and Unusual Herbs from the Amazon and China*. Gainesville, FL: The World Preservation Society, Inc., 1993.

Zadra, De, Adriana Alarco. *Perú—el Libro De Las Plantas Mágicas*, 2nd Ed. Lima: Concytec, 2000.

INDEX

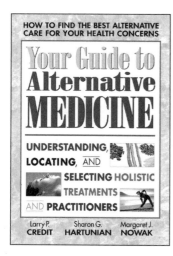

YOUR GUIDE TO ALTERNATIVE MEDICINE
Understanding, Locating, and Selecting Holistic Treatments and Practitioners
Larry P. Credit, Sharon G. Hartunian, and Margaret J. Nowak

The growing world of complementary medicine offers safe and effective solutions to many health disorders, from backache to headache. You may already be interested in alternative care approaches, but if you're like most people, you have a hundred and one questions you'd like answered before you choose a treatment. "Will I feel the acupuncture needles?" "What is a homeopathic remedy?" "Does chiropractic hurt?" *Your Guide to Alternative Medicine* provides the fundamental facts necessary to choose an effective complementary care therapy and begin treatment.

This comprehensive reference clearly explains numerous approaches in an easy-to-read format. For every complementary care option discussed, there is a description and brief history; a list of conditions that respond; information on the cost and duration of treatment; credentials and educational background for practitioners; and more. To find those therapies most appropriate for a specific condition, there is even a unique troubleshooting chart.

$11.95 US / $17.95 CAN • 208 pages • 6 x 9-inch paperback • ISBN 0-7570-0125-4

THE WHOLE HERB
For Cooking, Crafts, Gardening, Health, and Other Joys of Life
Barbara Pleasant

Herbs are nature's pure and precious gifts. They provide sustenance for both our bodies and our souls. They have been our medicine and our food. Their fragrance and beauty have warmed our hearts and delighted our senses.

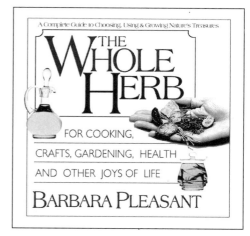

The Whole Herb is a complete, practical, and easy-to-follow guide to the many uses of these wonderful treasures of the earth. It presents their fascinating history, as well as their many uses, including herbs and health, herbs and cooking, herbs around the house, and herbs in the garden. A comprehensive A-to-Z reference profiles over fifty commonly used and affordable herb varieties. Each entry provides specific information on the herb's background, benefits, and uses, along with helpful buying guides, growing instructions, preservation methods, and safety information. Whether you want to use herbs to create better health, better meals, unforgettable fragrances, impressive crafts, or a beautiful garden, *The Whole Herb* is here to help.

$14.95 US / $22.50 CAN • 252 pages • 7.5 x 7.5-inch paperback • ISBN 0-7570-0080-0

For more information about our books,
visit our website at www.squareonepublishers.com